Prevalence and Control of Bovine Tuberculosis

Prevalence and Control of Bovine Tuberculosis

Editor: Owen Collins

MURPHY & MOORE
www.murphy-moorepublishing.com

www.murphy-moorepublishing.com

MURPHY & MOORE

Cataloging-in-Publication Data

Prevalence and control of bovine tuberculosis / edited by Owen Collins.
p. cm.
Includes bibliographical references and index.
ISBN 978-1-63987-763-8
1. Tuberculosis in cattle. 2. Tuberculosis in cattle--Transmission. 3. Tuberculosis in cattle--Prevention.
I. Collins, Owen.
SF808 .P74 2023
636.208 999 5--dc23

Murphy & Moore Publishing
1 Rockefeller Plaza,
New York City,
NY 10020, USA

ISBN 978-1-63987-763-8

Contents

Preface

Bovine tuberculosis is bacterial disease that occurs in cattle, domestic animals and wild animals. Mycobacterium bovis is the cause of this disease and can affect various animals, such as goats, deer, dogs, pigs, equines, cats and sheep. In the infected animals, evidence of the bacterium Mycobacterium bovis can be found in the throat and lungs. The other animals that come into contact with the breath or the discharges of the mouth or nose of an infected animal can contract bovine tuberculosis. There is no effective treatment for this disease and the animals which get infected with this disease are ultimately killed. The only way to control bovine tuberculosis is to isolate the healthy animals of the herd from the infected animals. This book elucidates the important perspectives on the prevalence and control of bovine tuberculosis. It presents researches and studies performed by experts across the globe. Those in search of information to further their knowledge will be greatly assisted by this book.

This book is a comprehensive compilation of works of different researchers from varied parts of the world. It includes valuable experiences of the researchers with the sole objective of providing the readers (learners) with a proper knowledge of the concerned field. This book will be beneficial in evoking inspiration and enhancing the knowledge of the interested readers.

In the end, I would like to extend my heartiest thanks to the authors who worked with great determination on their chapters. I also appreciate the publisher's support in the course of the book. I would also like to deeply acknowledge my family who stood by me as a source of inspiration during the project.

Editor

1

Can we Breed Cattle for Lower Bovine TB Infectivity?

Smaragda Tsairidou [1], Adrian Allen [2], Georgios Banos [1,3], Mike Coffey [3], Osvaldo Anacleto [1,4], Andrew W. Byrne [2], Robin A. Skuce [2], Elizabeth J. Glass [1], John A. Woolliams [1] and Andrea B. Doeschl-Wilson [1]*

[1] The Roslin Institute and Royal (Dick) School of Veterinary Studies, University of Edinburgh, Edinburgh, United Kingdom, [2] Agri-Food and Biosciences Institute, Belfast, United Kingdom, [3] Scotland's Rural College, Midlothian, United Kingdom, [4] Institute of Mathematical and Computer Sciences, University of São Paulo, São Paulo, Brazil

***Correspondence:**
Smaragda Tsairidou
smaragda.tsairidou@roslin.ed.ac.uk

Host resistance and infectivity are genetic traits affecting infectious disease transmission. This Perspective discusses the potential exploitation of genetic variation in cattle infectivity, in addition to resistance, to reduce the risk, and prevalence of bovine tuberculosis (bTB). In bTB, variability in *M. bovis* shedding has been previously reported in cattle and wildlife hosts (badgers and wild boars), but the observed differences were attributed to dose and route of infection, rather than host genetics. This article addresses the extent to which cattle infectivity may play a role in bTB transmission, and discusses the feasibility, and potential benefits from incorporating infectivity into breeding programmes. The underlying hypothesis is that bTB infectivity, like resistance, is partly controlled by genetics. Identifying and reducing the number of cattle with high genetic infectivity, could reduce further a major risk factor for herds exposed to bTB. We outline evidence in support of this hypothesis and describe methodologies for detecting and estimating genetic parameters for infectivity. Using genetic-epidemiological prediction models we discuss the potential benefits of selection for reduced infectivity and increased resistance in terms of practical field measures of epidemic risk and severity. Simulations predict that adding infectivity to the breeding programme could enhance and accelerate the reduction in breakdown risk compared to selection on resistance alone. Therefore, given the recent launch of genetic evaluations for bTB resistance and the UK government's goal to eradicate bTB, it is timely to consider the potential of integrating infectivity into breeding schemes.

Keywords: disease resistance, disease control, animal breeding, infectivity, bovine Tuberculosis

INTRODUCTION

Bovine tuberculosis (bTB) is a zoonotic disease, which can compromise both human health and international livestock trade. Zoonotic TB caused by *Mycobacterium bovis*, is responsible for an estimated 10–15% of human TB cases (1) and was estimated in 2016 as causing 12,500 deaths globally (2, 3). Addressing bTB infection in humans has been embedded within the United Nations Sustainable Development Goals 2016–2030 and World Health Organisation's (WHO) End TB Strategy framework, which employs a "One Health" approach aiming to end the global TB epidemic by 2030 (2–4).

In the UK, bTB has been the most pressing animal health problem, with financial losses amounting to over £175 m per annum (5). Tackling bTB has been a persistent challenge for the livestock industry, veterinary profession and policy-makers, and also the research community. The current national bTB eradication strategy involves the systematic testing of herds to identify and then remove infected cattle, and uses the Single Intradermal Comparative Cervical Test (SICCT), complemented by abattoir carcass inspections and, with increasing frequency, interferon-gamma testing. This surveillance regime has been successful in reducing disease spread in areas where bTB is prevalent and many EU countries and regions, including Scotland, have achieved Officially bTB Free (OTF) status (6). However, bTB persists in several regions (7) and herd incidence has increased in Wales, and also in High Risk and Edge areas in England (March 2018), despite the decrease in the overall herd incidence in England (8). Therefore, the continuing difficulties in eradicating bTB necessitate further exploration of additional disease control interventions that can complement existing strategies.

Selective breeding can complement classic disease control strategies, reducing the requirement for biosecurity measures and movement restrictions which have a major economic impact for herds undergoing a bTB breakdown (9, 10). Within the last few decades, breeding programmes (genetic and genomic selection) in livestock have achieved a remarkable improvement in production, e.g., milk yield in dairy cattle (11), and fitness traits such as fertility (12). Expanding the breeding objectives to include health and welfare traits offers new opportunities for disease control (10). The focus of genetic disease control so far has been on selection for improved resistance to becoming infected or diseased after exposure to pathogens. For example, by exploiting heritable genetic variation in disease resistance it has been possible to reduce mastitis incidence in cattle (13, 14) and mortality caused by infectious pancreatic necrosis in Atlantic salmon (15). Many studies have presented overwhelming evidence for genetic variation in resistance to bTB in cattle (16–19), which supports inclusion of bTB resistance in cattle breeding objectives in countries where bTB is prevalent. Recent efforts to combine national bTB surveillance and genetic data have enabled the publication of cattle evaluations for resistance to bTB in the UK (TB Advantage), which are currently used by farmers on a voluntary basis (20).

Veterinarians and epidemiologists have long considered reducing host infectiousness as an effective means to decrease disease transmission (21, 22). Infectiousness can be defined as the product of the contact rate between the infected individual and non-infected individuals, the propensity to transmit infection once infected (termed "infectivity" herein), and the duration of the infectious period (23, 24). For bTB, the contact rate between infected and non-infected herds is reduced by the movement restrictions imposed on herds with a bTB breakdown status. The duration of the infectious period is reduced by the test-and-cull policy which removes detectable infected animals, albeit with moderate animal-level sensitivity. In principle, infectivity can be reduced by vaccination, however, currently there are no vaccines (or subsequent tests) commercially available that allow differentiating between naturally infected and vaccinated individuals (i.e., a DIVA test) and would hence enable the safe use of vaccination for bTB control. Phenotypic variation in infectiousness is supported by numerous epidemiological studies showing that the Pareto principle commonly applies in epidemics, such that 20% of individuals are responsible for 80% of transmission events (22, 25–28). The individual differences in disease transmission are often attributed to different shedding patterns which may indicate phenotypic variation in host infectivity.

Emerging evidence suggests that infectivity can be, at least to some extent, under host genetic control (21, 29–33). Resistance and infectivity are thus two potentially distinct host genetic traits affecting disease transmission (see **Table 1** for definitions and statistical and mechanistic distinctions between resistance and infectivity). Hence, if genetic variation in infectivity exists, can be estimated reliably, and has no significant impact on other desired traits, reduced infectivity could be a target for genetic improvement, in addition to disease resistance. Several authors have previously proposed (29, 34, 35) or demonstrated theoretically (36–39), that breeding livestock for both resistance and reduced infectivity can be an effective approach to reduce disease risk and prevalence.

In this Perspectives article, we (a) review existing evidence that cattle may genetically differ in their bTB infectivity, (b) outline data and methodology requirements for estimating genetic infectivity for bTB, (c) discuss the benefits from considering infectivity in genetic evaluations, and (d) identify key challenges and future research opportunities for incorporating infectivity, in addition to resistance, in cattle breeding programmes aiming to reduce bTB prevalence.

Emerging Evidence That Infectivity Is Genetically Controlled

In bTB, differences in shedding patterns of *M. bovis* have been reported in various studies, but those have been mostly attributed to phenotypic variation rather than host genetics. For example, the number and frequency of episodes of shedding of *M. bovis* in cattle, were found to be dose- and infection route-dependent (40). Even amongst controlled experimentally infected calves, significant variation in shedding patterns have been described amongst individuals when presented with the same dose and infection route (41). In wild boars, the intensity and shedding of mycobacteria from the *M. tuberculosis* complex were found to affect the probability of new infections, while shedding intensity was shedding-route-dependant (42). In badgers, heterogeneity in shedding was found between different social groups (43) which may indicate family, and hence genetic, differences in shedding. Other studies found that the type of tuberculous lesions developed can affect the potential of infected individuals for transmitting infection (44), while evidence suggests that cattle with and without confirmed lesions may constitute, at least to some extent, genetically different subpopulations (45). Heterogeneity in lesion formation and stability of infected individuals suggests variation

TABLE 1 | Mechanistic and statistical distinction between resistance and infectivity in the context of bTB.

	Resistance	Infectivity
Definition (generic)	Propensity of an individual to become infected, given exposure	Propensity of an individual, once infected, to transmit infection to non-infected group members
Interpretation (bTB context)	For a given uniform level of exposure, a more resistant cow has lower risk of becoming *M. bovis* infected than a cow with low resistance	Given uniform contact rates and duration of infectious period, group members exposed to an infected cow with high infectivity have a greater risk of becoming *M. bovis* infected than when exposed to an infected cow with low infectivity
Disease phenotypes used in statistical models to infer trait estimates	Individuals' bTB infection status, based on ante-mortem test results, measured at multiple time points throughout a breakdown, possibly combined with post-mortem test results	
Trait contribution to disease phenotype	Only affects a cow's own infection status (direct effect on own disease phenotype)	Can only affect the infection status of group members (indirect effect on disease phenotype of group member)
Underlying mechanisms	Unknown; Speculated to be related to mechanisms affecting bacterial entry, establishment and within-host replication	Unknown; Speculated to be related to mechanisms controlling bacterial shedding patterns

in mechanisms underlying infectivity rather than resistance, as less stable lesions are more prone to breaking open and thus to higher bacterial shedding. Human tuberculosis epidemiology is consistent with the existence of *M. tuberculosis* super-spreaders (46, 47), which may indicate the existence of individuals with high infectivity. In bTB epidemiological studies, the best model fit has been observed when accounting for *M. bovis* super-spreaders (48, 49), and super-spreading has been proposed for badgers and other wildlife species (7, 50, 51). However, there remains a controversy about the existence of super-spreaders in bTB (52).

In other diseases, genetic variation in infectivity was found to manifest itself in various ways, such as through genetic differences in the potential for, quantity and type of infectious material shed by infected hosts. For example, genetic variation was found in the fecal egg count of sheep artificially infected with the same gastro-intestinal parasite strain and dose (53, 54). Furthermore, in cases of hosts infected with more than one genotype of the same pathogen, host immune response can affect pathogen strain competition and diversity with subsequent effect on host infectivity (55). More direct evidence for genetic differences in host infectivity has been recently obtained from transmission experiments of viral and protozoal infections in fish (31, 33). In these studies fish were found to differ in their probability of becoming diseased depending on the family or genotype of the initially infected fish that seeded the infection.

In summary, phenotypic variation in host infectivity is a common phenomenon, and for some diseases, this was shown to encompass genetic variation. In bTB, phenotypic variation in *M. bovis* shedding has been demonstrated by a few studies, but the extent to which this variation is due to cattle genetics is currently unknown. It is possible that host disease resistance and infectivity share some common genetic pathways controlling pathogen replication and consequently shedding (**Table 1**). This raises the question as to what extent bTB infectivity and resistance are genetically correlated, and how combined resistance and infectivity can affect bTB transmission.

Data and Methodology Requirements for Estimating Genetic Effects for bTB Infectivity

Infectivity, referring to an individual's ability to transmit infection (**Table 1**), is difficult to measure directly from field data where transmission routes (who-infects-whom) are difficult to trace and many transmissions are not observed or detected. Infectivity phenotypes can be obtained by measuring individual shedding rates (56). Measuring shedding has only been practical in special cases, e.g., fecal egg count for nematodes, and is very challenging if carried out routinely on the scale of sample sizes needed to inform breeding programmes.

However, shedding is not the only phenotype that can be used to track infectivity. Instead, it is possible to estimate genetic variation in infectivity by monitoring the progression of infection, i.e., the infection status of individuals, in different herds over time. Recently, novel inference methods have been developed to simultaneously estimate and untangle genetic effects for resistance and infectivity from longitudinal data of individual infection status (**Table 1**) (34, 36, 57, 58).

Common requirements for estimating genetic variation in infectivity using these novel methods are that (i) genetically related individuals are spread over different epidemics (herds/breakdowns), (ii) individual epidemics occur in "closed" groups with minimum between-group transmission, and (iii) individual infection times differ, and are known or can be inferred. These requirements appear to be satisfied by bTB. The UK national bTB eradication scheme has generated systematic repeated records of SICCT test results for a large number of herds containing related animals. In addition, due to movement restrictions imposed on herds undergoing a breakdown, herds can be considered as closed groups during the breakdown period, and data collected can be used to infer infectivity. Although the exact time of cattle infection with *M. bovis* is unknown, the repeated SICCT testing during this period provides longitudinal measurements of individuals' infection status, from which infection times can be inferred using Bayesian inference and data augmentation methods (34, 58).

It remains to be tested with field bTB data, how various sources of uncertainty affect genetic infectivity estimates. For example, these methods assume knowledge of the true infection status of an individual, which raises the question whether SICCT and other monitoring records are appropriate for this purpose. Of these, SICCT is the most commonly available measurement but its relatively poor sensitivity is well documented, i.e., its ability to correctly identify infected individuals; published sensitivity estimates range from 26 to 91% (59–63). Whether the test result reflects the true infection status of an animal is under on-going investigation within the bTB research community. Nevertheless, the positive predictive value of the test, i.e., the proportion of individuals that test positively and truly have the disease, is sufficiently high that false positives are likely to be few amongst the observed reactors. The specificity of SICCT in officially tuberculosis free herds has been estimated to be 99.98% (64). Therefore, already recorded SICCT phenotypes can provide information to search for genetic effects associated with infectivity. Including information from culling associated with SICCT testing has proven adequate for obtaining sufficiently accurate estimated breeding values (EBVs) for bTB resistance in the current bTB genetic evaluations (20). Expanding these evaluations to consider both resistance and infectivity would be expected to be beneficial primarily in high bTB risk areas, where the positive predictive value of SICCT is higher due to the higher disease prevalence (65).

Expected Benefits From Implementing Infectivity as an Additional Disease Phenotype in Genetic Evaluations for bTB Control

bTB has been a seemingly intractable problem in the UK in recent decades and understanding how cattle genetics influences bTB spread is important for eradication. Under the hypothesis that some cattle infected with bTB are genetically more infectious than others, reducing the occurrence of cattle with higher genetic infectivity through selective breeding would (i) reduce bTB transmission between cattle by removing highly infectious individuals comprising a major risk factor for herds, (ii) reduce shedding of *M. bovis* and hence reduce a major source of infection for the environment (30) and wildlife vectors, e.g., indirectly reduce bTB spill over to badgers. Badgers are susceptible to *M. bovis* infection and reducing infectivity in cattle should also reduce the pathogen burden in the environment (shedding e.g., in milk, feces, air, etc.).

If we were to estimate infectivity effects, it would enable breeders and farmers to select bulls whose offspring are not only expected to be less likely to become infected (more resistant), but also less likely to transmit bTB infection, if infected. Selection on breeding values for resistance and infectivity is expected to reduce the population R_0 (37, 39), i.e., the expected number of secondary cases produced by a typical infectious individual in a completely susceptible population (66), hence contributing to disease control. However, bTB transmission occurs within and across different species. Hence the overall bTB R_0 is composed of $R_{0_{cattle}}$, $R_{0_{badgers}}$, $R_{0_{cattle-to-badgers}}$, and $R_{0_{badgers-to-cattle}}$ (67, 68), where the cross-species relationships warrant further investigation. Reducing cattle infectivity would be expected to reduce $R_{0_{cattle}}$ and $R_{0_{cattle-to-badgers}}$, as well as the infection feedback loop from $R_{0_{badgers-to-cattle}}$. A small reduction in each component may suffice to bring the overall R_0 to below 1 and make the risk of new breakdowns negligible (10, 69). Investigating individual differences in infectivity might shed light on the variation observed in herd bTB prevalence and the relationship of infectivity with detectable bTB status, and why in some herds bTB persists with recurrent/chronic breakdowns, while other herds appear to be able to rapidly clear infection. Investigating variation in infectivity would also shed light on the weather bTB super-spreaders exist, as animals at the tail of the distribution would be "super spreaders" relative to all others, and what is their role in bTB spread.

A genetic-epidemiological simulation model can be used to assess the relative benefits of using a selection index that includes both resistance and infectivity compared to selecting on resistance alone. For this purpose we extended a stochastic epidemiological Susceptible-Latent-Infectious-Test sensitive model for bTB that originally assumed genetic variation only in resistance (70) with parameter values from the British genetic evaluations for bTB resistance (20) to incorporate hypothetical additional variation in infectivity (34, 38). We then used this model to simulate bTB spread in each herd and predict the impact of selection on breakdown risk, defined by the proportion of simulated bTB epidemics where infected index cases generated secondary cases. This is pertinent as field characteristics of epidemics often show curvilinear responses to control strategies. We found that when adding infectivity alongside resistance to the breeding objective, the reduction of the risk of a bTB breakdown was substantial and more pronounced in the early generations (**Figure 1**) (34, 38). For example, assuming 50% selection on sires, moderate heritabilities and prediction accuracies for resistance and infectivity, and zero correlation between resistance and infectivity, the relative epidemic risk at generation 5 was ~0.2 with selection for resistance alone, but <0.1 for combined selection for both resistance and infectivity, even when external sources of infection were included (**Figure 1**). These simulations designed as proof-of-principle, provide a crude estimate of the predicted effects which will depend on e.g., the magnitude of the genetic variance in the objective traits and various demographic factors. However, these findings are indicative that by targeting both resistance and infectivity in combination, disease control benefits can be of larger magnitude (i.e., more effective) and more responsive (i.e., quicker to see results) (38).

The epidemiological benefits and additional gain expected from adding infectivity to the breeding goal depends on its genetic correlation with other traits of economic interest. A classic example of the impact of adverse correlated responses, is the reduction of cattle fertility following selection on milk yield, due to adverse genetic correlation with milk yield (12). Based on estimated genetic correlations among traits, genetic selection for enhanced bTB resistance is not expected to adversely affect other traits in the breeding goal (16, 20), and was found to be unlikely to change the probability of correctly identifying non-infected

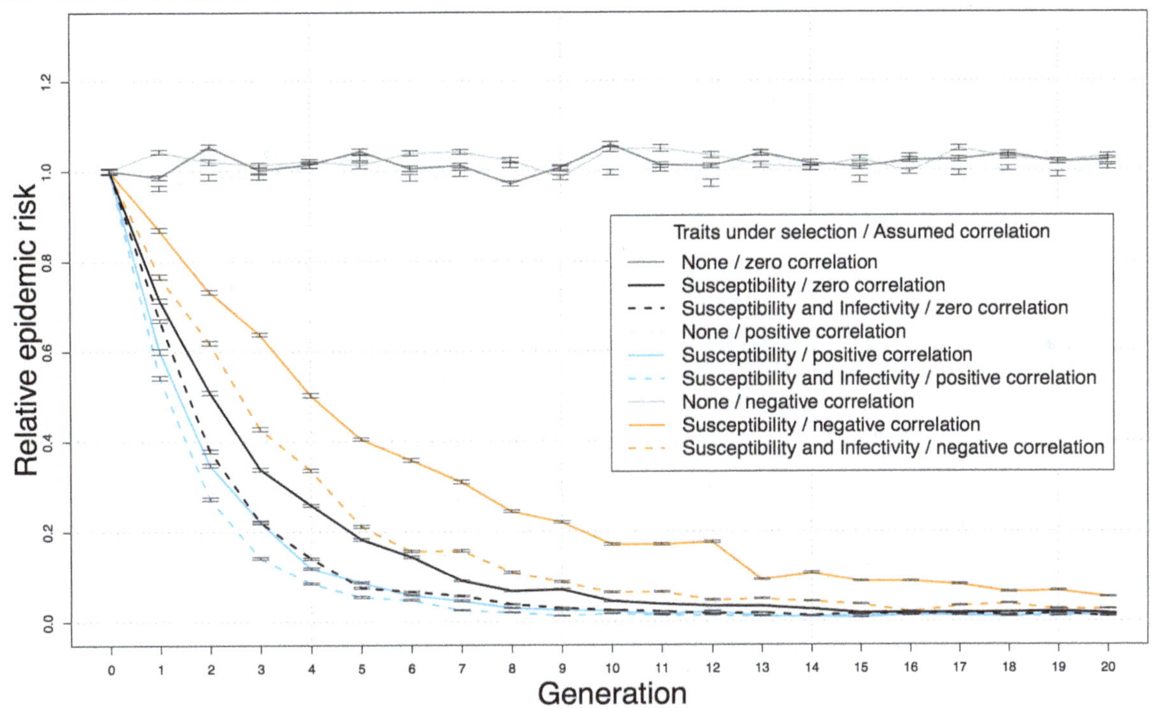

FIGURE 1 | Reduction in the predicted relative risk of bTB breakdown in a herd, following introduction of an infected cow, over 20 generations of selection for resistance and lower infectivity, or for resistance alone. Predictions from a stochastic genetic-epidemiological simulation model incorporating genetic variation in resistance and infectivity (38), comprising populations of 10,000 half-sib individuals randomly distributed into 100 herds of the same size. Means and standard errors were obtained over 50 replicates. The parameter values were based on the British genetic evaluations for bTB resistance (20) and a previous genetic-epidemiological model (70) as follows: bTB testing intervals of 60 days, SICCT sensitivity of 60%, 50% selection on the sires, accuracy of 0.5 and latent heritability of 0.6 [corresponding to heritability for the observed indicator traits of below 0.2 (70)] for both resistance and infectivity, economic values of one for both traits, and external force of infection of 5×10^{-5} (70). Each breakdown was initiated by one infectious individual, and variance and accuracy were assumed constant over generations. The correlation between resistance and infectivity was assumed to be zero, 0.5 or −0.5.

animals via the SICCT diagnostic test (71). However, genetic correlations between resistance and infectivity may affect the outcome of genetic bTB control. Indeed, based on the genetic-epidemiological bTB model described above (38) the strongest benefit of adding infectivity into the selection criterion compared to selecting on resistance alone is observed in the case of an adverse genetic correlation between the traits (**Figure 1**), and this is because the progress achieved by breeding schemes targeting only resistance would be delayed due to an indirect increase in infectivity. Considering breeding values for infectivity can help alleviate this delay and accelerate progress toward disease eradication (38).

Future Opportunities and Challenges

In principle, bTB surveillance schemes such as those implemented in the UK, RoI, and NZ, would permit researchers to pioneer the estimation of infectivity genetic effects without the need to collect new data. Current genetic evaluations for bTB resistance (20) use phenotype and pedigree information, with increasing amounts of genomic data. As the incidence of bTB reduces, the information obtained from pedigrees will also reduce. Therefore, genomic information becomes increasingly vital, and high-density genomic data can now be obtained cost-effectively by genotype imputation (72, 73). It has been shown that genomic prediction for bTB resistance using genomic information is feasible (18), and prediction accuracies can be improved by using larger training sets of genotyped animals and genome sequence information. This is pertinent for infectivity, as it has been shown in simulation studies that the prediction accuracy for infectivity is expected, at least initially, to be modest (34). This genomic information also allows investigation of the genetic architecture of bTB infectivity and the search for causal variants.

Challenges arising in the analysis of bTB data to uncover genetic infectivity include accounting for multiple and poorly understood transmission routes of *M. bovis*, and obtaining more reliable disease phenotypes. Separating the effects of the infectious dose from host response is extremely challenging in field situations where exposure may not be uniform (74). However, sophisticated Bayesian inference methods, coupled with phylodynamics and *M. bovis* genome sequence information, can help to infer transmission routes and obtain information on the networks of who-infects-whom (49, 75–78), which is useful for predicting infectivity (79). More reliable disease phenotypes could be obtained by quality control on individual tester performance to improve the consistency of data recording on the farms (80), and by developing improved diagnostics. Machine learning techniques (Deep Learning) hold the promise that sufficiently accurate disease phenotypes can be obtained in a cost-effective manner for large sample sizes using routinely collected mid infra-red spectral data from milk recording (Coffey M. personal communication October 2018). Together, continuous development of improved diagnostic and modeling tools provide promising prospects for genetic bTB control.

CONCLUSION

Host infectivity is an important trait for disease transmission and emerging evidence suggests that it may be under genetic control to some extent; however, the role of genetic infectivity of cattle in bTB spread remains to be explored. Infectivity might be difficult to capture from noisy field data; however, the UK bTB surveillance database and newly developed statistical methods provide the opportunity to estimate genetic effects for infectivity. Exploiting genetic variation in infectivity as a complementary bTB control method is a low-investment high-return approach, as it can be developed at minimal cost using data already available. Simulation studies suggest that breeding for both disease resistance and infectivity can complement and substantially enhance current disease control approaches toward bTB eradication. Using UK data to determine genetic regulation of disease transmission can create a platform for controlling bTB in other countries and for controlling other infectious diseases.

AUTHOR CONTRIBUTIONS

ST, AA, RS, GB, JW, and AD-W conceived the perspectives. ST drafted the manuscript, designed and carried out the simulations and participated in the interpretation of findings. JW and AD-W contributed to the initial draft and simulation designs. All authors contributed to later versions of the manuscript, read and approved the final manuscript.

ACKNOWLEDGMENTS

This work was carried out with funding from the Biotechnology and Biological Sciences Research Council Institute Strategic Programme grants BB/J004235/1 (ISP1) and BB/P013740/1 (ISP2) (OA, AD-W, GB and JW), and the European Union FP7 project FISHBOOST (KBBE - 7-613611) (ST). GB was also supported by the Rural and Environment Science and Analytical Services Division of the Scottish Government.

REFERENCES

1. Michel AL, Muller B, van Helden PD. *Mycobacterium bovis* at the animal-human interface: a problem, or not? *Vet Microbiol.* (2010) 140:371–81. doi: 10.1016/j.vetmic.2009.08.029
2. World Health Organization. *Roadmap for Zoonotic Tuberculosis* (2017). Available online at: http://www.fao.org/3/a-i7807e.pdf
3. Olea-Popelka F, Fujiwara PI. Building a multi-institutional and interdisciplinary team to develop a zoonotic tuberculosis roadmap. *Front Public Health* (2018) 6:167. doi: 10.3389/fpubh.2018.00167
4. Dean AS, Forcella S, Olea-Popelka F, Idrissi AE, Glaziou P, Benyahia A, et al. A roadmap for zoonotic tuberculosis: a one health approach to ending tuberculosis. *Lancet Infect Dis.* (2018) 18:137–8. doi: 10.1016/S1473-3099(18)30013-6
5. Abernethy DA, Upton P, Higgins IM, McGrath G, Goodchild AV, Rolfe SJ, et al. Bovine tuberculosis trends in the UK and the Republic of Ireland, 1995–2010. *Vet Rec.* (2013) 172:312. doi: 10.1136/vr.100969
6. DEFRA. *The Strategy for Achieving Officially Bovine Tuberculosis Free Status for England* (2014). Available online at: https://assets.publishing.service.gov.uk/government/uploads/system/uploads/attachment_data/file/300447/pb14088-bovine-tb-strategy-140328.pdf
7. Allen AR, Skuce RA, Byrne AW. Bovine tuberculosis in Britain and Ireland - a perfect storm? The confluence of potential ecological and epidemiological impediments to controlling a chronic infectious disease. *Front Vet Sci.* (2018) 5:109. doi: 10.3389/fvets.2018.00109
8. DEFRA. *Quarterly Publication of National Statistics on the Incidence and Prevalence of Tuberculosis (Tb) in Cattle in Great Britain – To End March 2018.* (2018) Available online at: https://www.gov.uk/government/statistics/incidence-of-tuberculosis-tb-in-cattle-in-great-britain
9. Bishop SC, Woolliams JA. Genomics and disease resistance studies in livestock. *Livest Sci.* (2014) 166:190–8. doi: 10.1016/j.livsci.2014.04.034
10. Bishop S, Axford R, Nicholas F, Owen J. *Breeding for Disease Resistance in Farm Animals.* 3rd Ed. Wallingford: CABI Publishing (2010).
11. Weigel KA, VanRaden PM, Norman HD, Grosu H. A 100-year review: methods and impact of genetic selection in dairy cattle-from daughter-dam comparisons to deep learning algorithms. *J Dairy Sci.* (2017) 100:10234–50. doi: 10.3168/jds.2017-12954
12. Wall E, Brotherstone S, Woolliams JA, Banos G, Coffey MP. Genetic evaluation of fertility using direct and correlated traits. *J Dairy Sci.* (2003) 86:4093–102. doi: 10.3168/jds.S0022-0302(03)74023-5
13. Heringstad B, Klemetsdal G, Ruane J. Selection for mastitis resistance in dairy cattle: a review with focus on the situation in the Nordic countries. *Livest Prod Sci.* (2000) 64:95–106. doi: 10.1016/S0301-6226(99)00128-1
14. Martin P, Barkema HW, Brito LF, Narayana SG, Miglior F. Symposium review: novel strategies to genetically improve mastitis resistance in dairy cattle. *J Dairy Sci.* (2018) 101:2724–36. doi: 10.3168/jds.2017-13554
15. Houston R, Bishop SC, Woolliams J, Haley C. *Marker-Assisted Selection to breed for resistance to Infectious Pancreatic Necrosis in Salmon* Research Excellence Framework (REF), impact case studies (2014). Available online at: http://impact.ref.ac.uk/CaseStudies/CaseStudy.aspx?Id=23913
16. Brotherstone S, White IM, Coffey M, Downs SH, Mitchell AP, Clifton-Hadley RS, et al. Evidence of genetic resistance of cattle to infection with *Mycobacterium bovis. J Dairy Sci.* (2010) 93:1234–42. doi: 10.3168/jds.2009-2609
17. Bermingham ML, Bishop SC, Woolliams JA, Pong-Wong R, Allen AR, McBride SH, et al. Genome-wide association study identifies novel loci associated with resistance to bovine tuberculosis. *Heredity* (2014) 112:543–51. doi: 10.1038/hdy.2013.137
18. Tsairidou S, Woolliams JA, Allen AR, Skuce RA, McBride SH, Wright DM, et al. Genomic prediction for tuberculosis resistance in dairy cattle. *PLoS ONE* (2014) 9:e96728. doi: 10.1371/journal.pone.0096728
19. Woolliams J, Brotherstone S, Coffey M. *A Preliminary Analysis of Existing Data to Provide Evidence of a Genetic Basis for Resistance of Cattle to Infection with M. bovis and for Reactivity to Currently Used Immunological Diagnostic Tests.* Defra, London, UK (2008).
20. Banos G, Winters M, Mrode R, Mitchell AP, Bishop SC, Woolliams JA, et al. Genetic evaluation for bovine tuberculosis resistance in dairy cattle. *J Dairy Sci.* (2017) 100:1272–81. doi: 10.3168/jds.2016-11897
21. Geenen PL, Van der Meulen J, Bouma A, De Jong MCM. Estimating transmission parameters of F4+ *E. coli* for F4-receptor-positive and-negative piglets: one-to-one transmission experiment. *Epidemiol Infect.* (2004) 132:1039–48.

22. Lloyd-Smith JO, Schreiber SJ, Kopp PE, Getz WM. Superspreading and the effect of individual variation on disease emergence. *Nature* (2005) 438:355–9. doi: 10.1038/nature04153
23. Keeling MJ, Rohani P. *Modeling Infectious Diseases in Humans and Animals.* Woodstock, NJ; Oxfordshire: Princeton University Press (2008).
24. Lipschutz-Powell D, Woolliams JA, Doeschl-Wilson AB. A unifying theory for genetic epidemiological analysis of binary disease data. *Genet Sel Evol.* (2013) 46:15. doi: 10.1186/1297-9686-46-15
25. Woolhouse MEJ, Dye C, Etard J-F, Smith T, Charlwood JD, Garnett GP, et al. Heterogeneities in the transmission of infectious agents: implications for the design of control programs. *Proc Natl Acad Sci USA.* (1997) 94:338–42.
26. Jankowski MD, Williams CJ, Fair JM, Owen JC. Birds shed RNA-viruses according to the pareto principle. *PLoS ONE* (2013) 8:e72611. doi: 10.1371/journal.pone.0072611
27. Gopinath S, Lichtman JS, Bouley DM, Elias JE, Monack DM. Role of disease-associated tolerance in infectious superspreaders. *Proc Natl Acad Sci USA.* (2014) 111:15780–5. doi: 10.1073/pnas.1409968111
28. Shen Z, Ning F, Zhou W, He X, Lin C, Chin DP, et al. Superspreading SARS events, Beijing, 2003. *Emerg Infect Dis.* (2004) 10:256–60. doi: 10.3201/eid1002.030732
29. Raszek MM, Guan LL, Plastow GS. Use of genomic tools to improve cattle health in the context of infectious diseases. *Front Genet.* (2016) 7:30. doi: 10.3389/fgene.2016.00030
30. Doeschl-Wilson AB, Davidson R, Conington J, Roughsedge T, Hutchings MR, Villanueva B. Implications of host genetic variation on the risk and prevalence of infectious diseases transmitted through the environment. *Genetics* (2011) 188:683–93. doi: 10.1534/genetics.110.125625
31. Doeschl-Wilson A, Anacleto O, Nielsen HM, Karlsson-Drangsholt TM, Lillehammer M, Gjerde B. New opportunities for genetic disease control: beyond disease resistance. In: *Proceedings of the World Congress on Genetics Applied to Livestock Production* (Auckland) (2018).
32. Lyall J, Irvine RM, Sherman A, McKinley TJ, Nunez A, Purdie A, et al. Suppression of avian influenza transmission in genetically modified chickens. *Science* (2011) 331:223–6. doi: 10.1126/science.1198020
33. Anacleto O, Cabaleiro S, Villanueva B, Saura M, Houston RD, Woolliams JA, et al. Genetic differences in host infectivity affect disease spread and survival in epidemics. *biorxiv[Preprint].* (2018). doi: 10.1101/483602
34. Anacleto O, Garcia-Cortés LA, Lipschutz-Powell D, Woolliams JA, Doeschl-Wilson AB. A novel statistical model to estimate host genetic effects affecting disease transmission. *Genetics* (2015) 201:871–84. doi: 10.1534/genetics.115.179853
35. Brooks-Pollock E, de Jong MCM, Keeling MJ, Klinkenberg D, Wood JLN. Eight challenges in modelling infectious livestock diseases. *Epidemics* (2015) 10:1–5. doi: 10.1016/j.epidem.2014.08.005
36. Biemans F, de Jong MCM, Bijma P. A model to estimate effects of SNPs on host susceptibility and infectivity for an endemic infectious disease. *Genet Sel Evol.* (2017) 49:53. doi: 10.1186/s12711-017-0327-0
37. Lipschutz-Powell D, Woolliams JA, Bijma P, Doeschl-Wilson AB. Indirect genetic effects and the spread of infectious disease: are we capturing the full heritable variation underlying disease prevalence? *PLoS ONE* (2012) 7:e39551. doi: 10.1371/journal.pone.0039551
38. Tsairidou S, Anacleto O, Raphaka K, Sanchez-Molano E, Banos G, Woolliams JA, et al. Enhancing genetic disease control by selecting for lower host infectivity. In: *Proceedings of the World Congress on Genetics Applied to Livestock Production* (Auckland) (2018).
39. Anche M, Jong M, Bijma P. On the definition and utilization of heritable variation among hosts in reproduction ratio R0 for infectious diseases. *Heredity* (2014) 113:364–74. doi: 10.1038/hdy.2014.38
40. McCorry T, Whelan AO, Welsh MD, McNair J, Walton E, Bryson DG, et al. Shedding of *Mycobacterium bovis* in the nasal mucus of cattle infected experimentally with tuberculosis by the intranasal and intratracheal routes. *Vet Rec.* (2005) 157:613–8. doi: 10.1136/vr.157.20.613
41. Kao RR, Gravenor MB, Charleston B, Hope JC, Martin M, Howard CJ. *Mycobacterium bovis* shedding patterns from experimentally infected calves and the effect of concurrent infection with bovine viral diarrhoea virus. *J R Soc Interface* (2007) 4:545–51. doi: 10.1098/rsif.2006.0190
42. Barasona JA, Torres MJ, Aznar J, Gortazar C, Vicente J. DNA detection reveals *Mycobacterium tuberculosis* complex shedding routes in its wildlife reservoir the Eurasian wild boar. *Transbound Emerg Dis.* (2017) 64:906–15. doi: 10.1111/tbed.12458
43. King HC, Murphy A, James P, Travis E, Porter D, Sawyer J, et al. Performance of a noninvasive test for detecting *Mycobacterium bovis* shedding in European badger (Meles meles) populations. *J Clin Microbiol.* (2015) 53:2316–23. doi: 10.1128/JCM.00762-15
44. Shaler CR, Horvath CN, Jeyanathan M, Xing Z. Within the enemy's camp: contribution of the granuloma to the dissemination, persistence and transmission of *Mycobacterium tuberculosis. Front Immunol.* (2013) 4:30. doi: 10.3389/fimmu.2013.00030
45. Wilkinson S, Bishop SC, Allen AR, McBride SH, Skuce RA, Bermingham M, et al. Fine-mapping host genetic variation underlying outcomes to *Mycobacterium bovis* infection in dairy cows. *BMC Genomics* (2017) 18:477. doi: 10.1186/s12864-017-3836-x
46. Walker TM, Ip CL, Harrell RH, Evans JT, Kapatai G, Dedicoat MJ, et al. Whole-genome sequencing to delineate *Mycobacterium tuberculosis* outbreaks: a retrospective observational study. *Lancet Infect Dis.* (2013) 13:137–46. doi: 10.1016/S1473-3099(12)70277-3
47. Ypma RJ, Altes HK, van Soolingen D, Wallinga J, van Ballegooijen WM. A sign of superspreading in tuberculosis: highly skewed distribution of genotypic cluster sizes. *Epidemiology* (2013) 24:395–400. doi: 10.1097/EDE.0b013e3182878e19
48. Trewby H, Wright DM, Skuce RA, McCormick C, Mallon TR, Presho EL, et al. Relative abundance of *Mycobacterium bovis* molecular types in cattle: a simulation study of potential epidemiological drivers. *BMC Vet Res.* (2017) 13:268. doi: 10.1186/s12917-017-1190-5
49. O'Hare A, Orton RJ, Bessell PR, Kao RR. Estimating epidemiological parameters for bovine tuberculosis in British cattle using a Bayesian partial-likelihood approach. *Proc Biol Sci.* (2014) 281:20140248. doi: 10.1098/rspb.2014.0248
50. Santos N, Almeida V, Gortázar C, Correia-Neves M. Patterns of *Mycobacterium tuberculosis*-complex excretion and characterization of super-shedders in naturally-infected wild boar and red deer. *Vet Res.* (2015) 46:129. doi: 10.1186/s13567-015-0270-4
51. Delahay RJ, Langton S, Smith GC, Clifton-Hadley RS, Cheeseman CL. The spatio-temporal distribution of *Mycobacterium bovis* (bovine tuberculosis) infection in a high-density badger population. *J Anim Ecol.* (2000) 69:428–41. doi: 10.1046/j.1365-2656.2000.00406.x
52. Bourne FJ, Donnelly CA, Cox DR, Gettinby G, McInerney JP, Morrison WI, et al. Re: TB policy and the ISG's findings. *Vet Rec.* (2007) 161:633–5. doi: 10.1136/vr.161.18.633-b
53. Bishop S, Jackson F, Coop R, Stear M. Genetic parameters for resistance to nematode infections in Texel lambs and their utility in breeding programmes. *Anim Sci.* (2004) 78:185–94. doi: 10.1017/S1357729800053972
54. Sallé G, Jacquiet P, Gruner L, Cortet J, Sauvé C, Prévot F, et al. A genome scan for QTL affecting resistance to *Haemonchus contortus* in sheep. *J Anim Ecol.* (2012) 90:4690–705. doi: 10.2527/jas.2012-5121
55. Read AF, Taylor LH. The ecology of genetically diverse infections. *Science* (2001) 292:1099–102. doi: 10.1126/science.1059410
56. Charpin C, Mahe S, Keranflec'h A, Belloc C, Cariolet R, Le Potier MF, et al. Infectiousness of pigs infected by the porcine reproductive and respiratory syndrome virus (PRRSV) is time-dependent. *Vet Res.* (2012) 43:69. doi: 10.1186/1297-9716-43-69
57. Anche MT, Bijma P, De Jong MC. Genetic analysis of infectious diseases: estimating gene effects for susceptibility and infectivity. *Genet Sel Evol.* (2015) 47:85. doi: 10.1186/s12711-015-0163-z
58. Pooley C, Bishop S, Marion G. Estimation of single locus effects on susceptibility, infectivity and recovery rates in an epidemic using temporal data. In *Proceedings of the 10th World Congress on Genetics Applied to Livestock Production* (Vancouver, BC)(2014).
59. de la Rua-Domenech R, Goodchild AT, Vordermeier HM, Hewinson RG, Christiansen KH, Clifton-Hadley RS. Ante mortem diagnosis of tuberculosis in cattle: a review of the tuberculin tests, gamma-interferon assay and other ancillary diagnostic techniques. *Res Vet Sci.* (2006) 81:190–210. doi: 10.1016/j.rvsc.2005.11.005

60. Clegg TA, Duignan A, Whelan C, Gormley E, Good M, Clarke J, et al. Using latent class analysis to estimate the test characteristics of the gamma-interferon test, the single intradermal comparative tuberculin test and a multiplex immunoassay under Irish conditions. *Vet Microbiol.* (2011) 151:68–76. doi: 10.1016/j.vetmic.2011.02.027
61. Bermingham ML, More SJ, Good M, Cromie AR, Higgins IM, Brotherstone S, et al. Genetics of tuberculosis in Irish Holstein-Friesian dairy herds. *J Dairy Sci.* (2009) 92:3447–56. doi: 10.3168/jds.2008-1848
62. Nunez-Garcia J, Downs SH, Parry JE, Abernethy DA, Broughan JM, Cameron AR, et al. Meta-analyses of the sensitivity and specificity of ante-mortem and post-mortem diagnostic tests for bovine tuberculosis in the UK and Ireland. *Prev Vet Med.* (2018) 153:94–107. doi: 10.1016/j.prevetmed.2017.02.017
63. Lahuerta-Marin A, Milne MG, McNair J, Skuce RA, McBride SH, Menzies FD, et al. Bayesian latent class estimation of sensitivity and specificity parameters of diagnostic tests for bovine tuberculosis in chronically infected herds in Northern Ireland. *Vet J.* (2018) 238:15–21. doi: 10.1016/j.tvjl.2018.04.019
64. Goodchild AV, Downs SH, Upton P, Wood JLN, de la Rua-Domenech R. Specificity of the comparative skin test for bovine tuberculosis in Great Britain. *Vet Rec.* (2015) 177:258. doi: 10.1136/vr.102961
65. Drewe JA. Bovine tuberculosis: how likely is a skin test reactor to be uninfected? *Vet Rec.* (2015) 177:256–7. doi: 10.1136/vr.h4760
66. Diekmann O, Heesterbeek JAP, Metz JAJ. On the definition and the computation of the basic reproduction ratio R0 in models for infectious diseases in heterogeneous populations. *J Math Biol.* (1990) 28:365–82. doi: 10.1007/BF00178324
67. Brooks-Pollock E, Wood JLN. Eliminating bovine tuberculosis in cattle and badgers: insight from a dynamic model. *Proc Biol Sci.* (2015) 282:20150374. doi: 10.1098/rspb.2015.0374
68. Heesterbeek JA, Roberts MG. The type-reproduction number T in models for infectious disease control. *Math Biosci.* (2007) 206:3–10. doi: 10.1016/j.mbs.2004.10.013
69. Aznar I, Frankena K, Byrne A, More S, De Jong M. Infection dynamics and effective control options of tuberculosis in cattle and badgers. In: *6th International M. bovis Conference*. Cardiff (2014).
70. Raphaka K. *Genetics of Bovine Tuberculosis Resistance in Dairy Cattle*. Ph.D. Thesis, The University of Edinburgh (2018).
71. Tsairidou S, Brotherstone S, Coffey M, Bishop SC, Woolliams JA. Quantitative genetic analysis of the bTB diagnostic single intradermal comparative cervical test (SICCT). *Genet Sel Evol.* (2016) 48:90. doi: 10.1186/s12711-016-0264-3
72. Burdick JT, Chen W-M, Abecasis GR, Cheung VG. *In silico* method for inferring genotypes in pedigrees. *Nat Genet.* (2006) 38:1002–4. doi: 10.1038/ng1863
73. Calus MP, Bouwman AC, Hickey JM, Veerkamp RF, Mulder HA. Evaluation of measures of correctness of genotype imputation in the context of genomic prediction: a review of livestock applications. *Animal* (2014) 8:1743–53. doi: 10.1017/S1751731114001803
74. Bishop SC, Doeschl-Wilson AB, Woolliams JA. Uses and implications of field disease data for livestock genomic and genetics studies. *Front Genet.* (2012) 3:114. doi: 10.3389/fgene.2012.00114
75. Brooks-Pollock E, Roberts GO, Keeling MJ. A dynamic model of bovine tuberculosis spread and control in Great Britain. *Nature* (2014) 511:228–31. doi: 10.1038/nature13529
76. Green DM, Kiss IZ, Mitchell AP, Kao RR. Estimates for local and movement-based transmission of bovine tuberculosis in British cattle. *Proc Biol Sci.* (2008) 275:1001–5. doi: 10.1098/rspb.2007.1601
77. Kao RR, Haydon DT, Lycett SJ, Murcia PR. Supersize me: how whole-genome sequencing and big data are transforming epidemiology. *Trends Microbiol.* (2014) 22:282–91. doi: 10.1016/j.tim.2014.02.011
78. Lam TT-Y, Wang J, Shen Y, Zhou B, Duan L, Cheung C-L, et al. The genesis and source of the H7N9 influenza viruses causing human infections in China. *Nature* (2013) 502:241–4. doi: 10.1038/nature12515
79. Lipschutz-Powell D, Woolliams JA, Bijma P, Pong-Wong R, Bermingham ML, Doeschl-Wilson AB. Bias, accuracy, and impact of indirect genetic effects in infectious diseases. *Front Genet.* (2012) 3:215. doi: 10.3389/fgene.2012.00215
80. Duignan A, Good M, More SJ. Quality control in the national bovine tuberculosis eradication programme in Ireland. *Rev Sci Tech.* (2012) 31:845–60. doi: 10.20506/rst.31.3.2166

2

Efficacy and Safety of BCG Vaccine for Control of Tuberculosis in Domestic Livestock and Wildlife

Bryce M. Buddle[1], Hans Martin Vordermeier[2], Mark A. Chambers[2,3] and Lin-Mari de Klerk-Lorist[4]*

[1] AgResearch, Hopkirk Research Institute, Palmerston North, New Zealand, [2] Animal and Plant Health Agency, Addlestone, United Kingdom, [3] Faculty of Health & Medical Sciences, School of Veterinary Medicine, University of Surrey, Guildford, United Kingdom, [4] Veterinary Wildlife Services, Kruger National Park, Department of Agriculture, Forestry and Fisheries, Pretoria, South Africa

***Correspondence:**
Bryce M. Buddle
bryce.buddle@agresearch.co.nz

Bovine tuberculosis (TB) continues to be an intractable problem in many countries, particularly where "test and slaughter" policies cannot be implemented or where wildlife reservoirs of *Mycobacterium bovis* infection serve as a recurrent source of infection for domestic livestock. Alternative control measures are urgently required and vaccination is a promising option. Although the *M. bovis* bacille Calmette-Guérin (BCG) vaccine has been used in humans for nearly a century, its use in animals has been limited, principally as protection against TB has been incomplete and vaccination may result in animals reacting in the tuberculin skin test. Valuable insights have been gained over the past 25 years to optimise protection induced by BCG vaccine in animals and in the development of tests to differentiate infected from vaccinated animals (DIVA). This review examines factors affecting the efficacy of BCG vaccine in cattle, recent field trials, use of DIVA tests and the effectiveness of BCG vaccine in other domestic livestock as well as in wildlife. Oral delivery of BCG vaccine to wildlife reservoirs of infection such as European badgers, brushtail possums, wild boar, and deer has been shown to induce protection against TB and could prove to be a practical means to vaccinate these species at scale. Testing of BCG vaccine in a wide range of animal species has indicated that it is safe and vaccination has the potential to be a valuable tool to assist in the control of TB in both domestic livestock and wildlife.

Keywords: BCG, cattle, diagnosis, goats, deer, tuberculosis, vaccination, wildlife

INTRODUCTION

Tuberculosis (TB) in domestic livestock and wildlife is caused by *Mycobacterium bovis*, *Mycobacterium caprae*, and other members of the *Mycobacterium tuberculosis* complex, including *M. tuberculosis* whose role in animal TB is being increasingly recognised, particularly in studies from Africa and Asia (1). Livestock TB continues to be a major economic animal health problem worldwide. It has been estimated that >50 million cattle are infected worldwide, costing US$3 billion annually (2). The disease is an important zoonosis, causing TB in humans, particularly through consumption of unpasteurised milk or through co-habitation with infected animals. The "test and slaughter" bovine TB control programmes introduced in many countries in the mid-twentieth century achieved dramatic results and a number of countries were able to eradicate this disease. However, these control programmes have not been affordable or socially acceptable in many developing countries, and more than 94% of the world's population live in countries in which control of TB in cattle or buffaloes is limited or absent (3). Furthermore, a confounding factor in the control of bovine TB in a number of countries has been the existence of wildlife reservoirs of *M. bovis* infection.

Wildlife serving as maintenance hosts for *M. bovis* include the Australian brushtail possum (*Trichosurus vulpecula*) in New Zealand, the European badger (*Meles meles*) in United Kingdom (UK) and Ireland, white-tailed deer (*Odocoileus virginianus*) in Michigan, USA [reviewed in (4)] and Eurasian wild boar (*Sus scrofa*) in the Iberian Peninsula, Spain (5). In addition, red deer (*Cervus elaphus*) in several parts of Europe (6), African buffalo (*Syncerus caffer*) in South Africa (7), and wood bison (*Bison bison athabascae*) and wapiti (*Cervus elephus manitobensis*) in Canada (8) serve as maintenance hosts for infection in hunting estates and national parks. These various maintenance hosts act as sources of infection for domestic species, and in national parks, infection can spill over to other unique wildlife species including Iberian lynx (*Lynx pardinus*), lions (*Panthera leo*), leopard (*Panthera pardus*), and wild dogs (*Lycaon pictus*). Partial control has been achieved for some of these maintenance hosts by minimising contact with livestock, reducing the density of animals or banning artificial feeding that causes local high densities of animals (9–11). However, few if any of these control measures can be implemented for some protected species or where interference of a natural regulated ecosystem is deemed undesirable. For these reasons, the development and use of vaccines for control of TB in both domestic livestock and wild animals is very appealing.

Although no TB vaccines are currently registered for protection against TB in domestic livestock, there is renewed interest in their use from the realisation of the financial impact of bovine TB on animal health and trade, and due to the difficulty controlling the disease. In addition, the use of vaccines to control the TB in wildlife reservoirs of infection could be very valuable in limiting the spread of infection to domestic livestock and *M. bovis* bacille Calmette-Guérin (BCG) was registered for intramuscular administration to badgers in the UK in 2010. Evidence of the use of a vaccine to control a disease in wildlife has been shown from the success of using vaccination to control rabies in foxes in Europe (12). BCG vaccine is the only registered TB vaccine for humans and was developed by Calmette and Guérin from a strain of *M. bovis* originally isolated by Nocard from a case of tuberculous mastitis. Following serial passage of the strain on ox bile glycerine-potato medium for 230 passages, between 1908 and 1919, this variant strain was shown to be attenuated in animals and conferred resistance to challenge of animals with virulent *M. bovis* and *M. tuberculosis* [reviewed in (13)]. The strain was distributed to many countries in the 1920s and continuing passage in differing conditions produced a considerable number of daughter strains, with varying antigenic profiles (14).

Vaccination of humans commenced in 1921 and in a meta-analysis, vaccination of newborns and infants significantly reduced the risk of TB by an average of over 50%, although efficacy ranged from 0 to 80% (15). Many field trials of BCG vaccination of cattle were conducted in the first half of the twentieth century and the major caveats that restricted the use of TB vaccines in cattle were that protection was not complete and vaccination could sensitise animals to respond in traditional TB diagnostic tests. These problems can now be potentially overcome by using vaccination integrated with other control measures and use of diagnostic tests which can differentiate infected from vaccinated animals (DIVA tests). Currently, there is very large effort to develop improved TB vaccines for humans, by developing vaccines which may replace BCG or those that could boost immunity following initial vaccination with BCG (16). Research to develop improved TB vaccines for livestock is following a similar path. Information on the efficacy of BCG in animals can be of assistance in the development of these new generation vaccines for use in multiple species. For most wildlife species, however, vaccination efforts are restricted to the use of a single-shot vaccine since access to the same individuals in order to deliver a booster is unrealistic. The focus of this paper is to provide a review of the efficacy and safety of BCG vaccine in domestic livestock and wildlife to assist in optimising the use of BCG vaccine in animals as well as providing a guide for the development of improved TB vaccines. TB vaccines that do not use BCG are being studied for some applications, such as a heat-inactivated *M. bovis* whole-cell vaccine for wild boar, but these are not the focus of this review.

VACCINATION OF CATTLE

Historical Studies of BCG

Studies of BCG vaccine in cattle were first reported by Calmette and Guérin (17) and showed that relatively high doses of BCG (20 mg) could induce protection in cattle against experimental challenge with *M. bovis*. In the studies of Calmette and Guérin (18), intravenous challenge of control calves with virulent *M. bovis* resulted in severe generalised TB by 30–60 days. In contrast, the BCG vaccinates which were challenged remained healthy, but virulent *M. bovis* could be isolated from their bronchial lymph nodes when the animals were killed at 3–4 months post-challenge. A number of other researchers reported similar results in experimental challenge studies where BCG vaccination did not induce absolute immunity, but moderated the severity of the infection [reviewed in (19)]. A comparison of routes of vaccination with BCG showed that intravenous, intradermal and oral routes conferred some resistance to feeding milk containing large doses of virulent *M. bovis*, although not greater than that conferred with subcutaneous vaccination (20). Field studies of BCG vaccination of cattle using either a subcutaneous or intravenous route of vaccination showed variable results which may in part have been influenced by the duration and the potency of the exposure. Promising results were shown by Rankin (21) with 86% (37 of 43) non-vaccinates with tuberculous lesions compared to 33% (22 of 66) for the BCG vaccinates by 8–10 months post exposure. Watson (22) undertook a study over a longer duration where new-born calves were vaccinated with BCG subcutaneously (50–100 mg dose), fed pasteurised milk for 1–2 months, and then exposed to *M. bovis* through ingestion of raw milk from infected cows or co-habitation with infected cattle.

The study demonstrated that there was good resistance in calves compared to controls by 1 year post-exposure, but resistance declined steadily up to reproductive age where there was little evidence of protection. A number of uncontrolled trials were undertaken to determine whether BCG vaccination could clear TB infection in heavily infected herds. Some studies reported that BCG vaccination eliminated disease over 7 years (23, 24), while others found this approach reduced the skin test reactivity and resulted in newly introduced unvaccinated animals ($n = 100$) remaining skin test negative over a 5 year post-vaccination period. This approach was judged to be impractical and slow (25).

These early studies indicated that BCG could induce some protection against TB, although protection was not absolute, appeared to wane after 1–2 years and vaccination could induce positive reactivity in the tuberculin test. It was concluded that TB could be eradicated faster and more efficiently using "test and slaughter" control programmes than relying only on vaccination with BCG. However, it was considered that BCG vaccination could possibly have a role in disease control in countries where "test and slaughter" programmes could not be implemented due to economic or social reasons and a number of trials were conducted in Malawi in the 1970s for this purpose. Ellwood and Waddington (26) showed that the development of tuberculous lesions and progressive infection was less in BCG vaccinates following experimental *M. bovis* challenge compared to controls, providing encouragement to proceed with a field study. In the field trial, 3–12 month old calves were injected with 10^7 colony forming units (CFU) of BCG (Glaxo strain) and revaccinated 6 months later, while alternate calves in each herd were sham inoculated (27). When the animals were slaughtered and necropsied 5 years after the commencement of study, no significant differences could be found in the number of animals with tuberculous lesions, 36 of 204 (17.7%) in the vaccinates and 44 of 210 (21.0%) in the controls. The numbers of cattle which were bacteriologically positive and those with lesions at more than one site were also similar for the two groups.

Possible reasons for the failure to protect in the field trials could include administration of high doses of BCG (1–100 mg parenterally), very high level of *M. bovis* exposure, exposure of young calves to *M. bovis* through consumption of milk from infected cows prior to vaccination, lack of long-term protection, and prior sensitisation to environmental mycobacteria or helminths. In relation to the dose of BCG, Griffin et al. (28) demonstrated in deer that parenteral vaccination of a high dose of BCG (10^8 CFU) was less effective than doses of 10^4-10^7 CFU BCG, whereas higher doses of BCG in badgers appearred more efficacious (29). This suggests the optimal dose of BCG to use in any given species will probably need to be determined empirically. Informative meta-analysis of field trials in cattle have not been undertaken due to varying doses, vaccination routes and strains of BCG used, together with different methods to measure protection and varying levels of exposure to *M. bovis*. Furthermore, robustly controlled designs and statistical analyses of results were rarely undertaken and in most studies, the vaccinated and non-vaccinated animals were kept on separate farms.

Recent Studies to Assess Factors Affecting BCG Vaccine Efficacy in Cattle

Over the past 25 years, a large number of vaccination/challenge trials have been undertaken in cattle using harmonised models, allowing comparisons between varying studies with BCG tested alone or in comparative studies with other vaccines. Challenge models have focused on using a relatively low challenge dose of *M. bovis* (10^3-10^4 CFU) administered via endobronchial/intratracheal inoculation or by aerosol (30, 31). This has resulted in the development of tuberculous lesions mimicking those from the natural disease in the lower respiratory tract. Similar BCG strains have been used (initially Pasteur, then BCG Danish 1331) and protection assessed by quantitative gross, histopathological, and microbiological findings.

It is important to determine factors which influence the efficacy of BCG to optimise the use of the vaccine and **Table 1** summarises many of these factors. Results from a number of studies have shown that doses of 10^4-10^6 CFU of BCG administered parenterally induced equivalent protection (30, 32), while higher doses (10^8 CFU) were required to induce protection when BCG was administered orally (33, 34). When BCG vaccine was administered at optimal doses, protection induced by the subcutaneous or oral route was very similar, although an advantage from oral administration of BCG was slightly lower tuberculin skin test reactivity. Combinations of BCG by parenteral and mucosal routes has provided mixed results with no enhancement of protection observed when BCG was administered subcutaneously and orally on the same day (35), but a small enhancement in protection with simultaneous administration of BCG by subcutaneous and endobronchial routes (36). Pasteur and Danish strains of BCG induced similar protection, although the kinetics of the cellular immune response varied with the two strains (37, 38). Calves vaccinated subcutaneously with the Phipps strain of BCG had lower mean rank for the total number of tuberculous lesions following a high challenge dose of *M. bovis* (10^5 CFU) delivered by aerosol compared to controls, although this difference was not significant (46). Neonatal or very young calves were protected at least as well as older calves (39, 40). In one study, natural pre-sensitisation to environmental mycobacteria appeared to have an adverse effect on subsequent immunity induced by BCG vaccine, with less protection induced compared to that for two other attenuated *M. bovis* vaccines (41). While in another study, there was evidence that *M. avium* exposure induced partial protection against *M. bovis* infection, which could possibly mask subsequent immunity induced by BCG (42). Studies in guinea pigs and mice have provided additional information on the effects of pre-sensitisation with environmental mycobacteria where some strains of *M. avium* masked or blocked any protective effect induced by BCG vaccination, while other strains had no effect (47, 48). Studies in Northern Ireland indicated that co-infection of cattle with a liver fluke, *Fasciola hepatica*, and BCG resulted in a suppression of Th1 type immune responses to BCG, potentially affecting immunity induced by BCG vaccination (49). Vaccination of cattle with BCG 3 weeks after an experimental challenge with *M. bovis*, did not produce a beneficial effect,

TABLE 1 | Experimental challenge studies to assess factors affecting the efficacy of BCG vaccine for protection of cattle against TB.

Factor		Age of vaccination	BCG strain	Vaccine dose (CFU)	Vaccine route	*M. bovis* challenge	Measure of disease[†]	Assessment BCG vs. Control	References
Dose of BCG	1.	5–6 months	Pasteur	6×10^4	S/C	I/T	Proportion with lesions	2/15 vs. 10/16*	(30)
		5–6 months	Pasteur	6×10^6	S/C	I/T	Proportion with lesions	4/15 vs. 10/16*	
	2.	5–6 months	Danish	2×10^5	S/C	E/B	Proportion with lung lesions	3/9 vs. 10/10*	(32)
		5–6 months	Danish	2×10^6	S/C	E/B	Proportion with lung lesions	2/9 vs. 10/10*	
	3.	6 months	Danish	2×10^7	Oral	I/T	Median total lesion score	5 (0, 8)[‡] vs. 11 (8, 13.5)*	(33)
		6 months	Danish	2×10^8	Oral	I/T	Median total lesion score	3.5 (0, 10.5) vs. 11 (8, 13.5)*	
	4.	6 months	Danish	1×10^6	Oral	I/T	Median LN lesion score	4 (1, 12) vs. 3.5 (0, 12)	(34)
		6 months	Danish	1×10^7	Oral	I/T	Median LN lesion score	4 (0, 12) vs. 3.5 (0, 12)	
		6 months	Danish	2×10^8	Oral	I/T	Median LN lesion score	1 (0, 9) vs. 3.5 (0, 12)*	
Route(s) of vaccination	1.	6 months	Danish	1×10^6	S/C	I/T	Median total lesion score	0 (0, 10) vs. 11 (8, 13.5)*	(33)
		6 months	Danish	2×10^8	Oral	I/T	Median total lesion score	3.5 (0, 10.5) vs. 11 (8, 13.5)*	
	2.	6 months	Pasteur	$10^6 + 10^9$	S/C + Oral	I/T	Median total lesion score	1 (0, 12) vs. 8 (0, 15)*	(35)
		6 months	Pasteur	10^6	S/C	I/T	Median total lesion score	1 (0, 8) vs. 8 (0, 15)*	
		6 months	Pasteur	10^9	Oral	I/T	Median total lesion score	0.5 (0, 7) vs. 8 (0, 15)*	
	3.	5–7 months	Danish	$5 \times 10^5 + 5 \times 10^5$	S/C + E/B	E/B	Median total lesion score	1 (0, 15) vs. 12 (0, 28)*	(36)
		5–7 months	Danish	1×10^6	S/C	E/B	Median total lesion score	3 (0, 15) vs. 12 (0, 28)	
		5–7 months	Danish	1×10^6	E/B	E/B	Median total lesion score	1 (0, 27) vs. 12 (0, 28)	
Strain of BCG	1.	6 months	Pasteur	10^6	S/C	I/T	Median total lesion score	6 (0, 21) vs. 13.5(4, 17)*	(37)
		6 months	Danish	10^6	S/C	I/T	Median total lesion score	7 (0, 13) vs. 13.5(4, 17)*	

(Continued)

TABLE 1 | Continued

Factor		Age of vaccination	BCG strain	Vaccine dose (CFU)	Vaccine route	*M. bovis* challenge	Measure of disease[†]	Assessment BCG vs. Control	References
	2.	6 months	Pasteur	2×10^6	S/C	I/T	Median total lesion score	2 (0, 18) vs. 16 (10, 20)*	(38)
		6 months	Danish	2×10^6	S/C	I/T	Median total lesion score	8 (4, 11) vs. 16 (10, 20)*	
Neonatal vaccination	1.	8 h	Pasteur	10^6	S/C	I/T	Proportion with lesions	0/10 vs. 10/10*	(39)
		6 weeks	Pasteur	10^6	S/C	I/T	Proportion with lesions	1/9 vs. 10/10*	
	2.	1 day	Danish	10^6	S/C	I/N	Median total lesion score	2 (0, 4) vs. 13 (0, 30)*	(40)
Pre-sensitisation with *M. avium* spp.	1	5–6 months	Pasteur	10^5	S/C	I/T	Proportion with LN lesions	14/18 vs. 7/9	(41)
		5–6 months	Atten.1 *M. bovis*	10^6	S/C	I/T	Proportion with LN lesions	3/9 vs. 7/9*	
		5–6 months	Atten.2 *M. bovis*	10^6	S/C	I/T	Proportion with LN lesions	3/9 vs. 7/9*	
	2	4–6 months	*M. avium*	10^6	S/C	I/N	Median total lesion score	4 (0, 9) vs. 9 (0, 15)	(42)
Duration of protection and revaccination	1.	2–4 weeks	Danish	10^6	S/C	E/B (12 mths)	Median total lesion score	8 (0, 16) vs. 16 (0, 38)*	(43)
						E/B (24 mths)	Median total lesion score	8 (5, 17) vs. 10 (8, 17)	
	2.	2–4 weeks	Danish	3×10^5	S/C	E/B (2.5 yrs)	Median total lesion score	7.5 (0, 17) vs. 10 (3, 17)	(44)
		2–4 weeks and 2 years	Danish	3×10^5	S/C	E/B (2.5 yrs)	Median total lesion score	4 (0, 10) vs. 10 (3, 17)*	
Vaccination pre- or post-challenge	1.	5–6 months	Danish	1×10^6 (pre-challenge)	S/C	E/B	Proportion with LN lesions	4/12 vs. 10/12*	(45)
				1×10^6 (3wks post-challenge)	S/C	E/B	Proportion with LN lesions	11/12 vs. 10/12	

[†]Measure of protection was standardized where possible and in some cases, recalculated from original data.
*[‡]Median (range); *$P < 0.05$.*
CFU, Colony Forming Unit; S/C, Subcutaneous; I/T, Intratracheal; E/B, Endobronchial; I/N, Intranasal.
Atten. 1 M. bovis and Atten. 2 M. bovis: Two attenuated strains of M. bovis.

nor increased tuberculous pathology (45). Protection against experimental challenge was shown to be effective at ≤12 months post-vaccination, but had waned by 24 months post-vaccination (43). Together these studies suggest that immunity wanes between 1 and 2 years post-vaccination when protection is measured in a stringent *M. bovis* challenge model.

Two studies report the effect of revaccination with BCG. In the first study, calves vaccinated within 8 h of birth or at 6 weeks of age showed a high level of protection against *M. bovis*, while those vaccinated within 8 h of birth and revaccinated at 6 weeks of age had reduced protection (39). The revaccinated calves with the lowest level of protection had the strongest antigen-specific IFN-γ responses post-initial vaccination, suggesting that revaccination had induced an inappropriate immune response. In neonatal calves, antigen-specific IFN-γ responses remain at elevated levels for longer than those seen in older calves, possibly due to a more active BCG infection and BCG revaccination of young calves may be contra-indicated. In contrast, calves vaccinated with BCG at 2–4 weeks of age and revaccinated at 2 years of age when immunity had waned, showed a significant level of protection when challenged 6 months later, while those receiving only the initial vaccine dose were not protected when challenged at the same time (44).

In the past decade a number of field BCG vaccination trials or experiments have been undertaken under natural transmission (in contact) conditions and have provided insights into the effectiveness of BCG vaccine under different levels of disease prevalence over varying time periods (**Table 2**). The field experiments in Mexico (50) and Ethiopia (51, 52) involved the exposure of vaccinated and non-vaccinated calves to herds of cows which had reactor rates of 40% in the Mexican experiment and 100% in the two experiments in Ethiopia. In the Mexican experiment, vaccination induced a significant level of protection against TB and the vaccine efficacy was estimated to be 59.4%. The level of exposure in the experiments in Ethiopia was very high with ~85% of the non-vaccinated calves developing tuberculous lesions. Despite this high level of exposure, the vaccine efficacy in the first experiment was considered to be similar to that in the Mexican experiment and there were significantly fewer vaccinated animals with lesions and culture positive for *M. bovis* as well as significantly more vaccinated animals that would have passed slaughterhouse meat inspection than that for the controls (51). The vaccine efficacy in the second experiment conducted in Ethiopia when measured by comparing lesioned, culture or histology-positive animals in the BCG-vaccinated group with naïve controls was relatively low (around 30%) (52). However, in this last experiment, the severity of pathology and dissemination of *M. bovis* was significantly lower in the vaccinated, infected animals compared to that for the non-vaccinated animals, which could relate to a lower ability to transmit disease (onward transmission). The difference between the two Ethiopian experiments was attributed to a higher prevalence of overt clinical signs of TB in the infected herd in the second experiment.

A large field trial was undertaken in New Zealand to evaluate the efficacy of BCG vaccine administered orally (53). Free-ranging, vaccinated and non-vaccinated cattle were stocked at low densities and were naturally exposed to *M. bovis* for periods of 1–4 years from tuberculin reactor cattle (reactor herd prevalence of 5–10%) and a wildlife reservoir of infection (brushtail possums). BCG vaccine was administered orally to cattle in an attempt to reduce tuberculin skin test reactivity. This trial included 1,286 cattle and at slaughter the prevalence of infection was 4.8% among vaccinates and 11.9% in non-vaccinates. The overall vaccine efficacy was estimated to be 67.4%, but higher for those killed within 2 years post-vaccination (77.4%). Vaccination also appeared to slow the progression of TB, with infected vaccinates more likely to have no visible lesions and less likely to have a high lesion score.

In summary, the field experiments and trials have shown that BCG vaccination can markedly reduce the number of cattle infected with *M. bovis*, which is different to that seen in the experimental challenge trials where vaccination only reduced the severity of the disease. However, an exception was in the field trial when there was a very high exposure to *M. bovis* (52). With the longer exposure periods, there appeared to be a waning of immunity after 2 years (53).

Differentiating Infected From Vaccinated Animals (DIVA) Tests

It is well-established that vaccination with BCG can compromise the interpretation of the tuberculin skin test, which serves as the primary surveillance test for "test and slaughter" bovine TB control strategies. Using the single intradermal comparative cervical test, 80% of BCG-vaccinated calves were shown to react in the tuberculin skin test at 6 months post-vaccination, but decreasing to 10–20% by 9 months post-vaccination (54) and in a another study, the maximum skin test reactivity was observed after 5 weeks, but disappeared completely by 18 months after vaccination (55). Positive responses were also observed in the caudal fold skin test at 6 months after BCG vaccination compared to that for a corresponding control group, but there were no differences between the groups by 12 months after vaccination (44). DIVA tests will be required for countries intending to use BCG vaccination alongside conventional "test and slaughter" control strategies. DIVA tests have now been developed using antigens from the *M. tuberculosis* complex which are not expressed or secreted by BCG and can be used instead of bovine PPD in the whole blood IFN-γ or skin tests. Two of the antigens used in the DIVA tests are the ESAT-6 and CFP10 proteins, which are encoded in the RD1 region of *M. tuberculosis* and *M. bovis*, but not in BCG, which has lost this region of its genome (56–58), and a third antigen, Rv3615c, which is not located in the RD1 region, but its secretion is dependent on the esx-1 secretion system located in the RD1 region (59). A recent evaluation of the whole blood IFN-γ test incorporating ESAT-6, CFP10, and Rv3615c indicated that the sensitivity was similar to that with the comparative tuberculin readout using avian and bovine PPD. When tested in non-infected animals, both the DIVA and tuberculin readouts gave similar specificities of between 97 and 99%. The relative specificity of the DIVA blood test was also high (95%) in BCG-vaccinated cattle and was significantly greater than that observed for the tuberculin readout

TABLE 2 | Recent field trials to assess the efficacy of BCG for protection of cattle against TB.

Trial	Country	BCG strain	Vaccine dose	Vaccine route	Age at vaccination	Source of infection	In-contact (exposure) time	Measurement of disease	Assessment: BCG vs. Control	References
1.	Mexico	Tokyo	10^6	S/C	1–2 weeks	Infected herd (40% herd reactor prevalence)	10 months	Proportion positive in three tests: PPD skin test, PPD IFN-γ test, ESAT-6/CFP10 IFN-γ test	6/65 vs. 15/66* (9.2% vs. 22.8%) 59.4% efficacy	(50)
2.	Ethopia	Danish	10^6	S/C	2 weeks	Infected herd (100% herd reactor prevalence)	10–23 months	Proportion with lesions	5/13 vs. 12/14* (39% vs. 86%)	(51)
								Mean total pathology score (95% CI)	4.6 vs. 14.1* (0, 10.5) vs. (2.5, 24.6)	
3.	Ethopia	Danish	10^6	S/C	2 weeks	Infected herd (100% herd reactor prevalence)	1 year	Proportion with lesions	15/23 vs. 22/26 (65% vs. 85%)	(52)
								Mean total pathology score (95% CI)	4.0 (1.8, 6.1) vs. 7.8* 2.5, 13.1)	
4.	New Zealand	Danish	10^8	Oral	6–30 months	Infected herd and wildlife (5–10% herd reactor prevalence)	1–4 years	Proportion with TB lesions and/or *M. bovis* cultured	31/644 vs. 63/531* (4.8% vs. 11.9%) 67.4% efficacy	(53)

CFU, Colony Forming Units; S/C, Subcutaneous; CI Confidence interval; IFN-γ, Gamma-interferon; PPD, Purified protein derivative $^*P < 0.05$.

(71%) (60). One scenario to use the DIVA blood test would be to re-test tuberculin-positive cattle; alternatively, it is also possible to use these antigens in a skin test rather than the IFN-γ test. The DIVA skin test in cattle has now been shown to have a high sensitivity for *M. bovis*-infected cattle, to a similar level than that for the comparative cervical skin test in non-vaccinated cattle while not compromised by vaccination with BCG or with vaccines against Johne's disease (61, 62).

VACCINATION OF GOATS

TB infection of goats is caused by *M. bovis* or *M. caprae* and in the natural disease lesions are predominantly found in the lungs and associated lymph nodes, indicating an aerosol route of infection (63). The disease is responsible for economic losses in endemic areas and infected goats may be a source of TB for cattle or humans. Caprine TB is present in a number of European countries, but currently there are no caprine TB control campaigns in the European Union. To determine protective efficacy of vaccines, gross and microscopic lesions have been assessed by qualitative and quantitative analyses, together with mycobacterial culture from lung-associated lymph nodes. The precise determination of the total lung lesion burden related to total lung volume has been achieved using multi-detector computed tomography (64).

BCG Danish vaccine administered subcutaneously at a dose of 5×10^5 CFU was shown to be safe and no shedding of BCG was detected in the faeces of vaccinated kids or in the milk of vaccinated, lactating goats (65). BCG was isolated from a lymph node draining the site of vaccination from one kid at 8 weeks post-vaccination, but not from any goats at 24 weeks post-vaccination. A single dose of BCG vaccine administered subcutaneously to goats was shown to significantly induce protection against an endobronchial challenge with *M. caprae*, with reductions in pulmonary pathology and bacterial load. Vaccination with BCG appeared to prevent haematogenous dissemination of mycobacteria with extra-thoracic TB lesions only found in non-vaccinated goats (66). A comparison of parenterally administered BCG and heat-inactivated *M. bovis* vaccines showed that both vaccines provided similar levels of protection against a *M. caprae* experimental challenge, with a reduction in the volume of thoracic TB lesions and extra-pulmonary lesions compared to non-vaccinates (67). Use of mycobacterial DIVA reagents, ESAT-6 and CFP10, in the IFN-γ test was able to differentiate TB-infected from BCG-vaccinated goats. A field BCG vaccination trial was recently undertaken in a herd of goats infected with *M. caprae* (68). Twenty-three goat kids were vaccinated subcutaneously with 10^5 CFU of BCG Danish, with a further 22 kids serving as non-vaccinated controls. Two months later, the kids were mixed with a herd of goats which had a TB reactor rate of 79%. Sixteen months later, all trial goats were killed and necropsied. Vaccination significantly reduced the number of animals with TB lesions compared to that for non-vaccinates (35 and 77% respectively; representing a vaccine efficacy of 53%) and when extrapulmonary cases were considered, the reduction were even higher (17 and 68%, respectively; vaccine efficacy of 75%). Vaccination has been seen as a valuable long-term control prospect, reducing the TB prevalence prior to starting a test and slaughter eradication programme which would reduce economic costs for producers and the public sector.

VACCINATION OF SHEEP

Sheep have traditional been considered a rare host for the *M. tuberculosis* complex, but can be part of a multi-species system which may maintain TB in a region, at least in mixed farms where sheep cohabit with TB-infected cattle and/or goats (69). In a trial where lambs were vaccinated parenterally with BCG Danish and subsequently challenged endobronchially with *M. caprae*, the vaccinated lambs had a significant reduction in gross lesions compared to the non-vaccinated controls (70). All challenged lambs developed gross lesions in the respiratory system, which were similar to those observed in goats experimentally challenged with *M. caprae* at a similar dose.

VACCINATION OF DEER

TB in farmed and feral deer is predominantly caused by *M. bovis*, and in the USA and Spain, feral deer also serve as a wildlife reservoir of *M. bovis* infection, acting as a source of infection for domestic livestock (6, 10). Deer serve as important domestic livestock species, farmed predominantly for the production of venison, while feral deer are valued for hunting. Tuberculous lesions are commonly described as liquefied or abscess-like in contrast to the caseous nature of the lesions seen in cattle and goats (71, 72). The most frequent site of the tuberculous lesions is in the retropharyngeal lymph nodes, followed by lesions in the lungs and associated lymph nodes as well as in the mesenteric lymph nodes (73). BCG vaccination studies of deer has been undertaken to assess whether vaccination could be an effective method of protecting farmed deer from TB and in feral deer to prevent reinfection back into cattle herds.

Studies of BCG vaccine in red deer have shown that a single dose of BCG administered subcutaneously to 3 month old deer could reduce disease severity, while revaccinating deer at intervals of 8–16 weeks intervals induced protection against infection, but not at an interval of 43 weeks (74). Increasing the time period between booster dose and *M. bovis* challenge from 6 to 26 or 52 weeks had no significant effect on protection. Two doses of 10^4-10^7 CFU of BCG induced protection against TB, but less with a dose of 10^8 CFU and killed BCG in a mineral-in-oil adjuvant induced no protection (28). A study in red deer in Spain compared oral administration of BCG Danish (10^8 CFU) with oral administration of heat-inactivated *M. bovis*, 10^7 bacilli, followed by an experimental challenge with *M. bovis* (75). Only the heat-inactivated vaccine induced a significant reduction in lesion pathology compared to that for the non-vaccinates, however, the results were constrained by very small group sizes (5 animals/group). Neither vaccine induced a bovine PPD IFN-γ response post-vaccination. Parenteral BCG administered at a dose of 10^6 CFU or oral BCG at 10^8 CFU induced a similar degree of protection in white-tailed deer (76). Parenteral vaccination with either BCG Danish or Pasteur resulted in decreased disease severity, without sterile immunity (77). A booster dose 6 weeks later did not raise the level of protection (78). BCG was shown to persist for 3–9 months in lymphoid tissues of deer vaccinated parenterally or orally (79). Evidence has been provided of transmission of BCG from parenterally vaccinated deer to in-contact, non-vaccinated deer (77, 79). In another study, deer orally vaccinated with 10^9 CFU BCG Danish were housed with non-vaccinated deer for 27 weeks. There was immunological evidence of transmission of BCG to the non-vaccinated animals, but no BCG could be isolated from the tissues of either group of animals when killed 27 weeks after vaccination (80). There was no evidence (immunologically or by culture) of transmission of BCG to the cattle which were exposed to the room previously occupied by the vaccinated deer. Complications can occur with the delivery of oral vaccine baits to feral deer as the provision of supplementary feed to feral deer can lead to large numbers of deer congregating together resulting in the spread of TB (81), also there are concerns about non-target uptake of live vaccine baits, particularly by cattle. Simulation modelling has examined the potential role that vaccination could play in control programmes to minimise cattle herd breakdowns (82). Vaccination of 50–90% of susceptible deer within a 5 km radius of cattle farms was predicted to result in a 95% probability of having no cattle herd breakdowns in 15–18 years.

BCG VACCINATION OF WILDLIFE

The requirements for a vaccine for wildlife differ to those for domestic livestock in that preferentially, the vaccine would be self-administered via an oral route and animals would only receive a single vaccination. Vaccination should prevent the spread of infection to other wildlife or livestock, but complete protection against infection would not be necessary. Recent studies in multiple wildlife species have shown that BCG vaccine can fulfil these requirements and provide protection against TB (**Table 3**).

Vaccination of Brushtail Possums

The brushtail possum is the major wildlife reservoir of *M. bovis* infection in New Zealand as well as declared as a noxious pest. Possums are highly susceptible to *M. bovis* infection and lesions are found predominantly in the lungs and superficial lymph nodes. Culling of possums by trapping and poisoning has been a major contributor to the dramatic reduction in the numbers of infected cattle over the past 20 years (11). Vaccination of possums against TB has the potential to be an effective TB control measure when it is not suitable to cull possums such as near urban areas.

BCG vaccination of possums via a number of different routes including subcutaneous, intranasal and oral have induced a significant level of protection against experimental *M. bovis* challenge by intratracheal and aerosol routes (83, 93). Oral administration of BCG via baits would be the preferred route of administration of BCG vaccine to wild possums, but it was shown that direct administration of BCG intragastrically was less effective compared to administered by the same route and mixed with a drug to reduce gastric acidity or when administered intraduodenally (94, 95). To increase the efficacy of oral administered BCG vaccine, the BCG bacilli were encapsulated in a lipid matrix which protected the bacteria from degradation in the acidic stomach environment, resulting in improved protection against a *M. bovis* challenge as well as increasing shelf life of the vaccine in the field (83, 96). Vaccine-induced immunity was shown to wane between 6 and 12 months post-vaccination following oral vaccination and there were no differences between BCG doses of 10^7 and 10^8 CFU or between Danish and Pasteur strains of BCG (97). A more recent study indicated that protection against an experimental *M. bovis* infection extended out to

TABLE 3 | Summary of BCG vaccine efficacy studies in wildlife.

Species/Country	Route†	Challenge type	Vaccine efficacy‡	Notes/Particular issues	Key references
Bushtail possum/New Zealand	O,M, P	Aerosol,	+	High vaccine cost compared to that for poisons	(83)
		natural exposure	+		(84)
European badger/ UK, Ireland	O,M, P	Endobronchial, Natural exposure	+ +	Parenteral vaccine licensed (BadgerBCG). For an oral vaccine: demonstration of consistent protection	(29, 85) (86–88)
White-tailed deer/ USA	O,P	Intratonsilar	+	BCG persistence in tissues, bans on supplementary baiting, non-target bait uptake	(76, 77)
Eurasian wild boar/Spain	O	Oral	+	Non-target bait uptake	(89)
		Natural exposure	±	Regulatory issues	(90)
Ferret/New Zealand	O,P	Oral	±	Rarely maintenance host for *M. bovis*	(91, 92)
African buffalo/ South Africa	P	Intratonsilar	–	Practicality of vaccine delivery in the field	(7)

†*Vaccination route, O, oral; M, other mucosal; P, parenteral.*
‡*Vaccine efficacy, + protection, ± partial protection, – no protection.*

28 months post-vaccination (98). BCG bacilli were shown to be stable in the lipid matrix for 7 weeks under room temperature conditions and 3–5 weeks under field conditions in a forest/pasture habitat, when maintained in weather-proof, bait-delivery sachets. Furthermore, uptake of oral bait placebo vaccines was shown to be high with 85–100% of wild possums accessing baits at bait densities of 40–80 sachets/hectare (96). Possums consuming oral bait BCG vaccine, containing 10^8 CFU of BCG, displayed no adverse clinical signs, but shed relatively low concentrations of BCG in their faeces, 10^2-10^4 CFU/g faeces, for up to a week and BCG could be isolated from their mesenteric lymph nodes for up to 8 weeks post vaccination (99).

Two field trials have been undertaken in possums to determine efficacy of BCG vaccine against natural exposure to *M. bovis* infection. In the first trial, BCG vaccine was administered intranasally and intraconjunctivally (total dose of 10^6 CFU of BCG Pasteur) to possums trapped in the field, with an equivalent number left non-vaccinated. After vaccination, the animals were released back into the field site, which was endemic for TB in wildlife (100). The animals were trapped, examined for clinical TB and released again every 2 months. Two years after the start of the study, possums were recaptured, killed and examined for TB lesions. Vaccination significantly reduced the proportion of possums infected with *M. bovis* (4/149 for vaccinates and 13/151 for non-vaccinates), with a vaccine efficacy of 69% for prevention of TB. The second field study was of a similar design, but with BCG vaccine administered orally in a lipid matrix (total dose 10^8 CFU BCG Danish). Again, there was a significant reduction in the proportion of infected possums in vaccinates (1/51) compared to that for the non-vaccinates (12/71), with a vaccine efficacy of 95% for prevention of TB (84). In contrast to the experimental challenge studies, protection against natural exposure to *M. bovis* vaccination resulted in protection against infection. The major constraint for the use of BCG vaccine in possums in New Zealand is cost of the vaccine compared to that for poisons, particularly when possums are considered as a noxious pest.

Vaccination of Badgers

The European badger is the major wildlife reservoir of *M. bovis* infection in Great Britain due to their relative abundance and ecology, the prevalence of infection and presentation of TB pathology compared to other sylvatic species (101, 102). Options for preventing the transmission of *M. bovis* from infected badgers to cattle are limited to minimising the potential for contact between them (biosecurity), reducing the number and density of infected badgers via selective and non-selective culling, and vaccination [reviewed in (103)]. Badgers are protected by law in the UK and Ireland which limits the public acceptability and practicality of culling and for disease control, and culling of badgers in England and Ireland has sometimes delivered conflicting results that likely reflect subtle differences in the epidemiology of the disease locally (104). Vaccination of badgers against TB has the potential to be an effective TB control measure, especially in combination with other control measures (105) and considerable progress has been made in testing the efficacy of BCG vaccine in badgers.

BCG vaccine has been administered to badgers via a variety of routes, including subcutaneous, intramuscular and mucosal (conjunctival and oral) and vaccination by all these routes has induced significant protection against experimental endobronchial challenge with *M. bovis* [reviewed in (103)]. The use of BCG to vaccinate badgers against TB in the UK by the intramuscular route was licensed by the UK Competent Authority (Veterinary Medicines Directorate) in 2010 as BadgerBCG and is available for use by veterinarians and trained lay vaccinators under prescription from a veterinarian. Licensing of BadgerBCG required evidence of vaccine safety and efficacy and laboratory and field studies showed that vaccination of badgers by injection with BCG was both safe and significantly reduced lesions of TB caused by *M. bovis* (29, 106). Protection was incomplete, in that *M. bovis* infection of vaccinated badgers still produced either visible pathology or *M. bovis* was isolated from organs at necropsy. Results from a 4-year field study of BCG in wild badgers were consistent with the direct protective effect of BCG observed in experimental studies. Individual badgers that initially tested negative to a panel of diagnostic tests, presumed uninfected, were significantly less likely to subsequently test positive to serological and immunological tests for TB following vaccination, compared to non-vaccinated control animals (86, 107). Furthermore, non-vaccinated cubs captured in vaccinated social groups were significantly less likely to test positive to TB when more members of their group had been previously vaccinated. The most plausible explanation for this result is that BCG had caused a herd immunity effect, with the rate of *M. bovis* transmission being more effectively reduced in social groups where a higher proportion of animals had been vaccinated.

A practical limitation to the extensive use of BadgerBCG is the need to trap badgers before the vaccine can be injected and the use of an oral bait delivery system would be advantageous. BCG has been incorporated in a wide variety of baits, including encapsulation in the same lipid matrix used to deliver BCG orally to possums. Administration of BCG orally to captive badgers, either directly to the back of the throat, or indirectly via ingested bait has been shown to protect badgers against experimental challenge with *M. bovis* and there was no difference in the levels of protection induced by Pasteur and Danish sub-strains of BCG (85, 108). To assess the vaccine safety, badgers were orally dosed with 10^9 CFU of BCG, followed 14 days later by a single oral dose of 10^7 CFU BCG (109). No adverse physical effects were observed, nor effects on the social behaviour and feeding habits of the vaccinated animals. BCG was cultured from the faeces of two of nine vaccinated animals (10^2 CFU/g) ~48 h after the higher dose of BCG was administered and by one of the nine vaccinated animal (80 CFU/g) ~24 h after receiving the lower dose of BCG. No evidence was found for the transmission of BCG to non-vaccinated, sentinel, badgers housed with the vaccinated animals despite the occasional excretion of BCG in faeces. The target dose of BCG for the oral vaccination of badgers is yet to be defined.

A field trial was recently completed in Ireland that provided the first estimate of oral BCG efficacy under field conditions (87). Lipid-encapsulated BCG was delivered to the back of the throat of anaesthetised badgers, whilst other badgers received only the lipid as placebo. The study area was divided into three equally representative zones with different proportions (0, 50, and 100%) of the badger population in each zone being vaccinated with either BCG or placebo. Attempts were made to capture badgers every 6 months and between the first two capture periods the vaccine efficacy was estimated to be 36%, while it was 84% for capture periods 3–6. Among the vaccinated badgers that seroconverted, the median time to seroconversion (413 days) was significantly longer when compared with non-vaccinated animals (230 days). In addition, there was a significant reduction in the proportion of animals presenting with *M. bovis* culture confirmed lesions in the fully (100%) vaccinated zone (9%), compared with the non-vaccinated (0%) zone (26%).

Vaccination of Wild Boar

Wild boar serve as the main wildlife reservoir of the *M. tuberculosis* complex (MTC) in the Mediterranean regions of the Iberian Peninsula, Spain and TB prevalence in wild boar has been associated with TB occurrence on cattle farms (110, 111). Wild boar are widespread in Eurasia and can be found in high densities, particularly on hunting estates (112). These animals are highly susceptible to MTC infection and lesions are most frequently found in the mandibular lymph nodes, although generalised disease is often seen, with involvement of the lungs and thoracic lymph nodes (113). Direct contact between wild boar and other species is thought to be very rare in Mediterranean habitats and inter-species transmission of MTC involving wild boar is considered to occur indirectly at locations such as waterholes (114). Although, transmission of TB between wild boar and cattle could be minimised by culling of wild boar and preventing inter-species contact, vaccination could be a more cost-effective and sustainable disease control measure.

Oral vaccination with BCG Danish (10^6 CFU/dose) vaccine has produced significant protection (70–80% lesion score reduction) in laboratory challenge trials (89, 115). The focus has been to vaccinate piglets as they are less likely to be infected and can be targeted by appropriate timing of bait delivery and with the use of a patented bait delivery system that reduces uptake by non-target species and excludes adult boar (116). In a recent safety study, wild boar were dosed with an oral bait containing 10^6 CFU of BCG and groups of vaccinated animals were killed at 1, 3, 5, and 9 months post-vaccination (117). No adverse clinical signs were observed and tissues collected from the animals were culture negative for BCG. A field trial undertaken from 2012 to 2016 tested the uptake rates and efficacy of orally delivered BCG and heat-inactivated *M. bovis* vaccines in high prevalence settings (40–80% wild boar infection prevalence) in Montes de Toledo, Spain (90). The two vaccines were tested at different sites, one managed and one natural (or unmanaged) site for each vaccine, with an additional 15 non-vaccinated control sites. Vaccine baits were deployed using selected piglet feeders and the uptake rates were 50–74% in natural sites and 89–92% in managed sites. A significant reduction in the TB prevalence was only seen from one vaccinated site: heat-inactivated *M. bovis* vaccine in the managed site; with a 34% reduction in the prevalence of animals with lesions. A limitation of the study was that vaccines were deployed at different sites and efficacy was measured by the change in TB lesion prevalence compared to time zero.

Vaccination of Ferrets

In New Zealand, ferrets (*Mustela furo*) can become infected with *M. bovis* via feeding on tuberculous carcasses, particularly possums and potentially can become a source of infection for other wildlife or cattle (118). In most circumstances, ferrets are simply spill-over hosts and as yet, there is no confirmation that ferrets act as true maintenance hosts in New Zealand. Rather, ferrets could be characterised as extended spill-over hosts in which *M. bovis* infection originally acquired from possums could occasionally cycle within a ferret population before disappearing (119). Vaccination has been considered as a possible control measure for ferrets and in the first of two vaccination trials, ferrets orally vaccinated with BCG incorporated into dietary meat were partially protected against oral challenge with virulent *M. bovis* (91). In the second trial, vaccination of ferrets with BCG by the subcutaneous route resulted in reduced severity of disease following experimental infection with *M. bovis* (92).

Vaccination of African Buffalo

M. bovis infection is currently endemic in the Greater Kruger National Park Complex and the Hluhluwe-iMfolozi Park (120, 121), as well as in several private farms and conservancies in South Africa (122). African buffaloes are likely to be major maintenance hosts of TB (123) and play an important role in spill-over infection to other wildlife species, and of particular importance is spread of infection to predators (lions), large browsers (white rhino) and other co-located species such as kudu, baboons, and warthogs (124). In addition, there has been "spill-back" to domestic cattle (125). As "test and cull" is not a viable option for free-ranging buffaloes due to logistical impracticality and the animals' extensive geographical range, vaccination remains the only realistic alternative.

A preliminary vaccine trial was undertaken in semi-free-range buffalo to assess the efficacy of BCG vaccine. Two doses of BCG were administered subcutaneously (10^7 CFU of BCG) and the buffaloes were challenged with virulent *M. bovis* via the intratonsilar route. The study did not reveal significant differences in the number of lesioned animals between the vaccinated and control groups (7). There were various contributing factors which could have played a role in the perceived negative results such as the age of vaccinated animals with the majority being older than 12 months at the start of the study, the route of vaccine application, challenge dose, exposure to non-tuberculous mycobacteria and stress on the animals with the grazing limitations. Future studies should aim to determine if BCG vaccination could reduce TB in vaccinated herds compared to non-vaccinated herds by targeting buffaloes <12 months old and monitoring over a period of 5–10 years in order to determine true disease status. If successful, vaccination could have a positive cascading effect, reducing *M. bovis* disease rates in other animal species. The available data does not suggest any risk to "off-target" species from BCG delivery, which reduces the ethical barriers to implementation.

SAFETY OF BCG VACCINE IN TARGET AND NON-TARGET SPECIES

BCG vaccine is one of the most widely used human vaccines, with 100 million children receiving the vaccine annually and remains one of the safest vaccines available. Reports of adverse reactions arising from BCG vaccination of children are relatively uncommon and a review of reactions to BCG vaccine in humans and animals has recently been provided by Murphy et al. (126). More severe reactions to BCG vaccine in humans were often the result of vaccination of immune-compromised individuals and factors influencing the development of adverse reactions included the potency and dose of the vaccine strain, route of delivery, age and immune status of the host and skill of the operator administering the vaccine. The most common reactions were local and regional reactions, which were generally self-limiting where suppurative lymphadenitis and abscesses were the most frequent occurring reactions.

BCG vaccine has been tested in a large number of animal species (**Table 4**) and relatively minor adverse clinical signs have been observed in some cases. In cattle, Francis (19) described local lesions arising following subcutaneous administration of large doses of BCG, similar to those seen with inoculation of large doses of dead bacilli, but no progressive lesions were produced and bacilli were gradually eliminated from the body. Repeat passaging of BCG vaccine in animal species is still to be undertaken to ensure no reversion to virulence, but the evidence from its use in humans for nearly a century has emphasised the safety of the vaccine.

Local abscesses or nodules have been observed following subcutaneous injections of BCG in a number of other animal species and these resolved relatively quickly (**Table 4**). No adverse effects have been observed after oral administration of BCG in animals other than cervical lymphadenitis observed in mice (127), similar to a reaction observed occasionally in young vaccinated children (126). Following oral dosing with BCG of possums and badgers, transient shedding of low numbers of BCG in faeces was observed (99, 109). Transmission of BCG from vaccinated animals to in-contact non-vaccinates has only been recorded in white-tailed deer (79). There is a risk that distribution of oral baits containing BCG for wildlife could lead to uptake by non-target animal species such as cattle, resulting in a subsequent positive tuberculin skin test response and therefore special care with regards to bait distribution is essential. The chance of cattle becoming infected with BCG from faecal contamination of pasture or feed from vaccinated wildlife would be very rare as tuberculin skin test reactivity following oral administration of BCG to cattle has only been recorded with high doses of BCG ($\geq 10^7$ CFU) (34). Similar to the situation in humans, BCG vaccine is considered to be a safe vaccine in all animal species tested.

TABLE 4 | Studies of safety of BCG vaccine of different strains in target and non-target animal species.

Animal species	BCG strain	Adverse clinical signs	Key references
Mouse	Pasteur	Cervical lymphadentitis—oral, None—S/C	(127)
Hamster	Tice	Pleural reaction—I/P high dose	(128)
Guinea pig	Tice	None—I/D	(129)
Rabbit	Phipps	Local abscess—I/D	(130)
Dog	Tice	Mild pleural reaction—I/P	(128)
Monkey	Pasteur	Axilliary lymphadenitis- high dose I/D	(131)
		Local draining abscess—medium dose S/C	
Sheep	Danish	None—S/C	(70)
Horse	Pasteur	None—intralesion injection	(132)
Goat	Danish	None—S/C, no shedding in milk or faeces	(65)
Cattle	Pasteur	Local swelling at injection site—S/C	(19)
White-tailed deer	Danish	None—S/C, Oral, BCG persisted in draining LNs (12 months), transmission to in-contacts	(79, 80)
Red deer	Pasteur	None—S/C, persisted in draining LNs (14 wks)	(133)
Possum	Danish	None—Oral, shedding in faeces (1 wk), persisted in mesenteric LNs (8 wks)	(99)
	Pasteur	None—Aerosol, S/C	(93)
Badger	Danish	None—Oral, single and repeat dosing, shedding in faeces (48 h)	(109)
	Danish	I/Mus, S/C, single, and repeat injection, local swelling at injection site	(106)
Wild boar	Danish	None—low dose oral, BCG not re-isolated	(117)
Ferret	Pasteur	None—Oral, S/C	(91, 92)
African buffalo	Pasteur	None—S/C	(7)

Vaccination route: I/D, intradermal; I/M, Intramuscular; I/P, Intrapleural; S/C, Subcutaneous.

CONCLUSIONS

Experimental challenge studies in domestic livestock including cattle, goats, sheep and farmed deer have demonstrated that BCG vaccination can moderate the severity of the disease, while field trials in cattle and goats have indicated that vaccination can also reduce infection. No single vaccine has been shown to be better than BCG in cattle, although combinations of BCG with various subunit TB vaccines have produced encouraging results and could have application in the future [reviewed in (2, 134)]. Vaccination of cattle with BCG would have greatest application in countries where "test and slaughter" strategies are not affordable or socially acceptable and in this situation, BCG could play a role in reducing the spread of bovine TB. It is well-recognised in humans that BCG confers some non-specific protective effects against other pathogens (135), but this has yet to be evaluated in cattle. Improvement in general health of animals *per se* and/or increased productivity post-BCG vaccination could potentially have benefits in developing countries. Strategic use of BCG vaccine for livestock could also be implemented in regions where wildlife serve as reservoirs of infection, particularly where it is not feasible to contain the spread of infection from wildlife. In these situations, DIVA tests, particularly skin tests utilising specific *M. bovis* antigens, could be used in livestock in association with vaccination to allow vaccination to be integrated with "test and slaughter" control measures.

A number of recommendations can be made from the experimental challenge and field experiments in cattle. Calves should be vaccinated with BCG as young as possible, optimally by 2–4 weeks of age, at doses of 10^5-10^6 CFU parenterally or 10^8 CFU orally and no differences have been detected in protection induced by two of the most commonly used BCG strains, Pasteur and Danish. Protection has been shown to wane between 1 and 2 years post-vaccination and revaccination is recommended every 1–2 years to maintain levels of immunity. BCG vaccine has been shown to be safe in cattle and vaccination of cattle pre-infected with *M. bovis* is not likely to exacerbate or cure infection. Vaccination is likely to produce false reactions in traditional TB diagnostic tests in the first 12 months post-vaccination and as protection induced by BCG is not complete, DIVA tests should be used if "test and slaughter" control policies are in place. It would be preferable to use BCG vaccination in association with other TB control measures such as minimising the chance of early exposure to *M. bovis* by feeding young calves with colostrum or milk from non-reactor cattle or with heated milk, segregating reactor and non-reactor cattle into separate herds and keeping vaccinated calves with the non-reactor animals.

The field testing of BCG vaccine in possums and badgers administered via oral or parenteral routes have resulted in the induction of significant reductions in infection of these animals and a parenteral BCG vaccine has now been licensed for use in badgers in the UK. In wild boar, feral deer and ferrets, BCG vaccine has been shown to induce significant levels of protection against experimental challenge with TB. Practical systems for delivery of oral bait TB vaccines to wildlife have now been established, but further research is necessary to improve oral bait formulations with appropriate attractants, systems for optimising bait distribution and avoiding bait uptake by non-target species. BCG vaccine has been shown to be safe in all animal species tested, although BCG has been isolated from lymph nodes draining vaccination sites and from faeces of animals for a short period following oral vaccination. There was evidence that vaccinated white-tailed deer could transmit BCG to non-vaccinated pen-mates, but not to cattle exposed to the room previously occupied by the vaccinated deer.

In summary, there have been major advances in the past 10–20 years in our understanding of the factors influencing BCG vaccine efficacy for domestic livestock and wild animals. To optimise the use of BCG vaccine, it will be important to continue to field test BCG vaccine in the various animal species in different environments, husbandry systems and in the presence of varying levels of disease prevalence as well as evaluating the practical application of DIVA tests. Although BCG vaccine may not provide complete protection against exposure to *M. bovis*, the protection should be sufficient to markedly reduce onward transmission to others animals. This feature could ensure that BCG vaccine could be particularly valuable for reducing infection in wildlife populations and in domestic animals where infection is currently very high and where "test and slaughter" control strategies are not able to be undertaken. There are numerous technical hurdles still to be overcome before an economically viable oral vaccine for use in badgers in the UK might be available. In the meantime it is beholden on stakeholders to make the best use of the existing tools available, this includes the intramuscular BadgerBCG vaccine. Cattle BCG vaccination in countries using "test and slaughter" control strategies also face significant hurdles. For example, a BCG vaccination-compatible DIVA test needs to be validated to allow vaccination to continue alongside traditional "test and slaughter" control programmes; currently BCG vaccination is prohibited under EU and some other countries' legislation and this would need to change; finally, cost-benefit analyses would decide whether deployment would proceed.

AUTHOR CONTRIBUTIONS

BB, HV, MC, and L-MdK-L wrote sections of the manuscript. All authors contributed to the manuscript revision, read and approved the submitted version.

ACKNOWLEDGEMENTS

The initiative to prepare this review arose from discussions at a workshop under the auspices of the Faculty of Medicine, Hebrew University, Israel which recognised that BCG vaccine could play an important role in control of bovine TB, but up to now its use has been limited. The authors wish to acknowledge the funding received from AgResearch New Zealand and the Department for Environment, Food, and Rural Affairs UK.

REFERENCES

1. Sweetline AN, Ronald BS, Kumar TM, Kannan P, Thangavelu A. Molecular identification of *Mycobacterium tuberculosis* in cattle. *Vet Microbiol.* (2017) 198:81–7. doi: 10.1016/j.vetmic.2016.12.013.
2. Waters WR, Palmer MV, Buddle BM, Vordermeier HM. Bovine tuberculosis vaccine research: historical perspectives and recent advances. *Vaccine* (2012) 30:2611–22. doi: 10.1016/j.vaccine.2012.02.018.
3. Cousins DV. *Mycobacterium bovis* infection and control in domestic livestock. *Rev Sci Tech.* (2001) 20:71–85. Available online at: https://www.oie.int/doc/ged/D9347.PDF
4. de Lisle GW, Bengis RG, Schmitt SM, O'Brien DJ. Tuberculosis in free-ranging wildlife: detection, diagnosis and management. *Rev Sci Tech.* (2002) 21:317–34. Available online at: https://pdfs.semanticscholar.org/5417/064a4772377003a12056ccf6e964f911ab1b.pdf
5. Naranjo V, Gortázar C, Vicente J, de la Fuente J. Evidence of the role of European wild boar as a reservoir of tuberculosis due to *Mycobacterium tuberculosis* complex. *Vet Microbiol.* (2008) 127:1–9. doi: 10.1016/j.vetmic.2007.10.002
6. Santos N, Almeida V, Gortázar C, Correia-Neves M. Patterns of *Mycobacterium tuberculosis* complex excretion and characterization of super-shedders in naturally-infected wild boar and red deer. *Vet Res.* (2015) 46:129. doi: 10.1186/s13567-015-0270-4
7. de Klerk LM, Michel AL, Bengis RG, Kreik NP, Godfroid J. BCG vaccination failed to protect yearling African buffaloes (*Syncerus caffer*) against experimental intratonsilar challenge with *Mycobacterium bovis*. *Vet Immunol Immunopathol.* (2010) 137:84–92. doi: 10.1016/j.vetimm.2010.04.013
8. Nishi JS, Shury T, Elkin BT. Wildlife reservoirs for bovine tuberculosis (*Mycobacterium bovis*) in Canada: strategies for management and research. *Vet Microbiol.* (2006) 112:325–38. doi: 10.1016/j.vetmic.2005.11.013
9. Griffin JM, Williams DH, Kelly GE, Clegg TA, O'Boyle I, Collins JD, et al. The impact of badger removal on the control of tuberculosis in cattle herds in Ireland. *Prev Vet Med.* (2005) 67:237–66. doi: 10.1016/j.prevetmed.2004.10.009
10. O'Brien DJ, Schmitt SM, Fitzgerald SD, Berry DE, Hickling GJ. Managing the wildlife reservoir of *Mycobacterium bovis*: the Michigan, USA, experience. *Vet Microbiol.* (2006) 112:313–23. doi: 10.1016/j.vetmic.2005.11.014
11. Livingstone PG, Hutchings SA, Hancox NG, de Lisle GW. Toward eradication: the effect of *Mycobacterium bovis* infection in wildlife on the evolution and future direction of bovine tuberculosis management in New Zealand. *N Z Vet J.* (2015) 63(Suppl. 1):4–18. doi: 10.1080/00480169.2014.971082
12. Pastoret PP, Brochier B. The development and use of a vaccinia-rabies recombinant oral vaccine for control of wildlife rabies; a link between Jenner and Pasteur. *Epidemiol Infect.* (1996) 116:235–40.
13. Oettinger T, Jørgensen M, Ladefoged A, Hasløv K, Andersen P. Development of the *Mycobacterium bovis* BCG vaccine: review of the historical and biochemical evidence for a genealogical tree. *Tuberc Lung Dis.* (1999) 79:243–50. doi: 10.1054/tuld.1999.0206
14. Behr MA, Wilson MA, Gill W P, Salamon H, Schoolnik GK, Rane S, et al. Comparative genomics of BCG vaccines by whole-genome DNA microarray. *Science* (1999) 284:1520–3. doi: 10.1126/science.284.5419.1520
15. Colditz GA, Berkey C S, Mosteller F, Brewer TF, Wilson ME, Burdick E, et al. The efficacy of bacillus Calmette-Guérin vaccination of newborns and infants in the prevention of tuberculosis: meta-analyses of the published literature. *Pediatrics* (1995) 96:29–35.
16. Wilkie ME, McShane H. TB vaccine development: where are we and why is it so difficult? *Thorax* (2015) 70:299–301. doi: 10.1136/thoraxjnl-2014-205202
17. Calmette A, Guérin C. Recherches expérimentales sur la defense del'organisme contre l'infection tuberculose. *Ann Inst Pasteur.* (1911) 25:625–41.
18. Calmette A, Guérin C. Vaccination des bovidés contre la tuberculose et methode nouvelle de prophylaxie de la tuberculose bovine. *Ann Inst Pasteur.* (1924) 38:371–98.
19. Francis J. *Bovine Tuberculosis.* London: Staples Press (1947). p. 220.
20. Haring CM, Traum J, Hayes FM, Henry BS. Vaccination of calves against tuberculosis with Calmette-Guérin culture, BCG. *Hilgardia* (1930) 4:307–94.
21. Rankin A. Rapport de la Commission de l'Alberta (Canada) sur le vaccine BCG (1927/28). *Ann Inst Pasteur.* (1929) 43:878–89.
22. Watson EA. Studies on bacillus Calmette-Guerin (B.C.G.) and vaccination against tuberculosis. *Can J Res.* (1933) 9:128–36.
23. Schellner H, Gaggermeier G. Vaccination of cattle in herds infected with TB with the 'strain P' tubercle bacillus described by Gräub. *Vet Bull.* (1955) 26:183 (Abstract 1117).
24. Rolle M, Wiethe H. Results of BCG vaccination in cattle in Bavaria. *Vet Bull.* (1956) 27:105 (Abstract 663).
25. Doyle TM, Stuart P. Vaccination of cattle with BCG. *Br Vet J.* (1958) 114:3–10.
26. Ellwood DC, Waddington FG. A second experiment to challenge the resistance to tuberculosis in BCG vaccinated cattle in Malawi. *Br Vet J.* (1972) 128:619–26.
27. Berggren SA. Field experiment with BCG vaccine in Malawi. *Br Vet J.* (1981) 137:88–96.
28. Griffin JF, MacKintosh CG, Slobbe L, Thomson AJ, Buchan GS. Vaccine protocols to optimise the protective efficacy of BCG. *Tuberc Lung Dis.* (1999) 79:135–43. doi: 10.1054/tuld.1998.0202
29. Lesellier S, Palmer S, Gowtage-Sequiera S, Ashford R, Dalley D, Davé D, et al. Protection of Eurasian badgers (*Meles meles*) from tuberculosis after intra-muscular vaccination with different doses of BCG. *Vaccine* (2011) 29:3782–90. doi: 10.1016/j.vaccine.2011.03.028
30. Buddle BM, de Lisle GW, Pfeffer A, Aldwell FE. Immunological responses and protection against *Mycobacterium bovis* in calves vaccinated with a low dose of BCG. *Vaccine* (1995) 13:1123–30. doi: 10.1016/0264-410X(94)00055-R
31. Palmer MV, Waters WR, Whipple DL. Aerosol delivery of virulent *Mycobacterium bovis* to cattle. *Tuberculosis* (2002) 82:275–82. doi: 10.1054/tube.2002.0341
32. Buddle BM, Hewinson RG, Vordermeier HM, Wedlock DN. Subcutaneous administration of a 10-fold-lower dose of a commercial human tuberculosis vaccine, *Mycobacterium bovis* Bacillus Calmette-Guérin Danish, induced levels of protection against bovine tuberculosis and responses in the tuberculin intradermal test similar to those induced by a standard cattle dose. *Clin Vaccine Immunol.* (2013) 20:1559–62. doi: 10.1128/CVI.00435-13
33. Wedlock DN, Aldwell FE, de Lisle GW, Vordermeier HM, Hewinson RG, Buddle BM. Protection against bovine tuberculosis induced by oral vaccination of cattle with *Mycobacterium bovis* BCG is not enhanced by co-administration of mycobacterial protein vaccines. *Vet Immunol Immunopathol.* (2011) 144:220–7. doi: 10.1016/j.vetimm.2011.09.005
34. Buddle BM, Wilson T, Aldwell FE, de Lisle GW, Vordermeier HM, Hewinson RG, et al. Low oral BCG doses fail to protect cattle against an experimental challenge with *Mycobacterium bovis*. *Tuberculosis* (2011) 91:400–5. doi: 10.1016/j.tube.2011.07.001
35. Buddle BM, Denis M, Aldwell FE, Vordermeier HM, Hewinson RG, Wedlock DN. Vaccination of cattle with *Mycobacterium bovis* BCG by a combination of systemic and oral routes. *Tuberculosis* (2008) 88:595–600. doi: 10.1016/j.tube.2008.01.005
36. Dean GS, Clifford D, Whelan AO, Tchilian E Z, Beverley PCL, Salguero FJ, et al. Protection induced by simultaneous subcutaneous and endobronchial vaccination with BCG/BCG and BCG/Adenovirus expressing antigen 85A against *Mycobacterium bovis*. *PLoS ONE* (2015) 10:e0142270. doi: 10.1371/journal.pone.0142270
37. Wedlock DN, Denis M, Vordermeier H M, Hewinson RG, Buddle BM. Vaccination of cattle with Danish and Pasteur strains of *Mycobacterium bovis* BCG induce different levels of IFN-γ post-vaccination, but induce similar levels of protection against bovine tuberculosis. *Vet Immunol Immunopathol.* (2007) 118:50–8. doi: 10.1016/j.vetimm.2007.04.005
38. Hope JC, Thom ML, McAulay M, Mead E, Vordermeier HM, Clifford D, et al. Identification of surrogates and correlates of protection in protective immunity against *Mycobacterium bovis* infection induced in neonatal calves by vaccination with *M. bovis* BCG Pasteur and *M. bovis* BCG Danish. *Clin Vaccine Immunol.* (2011) 18:373–9. doi: 10.1128/CVI.00543-10
39. Buddle BM, Wedlock DN, Parlane NA, Corner LA, de Lisle GW, Skinner MA. Revaccination of neonatal calves with *Mycobacterium bovis* BCG reduces the level of protection against bovine tuberculosis

induced by a single vaccination. *Infect Immun.* (2003) 71:6411–9. doi: 10.1128/IAI.71.11.6411-6419.2003

40. Hope JC, Thom ML, Villarreal-Ramos B, Vordermeier HM, Hewinson RG, Howard CJ. Vaccination of neonatal calves with *Mycobacterium bovis* BCG induces protection against intranasal challenge with virulent *M. bovis*. *Clin Exp Immunol.* (2005) 139:48–56. doi: 10.1111/j.1365-2249.2005.02668.x
41. Buddle BM, Wards BJ, Aldwell FE, Collins DM, de Lisle GW. Influence of sensitisation to environmental mycobacteria on subsequent vaccination against bovine tuberculosis. *Vaccine* (2002) 20:1126–33. doi: 10.1016/S0264-410X(010)00436-4
42. Hope JC, Thom ML, Villarreal-Ramos B, Vordermeier HM, Hewinson RG, Howard CJ. Exposure to *Mycobacterium avium* induces low-level protection from *Mycobacterium bovis* infection but compromises diagnosis of disease in cattle. *Clin Exper Immunol.* (2005) 141:432–9. doi: 10.1111/j.1365-2249.2005.02882.x
43. Thom ML, McAulay M, Vordermeier HM, Clifford D, Hewinson RG, Villarreal-Ramos B, et al. Duration of immunity against *Mycobacterium bovis* following neonatal vaccination with bacillus Calmette-Guérin Danish: significant protection against infection at 12, but not 24 months. *Clin Vaccine Immunol.* (2012) 19:1254–60. doi: 10.1128/CVI.00301-12
44. Parlane NA, Shu D, Subharat S, Wedlock DN, Rehm BH, de Lisle GW, et al. Revaccination of cattle with *Bacille Calmette-Guérin* two years after first vaccination when immunity has waned, boosted protection against challenge with *Mycobacterium bovis*. *PLoS ONE* (2014) 9:e106519. doi: 10.1371/journal.pone.0106519
45. Buddle BM, Shu D, Parlane NA, Subharat S, Heiser A, Hewinson RG, et al. Vaccination of cattle with a high dose of BCG vaccine 3 weeks after experimental infection with *Mycobacterium bovis* increased the inflammatory response, but not tuberculous pathology. *Tuberculosis* (2016) 99:120–7. doi: 10.1016/j.tube.2016.05.004
46. Canto Alarcon GJ, Rubio Venegas Y, Bojorquez Narvaez L, Pizano Martínez OE, García Casanova L, Sosa Gallegos S, et al. Efficacy of a vaccine formula against tuberculosis in cattle. *PLoS ONE* (2013) 8:e76418. doi: 10.1371/journal.pone.0076418
47. Palmer CE, Long MW. Effect of infection with environmental mycobacteria on BCG vaccination and tuberculosis. *Amer Rev Resp Dis.* (1966) 553–68.
48. Brandt L, Feino Cunha J, Weinreich Olsen A, Chilima B, Hirsch P, Appelberg R, et al. Failure of the *Mycobacterium bovis* BCG vaccine: some species of environmental mycobacteria block multiplication of BCG and induction of protective immunity to tuberculosis. *Infect Immun.* (2002) 70:672–8. doi: 10.1128/IAI.70.2.672-678.2002
49. Flynn RJ, Mannion C, Golden O, Hacariz O, Mulcahy G. Experimental *Fasciola hepatica* infection alters responses to tests used for diagnosis of bovine tuberculosis. *Infect Immun.* (2007) 75:1373–81. doi: 10.1128/IAI.01445-06
50. Lopez-Valencia G, Renteria-Evangelista T, Williams JdJ, Licea-Navarro A, Mora-Valle AD, Medina-Basulto G. Field evaluation of the protective efficacy of *Mycobacterium bovis* BCG vaccine against bovine tuberculosis. *Res Vet Sci.* (2010) 88:44–9. doi: 10.1016/j.rvsc.2009.05.022
51. Ameni G, Vordermeier M, Aseffa A, Young DB, Hewinson RG. Field evaluation of the efficacy of *Mycobacterium bovis* Bacillus Calmette-Guérin against bovine tuberculosis in neonatal calves in Ethiopia. *Clin Vaccine Immunol.* (2010) 17:1533–8. doi: 10.1128/CVI.00222-10
52. Ameni G, Tafess K, Zewde A, Eguale T, Tilahun M, Hailu T, et al. Vaccination of calves with *Mycobacterium bovis* Bacillus Calmette-Guérin reduces the frequency and severity of lesions of bovine tuberculosis under a natural transmission setting in Ethiopia. *Transbound Emerg Dis.* (2018) 65:96–104. doi: 10.1111/tbed.12618
53. Nugent G, Yockney I, Whitford J, Aldwell FE, Buddle BM. Efficacy of oral BCG vaccination in protecting free-ranging cattle from natural infection by *Mycobacterium bovis*. *Vet Microbiol.* (2017) 208:181–9. doi: 10.1016/j.vetmic.2017.07.029
54. Whelan AO, Coad M, Upadhyay BL, Clifford DJ, Hewinson RG, Vordermeier HM. Lack of correlation between BCG-induced tuberculin skin test sensitisation and protective immunity in cattle. *Vaccine* (2011) 29:5453–8. doi: 10.1016/j.vaccine.2011.05.057
55. Moodie PA. Tuberculin reactions in BCG. *Br Vet J.* (1977) 133:642–645.
56. Pollock JM, Andersen P. The potential of the ESAT-6 antigen secreted by virulent mycobacteria for specific diagnosis of tuberculosis. *J Infect Dis.* (1997) 175:1251–4.
57. van Pinxteren LA, Ravn P, Agger EM, Pollock J, Andersen P. Diagnosis of tuberculosis based on the two specific antigens ESAT-6 and CFP10. *Clin Diagn Lab Immunol.* (2000) 7:155–60. doi: 10.1128/CDLI.7.2.155-160.2000
58. Vordermeier HM., Whelan A, Cockle PJ, Farrant L, Palmer N, Hewinson RG. Use of synthetic peptides derived from the antigens ESAT-6 and CFP-10 for differential diagnosis of bovine tuberculosis in cattle. *Clin Diagn Lab Immunol.* (2001) 8:571–8. doi: 10.1128/CDLI.8.3.571-578.2001
59. Sidders B, Pirson C, Hogarth PJ, Hewinson RG, Stoker NG, Vordermeier HM, et al. Screening of highly expressed mycobacterial genes identifies Rv3615c as a useful differential diagnostic antigen for *Mycobacterium tuberculosis* complex. *Infect Immun.* (2008) 76:3932–9. doi: 10.1128/IAI.00150-08
60. Vordermeier HM, Jones GJ, Buddle BM, Hewinson RG. Development of immuno-diagnostic reagents to diagnose bovine tuberculosis in cattle. *Vet Immunol Immunopathol.* (2016) 181:10–4. doi: 10.1016/j.vetimm.2016.02.003
61. Whelan AO, Clifford D, Upadhyay B, Breadon EL, McNair J, Hewinson RG, et al. Development of a skin test for bovine tuberculosis for differentiating infected from vaccinated animals. *J Clin Microbiol.* (2010) 48:3176–81. doi: 10.1128/JCM.00420-10
62. Jones GJ, Whelan A, Clifford D, Coad M, Vordermeier HM. Improved skin test for differential diagnosis of bovine tuberculosis by the addition of Rv3020c-derived peptides. *Clin Vaccine Immunol.* (2012) 19:620–2. doi: 10.1128/CVI.00024-12
63. Pesciaroli M, Alvarez J, Boniotti MB, Cagiola M, Di Marco V, Marianelli C, et al. Tuberculosis in domestic animal species. *Res Vet Sci.* (2014) 97:S78–85. doi: 10.1016/j.rvsc.2014.05.015
64. Pérez de Val B, López-Soria S, Nofrarias M, Martin M, Vordermeier HM, Romera N, et al. Experimental model of tuberculosis in the domestic goat after endobronchial infection with *Mycobacterium caprae*. *Clin Vaccine Immunol.* (2011) 18:1872–81. doi: 10.1128/CVI.05323-11
65. Pérez de Val B, Vidal E, López-Soria S, Marco A, Cervera Z, Martín M, et al. Assessment of safety and interferon-gamma responses of *Mycobacterium bovis* BCG vaccine in goat kids and milking goats. *Vaccine* (2016) 34:881–6. doi: 10.1016/j.vaccine.2016.01.004
66. Pérez de Val B, Villarreal-Ramos B, Nofrarias M, López-Soria S, Romera N, Singh M, et al. Goats primed with *Mycobacterium bovis* BCG and boosted with a recombinant adenovirus expressing Ag85A show enhanced protection against tuberculosis. *Clin Vaccine Immunol.* (2012) 19:1339–47. doi: 10.1128/CVI.00275-12
67. Arrieta-Villegas C, Perálvarez T, Vidal E, Puighibet Z, Moll X, Canturri A, et al. Efficacy of parenteral vaccination against tuberculosis with heat-inactivated *Mycobacterium bovis* in experimentally challenged goats. *PLoS ONE* (2018) 13:e0196948. doi: 10.1371/journal.pone.0196948
68. Vidal E, Arrieta-Villegas C, Grasa M, Mercader I, Domingao M, Pérez de Val B. Field evaluation of the efficacy of *Mycobacterium bovis* BCG vaccine against tuberculosis in goats. *BMC Vet Res.* (2017) 13:252. doi: 10.1186/s12917-017-1182-5
69. Muñoz-Mendoza M, Romero B, Del Cerro A, Gortázar C, García-Marín JF, Menéndez S, et al. Sheep as a potential source of bovine TB: epidemiology, pathology and evaluation of diagnostic techniques. *Transbound Emerg Dis.* (2016) 63:635–46. doi: 10.1111/tbed.12325
70. Balseiro A, Altuzarra R, Vidal E, Moll X, Espada Y, Sevilla IA, et al. Assessment of BCG and inactivated *Mycobacterium bovis* vaccines in an experimental tuberculosis infection model in sheep. *PLoS ONE* (2017) 12:e0180546. doi: 10.1371/journal.pone.0180546
71. Beatson NS. Tuberculosis in Red Deer. In: Brown RD, editor. *Biology of Deer Production*. New York, NY: Springer Verlag (1985). p. 147–50.
72. Fitzgerald SD, Kaneene JB. Wildlife reservoirs of bovine tuberculosis worldwide: hosts, pathology, surveillance, and control. *Vet Pathol.* (2013) 50:488–99. doi: 10.1177/0300985812467472
73. Martín-Hernando MP, Torres MJ, Aznar J, Negro JJ, Gandía A, Gortázar C. Sampling strategy, lesion pattern and lesion distribution in naturally *Mycobacterium bovis* infected red deer and fallow deer. *J Comp Pathol.* (2010) 142:43–50. doi: 10.1016/j.jcpa.2009.07.003

74. Griffin JF, Mackintosh CG, Rodgers CR. Factors influencing the protective efficacy of a BCG homologous prime-boost vaccination regime against tuberculosis. *Vaccine* (2006) 24:835–45. doi: 10.1016/j.vaccine.2005.07.033
75. Thomas J, Risalde MA, Serrano M, Servilla I, Geijo M, Ortíz JA, et al. The response of red deer to oral administration of heat inactivated *Mycobacterium bovis* and challenge with a field strain. *Vet Microbiol.* (2017) 208:195–202. doi: 10.1016/j.vetmic.2017.08.007
76. Nol P, Palmer MV, Waters WR, Aldwell FE, Buddle BM, Triantis JM, et al. Efficacy of oral and parenteral routes of *Mycobacterium bovis* bacille Calmette-Guérin vaccination against experimental bovine tuberculosis in white-tailed deer (*Odocoileus virginianus*): a feasibility study. *J Wildl Dis.* (2008) 44:247–59. doi: 10.7589/0090-3558-44.2.247
77. Palmer MV, Thacker TC, Waters WR. Vaccination with *Mycobacterium bovis* BCG strains Danish and Pasteur in white-tailed deer (*Odocoileus virginianus*) experimentally challenged with *Mycobacterium bovis. Zoonoses Public Health* (2009) 56:243–51. doi: 10.1111/j.1863-2378.2008.01198.x
78. Palmer MV, Thacker TC, Waters WR. Vaccination of white-tailed deer (*Odocoileus virginianus*) with *Mycobacterium bovis* bacillus Calmette Guérin. *Vaccine* (2007) 25:6589–97. doi: 10.1016/j.vaccine.2007.06.056
79. Palmer MV, Thacker TC, Waters WR, Robbe-Austerman S, Lebepe-Mazur SM, Harris NB. Persistence of *Mycobacterium bovis* Bacillus Calmette-Guérin in white-tailed deer (*Odocoileus virginianus*) after oral or parenteral vaccination. *Zoonoses Public Health* (2010) 57:206–12. doi: 10.1111/j.1863-2378.2010.01329.x
80. Nol P, Rhyan JC, Robbe-Austerman S, McCollum MP, Rigg TD, Saklou NT, et al. The potential for transmission of BCG from orally vaccinated white-tailed deer (*Odocoileus virginianus*) to cattle (*Bos taurus*) through a contaminated environment: experimental findings. *PLoS ONE* (2013) 8:e60257. doi: 10.1371/journal.pone.0060257
81. Sorensen A, van Beest FM, Brook RK. Impacts of wildlife baiting and supplemental feeding on infectious disease transmission risk: a synthesis of knowledge. *Prev Vet Med.* (2014) 113:356–63. doi: 10.1016/j.prevetmed.2013.11.010
82. Ramsey DSL, O'Brien DJ, Cosgrove MK, Rudolph BA, Locher AB, Schmitt SM. Forecasting eradication of bovine tuberculosis in Michigan white-tailed deer. *J Wildl Manage.* (2014) 78:240–54. doi: 10.1002/jwmg.656
83. Aldwell FE, Keen D, Parlane N, Skinner MA, de Lisle GW, Buddle BM. Oral vaccination with *Mycobacterium bovis* BCG in a lipid formulation induces resistance to pulmonary tuberculosis in possums. *Vaccine* (2003) 22:70–6. doi: 10.1016/S0264-410X(03)00539-5
84. Tompkins DM, Ramsey DSL, Cross ML, Aldwell FE, de Lisle GW, Buddle BM. Oral vaccination reduces the incidence of bovine tuberculosis in a free-living wildlife species. *Proc Biol Sci.* (2009) 276:2987–95. doi: 10.1098/rspb.2009.0414
85. Chambers MA, Aldwell F, Williams GA, Palmer S, Gowtage S, Ashford R, Lesellier S. The effect of oral vaccination with *Mycobacterium bovis* BCG on the development of tuberculosis in captive european badgers (*Meles meles*). *Front Cell Infect Microbiol.* (2017) 7:6. doi: 10.3389/fcimb.2017.00006
86. Carter SP, Chambers M A, Rushton SP, Shirley M D F, Schuchert P, Pietravalle S, et al. BCG vaccination reduces risk of tuberculosis infection in vaccinated badgers and unvaccinated badger cubs. *PLoS ONE* (2012) 7:e49833. doi: 10.1371/journal.pone.0049833
87. Gormley E, Ní Bhuachalla D, O'Keeffe J, Murphy D, Aldwell FE. Oral vaccination of free-living badgers (*Meles meles*) with Bacille Calmette Guérin (BCG) vaccine confers protection against tuberculosis. *PLoS ONE* (2017) 12:e0168851. doi: 10.1371/journal.pone.0168851
88. Aznar I, Frankena K, More SJ, O'Keefe J, McGrath G, de Jong MCM. Quantification of *Mycobacterium bovis* transmission in a badger vaccine field trial. *Prev Vet Med.* (2018) 149:29–37. doi: 10.1016/j.prevetmed.2017.10.010
89. Gortázar C, Beltrán-Beck B, Garrido JM, Aranaz A, Sevilla I, Boadella M, et al. Oral re-vaccination of Eurasian wild boar with *Mycobacterium bovis* BCG yields a strong protective response against challenge with a field strain. *BMC Vet Res.* (2014) 10:96. doi: 10.1186/1746-6148-10-96
90. Díez-Delgado I, Sevilla I, Romero B, Tanner E, Barasona JA, White AR, et al. Impact of piglet vaccination against tuberculosis in endemic free-ranging wild boar populations. *Prev Vet Med.* (2018) 155:11–20. doi: 10.1016/j.prevetmed.2018.04.002
91. Qureshi T, Labes RE, Cross ML, Griffin JF, Mackintosh CG. Partial protection against oral challenge with *Mycobacterium bovis* in ferrets (*Mustela furo*) following oral vaccination with BCG. *Int J Tuberc Lung Dis.* (1999) 3:1025–33.
92. Cross ML, Labes RE, Young G, Mackintosh CG. Systemic but not intraintestinal vaccination with BCG reduces the severity of tuberculosis infection in ferrets (*Mustela furo*). *Int J Tuberc Lung Dis.* (2000) 4:473–80. Available online at: http://www.ingentaconnect.com/content/iuatld/ijtld/2000/00000004/00000005/art00013;jsessionid=fcfeo4ych6ru.x-ic-live-02
93. Aldwell FE, Keen DL, Stent VC, Thomson A, Yates GF, de Lisle GW, et al. Route of BCG administration in possums affects protection against bovine tuberculosis. *N Z Vet J.* (1995) 43:356–9. doi: 10.1080/00480169./1995.35920
94. Skinner MA, Keen DL, Parlane NA, Hamel KL, Yates GF, Buddle BM. Improving protective efficacy of BCG vaccination for wildlife against bovine tuberculosis. *Res Vet Sci.* (2005) 78:231–6. doi: 10.1016/j.rvsc.2004.07.007
95. Buddle BM, Aldwell FE, Keen DL, Parlane NA, Yates G, de Lisle GW. Intraduodenal vaccination of brushtail possums with bacille Calmette-Guérin enhances immune responses and protection against *Mycobacterium bovis* infection. *Int J Tuberc Lung Dis.* (1997) 1:377–83.
96. Cross ML, Henderson RJ, Lambeth MR, Buddle BM, Aldwell FE. Lipid-formulated BCG as an oral-bait vaccine for tuberculosis: vaccine stability, efficacy and palatability to New Zealand possums (*Trichosurus vulpecula*). *J Wildl Dis.* (2009) 45:754–65. doi: 10.7589/0090-3558-45.3.754
97. Buddle BM, Aldwell FE, Keen DL, Parlane NA, Hamel KL, de Lisle GW. Oral vaccination of brushtail possums with BCG: investigation into factors that influence vaccine efficacy and determination of duration of immunity. *N Z Vet J.* (2006) 54:224–30. doi: 10.1080/00480169.2006.36701
98. Tompkins DM, Buddle BM, Whitford J, Cross ML, Yates GF, Lambeth MR, et al. Sustained protection against tuberculosis conferred to a wildlife host by a single dose vaccination. *Vaccine* (2013) 31:893–9. doi: 10.1016/j.vaccine.2012.12.003
99. Wedlock DN, Aldwell FE, Keen DL, Skinner MA, Buddle BM. Oral vaccination of brushtail possums (*Trichosurus vulpecula*) with BCG: immune responses, persistence of BCG in lymphoid organs and excretion in faeces. *N Z Vet J.* (2005) 53:301–6. doi: 10.1080/00480169.2005.36564
100. Corner LA, Norton S, Buddle, BM, Morris RS. The efficacy of bacilli Calmette-Guérin vaccine in wild brushtail possums (*Trichosurus vulpecula*). *Res Vet Sci.* (2002) 73:145–52. doi: 10.1080/00480169.2002.36302
101. Delahay RJ, Smith GC, Barlow AM, Walker N, Harris A, Clifton-Hadley RS, et al. Bovine tuberculosis infection in wild mammals in the South-West region of England: a survey of prevalence and a semi-quantitative assessment of the relative risks to cattle. *Vet J.* (2007) 173:287–301. doi: 10.1016/j.tvjl.2005.11.011
102. Godfray HC, Donnelly CA, Kao RR, MacDonald DW, McDonald RA, Petrokofsky G, et al. A restatement of the natural science evidence base relevant to the control of bovine tuberculosis in Great Britain. *Proc Biol Sci.* (2013) 280:20131634. doi: 10.1098/rspb.2013.1634
103. Gormley E, Corner LA. Control strategies for wildlife tuberculosis in Ireland. *Transbound Emerg Dis.* (2013) 60(Suppl. 1):128–35. doi: 10.1111/tbed.12095
104. O'Connor CM, Haydon DT, Kao RR. An ecological and comparative perspective on the control of bovine tuberculosis in Great Britain and the Republic of Ireland. *Prev Vet Med.* (2012) 104:185–97. doi: 10.1016/j.prevetmed.2011.11.010
105. Abdou M, Frankena K, O'Keeffe J, Byrne AW. Effect of culling and vaccination on bovine tuberculosis infection in a European badger (*Meles meles*) population by spatial simulation modelling. *Prev Vet Med.* (2016) 125:19–30. doi: 10.1016/j.prevetmed.2015.12.012
106. Lesellier S, Palmer S, Dalley DJ, Davé D, Johnson L, Hewinson RG, et al. The safety and immunogenicity of Bacillus Calmette-Guérin (BCG) vaccine in European badgers (*Meles meles*). *Vet Immunol Immunopathol.* (2006) 112:24–37. doi: 10.1016/j.vetimm.2006.03.009
107. Chambers M, Rogers F, Delahay R, Lesellier S, Ashford R, Dalley D, et al. Bacillus Calmette-Guerin vaccination reduces the severity and progression of tuberculosis in badgers. *Proc Biol Sci.* (2011) 278:1913–20. doi: 10.1098/rspb.2010.1953
108. Murphy D, Costello E, Aldwell FE, Lesellier S, Chambers MA, Fitzsimons T, et al. Oral vaccination of badgers (*Meles meles*) against tuberculosis:

comparison of the protection generated by BCG vaccine strains Pasteur and Danish. *Vet J.* (2014) 200:362–7. doi: 10.1016/j.tvjl.2014.02.031

109. Perrett S, Lesellier S, Rogers F, Williams GA, Gowtage S, Palmer S, et al. Assessment of the safety of Bacillus Calmette-Guérin vaccine administered orally to badgers (*Meles meles*). *Vaccine* (2018) 36:1990–5. doi: 10.1016/j.vaccine.2018.02.101
110. Gortázar C, Che-Amat A, O'Brien D. Open questions and recent advances in the control of a multi-host infectious disease: animal tuberculosis. *Mammal Rev.* (2015) 45:160–75. doi: 10.1111/mam.12042
111. LaHue NP, Baños JV, Acevedo P, Gortázar C, Martínez-López B. Spatially explicit modelling of animal tuberculosis at the wildlife-livestock interface in Ciudad Real province, Spain. *Prev Vet Med.* (2016) 128:101–11. doi: 10.1016/j.prevetmed.2016.04.011
112. Massei G, Kindberg J, Licopp A, Gačic D, Šprem N, Kamler J, et al. Wild boar populations up, numbers of hunters down? A review of trends and implications for Europe. *Pest Manage Sci.* (2015) 71:492–500. doi: 10.1002/ps.3965
113. Martín-Hernando MP, Höfle U, Vicente J, Ruiz-Fons F, Vidal D, Barral M, al. Lesions associated with *Mycobacterium tuberculosis* complex infection in the European wild boar. *Tuberculosis* (2007) 87:360–7. doi: 10.1016/j.tube.2007.02.003
114. Santos N, Santos C, Valente T, Gortázar C, Almeida V, Correia-Neves M. Widespread environmental contamination with *Mycobacterium tuberculosis* complex revealed by a molecular detection protocol. *PLoS ONE* (2015) 10:e0142079. doi: 10.1371/journal.pone.0142079
115. Garrido JM, Sevilla IA, Beltrán-Beck B, Minguijón E, Ballesteros C, Galindo RC, et al. Protection against tuberculosis in Eurasian wild boar vaccinated with heat-inactivated *Mycobacterium bovis*. *PLoS ONE* (2011) 6:e24905. doi: 10.1371/journal.pone.0024905
116. Beltrán-Beck B, Romero B, Sevilla I, Barasona JA, Garrido JM, González-Barrio D, et al. Assessment of an oral *Mycobacterium bovis* BCG vaccine and an inactivated *M. bovis* preparation for wild boar in terms of adverse reactions, vaccine strain survival, and uptake by nontarget species. *Clin Vaccine Immunol.* (2014) 21:12–20. doi: 10.1128/CVI.00488-13
117. Nol P, Robbe-Austerman S, Rhyan JC, McCollan MP, Triantis JM, Beltrán-Beck B, et al. Determining the persistence of *Mycobacterium bovis* bacille Calmette-Guérin Danish in select tissues of orally vaccinated feral swine (*Sus scrofa* spp.) *Res Vet Sci.* (2016) 104:50–2. doi: 10.1016/j.rvsc.2015.11.007
118. Byrom AE, Caley P, Paterson BM, Nugent G. Feral ferrets (*Mustela furo*) as hosts and sentinels of tuberculosis in New Zealand. *N Z Vet J.* (2015). 63(Suppl. 1):42–53. doi: 10.1080/00480169.2014.981314
119. Caley P, Hone J. Estimating the force of infection; *Mycobacterium bovis* infection in feral ferrets *Mustela furo* in New Zealand. *J Anim Ecol.* (2002) 71:44–54. doi: 10.1046/j.0021-8790.2001.00573.x
120. Michel AL, Coetzee ML, Keet DF, Mare L, Warren R, Cooper D, et al. Molecular epidemiology of *Mycobacterium bovis* isolates from free-ranging wildlife in South African game reserves. *Vet Microbiol.* (2009) 133:335–43. doi: 10.1016/j.vetmic.2008.07.023
121. Hlokwe TM, Jenkins AO, Streicher EM, Venter EH, Cooper D, Godfroid J, et al. Molecular characterization of *Mycobacterium bovis* isolated from African buffaloes (*Syncerus caffer*) in Hluhluwe-iMfolozi Park in KwaZulu-Natal, South Africa. *Onderstepoort J Vet Res.* (2011) 78:1–6. doi: 10.4102/ojvr.v78i1.232
122. Hlokwe TM, De Klerk-Lorist LM, Michel AL. Wildlife on the move: a hidden tuberculosis threat to conservation areas and game farms through introduction of untested animals. *J Wildl Dis.* (2016) 52:837–43. doi: 10.7589/2015-10-281
123. Michel AL, Bengis RG. The African buffalo: a villain for inter-species spread of infectious diseases in southern Africa. *Onderstepoort J Vet Res.* (2012) 79:453. doi: 10.4102/ojvr.v79i2.453
124. Michel AL, Bengis RG, Keet DF, Hofmeyr M, Klerk LM, Cross PC, et al. Wildlife tuberculosis in South African conservation areas: implications and challenges. *Vet Microbiol.* (2006). 12:91–100. doi: 10.1016/j.vetmic.2005.11.035
125. Musoke J, Hlokwe T, Marcotty T, du Plessis BJ, Michel AL. Spillover of *Mycobacterium bovis* from wildlife to livestock, South Africa. *Emerg Infect Dis.* (2015) 21:448–51. doi: 10.3201/eid2103.131690
126. Murphy D, Corner LAL, Gormley E. Adverse reactions to *Mycobacterium bovis* bacille Calmette-Guerin (BCG) vaccination against tuberculosis in humans, veterinary animals and wildlife species. *Tuberculosis* (2008) 68:344–57. doi: 10.1016/j.tube.2007.11.010
127. Lagranderie M, Chavarot P, Balazuc AM, Marchal G. Immunogenicity and protective capacity of *Mycobacterium bovis* BCG after oral or intragastric administration to mice. *Vaccine* (2000) 18:1186–95. doi: 10.1016/S0264-410X(99)00386-2
128. Filardi MJ, Codish SD, Civerchia L, Howard RK, McKneally MF. Toxicity of intrapleural Bacillus Calmette-Guérin treatment in animals. *Cancer Res.* (1979) 39:3673–6.
129. Smith DW, Wiegeshaus E, Navalkar R, Grover AA. Host-parasite relationships in experimental airborne tuberculosis. I. Preliminary studies in BCG-vaccinated and nonvaccinated animals. *J Bacteriol.* (1966) 91:718–24.
130. Lurie MB, Zappasodi P, Cardona-Lynch E, Dannenberg AM Jr. The response to the intracutaneous inoculation of BCG as an index of native resistance to tuberculosis. *J Immunol.* (1952) 68:369–87.
131. Abolhassani M, Lagranderie M, Chavarot P, Balazuc AM, Marchal G. *Mycobacterium bovis* BCG induces similar immune responses and protection by rectal and parenteral immunization routes. *Infect Immun.* (2000) 68:5657–62. doi: 10.1128/IAI.68.10.5657-5662.2000
132. Klein WR, Bras GE, Misdorp W, Steerenberg PA, de Jong WH, Tiesjema RH, et al. Equine sarcoid: BCG immunotherapy compared to cryosurgery in a prospective randomised clinical trial. *Cancer Immunol Immunother.* (1986) 21:133–40.
133. Slobbe L, Lockhart E, O'Donnell MA, Mackintosh C, de Lisle G, Buchan G. An *in vivo* comparison of bacillus Calmette-Guérin (BCG) and cytokine-secreting BCG vaccines. *Immunology* (1999). 96:517–23. doi: 10.1046/j.1365-2567.1999.00702.x
134. Vordermeier HM, Jones GJ, Buddle BM, Hewinson RG, Villarreal-Ramos B. Bovine tuberculosis in cattle: vaccines, DIVA Tests, and host biomarker discovery. *Annu Rev Anim Biosci.* (2016) 4:87–109. doi: 10.1146/annurev-animal-021815-111311
135. Garly ML, Martins CL, Balé C, Baldé MA, Hedegaard KL, Gustafson P, et al. BCG scar and positive tuberculin reaction associated with reduced child mortality in West Africa. A non-specific beneficial effect of BCG? *Vaccine* (2003) 21:2782–90. doi: 10.1016/S0264-410X(03)00181-6

3

Bovine Tuberculosis Management in Northwest Minnesota and Implications of the Risk Information Seeking and Processing (RISP) Model for Wildlife Disease Management

Megan Cross[1*], *Alex Heeren*[2], *Louis J. Cornicelli*[3] *and David C. Fulton*[4]

[1] *Department of Fisheries and Wildlife, Michigan State University, East Lansing, MI, United States,* [2] *Sierra Nevada Research Institute, University of California, Merced, CA, United States,* [3] *Minnesota Department of Natural Resources, Division of Fish and Wildlife, St. Paul, MN, United States,* [4] *U.S. Geological Survey, Minnesota Cooperative Fish and Wildlife Research Unit, University of Minnesota, St. Paul, MN, United States*

Correspondence:
Megan Cross
crossmeg@msu.edu

Bovine tuberculosis (bTB) is an infectious, zoonotic disease caused by *Mycobacterium bovis* that can spread between domestic and wild animals, as well as to humans. The disease is characterized by the progressive development of lesions that compromise the victim's lungs and lymph system. The disease was first identified in northwest Minnesota in both cattle and white-tailed deer (*Odocoileus virginianus*) in 2005. Due to its risks to human and animal health, bTB has numerous implications related to population management, policy outcomes, stakeholder relations, and economic impacts. When dealing with complicated risks, like bTB, individuals often seek out and process information as a method to learn about, and cope, with the risk. We developed a questionnaire that adapted components of the Risk Information Seeking and Processing (RISP) model and surveyed northwest Minnesota deer hunters. Our objectives were to better understand how stakeholders perceive and act on information regarding disease management in wildlife and to understand the utility of the RISP model for such management contexts. We drew a random proportional sample of licensed deer hunters ($n = 2100$) from the area affected by bTB and conducted a multi-contact mail survey. We found that 43% of the variability in the information-seeking behaviors of respondents was explained by demographics, hunting importance, personal risk perceptions, attitudes, and subjective norms. However, these results are largely attributable to the factors in the RISP model encompassed by components of the Theory of Planned Behavior (i.e., attitudes, subjective norms, perceived behavioral control, and behavioral intentions). This information can help managers contextualize individuals' perceived risks to better frame communication efforts to address stakeholder concerns and develop best practices for disease communication. While the state of Minnesota is currently considered free of bTB, future outbreaks remain possible in Minnesota and elsewhere. Understanding the key factors in the processes through which deer hunters seek out information pertaining to the disease can help managers collect the data necessary to aid decisions about desired future management outcomes. In addition, testing RISP model performance in applied research improves its future use across a broad spectrum of topics throughout veterinary disease management.

Keywords: bovine tuberculosis, communication, disease management, information-seeking, risk information seeking and processing (RISP) model

INTRODUCTION

Bovine tuberculosis (*Mycobacterium bovis*, hereafter referred to as "bTB") is an infectious zoonotic disease that can spread among domestic and wild mammals and, in rare cases humans. Zoonotic diseases like bTB threaten agricultural economies, pose health risks to humans and wildlife, and disturb the social, political, and economic environments where they occur. In Minnesota, the appearance of bTB among wild white-tailed deer (*Odocoileus virginianus*) in 2005 was not only a health concern but also posed a risk to the state's deer hunt, a major economic industry, cultural event, and the primary method in which the state manages its deer population. Therefore, as bTB engaged numerous stakeholder groups, understanding how hunters viewed the risk, and whether their concerns impacted the decision to hunt, was of particular interest to management agencies.

The human dimensions of disease management in wildlife has increased in importance during recent years (1–5). Following Clarke (1), we used the Risk Information Seeking and Processing model (RISP) (6) as a core framework to discern the key considerations for understanding and better communicating with stakeholders about disease management in wildlife. In this study, we were interested in delineating the processes through which Minnesota deer hunters sought information about risks from bTB.

We addressed the following key questions:

1. How do hunters seek information about bTB?
2. What factors affect hunters' information seeking behaviors?
3. Is the RISP model useful for understanding well-established wildlife disease management issues?
4. What are the implications for natural resource management agencies and professionals?

Such information can help guide managers' decisions regarding the collection and analysis of information related to individuals' perceived risks and improve the development of communication best practices in instances of disease in wildlife.

The initial detection of bTB in northwest Minnesota occurred at a beef cattle operation in 2005 (7). Upon further testing, the disease was found in several other beef cattle operations and detected in wild white-tailed deer (*Odocoileus virginianus*) during fall 2005 hunter-harvested surveillance (7). Epidemiological evidence indicated the disease was introduced into a single beef cattle operation and from there it spilled over to deer (8, 9). Deer presumably served as a spillover host for the transmission of the disease among area livestock operations (8, 10, 11).

In response to the detection of bTB in cattle and deer, the Minnesota Department of Natural Resources (DNR) and the Minnesota Board of Animal Health took joint actions to decrease the likelihood of disease spread, eradicate the disease from cattle (and thus regain Accredited-free status within the United States Department of Agriculture's bTB eradication program), and reduce wild deer prevalence to undetectable levels. These strategies centered on preventative measures to reduce the likelihood of disease transmission. Example strategies included a temporary buy-out of cattle producers, construction of deer exclusion fencing around stored forage, prohibiting recreational deer feeding, and reducing the local deer population using hunting regulations, aerial gunning, ground sharpshooting, and deer shooting permits issued to landowners (8, 10, 12).

Although the disease was successfully eradicated in cattle and reduced to an undetectable level in deer by 2012, deer hunters considered the actions taken to achieve bTB-free status controversial (12). Among the general public, lethal control of deer (sharpshooting) is often contentious (12–14). Further, in instances of zoonotic disease affecting game species, hunters show more concern than the general public about game management (15, 16).

As it was being used in other studies the RISP model is the primary source for the conceptual framework used in our study, and data were collected following the methods outlined in Griffin et al. (6) work on RISP and recent adaptations to that model [see (1)]. The RISP model builds upon an earlier model, the Theory of Planned Behavior, by examining the relationship between information, knowledge, and risk perception (6). Multiple studies in the field of risk and threat perception have shown that information seeking and processing is an important component of how an individual perceives and responds to a risk (17–19).

According to the RISP model (**Figure 1**), an individual's perception of risk is driven by the degree to which they think they are informed about a threat and how he or she seeks out and processes information about the risk (6). Like many other risk perception models, Griffin's RISP model has been used to study health and personal risks. However, environmental risks have been a special emphasis of the RISP model research (18, 20, 21). Clarke (1) presented a modified RISP framework, which integrated values, to examine how individuals perceive zoonotic disease (such as bTB) as a threat to wildlife (**Figure 2**).

The central component that drives the RISP model is "information sufficiency" (6). In the process of developing the perception of a threat, an individual will assess how much information they currently have and evaluate that level based on how much information they think is necessary to

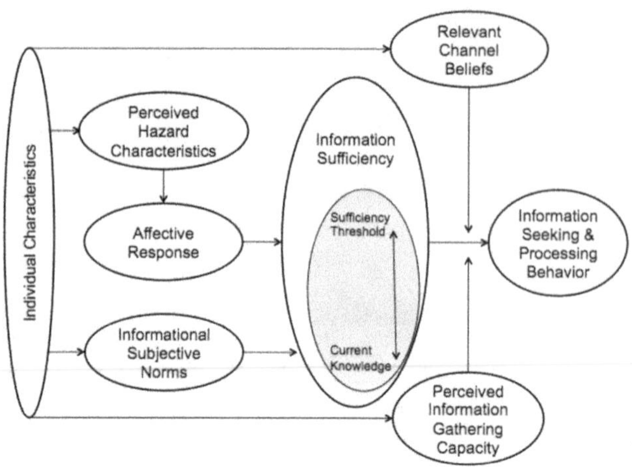

FIGURE 1 | Risk Information Seeking and Processing Model [adapted from (6)].

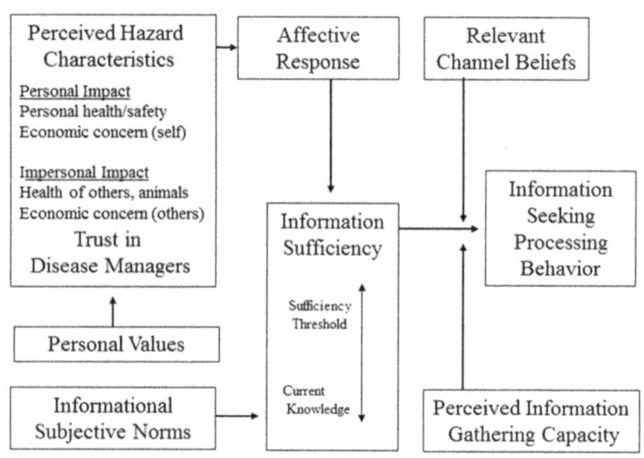

FIGURE 2 | Clarke's RISP framework for zoonotic diseases [adapted from (1)].

understand the threat. If the individual believes they have insufficient information, they will seek out and process additional information about the topic. Demographics, such as age, income, education level, and personal importance of hunting, and informational subjective norms (the social pressure to be informed) may influence individuals' information sufficiency thresholds.

Affective responses may also have an important influence on information sufficiency, and the common affective responses studied by RISP frameworks are worry and anxiety (17). However, fear and anger are also possible responses that could apply, with the degree of perceived personal control influencing with one expresses fear (low control) or anger (high control) to a situation (6, 20). Subjective norms, an individual's assessment of whether his or her peers expect him or her to be informed, can also lead to the information sufficiency stage regarding the threat (6). Even if an individual is not concerned about a risk, they may decide to learn more if they think it will give them more information to talk about with peers.

Another set of components, "perceived information gathering capacity," refers to whether the individual can understand (or comprehend) and access available information. Information that is too complicated or technical may discourage an individual from seeking more information about the risk. Relevant channel beliefs, which we did not collect data on, refer to the "channels," or sources of information, through which an individual learns about a risk (6). In the model, relevant channel beliefs do not interact with other predictor variables and subsequent work on RISP excludes relevant channel beliefs (22). The information sources or amount of information an individual has access to may affect desire to seek information about the source.

These variables are meant to measure an individual's heuristic and systematic processing of information, and in the model, are hypothesized to influence information seeking behavior through the information sufficiency and perceived information gathering capacity variables, which share a direct relationship with information seeking (1, 6, 23). Systematic processing refers to higher order processing, which requires effort on the part of the individual and, more likely than heuristic processing, may lead to attitudinal change (24, 25). Heuristic processing occurs at a comparatively shallow level and uses superficial cues for interpreting information (25). The two forms of information processing are a major field of social-psychological research (26–28). In the context of understanding perceptions about bTB, the distinction is important as hunters who engage in heuristic processing may be more easily discouraged from hunting due to concerns about bTB than those who engage in systematic processing.

In addition to Griffin et al. (6) RISP model, we adopted components of Clarke's (1) Zoonotic Disease Risk Information Seeking and Processing (ZDRISP) framework. Following Clarke (1), we measured hunters' perceptions of the impact of bTB to themselves, other people, and wildlife. The framework includes components that examine how personal impact (e.g., health and financial costs to the individual) and impersonal impact (e.g., health and financial costs to other people, wildlife species, and society) can be included in a traditional RISP model. Clarke (1) also emphasizes the importance of trust in the managing agency on information seeking and processing. Low trust of an agency might discourage, or frustrate people, from learning about the threat. Trust will also likely have an important role in whether an individual supports the agencies policies to manage the threat. Kahlor (19), building off similar communication processing frameworks, argued for a more integrated RISP model that was termed, "A Planned Risk Information Seeking Model" (PRISM). The key aspect of PRISM is the integration of the core RISP model with conceptual components from the Theory of Planned Behavior (24, 29). These components include: (1) positive/negative evaluations of a behavior (attitudes); (2) perceptions of social pressure to engage in a behavior (subjective norms); and (3) perceived ability to engage in a behavior (perceived behavioral control) (19).

Given the controversial nature of wildlife disease management, there is a need to understand how stakeholders perceive, gain, and distribute information. The RISP model hypothesizes that information sufficiency and perceived information gathering capacity directly influence information seeking behavior. Because of the direct relationship of these variables to information seeking in the model (**Figure 1**), we expect them to demonstrate the greatest influence on information seeking behavior relative to other variables. Previous studies conducted using the RISP framework and its variants (1, 19, 20) guided the development of the survey instrument used in this research. We also collaborated closely with the Minnesota DNR regarding their bTB strategy related to deer management. The adoption of this RISP model for evaluating perceived threats from wildlife disease aligns with bTB disease research in Michigan (30), and we were particularly interested in potential insights from the application of the model in the two similar contexts.

METHODS

Sampling

In Minnesota, deer are managed by permit area (n = 128) and hunters are asked to identify the areas they intend to hunt that year. Although hunters are not required to hunt only in the area they identify, previous research revealed that most return to the same location annually (31). We drew a proportional random sample from Minnesota's Electronic Licensing System license database of adult individuals who purchased a deer license and indicated they hunted in areas affected by bTB. Our survey followed a modified version of the Tailored Design Method (32). We mailed survey to 2,100 licensed hunters from the bTB affected permit areas (n = 7) and used three waves of mailing to maximize response rate. We collected data during late summer and fall of 2012 (University of Minnesota Institutional Review Board Study Number: 0609E92806).

Measurement Variables

Dependent Variable

Following the RISP model, we wanted to understand what variables influenced the likelihood of individuals to actively seek out bTB information. We used five items developed and tested in previous studies of the RISP framework to measure information seeking (**Table 1**). We used a five-point scale ranging from 1 = *"strongly disagree"* to 5 = *"strongly agree"* for each item. Questions that were phrased to report avoidance of information seeking were reverse coded for reliability and subsequent scale formation. We computed the latent dependent variable, "information seeking behavior" as the mean score of the 5 scale items.

Independent Variables

In addition to respondent demographics, we constructed seven latent independent variables as identified in the RISP (6) and ZDRISP (1) models. We measured (1) demographic variables such as age, education level, and importance of hunting, and following Clarke (1), (2) we assessed respondents' general perceptions of bTB impact concerns, or risk judgment (8 items) and personal impact concerns (4 items). Each item was measured on a five-point scale ranging from 1 = *"not at all"* to 5 = *"extremely" concerned.* We also measured the (3) individual affective responses (anger, worry, fear) of study participants to the discovery of bTB and the DNR's subsequent management of the disease on an 11-point scale ranging from 0 = *"none of this feeling"* to 10 = *"a lot of this feeling."* We measured (4) subjective norms using three items on a five-point scale from 1 = *"strongly disagree"* to 5 = *"strongly agree,"* and following Fishbein and Ajzen (29, 33), we used semantic differential scales to assess respondents' evaluation of seeking information about bTB management. Respondents were asked to evaluate (on a 7-point scale) whether their information seeking was worthless or valuable, foolish or wise, and unhelpful or helpful. We used six items to (5) define respondents' beliefs about their personal ability to obtain and understand bTB-related information. Responses related to information seeking capacity were also measured on a five-point style scale ranging from 1= *"strongly disagree"* to 5 = *"strongly agree."*

We also asked survey recipients about (6) their current knowledge and the amount of effort they dedicated to learning about bTB. We asked survey recipients to rate each on a scale ranging from 0 (no information) to 100 (all available information). Following Griffin et al. (20), we did not equate knowledge insufficiency as difference scores between these two measures but rather (7) regressed sufficiency threshold scores on initial knowledge scores to identify "information insufficiency" [as delineated in Cohen et al. (34)].

Data Analysis

Data were analyzed using the IBM Statistical Program for the Social Sciences (SPSS v. 20, 2013). (Any use of trade, firm, or product names is for descriptive purposes only and does not imply endorsement by the U.S. Government.) We grouped variables into their multi-item scales and tested internal consistency using Cronbach's alpha. Then we used hierarchical multiple regression models to examine the relationship between explanatory variables and the predictor, information seeking behavior as well as the ability of the RISP model to predict information seeking behaviors. We generated 7 separate models to test whether including each additional variable in our modified RISP framework improved the predictive ability of the model.

RESULTS

Response Rates and Respondent Characteristics

Of the 2,100 surveys mailed, 134 were undeliverable. For the remaining 1,966 surveys, 745 were completed and returned, resulting in a response rate of 38%. There was a wide distribution in the responses to survey items for variables included in the models, which suggested that our findings are likely to be representative of the sample population of hunters in all 7 deer permit areas impacted by bTB management. Most of survey respondents were male (93%) and half had completed

TABLE 1 | Measurement of variables.

Item	Mean	SD	alpha
(A) Dependent - Information seeking behavior[1]	0.77		
a) When the topic came up, I was likely to tune it out. (reverse coded)	3.79	0.89	
b) I'd go out of my way to avoid learning more about bovine TB management. (reverse coded)	4.08	0.84	
c) Gathering a lot of information about bovine TB management was a waste of time. (reverse coded)	3.83	0.93	
d) I tried to learn more about TB.	3.48	0.87	
e) I was likely to go out of my way to get more information about bovine TB management.	3.01	0.93	
(B) Independent			
1) Affective response[2]			NA
a) Anger	4.23	3.41	
b) Worry	4.65	3.36	
c) Fear	5.19	3.2	
2) Perceived impacts of bTB[3]			NA
a) Economic impacts to cattle producers	3.07	1.22	
b) Threats to the health of deer	3.81	1.03	
c) Reducing the deer population in the area	3.84	1.15	
d) Economic impacts to businesses that depend on deer hunting	3.23	1.16	
e) Threats to the health of other deer hunters from infected deer	2.74	1.32	
f) Reducing your deer hunting opportunity	3.72	1.2	
g) Threats to your personal health or family members from infected deer	2.68	1.4	
h) Financial costs to you personally	2.08	1.28	
3) Personal impact concerns[3]			0.71
a) Reducing the deer population in the area	0.48	0.65	
b) Reducing your deer hunting opportunity	0.58	0.59	
c) Threats to your personal health or family members from infected deer	0.45	0.68	
d) Financial costs to you personally	0.48	0.66	
4) Subjective norms[1]			0.74
a) People who are important to me thought I should stay on top of information about bovine TB	3.07	0.96	
b) People close to me expected me to get information about bovine TB	2.8	0.99	
c) Most of the people I know wanted to talk about bovine TB	2.99	1.18	
5) Perceived information gathering capacity[1]			0.74
a) I knew what questions to ask of the experts	2.77	0.96	
b) I knew where to go for information	3.39	0.95	
c) I could take the time to gather any information I needed	3.32	0.92	
d) Much of the information was too technical for me to understand (reverse coded)	3.44	0.87	
e) I could separate fact from fiction	3.86	0.86	
f) I could understand the information if I made the effort	2.77	0.7	
6) Attitude toward seeking information[4]			0.90
a) Worthless ... valuable	5.18	1.35	
b) Foolish ... wise	5.36	1.29	
c) Unhelpful ... helpful	5.16	1.25	
7) Trust in DNR[1]			0.93
a) I trust the Minnesota DNR to manage bovine TB	3.14	1.14	
b) DNR officials are concerned about minimizing the impacts of bovine TB on deer hunters	3.43	1.09	
c) The Minnesota DNR does a competent job of minimizing the impacts of bovine TB	3.22	1.06	
d) The DNR is open and honest in the things they do in say when managing bovine TB	2.92	1.12	
e) The DNR makes decisions about managing bovine TB in a way that is fair	2.87	1.08	
f) The DNR listens to deer hunters' concerns when managing bovine TB	2.76	1.13	

[1] *Response options ranged from "1 - Strongly disagree" to "5 - Strongly agree."*
[2] *Scale ranged from 0 to 10, where "0 - None of this feeling" to "10 - A lot of this feeling."*
[3] *Response options ranged from "1 - Not at all concerned" to "5 - Extremely concerned."*
[4] *Response options ranged from "1 - Extremely worthless/foolish/unhelpful" to "7 - Extremely valuable/wise/helpful."*

some education above the high school level (**Table 2**). Many respondents did not respond to the income question ($n = 211$), which is typically a component of personal characteristics in the RISP model. Income, however, did not appear to influence final model results and excluding it from the model provided a larger sample size for analysis. In a simple regression with income predicting information seeking behavior, the two variables were not strongly correlated, with $r_{(519)} = 0.008$, $p < 0.04$. For this reason, we did not use income as an independent variable in the analysis. The final usable response rate for modeling was 30% ($n = 598$) after removing individuals excluded due to incomplete responses to survey items other than income.

Scale Reliability and Model Results

Within the RISP framework, our reliability analyses supported the creation of the latent dependent variable (alpha = 0.77) and the independent latent variables (**Table 1**). Multiple regression demonstrated significant effects of attitudes, subjective norms, information seeking capacity and information insufficiency on the information seeking behaviors of northwest Minnesota deer hunters (**Tables 3, 4**). The final model in the hierarchical regression suggested the RISP framework explained 43% of the variability in northwest hunters' information seeking behaviors in response to bTB occurrence (**Table 3**).

Model 1 included only individual characteristics and explained a small amount of the variability in information seeking behaviors (6.5%) (**Table 3**). The addition of variables pertaining to personal impact, risk judgment, trust in DNR, and self-efficacy (Model 2) resulted in a ΔR^2 of 5.3% (**Table 3**). Affective response (Model 3) slightly increased the amount of explained variability in information seeking behaviors ($\Delta R^2 = 6.8\%$; $R^2 = 17.1\%$). Subjective norms and attitudes (Model 4) more than doubled the amount of explained variability in the RISP model ($\Delta R^2 = 19.9\%$; $R^2 = 37.0\%$). Current knowledge (Model 5) increased R^2 by 5.0%; whereas the addition of information insufficiency (Model 6) changed the amount of explained variability minimally ($\Delta R^2 = 0.1\%$). Each iteration of our global model was statistically significant.

In model 7, findings suggest only education, worry, subjective norm, information seeking capacity, and information insufficiency are statistically significant ($p < 0.05$) predictors of information seeking behaviors in the RISP model (**Table 3**). Information seeking capacity ($p < 0.001$) and information insufficiency ($p = 0.019$) were significant predictors of information seeking behaviors of northwest Minnesota deer hunters, after controlling for individual characteristics, perceived hazard characteristics, affective response, attitudes and informational subjective norms as the model suggests. As the variables most proximal to information seeking behavior in the RISP framework, the result is expected (**Figure 1**). However, while information insufficiency was significant ($p < 0.05$), the amount of additional variability it explains in the model was small (<1%). Changes in the amount of variability explained in the models are greatest with the addition of subjective norms and attitudes (19.9%) and affective response (6.8%) (**Table 3**).

In addition to the application of the RISP framework, we found that northwest Minnesota hunters reported their family, friends, and social network as their greatest source of information about bTB and bTB management, followed by statewide newspapers and news magazines. Respondents considered state agencies and public meetings as the least-utilized information source, except for the Minnesota Department of Natural Resources which had the third highest average response (**Table 4**).

TABLE 2 | Respondent characteristics.

	N	%
GENDER		
Male	675	93.0
Female	51	7.0
EDUCATION		
Grade school	7	1.0
Some high school	10	1.4
High school diploma or GED	151	20.9
Some vocational or technical school	65	9.0
Vocational or technical school (associate's)	126	17.5
Some college	118	16.4
Four-year college	164	22.7
Some graduate school	29	4.0

DISCUSSION

Our study aimed to better understand the information seeking behaviors of deer hunters regarding disease management. Specifically, we use the RISP model to investigate the relationships of individual variables on information seeking and processing behavior. To achieve this, we used hierarchical multiple regression analysis utilizing the RISP framework. Results revealed several discrepancies from the expectations of the RISP model and from studies using the RISP model in other contexts. These include research on topics ranging from environmental risks to the health communication sciences (19, 20, 30).

Unlike the findings of Kahlor's PRISM research (19), our application of the RISP model variable "information sufficiency" was statistically significant. However, its importance in predicting information seeking is diminished by its lack of predictive power. The addition of information sufficiency in the RISP model yielded almost no increase in variance in information seeking behavior explained (< 1%). Our finding differs from our original expectation—that variables most proximal to information seeking behaviors in the model would explain the greatest proportion of variation.

In our model of information seeking behaviors, we found that attitudes explained the greatest amount of variability in information seeking behaviors of northwest Minnesota hunters. We believe this relates to the time that elapsed between the survey implementation and the initial outbreak of bTB in MN. Bovine TB was originally detected in a wild deer in 2005, and this research was conducted in the summer of 2012. During that

TABLE 3 | RISP framework hierarchical regression models of self-reported information seeking behaviors in northwest Minnesota hunters, data from 2012.

Predictor	SE	Std. β	t	p	R^2	ΔR^2	F	p
Model 1					0.050		10.4	<0.001
Age	0.00	0.05	1.148	0.25				
Education	0.01	0.16	3.993	<0.001				
Hunting importance	0.03	0.16	4.012	<0.001				
Model 2					0.102		9.60	<0.001
						0.053	8.64	<0.001
Age	0.00	0.04	0.931	0.35				
Education	0.01	0.19	4.71	<0.001				
Hunting importance	0.03	0.13	3.18	0.00				
Personal Impact	0.03	0.15	3.57	<0.001				
Risk judgment	0.00	0.12	2.94	0.003				
Trust in DNR	0.03	0.09	2.20	0.029				
Self-efficacy	0.03	0.07	1.83	0.068				
Model 3					0.171		12.1	<0.001
						0.068	16.1	<0.001
Age	0.002	0.04	1.06	0.29				
Education	0.013	0.19	4.87	<0.001				
Hunting importance	0.031	0.10	2.40	0.02				
Personal impact	0.031	0.10	0.211	0.83				
Risk judgment	0.000	0.08	1.97	0.05				
Trust in DNR	0.027	0.10	2.58	0.01				
Self-efficacy	0.025	0.08	1.99	0.47				
Anger	0.009	0.06	1.16	0.25				
Worry	0.014	0.30	4.11	<0.001				
Fear	0.014	−0.04	−0.531	0.60				
Model 4					0.370		28.6	<0.001
						0.199	92.4	<0.001
Age	0.00	−0.02	−0.47	0.64				
Education	0.01	0.14	4.10	<0.001				
Hunting importance	0.03	0.07	2.02	0.04				
Personal impact	0.03	−0.06	−1.58	0.12				
Risk judgment	0.00	0.03	0.79	0.43				
Trust in DNR	0.02	0.03	0.69	0.49				
Self-efficacy	0.02	0.02	0.65	0.52				
Anger	0.01	0.01	0.17	0.87				
Worry	0.01	0.15	2.22	0.03				
Fear	0.01	−0.02	−0.25	0.81				
Subjective norm	0.03	0.26	6.71	<0.001				
Attitude	0.02	0.34	8.51	<0.001				
Model 5					0.420		32.5	<0.001
						0.050	50.7	<0.001
Age	0.00	0.01	0.322	0.75				
Education	0.01	0.09	2.71	0.01				
Hunting importance	0.03	0.06	1.79	0.07				
Personal impact	0.03	−0.04	-952	0.34				
Risk judgment	0.00	0.02	0.507	0.61				

(Continued)

TABLE 3 | Continued

Predictor	SE	Std. β	*t*	*p*	R^2	ΔR^2	F	*p*
Trust in DNR	0.02	0.02	0.557	0.58				
Self-efficacy	0.02	−0.01	−0.411	0.68				
Anger	0.01	−0.01	−0.323	0.75				
Worry	0.01	0.16	2.57	0.01				
Fear	0.01	0.01	0.092	0.93				
Subjective norm	0.03	0.20	5.32	<0.001				
Attitude	0.02	0.29	7.34	<0.001				
Capacity	0.04	0.25	7.12	<0.001				
Model 6					0.421		30.3	<0.001
						0.001	0.848	0.357
Age	0.00	0.01	0.24	0.81				
Education	0.01	0.09	2.70	0.01				
Hunting importance	0.03	0.06	1.76	0.08				
Personal impact	0.03	−0.04	−1.00	0.32				
Risk judgment	0.00	0.01	0.43	0.67				
Trust in DNR	0.02	0.02	0.67	0.50				
Self-efficacy	0.02	−0.01	−0.43	0.67				
Anger	0.01	−0.02	−0.43	0.67				
Worry	0.01	0.16	2.56	0.01				
Fear	0.01	0.01	0.16	0.87				
Attitude	0.03	0.20	5.10	0.00				
Subjective norm	0.02	0.29	7.32	0.00				
Capacity	0.04	0.25	6.83	0.00				
Current knowledge	0.00	0.03	0.921	0.35				
Model 7					0.427		28.9	<0.001
						0.006	6.02	0.014
Age	0.00	0.01	0.43	0.67				
Education	0.01	0.09	2.54	0.01				
Hunting importance	0.03	0.06	1.79	0.07				
Personal impact	0.03	−0.04	−0.97	0.33				
Risk judgment	0.00	0.01	0.25	0.80				
Trust in DNR	0.02	0.03	0.83	0.41				
Self-efficacy	0.02	−0.01	−0.20	0.84				
Anger	0.01	−0.02	−1.55	0.58				
Worry	0.01	0.16	2.50	0.01				
Fear	0.01	0.01	0.12	0.90				
Attitude	0.03	0.20	5.18	0.00				
Subjective norm	0.02	0.26	6.28	0.00				
Capacity	0.04	0.25	6.83	0.00				
Current knowledge	0.00	0.03	0.74	0.46				
Information insufficiency	0.00	0.09	2.45	0.01				

time, the Minnesota DNR implemented aggressive deer control efforts that resulted in a 60% decrease in the population, which likely increased negative attitudes toward bTB management and the agency in general.

Our findings pertaining to attitude and social norms exerting a strong influence on risk behaviors of individuals are similar to other applications of the model in the context of zoonotic disease risk perception [e.g., (30)].

TABLE 4 | Sources of information.

	N	Mean	SD
Radio news	718	2.43	0.955
Television news	712	2.33	0.943
Local newspapers	717	2.83	0.981
Statewide newspapers and news magazines	714	2.56	1.005
Internet sources	705	2.30	1.137
Minnesota DNR	716	2.74	1.005
Minnesota board of animal health	704	1.74	0.997
Family, friends, social network	719	2.86	0.888
Public meetings	707	1.65	0.951

Respondents were asked "From what sources did you get information about TB and bovine TB management?"
Responses were "1" (Not at all), "2" (Slightly), "3" (Moderately), "4" (Very Much).

Because the RISP model has been widely applied in other contexts and may be useful to natural resource managers in the future, it is important to understand its operation in an applied setting. This research suggests that using the complete RISP model to explain behaviors after the immediate onset of a threat, or once a threat has been eradicated, may be challenging. Information about the extent of disease was readily available by the time we surveyed hunters, and they were probably better informed about past risks (and the lack of present risk) from bTB than at the time of the initial disease detection. Model variables that are stable across time (e.g., demographics and attitudes) appear to be primary drivers (e.g., explain the greatest amount of variability). In particular, we believe that using the Theory of Planned Behavior (24) might provide a more parsimonious model in cases where the disease has been present for a substantial time, communication has been present, and attitudes, norms, and beliefs are likely the drivers of whether or not people will seek out and use information. In a case where the disease threat is relatively new and most people are unlikely to have had a lot of exposure to information about the threat, information insufficiency might be more of a driver soon after disease outbreak.

CONCLUSIONS, LIMITATIONS, AND IMPLICATIONS

Due to early detection of the disease and aggressive management actions, the prevalence of bTB in Minnesota never reached levels observed in Michigan, where bTB eradication from the wild population of white-tailed deer is unlikely (35). As such, Minnesota provides a case study for successful bTB management (if "success" is measured as no longer detecting positive animals). Although Minnesota received classification as a bTB-free state in 2011, the possibility of future occurrence of bTB or other wildlife disease outbreaks remains. Understanding how hunters perceive bTB and bTB management, as well as what motivates them to attend to information concerning the risks and management of bTB, is integral in creating socially acceptable policy to manage for future occurrences of bTB or similar zoonotic diseases affecting humans and wildlife (3, 35).

This project explores the use of the RISP model in the context of wildlife disease and management. The findings about the operation of the RISP theory in an applied context inform future research and management, indicating that in this instance attitudes and norms exert greater influence on hunters' information seeking behaviors than the RISP framework appears to suggest. Evidence suggests that successful natural resource management and policy implementation requires stakeholder support, especially from hunters and private landowners (12). Communicating zoonotic disease risks to the public, as in the case of bTB, proves challenging for managers (12). The findings from this study might appear to have little practical utility to wildlife management agencies that primarily focus on "scientific management" largely based in the biological sciences. The variables influencing risk perceptions and information seeking behaviors (attitudes and social norms) seem out of the control of managers. As noted by Riley et al. (36), however, effective wildlife management in the twenty-first century might require complex integration of biological and human dimensions information. Such integration is likely to move wildlife disease management decisions and actions away from only attempting to address the biological issues that appear to be under the control of "scientific management" toward also understanding and addressing the psychological and social phenomena associated with the stakeholders for whom agencies are managing the wildlife resource.

When this research is contextualized in this more complex management setting, its benefits to managers are more apparent. Clearly understanding the prevalent attitudes and subjective norms of stakeholder and communities impacted by bTB can assist in developing messages for communicating disease risks as well as management actions. In previous natural research management studies using the Theory of Reasoned Action or Theory of Planned Behavior, careful analysis of the beliefs influencing attitudes and norms have assisted with understanding stakeholders and developing messages and communication strategies. These studies have been conducted in diverse contexts including reintroduction of wolves (37), habitat conservation for endangered species (38), the lethal control of deer populations for conservation (13, 14) and support for limiting use of lead shot (39, 40). Our study demonstrates that the use of similar models holds promise for better understanding what influences stakeholder behaviors related to wildlife disease management. Decisions that clearly take into consideration the impacts to stakeholders may enhance the social acceptance of risk management actions and processing of communication, ultimately bettering relationships with stakeholders and improving policy outcomes.

We also noted several limitations of our study, mostly related to the time between initial detection (2005) and survey implementation (2012). Asking respondents to rate their affective responses when they initially heard about the outbreak limits our findings; there may have been inaccuracies in participants' recollections of their emotions upon hearing of bTB. We also expect that survey participants used hindsight to inform their responses related to perceptions of threats from bTB. We also asked people to recall in the past how they perceived threats of bTB after it had already been eradicated from the state. Had we surveyed hunters immediately following the onset of bTB, rather than after Minnesota was declared bTB free, respondents' likelihood of reporting perception of a threat from bTB may have been higher. Future research should attempt to minimize the duration between event and research. Additionally, while our response rate was not unusual for such surveys, the fact that most hunters (62%) we contacted did not respond to the survey may indicate a lack of concern, or apathy, about the topic.

AUTHOR CONTRIBUTIONS

DF and LC designed research. DF, LC, and AH performed research and collected data. MC, DF, LC analyzed data. All authors wrote and reviewed the paper.

REFERENCES

1. Clarke C. Seeking and processing information about zoonotic disease risk: a proposed framework. *Human Dim of Wildl.* (2009) 14:314–25. doi: 10.1080/10871200903096155
2. Heberlein TA, Stedman RC. Socially amplified risk: attitude and behavior change in response to CWD in Wisconsin deer. *Hum Dimen of Wildl.* (2009) 14:326–40. doi: 10.1080/10871200903115435
3. Holsman RH, Petchenik J, Cooney EE. CWD after "the fire": six reasons why hunters resisted Wisconsin's eradication effort. *Hum Dimen of Wildl.* (2010) 15:180–93. doi: 10.1080/10871201003718029
4. Vaske JJ, Shelby LB, Needham MD. Preparing for the next disease: the human-wildlife connection. In: Manfredo MJ, Vaske JJ, Brown PJ, Decker DJ, Duke EA, editors. *Wildlife and Society: The Science of Human Dimensions.* Washington, DC: Island Press (2009). p. 244–61.
5. Lyon KM, Vaske JJ. Predicting hunting participation in response to chronic wasting disease in four states. *Hum Dim Wildl.* (2010) 15:208–20. doi: 10.1080/10871201003770004
6. Griffin RJ, Dunwoody S, Neuwirth K. Proposed model of the relationship of risk information seeking and processing to the development of preventive behaviors. *Environ Res.* (1999) 80:S230–45.
7. Carstensen M, Pauly D, DonCarlos MW, Cornicelli L. Managing bovine tuberculosis in white-tailed deer in northwestern Minnesota: a 2007 progress report. In: *Michigan Bovine Tuberculosis Bibliography and Database* (2007). Available online at: http://digitalcommons.unl.edu/michbovinetb/19
8. Carstensen M, DonCarlos MW. Preventing the establishment of a wildlife disease reservoir: A case study of bovine tuberculosis in wild deer in Minnesota USA. *Vet Med Int.* (2011) 2011:413240. doi: 10.4061/2011/413240
9. Glaser L, Carstensen M, Shaw S, Robbe-Austerman S, Wunschmann A, Grear D, et al. Descriptive epidemiology and whole genome sequencing analysis for an outbreak of bovine tuberculosis in beef cattle and white-tailed deer in northwestern Minnesota. *PLoS ONE* (2016) 11:e0145735. doi: 10.1371/journal.pone.0145735
10. Muter BA, Gore ML, Riley SJ, Lapinski MK. Evaluating bovine tuberculosis risk communication materials in Michigan and Minnesota for severity, susceptibility, and efficacy messages. *Wildl Soc Bull* (2013) 37:115–21. doi: 10.1002/wsb.238
11. Ribeiro-Lima J, Carstensen M, Cornicelli L, Wells S, Forester J. Patterns of cattle farm visitation by white-tailed deer in relation to risk of disease transmission in a previously infected area with bovine tuberculosis in Minnesota US. *Trans Emerg Dis.* (2016) 64:1519–29. doi: 10.1111/tbed.12544
12. Carstensen M, O'Brien DJ, Schmitt SM. Public acceptance as a determinant of management strategies for bovine tuberculosis in free-Ranging US wildlife. *Vet Micro.* (2011) 151:200–4. doi: 10.1016/j.vetmic.2011.02.046
13. Fulton DC, Skerl K, Shank EM, Lime DW. Beliefs and attitudes toward lethal management of deer in Cuyahoga Valley National Park. *Wildl Soc Bull.* (2004) 32:1166–76. doi: 10.2193/0091-7648(2004)032[1166:BAATLM]2.0.CO;2
14. Dougherty EM, Fulton DC, Anderson DH. The influence of gender on the relationship between wildlife value orientations, beliefs, and the acceptability of lethal Deer control in Cuyahoga Valley National Park. *Soc Nat Res.* (2003) 16:603–23. doi: 10.1080/08941920309187
15. Stafford NT, Needham MD, Vaske JJ, Petchenik J. Hunter and nonhunter beliefs about chronic wasting disease in Wisconsin. *J Wildl Manage* (2007) 71:1739–44. doi: 10.2193/2006-557
16. Vaske JJ. Lessons learned from human dimensions of chronic wasting disease research. *Human Dim of Wildl.* (2010) 15:65–179. doi: 10.1080/10871201003775052
17. Griffin RJ, Neuwirth K, Dunwoody S, Giese J. Information sufficiency and risk communication. *Media Psych.* (2004) 6:23–61. doi: 10.1207/s1532785xmep0601_2
18. Kahlor L, Dunwoody S, Griffin RJ, Neuwirth K. Seeking and processing information about impersonal risk. *Sci Comm.* (2006) 28:163–94. doi: 10.1177/1075547006293916
19. Kahlor L. PRISM: A planned risk information seeking model. *Health Comm.* (2010) 25:345–56. doi: 10.1080/10410231003775172
20. Griffin RJ, Yang Z, ter Huurne E, Boerner F, Ortiz S, Dunwoody S. After the flood: anger, attribution, and the seeking of information. *Sci Comm.* (2008) 29:285–315. doi: 10.1177/1075547007312309
21. Kahlor LA. An augmented risk information seeking model: the case of global warming. *Media Psych.* (2007)10:414–35. doi: 10.1080/15213260701532971
22. ter Huurne EF, Griffin RJ, Gutteling JM. Risk information seeking among US and Dutch residents: an application of the model of risk information seeking and processing. *Sci Comm.* (2009) 31:215–37. doi: 10.1177/1075547009332653
23. Griffin RJ, Neuwirth K, Giese J, Dunwoody S. Linking the heuristic-systematic model and depth of processing. *Comm Res.* (2002) 29:705–32. doi: 10.1177/009365002237833
24. Ajzen I. *Attitudes, Personality, and Behavior.* Chicago, IL: Dorsey Press (1988).
25. Eagly AH, Chaiken S. *The Psychology of Attitudes.* Orlando, FL: Harcourt Brace Jovanovich College Publishers (1993).
26. Tversky A, Kahneman D. Judgment under uncertainty: heuristics and biases. *Science* (1974) 185:1124–31.
27. Chaiken S. Heuristic versus systematic information processing and the use of source versus message cues in persuasion. *J Pers Soc Psych.* (1980) 39:752–66. doi: 10.1037/0022-3514.39.5.752
28. Trumbo CW. Information processing and risk perception: an adaptation of the heuristic-systematic model. *J Comm.* (2002) 52:367–82. doi: 10.1111/j.1460-2466.2002.tb02550.x
29. Fishbein M, Ajzen I. *Predicting and Changing Behavior: The Reasoned Action Approach.* New York, NY: Psychology Press (2010).
30. Triezenberg HA, Gore ML, Riley SJ, Lapinski MK. Perceived risks from disease and management policies: an expansion and testing of a zoonotic disease risk perception model. *Hum Dim Wildl.* (2014) 19:123–38. doi: 10.1080/10871209.2014.844288
31. Cornicelli L, Fulton DC, Grund MD, Fieberg J. Hunter perceptions and acceptance of alternative deer management regulations. *Wild Soc Bull.* (2011) 35:323–9. doi: 10.1002/wsb.51
32. Dillman DA, Smyth JD, Christian LM. *Internet, Mail, and Mixed-Mode Surveys: The Tailored Design Method.* 3rd ed. New York, NY: Wiley (2009).

33. Fishbein M, Ajzen I. *Belief, Attitude, Intention, and Behavior: An Introduction to Theory and Research.* Reading, MA: Addison-Wesley Publishing (1975).
34. Cohen J, Cohen P, West SG, Aiken LS. *Applied Multiple Regression/Correlation Analysis for the Behavioral Sciences.* New York, NY: Routledge (2013).
35. Ramsey DS, O'Brien DJ, Cosgrove MK, Rudolph BA, Locher AB, Schmitt SM. Forecasting eradication of bovine tuberculosis in Michigan white-tailed deer. *J Wildl Manage* (2014) 78:240–54. doi: 10.1002/jwmg.656
36. Riley SJ, Decker DJ, Carpenter LH, Organ JF, Siemer WF, Mattfeld GF, et al. The essence of wildlife management. *Wildl Soc Bull.* (2002) 30:585–93. doi: 10.2307/3784519
37. Pate J, Manfredo MJ, Bright AD, Tischbein G. Coloradans' attitudes toward reintroducing the gray wolf into Colorado. *Wildl Soc Bull.* (1996) 24:421–8.
38. Sorice MG, Haider W, Conner JR, Ditton RB. Incentive structure of and private landowner participation in an endangered species conservation program. *Cons Bio.* (2011) 25:587–96. doi: 10.1111/j.1523-1739.2011.01673.x
39. Schroeder SA, Fulton DC, Penning W, DonCarlos K. Using persuasive messages to encourage hunters to support regulation of lead shot. *J Wildl Mgmt.* (2012) 76:1528–39. doi: 10.1002/jwmg.420
40. Schroeder SA, Fulton DC, DonCarlos K. Clarifying beliefs underlying hunter intentions to support a ban on lead shot. *Soc Nat Resour.* (2016) 29:852–67. doi: 10.1080/08941920.2015.1107792

4

Development of a Multidimensional Proteomic Approach to Detect Circulating Immune Complexes in Cattle Experimentally Infected with *Mycobacterium bovis*

Syeda A. Hadi[1], *Wade R. Waters*[2], *Mitchell Palmer*[2], *Konstantin P. Lyashchenko*[3] *and Srinand Sreevatsan*[1*]

[1] Department of Pathobiology and Diagnostic Investigation, College of Veterinary Medicine, Michigan State University, East Lansing, MI, United States, [2] National Animal Disease Center, Agricultural Research Service, United States Department of Agriculture, Ames, IA, United States, [3] Chembio Diagnostic Systems Inc., Medford, NY, United States

***Correspondence:**
Srinand Sreevatsan
sreevats@msu.edu

Objective: To evaluate a high-resolution method to identify pathogen-specific biomarkers in serum of calves infected with *Mycobacterium bovis*.

Methods: Serum samples from four calves infected with *M. bovis* were collected before and after infection at weeks 9, 14, 15, 31, and 36. Immune-complex-associated mycobacterial antigens in the serum were enriched using an immunochromatography method termed, dual path platform (DPP). All regions of antigen capture zones, that consisted of monospecific rabbit polyclonal antibodies raised against *M. tuberculosis* lysates, on DPP strips were excised and analyzed by multidimensional proteomics. The resulting proteins were then passed through 4 rigorous peptide quality filters-false-hits, decoys, non-*M. tuberculosis* complex proteins were all removed followed by individual quality check of those remaining. Peptides were then checked on NCBI's BLASTp for *M. tuberculosis* complex specificity.

Results: Proteins in 2 of the animals passed the multipronged-highly stringent peptide quality analysis. Animal#54 had 7 unique *M. tuberculosis* complex proteins at week 14 post-infection, while animal#56 had 4 at week 36 post-infection along with 1 immunoglobulin.

Conclusion: *M. tuberculosis* complex -specific peptides identified in this study were identified in 2 animals and at 2 separate time points post infection. Further studies with better enrichment protocols and using larger sample sizes and replications are required to develop a TB-specific diagnostic tool for bovine tuberculosis.

Keywords: bovine tuberculosis, dual path platform, immune-complexes, mass-spectrometry, *Mycobacterium bovis*, mycobacteria, biomarkers, diagnostics

INTRODUCTION

Mycobacterium bovis causes tuberculosis primarily in cattle but it is also zoonotic. Transmission to humans occurs through close contact with infected animals or via consumption of contaminated animal products (e.g., unpasteurized milk or dairy products) (1–3). The primary screening test used in the field is tuberculin-based skin test which is time-consuming, labor intensive and associated with low sensitivity and variable specificity. Variability in specificity is caused by species differences and technique being used (4, 5). Ultimately a false-positive can lead to a considerable financial burden on farmers deterring control measures. Thus, there is a need for highly specific rapid field tests that are cost effective.

Immune complexes are formed by the non-covalent binding of antigens with antibody molecules circulating real-time (6). Lyashchenko et al. (7), reported the presence of *Mycobacterium* specific immune complexes in cattle experimentally infected with *M. bovis* detectable by the dual-path platform (DPP) assay that utilizes polyclonal antibodies against *M. tuberculosis* whole-cell antigens. This provided an unprecedented opportunity to interrogate *M. tuberculosis* complex-specific antigens enriched by polyclonal tuberculosis-specific antibodies using high resolution technique of liquid chromatography followed by dual mass-spectrometry (LC-MS/MS). LC-MS/MS can detect proteins at abundances as low as 10^{-15} moles, thereby enabling discovery of circulating in infected animals. In the present study, high-resolution multidimensional mass spectrometry analysis of the DPP-captured immune complexes was evaluated for its ability to identify the captured *M. bovis*-specific peptides that may aid in the development of a highly accurate tuberculosis diagnostics for animals and humans.

MATERIALS AND METHODS

Seven Holstein calves obtained from a TB-free herd in IA and housed in a biosafety level 3 (BSL-3) facility at the National Animal Disease Center, Ames, IA were infected at 11 months of age with 8×10^3 CFU of virulent *M. bovis* (95-1315; USDA Animal Plant and Health Inspection Service [APHIS] designation) by aerosol. This strain of *M. bovis* was isolated from a white-tailed deer in Michigan, USA. Animals were sampled for serum at multiple time points pre- and post-infection over the next 11.5 months at which point they were euthanized (7, 8). Necropsy of all the calves revealed presence of gross lesions in multiple organs specific to bovine tuberculosis and bacterial culturing from infected tissues confirmed the presence of *M. bovis* in all 7 animals infected.

In this pilot study we focused on 4 out of the 7 calves present in the original study (7), since they had the highest levels of circulating immune complexes to increase the probability of biomarker discovery. Pre- and post-inoculation samples collected at weeks 9, 14, 15, 31, and 36 were used to identify mycobacterial specific peptides. To characterize the circulating immune complexes-associated with *M. tuberculosis* complex, a rapid DPP-Ag assay was performed (**Figure 1**). The DPP antigen capture zone (test line) was coated with rabbit polyclonal antibodies raised against *M. tuberculosis* whole-cell lysate to enable capture of mycobacterial antigen-antibody complexes (7, 8). Pre-infection (baseline) sera from these four animals served as negative controls. Triplicates of each time points from every animal were made pre and post-infection (which summed up to 27 DPP-Ag assay strips for analysis) for each week 0, 9, 14, 31 and 36. A 50 μL aliquot of serum sample was placed on three independent DPP-Ag strips for each time-point, to allow for antigen enrichment of molecules on the capture zone, which were then processed as one single sample to allow for maximum enrichment, enhanced sensitivity, efficient use of the LC-MS/MS and improved proteomics profile generation.

The immune-complex capture zone of 2 mm width was excised and analyzed by LC-MS/MS analysis performed at University of Minnesota's Center for Mass Spectrometry and Proteomics (CMSP). Triplicates of DPP-assays for every animal were pooled for analysis. A region 2 mm upstream of the antigen capture zone (or the DPP test line) was also analyzed by LC-MS/MS. The enormous volume of peptide data generated by LC-MS/MS was passed through a series of stringent filters before the final candidates were considered.

First, PEAKS (Bioinformatics Solutions Inc.) software was used to query peptides generated in each triplicate-pooled-sample through LC/MS-MS against a database that included all documented peptides from *M. tuberculosis* Complex, cattle and rabbit proteins. These results were then analyzed by Scaffold (version Scaffold_4.7.5, Proteome Software Inc., Portland, OR) to validate all MS/MS based peptide identifications and to allow combined visualization of all sample results. All identified peptides were compared against a decoy database (generated in Scaffold_4.7.5), consisting of randomized peptide sequences, to remove any spurious hits. Second, any protein that matched against the decoy database, was removed from further analysis. We focused only on the *M. tuberculosis* complex proteins because they offer highest possible specificity for bovine tuberculosis diagnostics. The third filter was based on an individual quality check of the proteins with in Scaffold. Peptide identifications were accepted in Scaffold if they could be established at greater than 95.0% probability by the Peptide Prophet algorithm (9) with Scaffold delta-mass correction. Protein identifications were accepted if they could be established at greater than 95.0% probability and contained at least 2 identified peptides. Proteins that contained similar peptides and could not be differentiated based on MS/MS analysis alone were grouped to satisfy the principles of parsimony. Peptides and proteins that were selected in the third filter had percent probabilities varying from 74 to 100%. The fourth and the last filter was the identification of *M. tuberculosis* complex specificity using the National Center for Biotechnology Information (NCBI)'s non-redundant database BLASTp (basic local alignment search tool for proteins) analysis where two aspects were investigated: (1) E-value ($<1e^{-10}$) and (2) the species match of the peptides. If the proteins matched with any other bacteria other than *M. tuberculosis* complex, they were excluded from further consideration. Additionally, if any peptides had an E-value higher than $1e^{-10}$, which suggested that the species match was likely non-random, they were also removed from further consideration. This last filter was excessively stringent as it eliminated most of peptide hits discovered after decoy database search. Some of the peptides eliminated may still be useful in a future validation study.

The same pipeline was followed for identifying cattle specific immunoglobulins, where immunoglobulins were passed through all the filters described for *M. tuberculosis* complex proteins. Additionally, the proteins that overlapped between pre-infection and post-infection test-lines were excluded as it suggested that they were not associated with the *M. bovis* infection, rather existed in the background.

RESULTS AND DISCUSSION

The peptides generated from LC-MS/MS analysis resulted in identification of 26,945 proteins. Forty-nine percent of these were eliminated after the decoy database search. Of these, 3.73% were identified with the *M. tuberculosis* complex repertoire, 26.02% proteins were of host (bovine) origin and 21.35% were of leporine origin. DPP strips of all post-infection samples, except at week 31, had *M. bovis* proteins. After analysis, 11 *M. tuberculosis* complex-specific proteins were identified in two *M. bovis*-infected animals (**Table 1**). At week 14 (post-infection) serum from animal #54 showed 7 proteins that corresponded to peptides in *M. tuberculosis* complex with a BLAST *E*-value lower than $1e^{-10}$ (**Table 2**). At week 36 post-infection, serum of animal #56 had 4 proteins that corresponded to *M. tuberculosis* complex with an E-value lower than $1e^{-10}$(**Table 2**).

At week 14 post-infection in animal #54 polyketide synthase was detected, which plays a role in the growth of the bacteria and is considered a potential virulence factor (10). The detection of this protein at such an early stage in *M. bovis* infection agrees with other studies (11, 12) where polyketide synthase was detected through different techniques but at similar time points. Lamont et al. (11), showed that polyketide synthase can be used as a useful marker for detecting *M. bovis* infection in a multi-cut off fashion, based on the prevalence of the disease.

Killer cell immunoglobulin-like receptor ($1e^{-18}$) in animal #56 at week 36 corresponded to cattle (*Bos taurus*) specific immunoglobulin, alone passed all analysis filters. Even though pre-infection DPP-assays from all 4 animals were pooled together to enhance the probability of capturing all mycobacterial circulating immune complexes at base-line to compare them with proteins detected post-infection, no immune-complexes were detected at base-line.

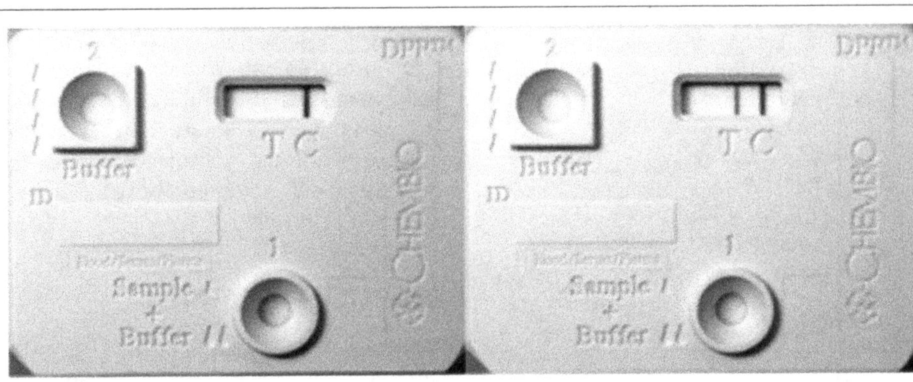

FIGURE 1 | Dual-path platform assay kit showing positive and negative controls. Dual-path platform assay was used to detect circulating antigen-antibody complexes in calves infected with *Mycobacterium bovis*. The rabbit polyclonal antibodies immobilized on the test line(T) acted as the capture reagent for the circulating immune-complexes in the infected animal's serum as well as signal detector when coated onto nano-gold-particles. DPP strip case: **Left**: Negative Control (serum from uninfected animals), **Right**: Positive control.

TABLE 1 | Enumeration of pathogen-derived proteins detected by mass spectrometry from DPP-Ag assay strips processed with serum samples from cattle experimentally infected with *Mycobacterium bovis*.

Animal ID	Pre-infection			*Mycobacterium bovis* infection			
	DPPAg result[a])	*Mycobacterium bovis* proteins identified[b]	Cattle specific immunoglobulins	Week post-inoculation	DPP-Ag result[a]	*Mycobacterium bovis* proteins identified	Cattle specific immunoglobulins
51	0	0	0	9	124	0	0
54	0	0	0	14	788	7	0
				15	772	0	0
56	0	0	0	36	485	4	1
57	0	0	0	31	447	0	0

[a]*DPP reader data (reflectance) in relative light units obtained as described (7).*
[b]*Pooled DPP-Ag strips processed with pre-infection sera from four calves.*

TABLE 2 | List of Mycobacterium tuberculosis complex-specific high confidence proteins at week 14 and week 36 and cattle immunoglobulin at week 36 that passed exclusion criteria.

***Mycobacterium tuberculosis* complex proteins at wk14**	**Peptide sequences used for BLASTp analysis**
Acyltransferase	QDGSASYDAAVR-MLKAGELVGVYPEATISR
Esterase	VFGAADPR-FACVVRAFASMFPGR
LLM class F420-dependent oxidoreductase	QKDYDEYGYR-FGTAGSRLDDLAAPLPR
Transposase, partial	MDPTEDQARALAR-VTGIGTVKPSLRVLR
Transcriptional regulatory protein embr2	FGILGPLEISAGFRSLPLGTPK-SPLGRLPLR
Hypothetical protein Mb3478	GASPATAAR-LPPALNPDDADALPTTDRLTTR
Polyketide synthase	DGDRVLAIVR-LVDAPLPSWTHRTLMLSR-MFNSLGIQYGPAFSGLVAVHTAR-LFVVTRSAASVLPSDLANLEQAGMR
***Mycobacterium tuberculosis* complex proteins at wk36**	**Peptide sequences used for BLASTp analysis**
Helicase helz	VYAHHGGARLHGEALRDHLER-RGNVLAAMAKLK-IDEMIEEKKALADLVVTDGEGWLTELST
Hypothetical protein Mb1791	FGVTINDVVVALCAGALRR-VPSQISDPAQR
Hypothetical protein Mb2390c	HGHGRDVAAHR-TGGHRQASSRIK-HQKPGDVPRDPRC
Chromosome partition protein Smc	LDTMAANLARLTDLTTELR-LAVRTAEER
Cattle Immunoglobulin at week 36	**Peptide sequences used for BLASTp analysis**
PREDICTED: killer cell immunoglobulin-like receptor, three domains, long cytoplasmic tail, 2 isoform X2	GEMLTSGHAPADFVIGPMTLASAGTYR

The proteins that did not comply with exclusion criteria were removed such as non-Mycobacterium tuberculosis complex proteins, decoy proteins, low quality proteins and proteins that did not identify with Mycobacterium tuberculosis complex when NCBI's non-redundant database BLASTp (basic local alignment search tool for proteins) analysis was used. The same pipeline was used to identify cattle immunoglobulins. The hyphen represents the space given in NCBI's BLASTp search that allowed to account for the presence of other amino acids in between the peptides that formed the proteins.

The panel of mycobacterial proteins and cattle specific immunoglobulin reported in the present study may be specific to the infection stage at which they were detected, as the proteins seen at week 14 did not overlap with those detected at week 36 post infection. Alternatively, since these distinct proteins sets were found in two different animals, they could be a result of animal-to-animal variation in host response to the infection.

A major limitation of our study was sample size. Since the LC/MS-MS analysis itself was expensive and limited amounts of infected animal sera were available, multiple replications on the same animals were not possible. Additionally, multiple logistical and financial issues precluded us working with larger sample sizes: (1) working with agricultural animals for experimental infection with a BSL-3 pathogen and (2) Expenses associated with a BSL-3 cost, animal costs as well as personnel. Thus, to compensate for this limitation triplication of every animal's sample was performed.

Furthermore, the use of an antiserum derived against *M. tuberculosis* may have compromised specificity of our approach to detect *M. bovis* specific antigens, although these organisms are genetically very closely related. Future analysis though should include multiple replications of experimental infections followed by DPP assay and LC-MS/MS to discover *M. bovis* specific peptides in a reproducible and accurate fashion. Furthermore, a field validation on multiple exposure levels in outbreaks would be necessary for this technology to be applicable in routine bovine TB diagnostics.

In conclusion, the panel of 11 proteins reported in this study are specific to *M. bovis*. Further studies with more robust enrichment methods and larger sample sizes would be required to confirm these findings. Further validation of the identified circulating immune-complexes in naturally infected cattle would enable us to effectively and broadly apply the DPP technology in field.

ETHICS STATEMENT

All studies were approved by the National Animal Disease Center Animal Care and Use and Institutional Biosafety committees and performed under appropriate project licenses within the conditions of the Animal Welfare Act.

AUTHOR CONTRIBUTION

WW and MP conducted the animal infection and testing studies. KL developed the DPP lateral flow devices. SS and SH developed protocols for extraction of total proteins from DPP devices, performed proteomics and data analysis. WW, SH, KL, and SS wrote the paper.

ACKNOWLEDGMENTS

We would like to thank University of Minnesota's Center of Mass Spectrometry and Proteomics, especially Mr. Todd W. Markowski for his input and guidance.

REFERENCES

1. Hlavsa MC, Moonan PK, Cowan LS, Navin TR, Kammerer JS, Morlock GP, et al. Human Tuberculosis due to *Mycobacterium bovis* in the United States, 1995-2005. *Clin Infect Dis.* (2008) 47:168–75. doi: 10.1086/589240
2. OIE (2015). *Manual of Diagnostic Tests and Vaccines- Chapter 2.4.6- Bovine Tuberculosis.* Paris: OIE. Available online at: www.oie.int/standard-setting/terrestrial-manual/access-online
3. Wilkins MJ, Meyerson J, Bartlett PC, Spieldenner SL, Berry DE, Mosher LB, et al. Human *Mycobacterium bovis* infection and bovine tuberculosis outbreak, michigan, 1994-2007. *Emerging Infect Dis.* (2008) 14:657–66. doi: 10.3201/eid1404.070408
4. Cousins DV, Florisson N. A review of tests available for use in the diagnosis of tuberculosis in non-bovine species. *Rev Sci Tech Off Int Epiz* (2005) 24:1039–59. doi: 10.20506/rst.24.3.1635
5. De la Rua-Domenech R, Goodchild AT, Vordermeier HM, Hewinson RG, Christiansen KH, and Clifton-Hadley RS. Ante mortem diagnosis of tuberculosis in cattle: a review of the tuberculin tests, gamma-interferon assay and other ancillary diagnostic techniques. *Res Vet Sci.* (2006) 81:190–10. doi: 10.1016/j.rvsc.2005.11.005
6. De Rycke L, Peene I, Hoffman IEA, Kruithof E, Union A, Meheus L, et al. Rheumatoid factor and anti-citrullinated protein antibodies in rheumatoid arthritis: diagnostic value, associations with radiological progression rate, and extra articular manifestations. *Ann Rheum Dis.* (2004) 63:1587–93. doi: 10.1136/ard.2003.017574
7. Lyashchenko KP, Greenwald R, Sikar-Gang A, Sridhara AA, Johnathan A, Lambotte P, Waters WR. Early detection of circulating antigen and igm-associated immune complexes during experimental *Mycobacterium bovis* infection in cattle. *Clin Vaccine Immunol.* (2017) 24:e00069-17. doi: 10.1128/CVI.00069-17
8. Waters WR, Vordermeier HM, Rhodes S, Khatri B, Palmer MV, Maggioli MF, et al. Potential for rapid antibody detection to identify tuberculous cattle with non-reactive tuberculin skin test results. *BMC Vet Res.* (2017) 13:164. doi: 10.1186/s12917-017-1085-5
9. Keller A, Nesvizhskii AI, Kolker E, and Aebersold R. Empirical statistical model to estimate the accuracy of peptide identifications made by MS/MS and database search. *Anal Chem.* (2002) 74:5383–92. doi: 10.1021/ac025747h
10. Forrellad MA, Klepp LI, Gioffré A, García JSY, Morbidoni HR, Santangelo MP, Bigi F. Virulence factors of the Mycobacterium tuberculosis complex. *Virulence* (2013) 4:3–66. doi: 10.4161/viru.22329
11. Lamont EA, Janagama HK, Ribeiro-Lima J, Vulchanova L, Seth M, and Yang M. Circulating *Mycobacterium bovis* peptides and host response proteins as biomarkers for unambiguous detection of subclinical infection. *J Clin Microbiol.* (2014) 52:536–43. doi: 10.1128/JCM.02433-13
12. Wanzala SI, Palmer MV, Waters WR, Thacker TC, Carstensen M, Travis DA, et al. Evaluation of pathogen specific biomarkers for the diagnosis of tuberculosis in white-tailed deer (*Odocoileus virginianus*). *Am J Vet Res.* (2017) 78:729–34. doi: 10.2460/ajvr.78.6.729

5

Bovine Tuberculosis in Britain and Ireland – A Perfect Storm? The Confluence of Potential Ecological and Epidemiological Impediments to Controlling a Chronic Infectious Disease

A. R. Allen†, R. A. Skuce and A. W. Byrne†*

Veterinary Science Division, Agri-Food and Biosciences Institute, Belfast, United Kingdom

Correspondence:
A. R. Allen
adrian.allen@afbini.gov.uk
†These authors have contributed equally to this work

Successful eradication schemes for bovine tuberculosis (bTB) have been implemented in a number of European and other countries over the last 50 years. However, the islands of Britain and Ireland remain a significant aberration to this trend, with the recent exception of Scotland. Why have eradication schemes failed within these countries, while apparently similar programs have been successful elsewhere? While significant socio-economic and political factors have been discussed elsewhere as key determinants of disease eradication, here we review some of the potential ecological and epidemiological constraints that are present in these islands relative to other parts of Europe. We argue that the convergence of these potential factors may interact additively to diminish the potential of the present control programs to achieve eradication. Issues identified include heterogeneity of diagnostic testing approaches, the presence of an abundant wildlife reservoir of infection and the challenge of sustainably managing this risk effectively; the nature, size, density and network structure of cattle farming; potential effects of *Mycobacterium bovis* strain heterogeneity on disease transmission dynamics; possible impacts of concurrent endemic infections on the disclosure of truly infected animals; climatological differences and change coupled with environmental contamination. We further argue that control and eradication of this complex disease may benefit from an ecosystem level approach to management. We hope that this perspective can stimulate a new conversation about the many factors potentially impacting bTB eradication schemes in Britain and Ireland and possibly stimulate new research in the areas identified.

Keywords: *Mycobacterium bovis*, Britain and Ireland, eradication, persistence, epidemiology

INTRODUCTION

Bovine tuberculosis (bTB) caused by *Mycobacterium bovis* is a zoonotic disease, primarily affecting livestock, which is of economic importance to the European Union (EU) due to its impact on trade. Indeed, at the inception of the European project, as the European Economic Community (EEC), the first legal initiatives were taken to combat the disease in 1964 with the drafting of council directive 64/432/EEC (1). The latter document foresaw that there was a requirement for animal health legislation to underpin intra-community trade in livestock and introduced the concept / definition of being "officially tuberculosis free" (OTF), defined as the percentage of herds confirmed as bTB infected not exceeding 0.1% per year for six consecutive years (2). The legislation also defined the goal of the EEC to be disease eradication as opposed to control. Further legislation followed which enshrined the need for member states of the EEC to fund and facilitate test and slaughter schemes for the purposes of bTB eradication (3). In many member states, eradication programmes proceeded effectively, resulting in the granting of OTF status to Denmark in 1980, the Netherlands in 1995, Germany and Luxembourg in 1997, Austria in 1999, France in 2001 and Belgium in 2002 (2). Other states were granted OTF status upon joining the EU – Finland and Sweden 1995 and Czech Republic 2004 (2). In 2009, Poland and Slovenia also attained OTF status, whilst non-member state Norway was recognised as meeting all EU standards around OTF status (4).

Against this backdrop of successful eradication is the contrasting situation observed in the islands at the western fringe of the European continent – Britain and Ireland. Despite dramatic initial success in controlling bTB, England, Wales and Northern Ireland have suffered increasing incidence since the late 1980s. The Republic of Ireland experienced a relatively less dramatic initial reduction in incidence and continues to exhibit an ongoing problem in eradicating bTB, however, recent figures suggest that the situation has stabilised. Scotland is the notable exception, having been granted OTF status in 2009 (4). Data from 2009 indicated that 5–6% of herds from both islands tested positive for the presence of *M. bovis* (4). A contributing factor to the rise in herd incidence in England and Wales can be attributed to the suspension of bTB testing during the 2001 outbreak of foot and mouth disease (5, 6). However it has been recognised that even before the foot and mouth epidemic, bTB herd incidence was on the rise and foot and mouth disease merely exacerbated an already existing problem consistent with an upward trend in incidence since 1986 (6). Indeed, data from the Department of the Environment Food and Rural Affairs (DEFRA) in Britain indicates that '*since 2003 the total number of new bTB breakdowns identified (every quarter) in GB has been doubling at a rate of every 10 years. Prior to the Foot and Mouth Disease epidemic of 2001, the doubling rate was every 5.2 years*' (7). More recently, England, Wales and Northern Ireland have exhibited a rise in herd incidence whilst the Republic of Ireland has experienced a fall (6). Whilst mainland Europe still has a substantial bTB problem in the Iberian peninsula (Spain herd incidence 1.4% in 2009), this pales in comparison to the problems observed in the UK and Republic of Ireland (4).

This begs the question – why, in comparison to continental neighbours, have the territories of the United Kingdom and Republic of Ireland struggled to eradicate bTB? In Europe, diagnostic testing using some variant of the tuberculin skin test methodologies is highly standardised (8–10) following international protocols laid down by EU Council Directive 64/432. Debate around the efficacy of the skin tests are an ongoing matter of concern, with traditional epidemiological approaches estimating wide ranges of sensitivity of 52–100% - median 80% (8). More recently, Bayesian non-gold standard methods applied to data from Ireland have suggested skin test sensitivity is in the region of 50–60% (11), which has been further supported by a Bayesian meta-analysis from studies in the literature from 1934 to 2009 (12). Such relatively poor diagnostic performance may explain a failure to eradicate disease since many truly infected animals will be mis-classified as disease free. However, similar testing schemes using standardised reagents, presumably with similar test performance characteristics, have been used across Western Europe and indeed other parts of the world such as Australasia (13, 14), resulting in disease freedom. Furthermore, the performance improves at the herd-level as a screening test to identify infection, depending on the herd-size (numbers tested) and true within-herd prevalence (15). Also, once infection is identified, supplemental testing with more sensitive tests can be used to clear the within-herd infection (16). One could come to the perhaps overly simplistic conclusion therefore, that even with a poor individual test sensitivity, eventual eradication can be attained. However if this is true, what is confounding progress in Britain and Ireland? Undoubtedly, despite widespread standardisation in the basic diagnostic approach of using injectable tuberculins, there are individual differences in the application of eradication programmes subject to the variations of differing national policies, politics, behaviours and country specific factors (6). Indeed some of these socio-political factors may be some of the most important factors to account for the difficulties encountered in Britain and Ireland (17). Even with such heterogeneity of approach across time and national boundaries, it remains startling that particularly in Britain, which came close to achieving eradication in the 1960 and 1970s (8, 18), bovine TB is resurgent (as discussed above). Therefore, alongside issues of differing diagnostic test application protocols, we propose it is also timely to consider other potential additional factors whose current impact is unknown, but which may be additively preventing progress towards eradication.

Specifically, we hypothesise that there may exist a convergence of detrimental risk factors unique to GB and Ireland that is undermining the bTB eradication effort in these territories. If certain factors do contribute to this hypothesised "perfect storm" underpinning a failure to eradicate bTB, what are they likely to be? Below we discuss some of the likely ecological and epidemiological candidates given current knowledge. These proposed factors are not meant to be a definitive or exhaustive list; indeed we fully recognise that there may be many "unknown unknowns". Rather our intention is to attempt to address the current impasse in bTB control in these islands by adopting a novel perspective which seeks to address the likely multi-factorial problems which afflict our national eradication programmes. We hope that in so doing, we can start a debate on how this *perfect storm* can be investigated and addressed through innovative approaches and methodologies.

THE FACTORS

Heterogeneity in bTB Diagnostic Approaches and Control Programmes

In the late nineteenth century, tuberculins, derived from the culture filtrate of TB causing bacilli (10), were initially produced as potential therapeutic agents by the discoverer of the tubercle bacllius, Robert Koch (10). Their lack of efficacy for this particular task, was superseded by the discovery they could be used in the diagnosis of tuberculosis

(8, 10). In the twentieth century it was discovered that intradermal injection and measurement before and after of skin thickness could be used to detect the delayed type hypersensitivity (DTH) reaction, indicative of bTB infection (8, 10). Since then, "repetitive use of tuberculin tests remains the basis of all bTB control programs to this day" in areas with endemic disease (10), following strict standards laid down by EU council directive 64/432.

Despite such standardisation, there remain differences in application of skin tests and in the programs they support across the EU. We address an overview of these below:

Different Tuberculins and Divergent Potencies

Tuberculin potency for use in all skin tests used in Europe is tightly regulated by EU Council Directive 64/432. It is however recognised that changes in manufacturing and production procedures can result in batch to batch variation in potency (10). Indeed, even with strict regulation, tuberculins of lower potency have been released before (10). Such batch to batch variation and low potency would affect sensitivity of the skin test by reducing the DTH response / skin swelling that underpins diagnosis. Could such heterogeneity underpin the divergent outcomes in Britain and Ireland's TB control programmes compared to mainland Europe? An understanding of the history of tuberculin production may help to partially address this issue. Prior to 1975, the UK produced tuberculin derived from three *M. tuberculosis* strains, which was used in both Britain and Ireland [(8), M. Good personal communication]. Use of this tuberculin, derived from the human pathogen, coincided with the lowest prevalence of bTB in GB suggesting that the testing scheme was very effective. In 1975, both the United Kingdom and Republic of Ireland switched from using an *M. tuberculosis* derived PPD to one derived from the GB AN5 strain of *M. bovis* (8) as this exhibited superior sensitivity and specificity to the *M. tuberculosis* PPD (8, 19, 20). During the period after the 1970s, England and Wales experienced the well documented rise in bTB prevalence despite using this apparently superior Weybridge tuberculin (6). In 1980 the Republic of Ireland switched to using tuberculin produced from the AN5 strain in Lelystad (M. Good personal communication) with the UK following suit in 2008 (21). Downs et al. (21) went on to compare Weybridge and Lelystad tuberculins for bTB breakdown data in GB between 2005 and 2009, finding that the Weybridge formulation exhibited a slightly higher sensitivity and lower specificity. Given this data, in the context of increasing prevalence of bTB in the UK, the Weybridge tuberculin could have resulted in the reduction of false negative animal / herd detection whilst increasing the false positive rate – a combination in conflict with the hypothesis that tuberculin differences underpin the prevalence rise in GB. Whilst it is impossible to know the quality of all Weybridge tuberculin batches produced between 1977 and 2009, it is pertinent to note that batch to batch variation is not just a feature of GB production from the 1970s onwards (21, 22).

Differing Test Formats Across Europe

The most obvious difference is related to the exact test used. In Continental Europe, the single intradermal test (SIT) / cervical intradermal test (CIT) is used, involving the inoculation of *M. bovis* derived purified protein derivative (PPD) to detect skin thickness increases indicative of infection (8, 9). Conversely, in Britain and Ireland, owing to problems with environmental members of the *Mycobacterium avium* complex of bacilli cross reacting with *M. bovis* PPD and reducing specificity (increasing false positives), a comparative test is used (8). The single intradermal comparative cervical test (SICCT) injects both *M. bovis* and *M. avium* derived PPD into separate locations of an animal's neck, and uses the resulting difference in skin thickness between both sites as a diagnostic metric (8). The SIT has been noted to have an increased sensitivity (fewer false negatives) compared to the SICCT (23): SIT sensitivity range 80.2–91.2%; SICCT sensitivity range 52–93.5% (8). It is possible that this difference in sensitivity in the test used in Britain and Ireland may contribute to the comparative difficulty in clearing infection these islands experience, compared to continental neighbours. However, if this were the sole cause of the latter stark difference, it fails to explain why the Republic of Ireland and the United Kingdom exhibit such divergent contemporary and historic herd prevalences (6) despite having used similar tuberculin preparations (see above).

Differing Approaches to bTB Programs Across Europe

In continental European countries, which do not have the same problem as Britain and Ireland, bTB testing programs can have radically different outcomes. For example herd de-population upon the detection of reactor animals was common in France (9) – effectively using skin test as a herd screening test (8). In the continental context however, there is now a move away from whole herd de-population measures because of the costs involved and also animal welfare concerns (9). Economic consequences of whole herd depopulation in Britain and Ireland are of even greater significance owing to the much higher infection prevalence in these regions, and consequently are generally rarely deployed (with notable exceptions: (24, 25). A movement towards more pre-movement testing, to prevent spread of infection to new areas, has been proposed as an alternative to depopulation (9), Pre-movement testing in the Republic of Ireland was a required part of the TB eradication scheme up until 1996 (20). Since then, an evaluation of reviving the practice in 2005 revealed no significant cost benefit, with the suggestion being that very few outbreaks were being caused by onward movement of animals (20). In Britain, pre and post movement testing was introduced in 2006 (APHA, 2017) at direct cost to individual farmers. In Northern Ireland, pre-movement testing has been considered (26), but is currently not an active part of the eradication scheme.

Deployment of gamma interferon, as a higher sensitivity ancillary test, in Britain and Ireland is variable – in Northern Ireland, participation in testing has been voluntary, with no statutory powers in place to remove test positive animals (16). In the Republic of Ireland and in Britain gamma interferon is now conventionally used in problematic herds to increase sensitivity in an attempt to clear infection, but their application and the basis for animal removal has varied widely (6).

Other European countries such as Switzerland also use the practice of taking inconclusive reactors from skin test positive herds (9); however it should be noted, Switzerland who undertook biennial testing (1960–1980), now resort to passive abattoir surveillance from 1980 onwards (9). Such inconclusive reactor animals have been shown to be at elevated risk of developing infection in the future (27) and could potentially lead to the retention on farm of high risk animals. The economic cost in removing all inconclusive reactor animals is an order of magnitude greater in countries like Britain and Ireland which have a higher disease prevalence.

Compartmentalisation of regions within European countries, based on relative prevalence has been used to contain infection and prioritise resources (2). However, the restrictions used to control spread of infection across these has not been implemented uniformly. Over a number of years, Italy compartmentalized some regions with higher prevalence (28), applying greater movement restrictions between regions on the basis of risk. In Britain, compartmentalization has only been implemented in recent years, and has does not completely prevent movement – relying on pre and post movement tests (29, 30). It is notable, this regionalization approach is not effective in places which have widespread infection without a single locus, such as the island of Ireland (31).

It is conceivable that the program differences discussed above have compounded the ongoing problem Britain and Ireland have with bTB, however it is currently difficult to quantify the magnitude of these impacts.

Summary

In summary, these differences in tuberculin potency, application of skin test formats and heterogeneity in downstream choices in program management could have had a divergent effect on the bTB outcomes observed in Britain and Ireland vs Continental Europe. However, it is extremely difficult to untangle their relative importance (as is the case for all of the hypothesised factors), especially against the background of such differing epidemiological (and ecological) contexts. Future research efforts, including "big data", could assess differing interventions in settings with similar prevalence. Such approaches are predicated on better data harmonisation and sharing.

WILDLIFE

Wildlife Hosts Are a Significant Impediment to Eradication

The presence of wildlife hosts of bTB has been found to be a major impediment to eradication in a number of countries worldwide [e.g., Michigan, USA, New Zealand, UK and Ireland; (32)]. Spill-back infection from wildlife to cattle can seed infection into cattle herds (33). In Michigan the wildlife host is the white tailed deer [*Odocoileus virginianus*; (34)], while in New Zealand there is a multi-host problem with the most significant reservoir being the non-native brushtail possum [*Trichosurus vulpecula*; (14)]. In continental Europe, recent research has suggested that wild boar may act as a reservoir of infection, causing increased risk to cattle herds in parts of France and Spain (35–37). Deer may be a widespread, but relatively localised, problem in a number of countries across Europe (38). It has been suggested that European badgers may also play a role in the epidemiology of bTB in cattle in Spain and France (39, 40), however, it is only in Britain and Ireland where there is strong evidence of their impact on the control of bTB in cattle (41–44).

Evidence That Badgers Are Implicated in the Epidemiology of bTB in Cattle - Culling

Badgers are a host species for *M. bovis*, and have been implicated in the epidemiology of cattle bTB in UK and Ireland (41, 42, 44)]. Culling trials have demonstrated significant reduction in risk to cattle herds in areas where badger densities were significantly reduced (41–44). The magnitude of this effect has been shown to be larger in the ROI than in (Randomised badger cull) trials in GB [compare (43, 45) with (41, 42)]. In GB, badger culling was associated with a temporarily increased risk also to herds found at the periphery of cull sites (41). This was hypothesised (the "perturbation effect" hypothesis) to be as a result of increasing frequency-dependent transmission amongst badger populations, causing increased spill back infection to cattle herds (41). This suggests that badgers can play a significant role in spilling back infection to cattle over short duration. However, this peripheral increased risk was transient [<2 years post-cull (46)]; and was not demonstrated during badger cull trials or government-led culling operations in ROI (43, 44, 47, 48). The apparent beneficial effects of proactive culling to farms in cull areas have been maintained for up to 5–11 years after GB cull trials (49–52), and up to 10 years post-cull trial in ROI (53).

Cattle and Badgers Share bTB Pathogen Strains Which Cluster in Time and Space - Strain Typing and Whole Genome Sequencing

Strain typing of *M. bovis* has demonstrated that both badgers and cattle share similar strains with geographic clustering across hosts indicative of interspecific transmission at local scales (48, 54–56). The best evidence for this ongoing transmission has been demonstrated at the genomic level (57, 58). Biek et al. (57) demonstrated that at the farm level, badgers and cattle shared the same or highly similar pathogen sequence type consistent with frequent and recent transmission events – however, the direction of transmission could not be established during that study. It is likely that transmission occurs in both directions (53, 59, 60); however, the force of infection may be greater from badgers-to-cattle than cattle-to-badgers owing to the continual removal of infected cattle through test-and-slaughter (61–63). It is conceivable there may be regional variation in the latter as a result of animal and wildlife densities. Furthermore, culling experiments (see above) have demonstrated that the cycling of infection can be interrupted with beneficial effects for reducing bTB prevalence in the target host population.

Britain and Ireland Have Higher Average Badger Densities Than Elsewhere in Europe

The islands of Britain and Ireland have the highest average recorded density of badgers compared to any other country in Europe (64). Median badger densities across badger study sites suggest a median density of 4.3–5.4 badger km^{-2} for the

British Isles, while studies from across Europe suggest that median badger densities are 0.29–0.55 badger km^{-2} [(64, 65), Byrne, unpublished]. Furthermore, in England and Wales there has been a significant increase in badger social group and population densities in recent decades (66, 67). These figures mask the wide variation in density at lower spatial scales (66, 68–70) – for example, badger densities in Spain can vary from <0.3 to 3.4 badgers km^{-2} across habitat types (71). Similarly, badger densities in Ireland can vary from 0.7 badgers km^{-2} in poor upland habitat (72); in ideal conditions on a wooded island, densities up to 37 badgers km^{-2} have been recorded (64). However, what is important is that badgers benefit from a benign temperate climate in the British Isles (73, 74), and have thrived in areas where woodland and pasture abound (66, 68–70). These habitats can maintain badgers at mean densities of 3–5 badgers km^{-2} in Britain and Ireland (64, 75) and are also the contact point for potential direct and indirect interaction between badgers and grazing cattle (76). While badger density *per se* may not be related directly to risk in a linear fashion, large-scale epidemiological studies in the Republic of Ireland (53), Northern Ireland (77) and in Great Britain (78) have found significant and positive associations between metrics of badger density and increased bTB herd breakdown risk.

There is considerable variation in the societal attitudes to the management of wildlife across Europe [e.g., see (65, 79–84)], and this results in significant variation in the actual management practices implemented across Europe. This may relate to the apparent conflict between conservation, animal welfare, and management goals, as well as cultural differences in the acceptability of pursuits such as hunting. Hunting is more common, and arguably more socially acceptable in many continental European countries [e.g., (82, 83)] than it is in the UK and Ireland. Badger hunting is widespread and relatively intense in a number of countries across continental Europe (65), despite the badger being listed under the Bern convention. In Germany, the annual recorded hunting bag for badgers has been between 50–70,000 per annum, within an increasing trend in the hunt bag in recent years – for example, the bag for 2016 was 71,168, a 11.98% increase from 2015 (85). Similarly, in Finland 8,600–14,000 badgers have been reported in the national hunting records per annum (86, 87) and an increasing trend is reported in Poland where recent game bags are in excess of 4,000 badgers (88). Badger hunting is common and widespread in France, though there are limited available data on the national badger status (89), but hunters have been used recently in bTB outbreaks to sample badgers (39, 90). In Britain and Ireland, the badger has been protected by legislation since the 1970's. It is likely that this protection status has had beneficial effects on population size (68, 70, 91, 92) and may have influenced the considerable variation in the estimated densities of badgers across European countries, and between the British Isles and continental Europe. Furthermore, this broader issue of the "palatability" of wildlife management within society, and the relationship between this effect and the interventions undertaken may have been a significant factor in the bTB epi-system within the UK and Ireland (93).

Badgers Exhibit Significant TB Prevalence

Prevalence of *M. bovis* infection in badger populations may be sought as base-line data, although it is likely to vary by region and over time and is recognised as being difficult to quantify accurately (94–96). Standard pathology investigations have limited sensitivity (42, 97, 98) with the result that prevalence is likely to be underestimated.

Recent investigations indicate that more detailed post-mortem examinations result in the detection of microscopic lesions that would otherwise evade detection by standard procedures (97–99). Badgers killed in road traffic accidents (RTA) have proven to be a useful source of data in attempting to determine badger TB prevalence at a county-wide scale (42, 56, 100). The ISG reported that standard post mortem examination revealed that 15% of GB RTA badgers had TB (42). The ISG cautioned, however, that at a localised level below county size, owing to reduced availability of RTA badgers, this method may not be sufficient for surveillance (42). Similar RTA data collected in NI indicated that ~15% of badgers were infected (101). In GB, the ISG reported that in proactive cull regions, 16.6% of badgers were tuberculous (42) whilst in reactive cull regions this figure was 14.9% (102).

Similarly, studies in the ROI indicated that, by the standard protocol, culled badger TB prevalence was 12.1% (98) and largely in agreement with RTA figures. More thorough post mortem examination of culled badgers led to the detection of an increased number of infected animals. Cranshaw et al. (97) demonstrated that, in GB, proactively culled RBCT badgers had a true prevalence of TB infection of 24.2%. Similarly, in the ROI, more detailed post-mortem examination of culled badgers from across the country revealed a prevalence of 36.3% (98). However, other studies found higher prevalence up to 43%, indicating the variation in estimates depending on sampling and laboratory methods (103). Using cage trapping, anaesthesia and live sampling of badgers Drewe et al. (104) used latent class analysis to estimate the outcome of multiple tests on live badgers (culture, gamma interferon and Stat-Pak ELISA), in the absence of a perfect gold standard diagnosis. Sensitivity of diagnostic testing was estimated at ~93% and badger TB prevalence was estimated subsequently as 20.8% in Woodchester Park, Gloucester (104). Intra-regional, inter-regional and temporal differences in badger TB prevalence are to be expected owing to the potential differences in ecology and population dynamics of both cattle and badgers in different areas as illustrated recently in the ROI (105). Indeed, Byrne et al. (74) demonstrated large spatial variation in badger infection risk based on a sample of over 5,000 badgers across the Republic of Ireland. Using standard PM techniques and bacteriological culture confirmation, there was an order of magnitude difference in the worst infected counties to the lowest prevalence counties. Furthermore, there was a significant decrease in prevalence from 26 to 11% positive, at a period where TB was declining in the local cattle populations.

Regardless of "true" prevalence, these studies indicate that a significant component of the badger population across the UK and Republic of Ireland is infected with *M. bovis*, where bTB is also prevalent in cattle.

CATTLE AND HUSBANDRY

Britain and Ireland Have Some of the Highest National Cattle Densities in Europe

As has been described above for the European badger, the density of host organism available for infection by the TB causing bacilli seems to be of critical importance to ongoing transmission of disease and persistence. By analogy to bTB, Human tuberculosis, caused by *M. bovis*' close relative, *Mycobacterium tuberculosis*, is typically associated with overcrowding in confined spaces (106, 107). It is not surprising therefore that as with badgers, cattle densities will probably have an influence on bTB transmission dynamics. The countries that make up the islands of Britain and Ireland have notably high cattle densities in comparison with other European countries. In 2010, out of 27 countries within the EU, Northern Ireland had the highest mean cattle density of any country at 112 cattle per km^2 (108, 109). The Republic of Ireland was third (84 cattle per km2), with Wales and England ranking 6 and 7th respectively (54 and 40 cattle per km2). Scotland, who are now officially bTB free, are ranked 13th with a mean density of 22 cattle per km2. To illustrate the differences amongst countries, the national herds are large relative to their area in Britain and Ireland, for example, both the Republic of Ireland and Spain have approximately 6 million cattle (109), yet Spain is 7.2 times the size of ROI (504,645 Spain/70,273 ROI km^2). Research suggests that both the size of herds [e.g., (53)] and the intensity of farming (110) can be associated with increased risk of bTB breakdown in endemic countries [for reviews see (54, 111, 112)]. Larger herds may constitute greater risk as it may be more difficult to clear infection, once identified within the herd, due to the poor sensitivity of skin tests (113). The density of cattle within farms can be a proxy measure for the intensity of agricultural production, and has been associated with increased risk of bTB (110). At a macro-scale the risk of bTB increases with increasing intensity (111), primarily due to closer proximity between animals and potential infectious contacts (110, 112). In Britain and Ireland there has been a move towards intensification, with a trend towards larger farm sizes, yet a decline in the absolute number of farms (113, 114). Recent changes in dairy production at the EU level may exacerbate this pattern in the future. However, interestingly, Acevedo et al. (115) did not find a relationship between host density and bTB prevalence when investigating European island as discrete bTB ecosystems.

Britain and Ireland Have Farming Characteristics That May Cause Difficulties in Managing Infectious Disease

Trade is a significant characteristic of cattle farming in the UK and Ireland, with significant patterns of movement that transcend national boundaries (116, 117). Indeed, for example, in 2015 there were 55,285 live animal exports from ROI to Northern Ireland (118). Gilbert et al. (116) showed that, at a GB level, there were significant flows of animals traded over long distances, and also showed that movement metrics were a significant risk factor for bovine TB. Ashe et al. (117) visualised the movement of a cohort of animals from one county in one year in Ireland; a remarkable pattern of movement that encompassed all regions of the island was apparent. However, cattle movement and trade is a scale dependent phenomenon. While long distance movements occur and can potentially link disparate areas epidemiologically, the majority of trade moves are local (119) – the movement kernel is long tailed (120). Recent analysis of trade networks in Northern Ireland has demonstrated that farms are extremely well connected, forming a robust network that is resistant to random and targeted node removal. Essentially, this indicates that the interconnectedness of this herd network makes it difficult to manage spread on an individual basis.

Small movement networks can contribute to the local risk of bTB (121), however they also may explain the strong clustering of pathogen genotype patterns at a local level in Northern Ireland (54). Furthermore, there is a phenomenon of farm fragmentation, whereby herds are made up of a number of spatial fragments. These fragments can have large footprints (122), relative to the home premises, allowing for increased exposure to neighbours or environmental reservoir risk. The long-established practice of seasonal rented grazing, known in Northern Ireland as "conacre," adds to the potential impacts of fragmentation. Furthermore, there are little data available to assess within herd movements of animals – a potential for dispersal of infection both to neighbouring herds, but also spread of infection into the environment, including wildlife hosts. The movement of animals, the spreading of slurry and the sharing of farm equipment could all increase the likelihood of maintenance of TB (92), furthermore the constituent nodes within these networks (e.g., specific farms, marts, auctions) can have disproportionate effects on diseases spread (120, 123). On the other hand, the fact that islands are disconnected to the continent, raises the perspective that this insularity could prove beneficial towards the longer term control of the pathogen (115). Currently, there is a lack of harmonisation of data pertaining to animal movements within Western Europe, to allow direct comparisons between EU member states in terms of network structure and connectivity. Attaining this harmonisation should be a major research goal going forward. Anecdotally, the very dense within and between herd movement networks in Ireland and the UK, are different compared to the rest of Europe. However, without detailed comparative data, this makes direct comparisons challenging.

THE PATHOGEN: *M. BOVIS*

M. Bovis Strain Heterogeneity

The population genetics of the *M. bovis* bacillus in these islands is relevant to investigate the current epidemic and is an ongoing source of interest for many researchers. From a phylo-geographic point of view, such research can inform on the population history and can potentially inform on probable routes of entry into Britain and Ireland in the distant past (124). From a more practical and less academic point of view, phylo-geographic differences in pathogen demographics and evolution may have an outcome that is of importance to disease control and epidemiology. Such region-specific evolution and adaptation can result in differing pathogen phenotypes that result in differing disease outcomes and dynamics as has been well-documented for *M. tuberculosis* infection in humans (125–128). For example, in Vietnamese populations, specific strains of a Beijing lineage of *M. tuberculosis* have been observed in a number of cases to result in a meningeal form of the disease, rather than the expected pulmonary disease pattern (129). Indeed the Beijing lineage of *M. tuberculosis* is recognised as exhibiting a hypervirulent phenotype distinct from other phylogeographically distinct lineages (130). The latter evidence indicates that certain lineages of a tuberculosis-causing bacillus can vary in their phenotype in epidemiologically meaningful ways. So, the obvious question arises, could something similar happen with bovine tuberculosis caused by *M. bovis?*

Consequently, it is pertinent to attempt to understand the population structure and history of *M. bovis* in Britain and Ireland. The extant *M. bovis* population is almost exclusively dominated by a single clonal complex – the Eu1 clonal complex (124). This is indicative of a genetic bottleneck occurring at some point in the pathogen's history on these islands, an event which led to a contraction in diversity, resulting in greater homogeneity. Such bottlenecks are features of clonal pathogens like *M. bovis* (131). Whether this bottleneck occurred at the time of colonisation or subsequently is unknown. While this Eu1 lineage is present on other parts of Western Europe it is nowhere near as dominant as it is on these islands (124). Eu1 is also found globally among former trading partners and members of the British Empire, suggesting wider dissemination during colonial times (124). It has been shown that this Eu1 lineage spread throughout Britain and Ireland, leading to a homogenised *M bovis* population potentially brought about by the free movement of infected animals between territories (132). More recent cattle movement controls as part of national TB eradication schemes may have subsequently isolated regions one from another and driven more local evolution of specific strain types (132). Previously, Smith et al. (133) had sought evidence to support a hypothesis that a test and slaughter bottleneck of the *M. bovis* population in the 1950 and 1960s may have constituted selection pressure for the evolution and clonal expansion of a "fitter" clone that exhibited some form of advantage with respect to evading the test and slaughter scheme. Quite what the latter advantage could be, if it existed, is still a matter of debate. An ability to evade diagnostic testing is one possibility whilst invasion of / adaptation to a new host / niche such as a wildlife reservoir is another possibility (133).

The host range of the TB- causing bacilli is an intriguing puzzle (134). The human pathogen, M. tuberculosis, disseminates in human populations but appears not to be transmissible between non-human animals (134–136). Conversely, *M. bovis* appears to be able to disseminate among many non-human animal species, but humans are generally a dead end host (134–136). However, there is an interesting exception. Recently, Gonzalo Ascenzio *et al.* (137) demonstrated that a subtle mutation in the virulence genes of *M. bovis* can cause it to freely disseminate in humans. This is evidence that a small genetic change in a pathogen can radically expand maintenance host range. Could the Eu1 lineage of *M. bovis* have undergone a similar transition to become a better host generalist? It is noticeable that wherever Eu1 strains are found around the globe, there is a wildlife reservoir problem (124, 134). However, some caution is required here. This may just be an effect of recent demography and trade (124). The Eu1 lineage may just be a "lucky clone", dispersed by chance events. Additionally, the countries which inherited its diaspora are mostly developed world nations likely to have good disease surveillance infrastructure. Therefore, perhaps apparent increased propensity for wildlife adaptation is purely confirmation bias? The fact that many of these countries have had much greater success in bovine TB eradication than Britain and Ireland is also perhaps indicative that there is nothing obviously fitter about the Eu1 clonal complex, and that the wide dissemination of this lineage may purely be a matter of demography and international trade (124). Additionally, other European lineages of *M. bovis*, distinct from Eu1, have been observed to infect cattle and wildlife populations in Spain (138), Portugal (139) and France (140). However, in the absence of empirical comparisons between multiple *M. bovis* lineages, the pathology they induce across multiple hosts and their epidemiological characteristics, it is perhaps premature to rule out the hypothesis of the Eu1 lineage being in some way fitter. This bears further investigation (134). It is not inconceivable that whilst multiple *M. bovis* lineages have similar host ranges, the relative efficacy and virulence within similar hosts may be different owing to genotypic and phenotypic divergence as has been seen with *M. tuberculosis* lineages (127). Similarly, whilst the global diaspora of Eu1 *M. bovis* strains arising from historical trade and colonialism (124) are undoubtedly genetically similar, there remains the potential for region specific evolution since introduction. Different ecological contexts and applications of control schemes could have resulted in phenotypic divergence from a similar ancestral stock of bacilli.

Further work looking for an *M. bovis* strain phenotype in Northern Ireland has yielded limited evidence of an advantageous adaptation with regard to ability to evade detection. Wright et al. (141) demonstrated that field isolates of differing strain type exhibited no significant difference in response to the tuberculin skin test at the animal level. Allen et al. (132) raise the caveat that Wright *et al's* study was confined solely to Northern Ireland which contains strains from only the Eu1 lineage, and a geographically distinct sub population of Eu1 at that. Given the likely genetic homogeneity, would one reasonably expect to find stark differences in disease outcome / pathogen phenotype in such a setting (132)? Ideally, comparison of the epidemiological characteristics of strains extant in the recent past, predating test and slaughter schemes, within Britain and Ireland would also have been very interesting. However these strains are unavailable as their presence predates molecular characterisation and sample storage. Indeed, our knowledge of the *M. bovis* population in these islands is currently limited to that which is extant, and we have no definitive way of knowing whether Eu1 strains have always predominated or supplanted another lineage(s) of the bacillus. The fact that Eu1 strains were exported during the time of Empire suggests this lineage may have been at the very least, common for a considerable period of time in Britain and Ireland. Therefore any speculation on a fitter phenotype evolving within Britain and Ireland may be moot. Allen et al. (132) suggest that casting the net wider and comparing Eu1 to non Eu1 lineages in Western Europe or further afield may yield more fruit in this endeavour. In line with this hypothesis, it is perhaps telling that differences in disease outcome in *M. tuberculosis* have been observed at the level of major lineages – see previous. It is of note however that in a study, again confined to Northern Ireland and Eu1 only strains, Wright et al. (142) did find evidence for a difference in strain virulence, and Milne et al. (143) have observed that certain strains are associated with chronic, ongoing infections in certain herds over many years.

Given the contrasting views and evidence discussed above, the null hypothesis, in which there is nothing inherently "special" about *M. bovis* strains in Britain and Ireland, remains inherently plausible, but worthy of greater study. Much of the argument that Eu1 is not special seems to hinge on anecdote in the absence of data. Where empirical evidence is available, there are limitations in our ability to infer wider trends from geographically restricted findings as discussed previously. It would therefore in our view, be pertinent to attempt to address issues of pathogen lineage and its potential effects on bovine TB diagnosis and host range with well-designed studies and analyses. Regarding effects on TB diagnosis, we have already suggested above that intra lineage comparison across a wider geographic area is a better way to definitively settle this question. Overall then, it is our opinion that it would be better to empirically affirm or reject these hypotheses around evasion of diagnosis and host adaptation rather than dismiss them on the basis of gut feeling in the absence of hard evidence. If either or both hypotheses proved to be have some grounding in fact, then this could have implications for the application of control schemes in Britain and Ireland.

CO-INFECTION – EFFECTS ON BTB DIAGNOSIS

Co-infection dynamics are increasingly being recognised as a driver of the heterogeneous response of hosts to infection, and for persistence of diseases over time (144, 145). *Mycobacterium bovis* infection may be modulated by the presence of other infections (146–148), especially where severe infections immunocompromise the host. There is some evidence that *Mycobacterium bovis* infection progression can be impacted by viral infections such as Bovine Viral Diarrhoea (BVD), with the immunological response compromising tests used to disclose infected animals (149, 150), but see (151). Similarly, exposure to other infectious *Mycobacterium* species such as *M. avium paratuberculosis* (MAP or Johne's disease) can confound the immunological diagnosis of bTB through cross-reactivity (151–153). Furthermore, environmental mycobacteria can also affect the performance of bTB immunological tests, for example *M. hiberniae* (154, 155). Some of these environmental mycobacteria have been closely associated with bogs and peaty soils and subsoils (156), which is a significant habitat type within the British Isles (157), and could potentially impact on tuberculin skin test performance. Indeed, the potential for cross reaction is one of the reason why in Britain and Ireland the comparative skin test is used (bovine and avian tuberculin), which is not the case in other jurisdictions where such cross-reactions are rare (8).

MAP is now endemic in Ireland and Britain (158, 159), and suffers from similar diagnostic problems to bTB. Recent research from Ireland has highlighted the potential nexus between MAP and bTB (151, 160, 161). MAP exposure can affect the correct diagnosis of bTB, hindering the disclosure of truly-infected animals. However, it should be noted that MAP is now widely distributed in Western Europe, and similar problems have been described there [e.g., Spain; (162)]. Britain and Ireland may be particularly vulnerable to interference owing to the fact both territories use the comparative tuberculin test.

Recently, liver fluke (*Fasciola hepatica*) infection has been associated with a negative impact on the disclosure of bTB using the experimentally-infected cattle model and SCIT testing (146–148, 163). The prevalence of fluke infection in GB has also been associated negatively with the probability of dairy herds breaking down for bTB after whole herd tests. The size effect was large, with an estimated under-ascertainment of 33% (148). Co-infection, therefore, represents a mask potentially hiding the true infection status of both animals and herds, making clearance and ultimately eradication very difficult.

Liver fluke is endemic in Britain and Ireland, with high prevalence of infection (148, 164–166). At farm level, prevalence has been estimated as 86% in Wales, 83% in Ireland and 48% in England (164, 165). At the animal level, >60% animals exhibit some evidence of fluke damage in the livers of slaughtered cattle in Ireland (167). Using surveillance data, Byrne et al. (166) showed that >60% of herds had some infected animals in Northern Ireland, while herd prevalence approached 100% where at least 100 animals were sampled over a three year period. Given the results of Claridge et al. (148), these levels of infection may have a significant impact on the disclosure of bTB-exposed animals using immunological tests like SCITT. However, recent research from Northern Ireland failed to show a large size effect of co-infection on tuberculin reactions from field data (161), but did find associations between fluke co-infection and TB pathology mirroring other studies (146, 161, 168). But how different are the British Isles than other countries in Europe in terms of fluke exposure?

Recent spatial analyses and comparative studies across Europe have suggested that there are significantly lower levels of infection in continental Europe than in the British Isles (169–171), with particularly high levels of infection in cattle throughout the island of Ireland (170).

The distribution and abundance of liver fluke in the environment is strongly affected by climate and habitat types, through exposure and survival of intermediate hosts (164). This is in part due to the wet, temperate climate within the north-western Europe (169, 170). The exposure of livestock in the British Isles is also affected by farming practice (field based grazing), soil type, high soil moisture level and the abundant access to fresh water sources (172, 173).

While recent research has found equivocal evidence for the mechanism (168), there has been no comparative analysis of data derived from low and high fluke prevalence areas (i.e., international comparisons). One suggested hypothesis in Ireland is that such a high proportion of animals are exposed that there is a general depression of tuberculin reaction sizes (161).

CLIMATE AND ENVIRONMENT

Climate Adaptation and Change - Effects on Fluke

Future forecasts of fluke infection risk paint a depressing picture for parts of Europe, with especially significant predicted increases in risk for Britain and Ireland (169, 174). These forecasts have been primarily derived from climate projections, which for the most part are suggesting that Britain and Ireland will become warmer and wetter on average, but also more climatologically variable. Fox et al. (174) forecast significant increases in fluke in all regions of the United Kingdom, with a projected epidemic for parts of Wales by 2050. Similarly, Caminade et al. (169) also forecast significant future risk for increasing fluke in Ireland and Britain up to the year 2080, but also increasing risk for north-western parts of continental Europe. This increasing parasitic risk, coinciding with the troubling emergence of fluckicide resistance, indicates that screening tests such as the SCITT and surveillance data based on post-mortem pathology for bTB, may become even less robust for disclosure of infected animals.

Environmental Contamination with *M.bovis*

Despite recent advances in epidemiological analyses, molecular typing and whole genome sequencing of *M. bovis* (54, 57, 60), surprisingly little is known about the exact transmission mechanisms that spread infection within and between cattle and wildlife populations. Previously, owing to the work of UK government appointed ISG, who administered the Randomised Badger Culling Trial (RBCT) in Britain, it was assumed that direct contact between animals was required to facilitate disease transmission by aerosolised *M. bovis* bacilli leaving the respiratory tract (42).The cited evidence for the primacy of this suspected transmission route was the preponderance of tuberculous lesions observed in the upper respiratory tracts of both badgers and cattle that underwent post mortem examination (42, 175). However, more recently, studies which made use of proximity logger collars fitted to sympatric (42) cattle and badgers in Northern Ireland and England, failed to detect very close contact between species that would facilitate direct respiratory transmission (176–179). These findings do not preclude the hypothesised existence of super-spreaders in cattle and badgers. The ISG however were sceptical that many such super spreader badgers existed (42). The latter may however be controversial, with some evidence of badger super-shedding in a high density English badger population (96), and indeed the precedent of super shedding in other wildlife species (180). The latter opinion, in concert with the apparent lack of meaningful direct contact between species, has raised the possibility that a contaminated environment may potentially be playing some indirect role in disease transmission between species (42, 177, 179, 181, 182). This hypothesis has been raised before, with studies in the past focusing on the potential role badger urine and faeces may play in contaminating soil, pasture and feed (76). Renal lesions have been observed to be the second most common type of tuberculous pathology in infected badgers in some earlier localised studies (183, 184). More recently, 13–14% of culled badgers exhibited such lesions in GB (185), with a similar 15% lesion presentation rate seen in Northern Ireland (101). Badger urine has been observed on occasion to contain 250,000–300,000 bacilli per millilitre (186, 187). Badger faeces deposited at latrines close to territorial boundaries have also been observed to be potential sources of *M. bovis* in the environment (188). These bacilli are believed to enter the GI tract via ingestion of respiratory mucus (51). In one gram of badgers faeces, 75 colony forming units have been observed (187). It is conceivable that badgers and cattle inspecting urine trails or faecal latrines left for territorial marking (75, 188) could aerosolise bacilli from these sources and seed a respiratory tract infection. Other prominent veterinary pathogens have been observed to be aerosolizable from an environmental source - *Coxiella burnetii*, which causes of Q Fever, has been observed to infect animals and humans exposed to contaminated wool (189) and *Mycobacterium avium paratuberculosis*, the causative agent in Johne's Disease has been observed to be aerosolised in dust particles derived from bovine faecal material in animal housing (190). An intriguing recent study demonstrated that *M. canettii*, a pathogen predicted to be a common ancestor for the *M. tuberculosis* Complex, could produce pulmonary infection, indistinguishable from aerosol-mediated pulmonary infection, in mice fed spiked material (191).

A crucial question for the viability of this hypothesis is how long can *M. bovis* persist in the environment? Previously, bacilli in badger urine were observed to survive on pasture for ~3 days in the summer and ~14 days in the winter (186) potentially due to the differing intensity of solar UV radiation, which can kill the bacilli. A number of studies in different countries indicate that the survival of *M. bovis* in environmental matrices is variable (192). *M. bovis* in faeces or faeces-contaminated soil appears to remain viable for up to ~6 months in some studies (193, 194). More recently, Barbier et al. (195) have undertaken *in vitro* experiments in which differing soil types were seeded with *M. bovis* and incubated at 4 and 22°C. Their findings indicated that *M. bovis* persisted for longer (up to 150 days) at the cooler temperature, whilst results for differing soil types were inconclusive (195). It may also be worth investigating whether *M. bovis* strain variation may have a role to play in adaptation to environmental persistence. Within the Eu1 major lineage that dominates the UK and Ireland (as discussed above), it has been noted that there is considerable heterogeneity in cell wall content as detected by Fourier Transform Infra-Red Spectroscopy (196). Indeed, the major genetic deletion which is a hallmark of the Eu1 lineage removes a gene responsible for trehalose biosynthesis – an important component of the glycolipid rich hydrophobic cell wall (124). Recently it has been observed that hydrophobic cell wall components, which are a feature of the pathogenic bacilli in the *Mycobacterium tuberculosis* complex, aid aerosolisation and pathogenicity (197). Conversely, environmental mycobacteria appear to have more hydrophilic cell wall components (197). Could the Eu1 lineage, or some of its descendants have evolved a phenotype that retained pathogenicity but permitted environmental persistence? Comparison to other lineages in the type of experiments Barbier et al. (195) have performed may be a useful way of addressing this hypothesis.

Current and Future Climate Effects on *M. Bovis* Persistence in the Environment

Also pertinent to this debate is the climate of the UK and Ireland compared to continental Europe. Britain and Ireland inhabit a zone of the globe whose predominant weather tends to be mild and wet without experiencing extremes in temperature – classified under the Köppen system as a Cfb climate; temperate with no dry season and 10 or more months of the year exhibiting temperatures above 10 °C (198). Much of Western Europe, including northern Spain, most of France, Germany, Belgium and Holland are also categorised as belonging to this Köppen climate category (198). However, it is noted that whilst the Köppen system is useful for broad inferences of year on year regional climate (199), it can miss intra-regional variation, particularly in European locales (198). Britain and Ireland are a case in point. Both territories are islands, surrounded on all sides by the Atlantic Ocean and various seas. Indeed, the North Atlantic Oscillation is the primary driver of the maritime climate niche within the broader Cfb category that Britain and Ireland occupy (200). Whilst there is variation across Britain and Ireland in climate - a general west to east cline in temperature, precipitation and sunlight is observed (200) - the general trend (even for south east Britain, which is most like the continent) is that both islands exhibit milder winters and cooler summers than continental neighbours (201). Indeed, records show that these islands receive less sunshine (202) and more precipitation (203) than other Western European countries. Given what we have discussed above about the factors effecting viability of *M. bovis* in the environment, could these contemporary conditions influence *M. bovis* survival in the environment of these islands, or specific regions of them, compared to continental nations? The obvious counterpoint to this is that Britain in particular came close to eradicating bTB through the 1950 and 1960s (18). So, if a contaminated environment was important for regional persistence, shouldn't that have prevented the scale of decline in prevalence during that period? It depends on the likely scale of importance an environmental reservoir would constitute, and whether that importance has changed with time. Perhaps the changing circumstances in wildlife abundance, farming practices, strain effects etc since the 1970s could have conspired to make a contaminated environment more of a contemporary problem in contrast to the past? Alternatively, if the role of environmental contamination is relatively small regardless of the point in time it occurs in, then it could still be an important factor in regional persistence. For instance, Britain did not completely eradicate bTB after initial success in reducing prevalence throughout the 1950 and 1960 s. Low level infection in cattle remained a problem with eventual recrudescence through the 1970–2000 s leading to the current impasse (18). It is plausible that an environmental reservoir may have played a role, alongside other factors, in preventing that final push to complete eradication.

With changing climate in the future, the UK and Ireland are predicted to see even milder, wetter weather (204, 205), with intra-regional variation in exact outcomes. Predicted general trends are for drier, hotter summers (205, 206), potentially with less cloud cover in southern Britain (205), and milder, wetter winters with increased probability of extreme precipitation events [Sweeney et al, 2001; (205)]. It would be pertinent therefore to begin to address whether contemporary climate effects and predicted future effects are likely to have any impact on the survivability of *M. bovis* in the British and Irish environment. These questions could perhaps be addressed in the future using field data and *in vitro* experimentation. The effect of weather conditions have been correlated with variation in *M. bovis* risk in cattle (116, 207–209), and such weather variation has significant impact on the population dynamics of wild reservoirs also (74, 210) potentially impacting patterns of infection (95), adding to the complexity.

Emerging Environmental Hosts

Alongside general environmental contamination with *M. bovis*, and potentially contributing to it, is the role that soil based organisms may play in dissemination of bacilli and their persistence. Specifically, protozoa have been implicated as potential reservoirs of *M. bovis*. It has in the past been hypothesised that the benign environmental bacteria that went on to become virulent, intracellular pathogens, may have evolved many of their intracellular persistence apparatus within the "nurseries" of environmental protozoa (211–214). Initially, Mardare et al. (215) had suggested that amoeba predation of bacilli was more likely to result in inactivated bacilli and reduced persistence in environmental samples. However, more recently it has been shown that protozoa containing TB causing bacilli, when fed to mice can result in active tuberculous infection (216).

Earthworms have also recently been observed to ingest *M. bovis* from cattle faeces and disseminate bacilli in castings across the wider landscape (217). From regional sampling and regression of soil content data, predicted earthworm abundance and species diversity across Europe have recently been determined (218). These data demonstrate that earthworm abundance is greatest in Denmark, Holland, Britain and Ireland compared to other Western European countries and that Ireland and Britain display one of the highest diversities of species across the continent (218). Earthworms have also been noted as a major component of the diet of badgers, particularly in Britain (219) and to a lesser extent in Ireland (220). Greater investigation of the potential role these ecosystem engineer species play in the epidemiology of bTB may shed light on environmental persistence and transmission dynamics.

What About Scotland? Is It the Exception That Proves the Rule?

Scotland poses an apparent challenge to the paradigm we have attempted to develop within this manuscript as an Officially TB Free (OTF) territory within Britain – it is part of the British isles, badgers reside there (there are also other potential wildlife hosts, with relatively large deer populations) especially in the lowlands, there is a significant cattle industry, and similar tests and testing regimes have been employed as in the rest of the British Isles. However, the relative magnitude of these characteristics is worth dwelling upon.

Badger density is significantly lower than in the rest of the British Isles (66, 67, 69, 70, 221). Badger abundance can be estimated using the density of main setts, representing the number of social groups within an area, allowing for reasonable estimation of abundance at large national scales (222). Comparing the mean social group density across countries of the British Isles, Scotland has the lowest mean density of 0.11 social groups km^{-2} (to the nearest thousand, 9,000 social groups (221), whereas in England and Wales the average value is 0.49 km^{-2} [72,000 social groups (66)], the Republic of Ireland has 0.25 km^{-2} [(19,000 social groups (69)]; and Northern Ireland, with the highest estimated density, of 0.58 km^{-2} [8,000 social groups (70)]. While there is debate as to the linearity of the relationship between social group density and abundance [(223); but see (222)] the magnitude of the difference would suggest a significant difference in average badger population density between the countries (69). This is most likely related to the low proportion of the most suitable badger habitat in Scotland (much of Scotland is exposed, and/or upland).

Similarly, Scotland's cattle density is significantly lower than other countries within the British Isles [see above (6)]. However, the cattle industry is concentrated in the lowlands, meaning that similar intensity of farming may be occurring at local scales, with large herd sizes being reported (6). Scotland has a lower proportion of dairy farms, relative to the rest of the UK and ROI, and dairy herds can represents an increased risk relative to other farming types [(6, 224); but see (225)].

Furthermore, there are significant trade links between Scotland and the rest of the UK and ROI, including from relatively high TB risk areas (225, 226). This trade represents a risk for Scottish farmers who trade in from high incidence areas (225, 226), but the relative risk has been diminished significantly through the introduction of pre- and post-movement testing of traded animals (226). These restrictions have reduced the amount of international trade and also reduced the risk to infection (re)introduction (226).

In terms of liver fluke, recent spatial models would suggest that much of Scotland (especially the highlands) is high risk and future climate changes may exacerbate this problem (174). The confounding effects of co-infection in low prevalence situations seem not to mitigate against the maintenance of disease freedom.

Scotland is on a quadrennial testing regime, with herds tested at least once every four years (225), therefore, the testing regime is at a lower frequency than much of the rest of the UK and Ireland.

An argument could be made that Scotland reduced historic bTB levels to a low enough level to allow cattle measures alone to achieve freedom. Perhaps then, the historical reduced wildlife and cattle densities were then sufficient to act as a bulwark against recrudescence and the establishment of endemic disease? In fact, GB was very close to eradication in the 1980s before bTB re-emerged significantly in the 30 years since (18). During this period high bTB levels were largely confined to the south and south east of Britain, from where the epidemic has slowly expanded (227). In the intervening period badger population density has increased significantly (66–68), the intensity of cattle farming may also have increased, coinciding with policy changes, and there may be potential interactive effects of concurrent infections, all of which would have been exacerbated by the 2001 foot and mouth crisis (6).

CONCLUSIONS

In this article we have attempted to propose potential reasons why the British and Irish experience in eradicating bovine tuberculosis has been so fraught compared to that of other jurisdictions in recent times. Our suggestions have arisen from a broad comparative approach which contrasts landscape, ecological, animal husbandry and molecular epidemiological characteristics within Britain and Ireland to those primarily observed on the wider European Continent. We note, with caution, that correlation is not causation. However for all proposed factors, we have endeavoured to present a coherent narrative, supported by published evidence, which links each to pertinent aspects of bTB epidemiology. We do not propose that these potential factors are exhaustive, merely that they may be worthy of further investigation, and individually or collectively may constitute novel hypotheses that go some way to explaining the comparative lack of progress in bTB eradication in these islands.

Our hypothesis is that owing to their history, ecology and geography, Britain and Ireland may occupy a "goldilocks zone" for bovine TB. Factors highlighted in this review include the presence of a sufficient wildlife reservoir, a potentially amenable environment for *M. bovis* maintenance, a number of endemic infections that could impact on the diagnosis and transmission of bTB, an evolutionary lineage of the pathogen unique to Western Europe and a large, highly connected, dense network of farms where the movement of infected animals could be facilitated, partially due to the limitations of the statutory test at the individual level.

As regards further investigation, we propose a wider scale comparison of all listed factors across Britain and Ireland, and their association with risk of bTB persistence and other pertinent epidemiological outcomes, contrasted to territories / regions with lower bTB prevalence. The latter may help to ascertain if any of the factors have a significant impact on bTB eradication efforts and also to quantify their relative importance. The latter type of investigation could be achieved in two ways:

1. Aggregating all retrospective information for the listed factors across multiple patches of interest across Britain and Ireland into a single data resource that could contrast intra-regional differences and find potential associations and effects – in effect a meta-analysis.
2. Prospectively, across Britain, Ireland and Western European countries, identify regions with varying burdens of disease and actively measure / catalogue the stated factors for statistical analyses.

A caveat is that both strategies would bring their own inherent problems. Both would require harmonisation of retrospectively and prospectively collected data, to control for differences in bTB eradication scheme administration and data collection methods.

However, efforts to survey broader vistas of the bTB landscape may make these efforts more worthwhile, identifying novel mechanisms amenable to control. There may have been a tendency to restrict one's horizons when investigating bTB persistence in Britain and Ireland – a parochial approach, that whilst understandable with a complex disease affecting many herds and animals on a national scale – may miss some important epidemiological drivers. Owing to potential intra-national homogeneity in the characteristics of risk factors, their relative importance at a wider scale could be masked – for example: since the lineage of *M. bovis* found in Britain and Ireland lacks diversity, intra-national comparison of potential effects of strain variation would be difficult to detect, since everything seems so genetically similar.

A potential criticism of our focus on some of these factors, is that even if they did have a significant effect on bTB epidemiology, that effect may be very small and therefore, any intervention would potentially not be practical or cost efficient. However, in the absence of firm evidence either way, this criticism could appear to be somewhat pessimistic. The reproductive index (R0) for bovine TB between cattle in Britain has been estimated to be low – 1.1 (228). Between badgers, R0 has also been observed to be low – ranging from 1.03 to 1.19 (223). Between species R0 has recently been estimated to be in the region of 0.05 (60). These results suggest that not much effort may be needed to tip the R0 (of the two-host system) below one and drive the epidemic to extinction. It may well be that targeted intervention on multiple factors of small effect, when combined with the larger effects of the nationally managed eradication schemes, could help achieve this goal. In effect, we are suggesting that addressing some of the potential factors identified here, may result in an aggregation of marginal gains that takes the standard eradication scheme protocol as its base line, and applies an ecosystem management approach to drive down remaining infection.

AUTHOR CONTRIBUTIONS

AA and AB came up with the concept for the manuscript and drafted it. RS made additions to the text, edited existing text and gave advice.

REFERENCES

1. Anon. "Council Directive 64/432/EEC". *Off J Eur Comm* (1964).
2. Reviriego Gordejo FJ, Vermeersch JP. Towards eradication of bovine tuberculosis in the European Union. *Vet Microbiol* (2006) 112(2-4):101–9. doi: 10.1016/j.vetmic.2005.11.034
3. Anon. in: L145. *Off J Eur Comm* (1977).
4. European Food Safety AuthorityEuropean Centre for Disease Prevention and Control. "SCIENTIFIC REPORT OF EFSA AND ECDC - The European Union summary report on trends and sources of zoonoses, zoonotic agents and food-borne outbreaks in 2009". *EFSA Journal: European Food Standards Agency* (2011) 9(3):2090.
5. Vial F, Miguel E, T. Johnston W, Mitchell A, Donnelly CA. Bovine tuberculosis risk factors for british herds before and after the 2001 foot-and-mouth epidemic: what have we learned from the TB99 and CCS2005 studies? *Transbound Emerg Dis* (2015) 62(5):505–15. doi: 10.1111/tbed.12184
6. Abernethy DA, Upton P, Higgins IM, Mcgrath G, Goodchild AV, Rolfe SJ, et al. Bovine tuberculosis trends in the UK and the Republic of Ireland, 1995–2010. *Vet Rec* (2013) 172(12):312. doi: 10.1136/vr.100969
7. Anon. *Bovine TB Eradication programme for England.* London: DEFRA (2011).
8. de La Rua-Domenech R, Goodchild AT, Vordermeier HM, Hewinson RG, Christiansen KH, Clifton-Hadley RS. Ante mortem diagnosis of tuberculosis in cattle: a review of the tuberculin tests, γ-interferon assay and other ancillary diagnostic techniques. *Res Vet Sci* (2006) 81(2):190–210. doi: 10.1016/j.rvsc.2005.11.005
9. Schiller I, Raywaters W, Vordermeier HM, Jemmi T, Welsh M, Keck N, et al. Bovine tuberculosis in Europe from the perspective of an officially tuberculosis free country: trade, surveillance and diagnostics. *Vet Microbiol* (2011) 151(1-2):153–9. doi: 10.1016/j.vetmic.2011.02.039
10. Good M, Bakker D, Duignan A, Collins DM. The history of *in vivo* tuberculin testing in bovines: tuberculosis, a "one health" issue. *Front Vet Sci* (2018) 5:59. doi: 10.3389/fvets.2018.00059
11. Clegg TA, Duignan A, Whelan C, Gormley E, Good M, Clarke J, et al. Using latent class analysis to estimate the test characteristics of the γ-interferon test, the single intradermal comparative tuberculin test and a multiplex immunoassay under Irish conditions. *Vet Microbiol* (2011) 151(1-2):68–76. doi: 10.1016/j.vetmic.2011.02.027
12. Nuñez-Garcia J, Downs SH, Parry JE, Abernethy DA, Broughan JM, Cameron AR, et al. Meta-analyses of the sensitivity and specificity of ante-mortem and post-mortem diagnostic tests for bovine tuberculosis in the UK and Ireland. *Prev Vet Med* (2018) 153:94–107. doi: 10.1016/j.prevetmed.2017.02.017
13. Radunz B. Surveillance and risk management during the latter stages of eradication: experiences from Australia. *Vet Microbiol* (2006) 112(2-4):283–90. doi: 10.1016/j.vetmic.2005.11.017
14. Livingstone PG, Hancox N, Nugent G, de Lisle GW. Toward eradication: the effect of *Mycobacterium bovis* infection in wildlife on the evolution and future direction of bovine tuberculosis management in New Zealand. *N Z Vet J* (2015) 63 Suppl 1:4–18. doi: 10.1080/00480169.2014.971082
15. Martin SW, Shoukri M, Thorburn MA. Evaluating the health status of herds based on tests applied to individuals. *Prev Vet Med* (1992) 14(1-2):33–43. doi: 10.1016/0167-5877(92)90082-Q
16. Lahuerta-Marin A, Gallagher M, Mcbride S, Skuce R, Menzies F, Mcnair J, et al. Should they stay, or should they go? Relative future risk of bovine tuberculosis for interferon-gamma test-positive cattle left on farms. *Vet Res* (2015) 46(1):90. doi: 10.1186/s13567-015-0242-8
17. Robinson PA. Framing bovine tuberculosis: a 'political ecology of health' approach to circulation of knowledge(s) about animal disease control. *Geogr J* (2017) 183(3):285–94. doi: 10.1111/geoj.12217
18. Goodchild T, Clifton-Hadley R, Thoen CO, Steele JH, Gilsdorf MJ. "The fall and rise of bovine tuberculosis in Great Britain". In: *Mycobacterium bovis Infection in Animals and Humans.* 2nd ed. Wiley-Blackwell (2008).
19. Lesslie IW, Herbert CN, Burn KJ, MacClancy BN, Donnelly WJ. Comparison of the specificty of human and bovine tuberculin PPD for testing cattle. 1-Republic of Ireland. *Vet Rec* (1975) 96(15):332–4. doi: 10.1136/vr.96.15.332
20. Good M. Bovine tuberculosis eradication in Ireland. *Ir Vet J* (2006) 59:154–62.
21. Downs SH, Clifton-Hadley RS, Upton PA, Milne IC, Ely ER, Gopal R, et al. Tuberculin manufacturing source and breakdown incidence rate of bovine tuberculosis in British cattle, 2005-2009. *Vet Rec* (2013) 172(4):98. doi: 10.1136/vr.100679
22. Good M, Clegg TA, Murphy F, More SJ. The comparative performance of the single intradermal comparative tuberculin test in Irish cattle, using tuberculin PPD combinations from different manufacturers. *Vet Microbiol* (2011) 151(1-2):77–84. doi: 10.1016/j.vetmic.2011.02.028
23. Praud A, Boschiroli ML, Meyer L, Garin-Bastuji B, Dufour B. Assessment of the sensitivity of the gamma-interferon test and the single intradermal comparative cervical test for the diagnosis of bovine tuberculosis under field conditions. *Epidemiol Infect* (2015) 143(01):157–66. doi: 10.1017/S0950268814000338
24. Good M, Clegg TA, Duignan A, More SJ. Impact of the national full herd depopulation policy on the recurrence of bovine tuberculosis in Irish herds, 2003 to 2005. *Vet Rec* (2011b) 169(22):581. doi: 10.1136/vr.d4571
25. Karolemeas K, de La Rua-Domenech R, Cooper R, Goodchild AV, Clifton-Hadley RS, Conlan AJ, et al. Estimation of the relative sensitivity of the comparative tuberculin skin test in tuberculous cattle herds subjected to depopulation. *PLoS One* (2012) 7(8):e43217. doi: 10.1371/journal.pone.0043217
26. Abernethy DA, Denny GO, Menzies FD, Mcguckian P, Honhold N, Roberts AR. The Northern Ireland programme for the control and eradication of Mycobacterium bovis. *Vet Microbiol* (2006) 112(2-4):231–7.
27. Clegg TA, Good M, Duignan A, Doyle R, Blake M, More SJ. Longer-term risk of *Mycobacterium bovis* in Irish cattle following an inconclusive diagnosis to the single intradermal comparative tuberculin test. *Prev Vet Med* (2011) 100(3-4):147–54. doi: 10.1016/j.prevetmed.2011.02.015
28. Marangon S, Martini M, Dalla Pozza M, Neto F. A case-control study on bovine tuberculosis in the Veneto Region (Italy). *Prev Vet Med* (1998) 34(2-3):87–95. doi: 10.1016/S0167-5877(97)00087-1
29. DEFRA. *Strategy for Achieving Officially Bovine Tuberculosis Free Status for England: The 'edge area' strategy.* (2014). Available at: https://assets.publishing.service.gov.uk/government/uploads/system/uploads/attachment_data/file/300447/pb14088-bovine-tb-strategy-140328.pdf

30. TB Hub. *Working towards bovine TB free status in England.* (2017). Available at: http://www.tbhub.co.uk/wp-content/uploads/2017/09/infographic-TB-measures.pdf
31. Mcgrath G, Abernethy D, Stringer L, More SJ. An all-island approach to mapping bovine tuberculosis in Ireland. *Ir Vet J* (2009) 62(3):192–7. doi: 10.1186/2046-0481-62-3-192
32. Palmer MV. *Mycobacterium bovis* : characteristics of wildlife reservoir hosts. *Transbound Emerg Dis* (2013) 60(Suppl. 15):1–13. doi: 10.1111/tbed.12115
33. Nugent G. Maintenance, spillover and spillback transmission of bovine tuberculosis in multi-host wildlife complexes: a New Zealand case study. *Vet Microbiol* (2011) 151(1-2):34–42. doi: 10.1016/j.vetmic.2011.02.023
34. O'Brien DJ, Schmitt SM, Fierke JS, Hogle SA, Winterstein SR, Cooley TM, et al. Epidemiology of Mycobacterium bovis in free-ranging white-tailed deer, Michigan, USA, 1995–2000. *Prev Vet Med* (2002) 54(1):47–63. doi: 10.1016/S0167-5877(02)00010-7
35. Gortazar C, Vicente J, Boadella M, Ballesteros C, Galindo RC, Garrido J, et al. Progress in the control of bovine tuberculosis in Spanish wildlife. *Vet Microbiol* (2011) 151(1-2):170–8. doi: 10.1016/j.vetmic.2011.02.041
36. Vicente J, Höfle U, Garrido JM, Fernández-de-Mera IG, Juste R, Barral M, et al. Wild boar and red deer display high prevalences of tuberculosis-like lesions in Spain. *Vet Res* (2006) 37(1):107–19. doi: 10.1051/vetres:2005044
37. Richomme C, Boschiroli ML, Hars J, Casabianca F, Ducrot C. Bovine tuberculosis in livestock and wild boar on the Mediterranean Island, Corsica. *J Wildl Dis* (2010) 46(2):627–31. doi: 10.7589/0090-3558-46.2.627
38. Gortázar C, Delahay RJ, Mcdonald RA, Boadella M, Wilson GJ, Gavier-Widen D, et al. The status of tuberculosis in European wild mammals. *Mamm Rev* (2012) 42(3):193–206. doi: 10.1111/j.1365-2907.2011.00191.x
39. Payne A, Boschiroli ML, Gueneau E, Moyen JL, Rambaud T, Dufour B, et al. Bovine tuberculosis in "Eurasian" badgers (Meles meles) in France. *Eur J Wildl Res* (2013) 59(3):331–9. doi: 10.1007/s10344-012-0678-3
40. Balseiro A, González-Quirós P, Rodríguez Óscar, Francisca Copano M, Merediz I, de Juan L, et al. Spatial relationships between Eurasian badgers (Meles meles) and cattle infected with Mycobacterium bovis in Northern Spain. *Vet J* (2013) 197(3):739–45. doi: 10.1016/j.tvjl.2013.03.017
41. Donnelly CA, Woodroffe R, Cox DR, Bourne FJ, Cheeseman CL, Clifton-Hadley RS, et al. Positive and negative effects of widespread badger culling on tuberculosis in cattle. *Nature* (2006) 439(7078):843–6. doi: 10.1038/nature04454
42. Bourne FJ, Donnelly CA, Cox DR, Gettinby G, Mcinerney JP, Morrison WI, et al. Re: TB policy and the ISG's findings. *Vet Rec* (2007) 161(18):633–5. doi: 10.1136/vr.161.18.633-b
43. Eves JA. Impact of badger removal on bovine tuberculosis in east County Offaly. *Ir Vet J* (1999) 52:199–203.
44. Griffin JM, More SJ, Clegg TA, Collins JD, O'Boyle I, Williams DH, et al. Tuberculosis in cattle: the results of the four-area project. *Ir Vet J* (2005) 58(11):629–36. doi: 10.1186/2046-0481-58-11-629
45. Griffin JM, Williams DH, Kelly GE, Clegg TA, O'Boyle I, Collins JD, et al. The impact of badger removal on the control of tuberculosis in cattle herds in Ireland. *Prev Vet Med* (2005) 67(4):237–66. doi: 10.1016/j.prevetmed.2004.10.009
46. Jenkins HE, Woodroffe R, Donnelly CA. The duration of the effects of repeated widespread badger culling on cattle tuberculosis following the cessation of culling. *PLoS One* (2010) 5(2):e9090. doi: 10.1371/journal.pone.0009090
47. Kelly GE, Condon J, More SJ, Dolan L, Higgins I, Eves J. A long-term observational study of the impact of badger removal on herd restrictions due to bovine TB in the Irish midlands during 1989–2004. *Epidemiol Infect* (2008) 136(10):1362–73. doi: 10.1017/S0950268807000027
48. Olea-Popelka FJ, Fitzgerald P, White P, Mcgrath G, Collins JD, O'Keeffe J, et al. Targeted badger removal and the subsequent risk of bovine tuberculosis in cattle herds in county Laois, Ireland. *Prev Vet Med* (2009) 88(3):178–84. doi: 10.1016/j.prevetmed.2008.09.008
49. Clifton-Hadley RS, Wilesmith JW, Richards MS, Upton P, Johnston S. The occurrence of Mycobacterium bovis infection in cattle in and around an area subject to extensive badger (Meles meles) control. *Epidemiol Infect* (1995) 114(01):179–93. doi: 10.1017/S0950268800052031
50. Krebs J. *Bovine TB in cattle and badgers.* London: UK Government: *MAFF* (1997).
51. Gallagher J, Clifton-Hadley RS. Tuberculosis in badgers; a review of the disease and its significance for other animals. *Res Vet Sci* (2000) 69(3):203–17. doi: 10.1053/rvsc.2000.0422
52. Donnelly CA, Jenkins HE, Woodroffe R. *Analysis of further data (to August 2011) on the impacts on cattle TB incidence of repeated badger culling.* (2011).
53. Byrne AW, White PW, Mcgrath G, O'Keeffe J, Martin SW. Risk of tuberculosis cattle herd breakdowns in Ireland: effects of badger culling effort, density and historic large-scale interventions. *Vet Res* (2014) 45(1):109. doi: 10.1186/s13567-014-0109-4
54. Skuce RA, Mallon TR, McCormick C, Mcbride SH, Clarke G, Thompson A, et al. Bovine tuberculosis: herd-level surveillance of *Mycobacterium bovis* genotypes in Northern Ireland (2003-2008). *Adv Anim Biosci* (2010) 1(01):112. doi: 10.1017/S2040470010002554
55. Kelly GE, More SJ. Spatial clustering of TB-infected cattle herds prior to and following proactive badger removal. *Epidemiol Infect* (2011) 139(08):1220–9. doi: 10.1017/S0950268810002323
56. Goodchild AV, Watkins GH, Sayers AR, Jones JR, Clifton-Hadley RS. Geographical association between the genotype of bovine tuberculosis in found dead badgers and in cattle herds. *Vet Rec* (2012) 170(10):259–259. doi: 10.1136/vr.100193
57. Biek R, O'Hare A, Wright D, Mallon T, Mccormick C, Orton RJ, et al. Whole genome sequencing reveals local transmission patterns of mycobacterium bovis in sympatric cattle and badger populations. *PLoS Pathog* (2012) 8(11):e1003008. doi: 10.1371/journal.ppat.1003008
58. Trewby H, Wright D, Breadon EL, Lycett SJ, Mallon TR, Mccormick C, et al. Use of bacterial whole-genome sequencing to investigate local persistence and spread in bovine tuberculosis. *Epidemics* (2016) 14:26–35. doi: 10.1016/j.epidem.2015.08.003
59. Allen A, Skuce R, McDowell S. *"Bovine TB: a review of badger to cattle transmission".* Belfast: UK: Department of Agriculture and Rural Development (DARD) (2011).
60. Brooks-Pollock E, Wood JL. Eliminating bovine tuberculosis in cattle and badgers: insight from a dynamic model. *Proc Biol Sci* (2015) 282(1808):20150374. doi: 10.1098/rspb.2015.0374
61. Barlow ND. "Critical Evaluation of Wildlife Disease Models". In: Grenfell BT, Dobson AP, editors. *Ecology of Infectious Diseases in Natural Populations.* Cambridge, UK: Cambridge University Press (1995). p. 230–59.
62. Corner LAL, Murphy D, Gormley E. Mycobacterium bovis infection in the Eurasian badger (Meles meles): the disease, pathogenesis, epidemiology and control. *J Comp Pathol* (2011) 144(1):1–24. doi: 10.1016/j.jcpa.2010.10.003
63. Donnelly CA, Nouvellet P. The contribution of badgers to confirmed tuberculosis in cattle in high-incidence areas in England. *PLoS Curr* (2013) 5. doi: 10.1371/currents.outbreaks.097a904d3f3619db2fe78d24bc776098
64. Byrne AW, Sleeman DP, O'Keeffe J, Davenport J. The ecology of the European badger (Meles meles) in Ireland: a review. Biology and Environment. *Proceedings of the Royal Irish Academy.* . (2012). p. 112B. (105–32.
65. Griffiths HI. *On the hunting of badgers: an inquiry into the hunting and conservation of the Eurasian badger Meles meles (L.) in the western part of its range.* Brynna, Wales, UK: Piglet Press (1991).
66. Judge J, Wilson GJ, Macarthur R, Delahay RJ, Mcdonald RA. Density and abundance of badger social groups in England and Wales in 2011–2013. *Sci Rep* (2015) 4(1):3809. doi: 10.1038/srep03809
67. Judge J, Wilson GJ, Macarthur R, Mcdonald RA, Delahay RJ. Abundance of badgers (Meles meles) in England and Wales. *Sci Rep* (2017) 7(1):276. doi: 10.1038/s41598-017-00378-3
68. Wilson G, Harris S, McLaren G. *"Changes in the British badger population, 1988 to 1997".* London, UK: Peoples' Trust for Endangered Species (1997).
69. Byrne AW, Acevedo P, Green S, O'Keeffe J. Estimating badger social-group abundance in the Republic of Ireland using cross-validated species distribution modelling. *Ecol Indic* (2014) 43:94–102. doi: 10.1016/j.ecolind.2014.02.024
70. Reid N, Etherington TR, Wilson GJ, Montgomery WI, Mcdonald RA. Monitoring and population estimation of the European badger *Meles meles* in Northern Ireland. *Wildlife Biol* (2012) 18(1):46–57. doi: 10.2981/11-016
71. Acevedo P, González-Quirós P, Prieto JM, Etherington TR, Gortázar C, Balseiro A. Generalizing and transferring spatial models: a case study to predict Eurasian badger abundance in Atlantic Spain. *Ecol Modell* (2014) 275:1–8. doi: 10.1016/j.ecolmodel.2013.12.011

72. Feore S, Montgomery WI. Habitat effects on the spatial ecology of the European badger (Meles meles). *J Zool* (1999) 247(4):537–49. doi: 10.1111/j.1469-7998.1999.tb01015.x
73. Johnson DDP, Jetz W, Macdonald DW. Environmental correlates of badger social spacing across Europe. *J Biogeogr* (2002) 29(3):411–25. doi: 10.1046/j.1365-2699.2002.00680.x
74. Byrne AW, Fogarty U, O'Keeffe J, Newman C. *In situ* adaptive response to climate and habitat quality variation: spatial and temporal variation in European badger (*Meles meles*) body weight. *Glob Chang Biol* (2015) 21(9):3336–46. doi: 10.1111/gcb.12939
75. Roper T. *Badger*. London: Harper Collins (2010).
76. Hutchings MR, Harris S. Quantifying the risks of TB infection to cattle posed by badger excreta. *Epidemiol Infect* (1999) 122(1):167–74. doi: 10.1017/S0950268898001897
77. Wright DM, Reid N, Ian Montgomery W, Allen AR, Skuce RA, Kao RR. Herd-level bovine tuberculosis risk factors: assessing the role of low-level badger population disturbance. *Sci Rep* (2015) 5(1):13062. doi: 10.1038/srep13062
78. Bessell PR, Orton R, White PCL, Hutchings MR, Kao RR. Risk factors for bovine Tuberculosis at the national level in Great Britain. *BMC Vet Res* (2012) 8(1):51. doi: 10.1186/1746-6148-8-51
79. Cassidy A. Vermin, victims and disease: UK framings of badgers in and beyond the bovine TB controversy. *Sociol Ruralis* (2012) 52(2):192–214. doi: 10.1111/j.1467-9523.2012.00562.x
80. Enticott G. Public attitudes to badger culling to control bovine tuberculosis in rural Wales. *European Journal of Wildlife Research* (2015) 61(3):387–98. doi: 10.1007/s10344-015-0905-9
81. Dandy N, Ballantyne S, Moseley D, Gill R, Peace A, Quine C. Preferences for wildlife management methods among the peri-urban public in Scotland. *European Journal of Wildlife Research* (2011) 57(6):1213–21. doi: 10.1007/s10344-011-0534-x
82. Andersone Žanete, Ozolinš J. Public perception of large carnivores in Latvia. *Ursus* (2004) 15(2):181–7. doi: 10.2192/1537-6176(2004)015<0181:PPOLC I>2.0.CO;2
83. Kaltenborn BP, Andersen O, Linnell JDC. Is hunting large carnivores different from hunting ungulates? Some judgments made by Norwegian hunters. *J Nat Conserv* (2013) 21(5):326–33. doi: 10.1016/j.jnc.2013.05.004
84. Proulx G, Abramov AV, Adams I, Jennings A, Khorozyan I, Rosalino LM, et al. World distribution and status of badgers–A review. In: *Badgers: Systematics, Biology, Conservation and Research Techniques*. Sherwood Park, Alberta, Canada: Alpha Wildlife Publications (2016). p. 31–116.
85. DVR - German Hunting Association Ev. Association of german national hunting associations for the protection of Wild, H.a.N.D.J. (2017). Available at: http://www.jagdverband.de/node/3304
86. Kauhala K, Holmala K. Landscape features, home-range size and density of northern badgers (*Meles meles*). *Ann Zool Fennici* (2011) 48(4):221–32. doi: 10.5735/086.048.0403
87. Finland OSO. *"Hunting 2013"*. Helsinki: Finnish Game and Fisheries Research Institute (2014).
88. Kauhala K, Kowalczyk R. "The raccoon dog (Nyctereutes procyonoides) in the community of medium-sized carnivores in Europe: its adaptations, impact on native fauna and management of the population". In: Álvares FI, Mata GE, editors. *Carnivores: Species, Conservation, and Management*. (2012). p. 49–77.
89. Fédération Départementale des Chasseurs du Finistère. Blaireau Euopeen, gestion et regulation. *FDC* (2014) 29:1–10.
90. Zanella G, Bar-Hen A, Boschiroli M-L, Hars J, Moutou F, Garin-Bastuji B, et al. Modelling transmission of bovine tuberculosis in red deer and wild boar in Normandy, France. *Zoonoses Public Health* (2012) 59(Suppl 2):170–8. doi: 10.1111/j.1863-2378.2011.01453.x
91. Reason P, Harris S, Cresswell P. Estimating the impact of past persecution and habitat changes on the numbers of Badgers Meles meles in Britain. *Mamm Rev* (1993) 23(1):1–15. doi: 10.1111/j.1365-2907.1993.tb00413.x
92. Griffiths DH, Thomas HJ. The status of the badger in Europe. *Mam Rev* (1993) 23:17–58.
93. O'Connor CM, Haydon DT, Kao RR. An ecological and comparative perspective on the control of bovine tuberculosis in Great Britain and the Republic of Ireland. *Prev Vet Med* (2012) 104(3-4):185–97. doi: 10.1016/j.prevetmed.2011.11.010
94. Society for General Microbiology (SGM). *Independent Overview of Bovine Tuberculosis Research in the United Kingdom*. London: DEFRA (2008).
95. Byrne AW, Kenny K, Fogarty U, O'Keeffe JJ, More SJ, Mcgrath G, et al. Spatial and temporal analyses of metrics of tuberculosis infection in badgers (Meles meles) from the Republic of Ireland: Trends in apparent prevalence. *Prev Vet Med* (2015) 122(3):345–54. doi: 10.1016/j.prevetmed.2015.10.013
96. Delahay RJ, Langton S, Smith GC, Clifton-Hadley RS, Cheeseman CL. The spatio-temporal distribution of Mycobacterium bovis (bovine tuberculosis) infection in a high-density badger population. *J Anim Ecol* (2000) 69(3):428–41. doi: 10.1046/j.1365-2656.2000.00406.x
97. Crawshaw TR, Griffiths IB, Clifton-Hadley RS. Comparison of a standard and a detailed postmortem protocol for detecting Mycobacterium bovis in badgers. *Vet Rec* (2008) 163(16):473–7. doi: 10.1136/vr.163.16.473
98. Murphy D, Gormley E, Costello E, O'Meara D, Corner LAL. The prevalence and distribution of Mycobacterium bovis infection in European badgers (Meles meles) as determined by enhanced post mortem examination and bacteriological culture. *Res Vet Sci* (2010) 88(1):1–5. doi: 10.1016/j.rvsc.2009.05.020
99. Jenkins HE, Woodroffe R, Donnelly CA. The effects of annual widespread badger culls on cattle tuberculosis following the cessation of culling. *International Journal of Infectious Diseases* (2008) 12(5):457–65. doi: 10.1016/j.ijid.2008.04.001
100. Abernethy DA, Walton E, Menzies F, Coucier E, Robinson P. "Mycobacterium bovis surveillance in European badgers (Meles meles) killed by vehicles in Northern Ireland: an epidemiological evaluation". *International Conference on Animal Health Surveillance (ICAHS)*; Lyon, France (2011).
101. Courcier EA, Menzies FD, Strain SAJ, Skuce RA, Robinson PA, Patterson IAP, et al. Monitoring *Mycobacterium bovis* in Eurasian badgers (*Meles meles*) killed by vehicles in Northern Ireland between 1998 and 2011. *Vet Rec* (2018) 182(9):259. doi: 10.1136/vr.103934
102. Woodroffe R, Donnelly CA, Cox DR, Gilks P, Jenkins HE, Johnston WT, et al. Bovine tuberculosis in cattle and badgers in localized culling areas. *J Wildl Dis* (2009) 45(1):128–43. doi: 10.7589/0090-3558-45.1.128
103. Corner LAL, O'Meara D, Costello E, Lesellier S, Gormley E. The distribution of Mycobacterium bovis infection in naturally infected badgers. *Vet J* (2012) 194(2):166–72. doi: 10.1016/j.tvjl.2012.03.013
104. Drewe JA, Tomlinson AJ, Walker NJ, Delahay RJ. Diagnostic accuracy and optimal use of three tests for tuberculosis in live badgers. *PLoS One* (2010) 5(6):e11196. doi: 10.1371/journal.pone.0011196
105. Murphy D, Gormley E, Collins DM, Mcgrath G, Sovsic E, Costello E, et al. Tuberculosis in cattle herds are sentinels for Mycobacterium bovis infection in European badgers (Meles meles): the Irish Greenfield Study. *Vet Microbiol* (2011) 151(1-2):120–5. doi: 10.1016/j.vetmic.2011.02.034
106. Beggs CB, Noakes CJ, Sleigh PA, Fletcher LA, Siddiqi K. The transmission of tuberculosis in confined spaces: an analytical review of alternative epidemiological models. *Int J Tuberc Lung Dis* (2003) 7:1015–26.
107. Millet J-P, Moreno A, Fina L, del Baño L, Orcau A, de Olalla PG, et al. Factors that influence current tuberculosis epidemiology. *European Spine Journal* (2013) 22(Suppl 4S4):539–48. doi: 10.1007/s00586-012-2334-8
108. Hardstaff JL, Marion G, Hutchings MR, White PC. Evaluating the tuberculosis hazard posed to cattle from wildlife across Europe. *Res Vet Sci* (2014) 97:S86–S93. doi: 10.1016/j.rvsc.2013.12.002
109. Statistics, Eurostat - European Union. (2010). Available at: http://appsso.eurostat.ec.europa.eu/nui/show.do?dataset=apro_mt_lscatl&lang=en (accessed 26 Nov 2017).
110. Humblet M-F, Gilbert M, Govaerts M, Fauville-Dufaux M, Walravens K, Saegerman C. New assessment of bovine tuberculosis risk factors in Belgium based on nationwide molecular epidemiology. *J Clin Microbiol* (2010) 48(8):2802–8. doi: 10.1128/JCM.00293-10
111. Cosivi O, Grange JM, Daborn CJ, Raviglione MC, Fujikura T, Cousins D. Zoonotic tuberculosis due to Mycobacterium bovis in developing countries. *Emerg Infect Dis* (1998) 4(1):59–70. doi: 10.3201/eid0401.980108
112. Humblet M-F, Boschiroli ML, Saegerman C. Classification of worldwide bovine tuberculosis risk factors in cattle: a stratified approach. *Vet Res* (2009) 40(5):50. doi: 10.1051/vetres/2009033
113. Brooks-Pollock E, Keeling M. Herd size and bovine tuberculosis persistence in cattle farms in Great Britain. *Prev Vet Med* (2009) 92(4):360–5. doi: 10.1016/j.prevetmed.2009.08.022

114. Mee JF. Temporal trends in reproductive performance in Irish dairy herds and associated risk factors. *Ir Vet J* (2004) 57(3):158. doi: 10.1186/2046-0481-57-3-158
115. Acevedo P, Romero B, Vicente J, Caracappa S, Galluzzo P, Marineo S, et al. Tuberculosis Epidemiology in Islands: Insularity, Hosts and Trade. *PLoS One* (2013) 8(7):e71074. doi: 10.1371/journal.pone.0071074
116. Gilbert M, Mitchell A, Bourn D, Mawdsley J, Clifton-Hadley R, Wint W. Cattle movements and bovine tuberculosis in Great Britain. *Nature* (2005) 435(7041):491–6. doi: 10.1038/nature03548
117. Ashe S, More SJ, O'Keeffe J, White P, Mcgrath G, Aznar I. Survival and dispersal of a defined cohort of Irish cattle. *Ir Vet J* (2009) 62(1):44. doi: 10.1186/2046-0481-62-1-44
118. Bord bia. Cattle live exports – graphs (2017). Available at: https://www.bordbia.ie/industry/farmers/pricetracking/cattle/pages/liveexports.aspx
119. Christley RM, Robinson SE, Lysons R, French NP. Network analysis of cattle movement in Great Britain. In: *Proceedings of the Society of Veterinary Epidemiology and Preventive Medicine*. Scotland. (2005).
120. Brown E, Marshall AH, Mitchell H, Byrne AW. "Analysing cattle movements in Northern Ireland using social network analysis". In: Brennan M, Lindberg A, editors. *Society for Veterinary Epidemiology and Preventive Medicine – Proceedings*. Tallinn, Estonia: Society for Veterinary Epidemiology and Preventive Medicine (2018). p. 21–3.
121. Green DM, Kiss IZ, Mitchell AP, Kao RR. Estimates for local and movement-based transmission of bovine tuberculosis in British cattle. *Proceedings of the Royal Society B: Biological Sciences* (2008) 275(1638):1001–5. doi: 10.1098/rspb.2007.1601
122. Skuce RA, Allen AR, Mcdowell SW. Herd-level risk factors for bovine tuberculosis: a literature review. *Vet Med Int* (2012) 2012(2):621210–. doi: 10.1155/2012/621210
123. Robinson SE, Christley RM. Exploring the role of auction markets in cattle movements within Great Britain. *Prev Vet Med* (2007) 81(1-3):21–37. doi: 10.1016/j.prevetmed.2007.04.011
124. Smith NH, Berg S, Dale J, Allen A, Rodriguez S, Romero B, et al. European 1: a globally important clonal complex of Mycobacterium bovis. *Infection, Genetics and Evolution* (2011) 11(6):1340–51. doi: 10.1016/j.meegid.2011.04.027
125. Gagneux S, Small PM. Global phylogeography of Mycobacterium tuberculosis and implications for tuberculosis product development. *Lancet Infect Dis* (2007) 7(5):328–37. doi: 10.1016/S1473-3099(07)70108-1
126. Gagneux S, Small PM. "Molecular evolution of mycobacteria,". In: Kaufmann SH, Rubin E, editors. *Handbook of tuberculosis*. New Jersey, United States: Wiley (2008).
127. Gagneux S. Genetic diversity in Mycobacterium tuberculosis. *Curr Top Microbiol Immunol* (2013) 374:1–25. doi: 10.1007/82_2013_329
128. Warner DF, Mizrahi V. Translating genomics research into control of tuberculosis: lessons learned and future prospects. *Genome Biol* (2014) 15(11):514. doi: 10.1186/s13059-014-0514-z
129. Caws M, Thwaites G, Dunstan S, Hawn TR, Thi Ngoc Lan N, Thuong NTT, et al. The influence of host and bacterial genotype on the development of disseminated disease with Mycobacterium tuberculosis. *PLoS Pathog* (2008) 4(3):e1000034. doi: 10.1371/journal.ppat.1000034
130. Luo T, Comas I, Luo D, Lu B, Wu J, Wei L, et al. Southern East Asian origin and coexpansion of *Mycobacterium tuberculosis* Beijing family with Han Chinese. *Proc Natl Acad Sci USA* (2015) 112(26):8136–41. doi: 10.1073/pnas.1424063112
131. Smith NH, Gordon SV, de La Rua-Domenech R, Clifton-Hadley RS, Hewinson RG. Bottlenecks and broomsticks: the molecular evolution of Mycobacterium bovis. *Nat Rev Microbiol* (2006) 4(9):670–81. doi: 10.1038/nrmicro1472
132. Allen AR, Dale J, Mccormick C, Mallon TR, Costello E, Gordon SV, et al. The phylogeny and population structure of Mycobacterium bovis in the British Isles. *Infection, Genetics and Evolution* (2013) 20:8–15. doi: 10.1016/j.meegid.2013.08.003
133. Smith NH, Dale J, Inwald J, Palmer S, Gordon SV, Hewinson RG, et al. The population structure of Mycobacterium bovis in Great Britain: Clonal expansion. *Proc Natl Acad Sci USA* (2003) 100(25):15271–5. doi: 10.1073/pnas.2036554100
134. Allen AR. One bacillus to rule them all? – Investigating broad range host adaptation in Mycobacterium bovis. *Infection, Genetics and Evolution* (2017) 53:68–76. doi: 10.1016/j.meegid.2017.04.018
135. Berg S, Smith NH. Why doesn't bovine tuberculosis transmit between humans? *Trends Microbiol* (2014) 22(10):552–3. doi: 10.1016/j.tim.2014.08.007
136. Behr MA, Gordon SV. Why doesn't Mycobacterium tuberculosis spread in animals? *Trends Microbiol* (2015) 23(1):1–2. doi: 10.1016/j.tim.2014.11.001
137. Gonzalo-Asensio J, Malaga W, Pawlik A, Astarie-Dequeker C, Passemar C, Moreau F, et al. Evolutionary history of tuberculosis shaped by conserved mutations in the PhoPR virulence regulator. *Proc Natl Acad Sci USA* (2014) 111(31):11491–6. doi: 10.1073/pnas.1406693111
138. Rodríguez S, Romero B, Bezos J, de Juan L, Álvarez J, Castellanos E, et al. High spoligotype diversity within a *Mycobacterium bovis* population: clues to understanding the demography of the pathogen in Europe. *Vet Microbiol* (2010) 141(1-2):89–95. doi: 10.1016/j.vetmic.2009.08.007
139. Cunha MV, Matos F, Canto A, Albuquerque T, Alberto JR, Aranha JM, et al. Implications and challenges of tuberculosis in wildlife ungulates in Portugal: a molecular epidemiology perspective. *Res Vet Sci* (2012) 92(2):225–35. doi: 10.1016/j.rvsc.2011.03.009
140. Hauer A, de Cruz K, Cochard T, Godreuil S, Karoui C, Henault S, et al. Genetic evolution of *Mycobacterium bovis* causing tuberculosis in livestock and wildlife in France since 1978. *PLoS One* (2015) 10(2):e0117103. doi: 10.1371/journal.pone.0117103
141. Wright DM, Allen AR, Mallon TR, Mcdowell SWJ, Bishop SC, Glass EJ, et al. Detectability of bovine TB using the tuberculin skin test does not vary significantly according to pathogen genotype within Northern Ireland. *Infection, Genetics and Evolution* (2013) 19:15–22. doi: 10.1016/j.meegid.2013.05.011
142. Wright DM, Allen AR, Mallon TR, Mcdowell SWJ, Bishop SC, Glass EJ, et al. Field-isolated genotypes of Mycobacterium bovis vary in virulence and influence case pathology but do not affect outbreak size. *PLoS One* (2013) 8(9):e74503. doi: 10.1371/journal.pone.0074503
143. Milne G, Graham J, Allen A, Lahuerta-Marin A, McCormick C, Presho E et al. "Herd characteristics, wildlife risk and bacterial strain genotypes in persistent breakdowns of bovine tuberculosis in Northern Irish cattle herds". In: Brennan M, Lindberg A, editors. *Society for Veterinary Epidemiology and Preventive Medicine – Proceedings*. Tallinn, Estonia: Society for Veterinary Epidemiology and Preventive Medicine (2018). p. 21–3.
144. Osborne LC, Monticelli LA, Nice TJ, Sutherland TE, Siracusa MC, Hepworth MR, et al. Coinfection. Virus-helminth coinfection reveals a microbiota-independent mechanism of immunomodulation. *Science* (2014) 345(6196):578–82. doi: 10.1126/science.1256942
145. Woolhouse MEJ, Thumbi SM, Jennings A, Chase-Topping M, Callaby R, Kiara H, et al. Co-infections determine patterns of mortality in a population exposed to parasite infection. *Sci Adv* (2015) 1(2):e1400026. doi: 10.1126/sciadv.1400026
146. Flynn RJ, Mannion C, Golden O, Hacariz O, Mulcahy G. Experimental Fasciola hepatica infection alters responses to tests used for diagnosis of bovine tuberculosis. *Infect Immun* (2007) 75(3):1373–81. doi: 10.1128/IAI.01445-06
147. Flynn RJ, Mulcahy G, Welsh M, Cassidy JP, Corbett D, Milligan C, et al. Co-Infection of cattle with *Fasciola hepatica* and *Mycobacterium bovis*-immunological consequences. *Transbound Emerg Dis* (2009) 56(6-7):269–74. doi: 10.1111/j.1865-1682.2009.01075.x
148. Claridge J, Diggle P, Mccann CM, Mulcahy G, Flynn R, Mcnair J, et al. Fasciola hepatica is associated with the failure to detect bovine tuberculosis in dairy cattle. *Nat Commun* (2012) 3(1):853. doi: 10.1038/ncomms1840
149. Charleston B, Hope JC, Carr BV, Howard CJ. Masking of two in vitro immunological assays for Mycobacterium bovis (BCG) in calves acutely infected with non-qctopathic bovine viral diarrhoea virus. *Vet Rec* (2001) 149(16):481–4. doi: 10.1136/vr.149.16.481
150. Kao RR, Gravenor MB, Charleston B, Hope JC, Martin M, Howard CJ. *Mycobacterium bovis* shedding patterns from experimentally infected calves and the effect of concurrent infection with bovine viral diarrhoea virus. *J R Soc Interface* (2007) 4(14):545–51. doi: 10.1098/rsif.2006.0190
151. Byrne AW, Graham J, Brown C, Donaghy A, Guelbenzu-Gonzalo M, Mcnair J, et al. Bovine tuberculosis visible lesions in cattle culled during herd breakdowns: the effects of individual characteristics, trade movement and co-infection. *BMC Vet Res* (2017) 13(1):400. doi: 10.1186/s12917-017-1321-z
152. Waters WR, Nonnecke BJ, Palmer MV, Robbe-Austermann S, Bannantine JP, Stabel JR, et al. Use of recombinant ESAT-6:CFP-10 fusion protein for differentiation of infections of cattle by Mycobacterium bovis and by M. avium

subsp. avium and M. avium subsp. paratuberculosis. *Clinical and Vaccine Immunology* (2004) 11(4):729–35. doi: 10.1128/CDLI.11.4.729-735.2004

153. Álvarez J, de Juan L, Bezos J, Romero B, Sáez JL, Gordejo FJR, Reviriego Gordejo FJ, et al. Interference of paratuberculosis with the diagnosis of tuberculosis in a goat flock with a natural mixed infection. *Vet Microbiol* (2008) 128(1-2):72–80. doi: 10.1016/j.vetmic.2007.08.034
154. Cooney R, Kazda J, Quinn J, Cook B, Muller K, Monaghan M. Environmental mycobacteria in Ireland as a source of non-specific sensitisation to tuberculins. *Ir Vet J* (1997) 50:370–3.
155. Hughes MS, Ball NW, Mccarroll J, Erskine M, Taylor MJ, Pollock JM, et al. Molecular analyses of mycobacteria other than the M. tuberculosis complex isolated from Northern Ireland cattle. *Vet Microbiol* (2005) 108(1-2):101–12. doi: 10.1016/j.vetmic.2005.03.001
156. Kazda J, Pavlik I, Falkinham Iii JO, Hruska K. *The Ecology of Mycobacteria: Impact on Animal's and Human's Health*. Berlin, Germany: Springer-Verlag (2010).
157. Montanarella L, Jones RJA, Hiederer R. The distribution of peatland in Europe. *Mires and Peat* (2006) 1:1.
158. Mcaloon CG, Doherty ML, Whyte P, O'Grady L, More SJ, Messam LLM, et al. Bayesian estimation of prevalence of paratuberculosis in dairy herds enrolled in a voluntary Johne's Disease Control Programme in Ireland. *Prev Vet Med* (2016) 128:95–100. doi: 10.1016/j.prevetmed.2016.04.014
159. Woodbine KA, Schukken YH, Green LE, Ramirez-Villaescusa A, Mason S, Moore SJ, et al. Seroprevalence and epidemiological characteristics of Mycobacterium avium subsp. paratuberculosis on 114 cattle farms in south west England. *Prev Vet Med* (2009) 89(1-2):102–9. doi: 10.1016/j.prevetmed.2009.02.005
160. Kennedy AE, Byrne N, O'Mahony J, Sayers RG. Investigations and implications of associations between mycobacterial purified protein derivative hypersensitivity and MAP-antibody ELISA in Irish dairy cows. *Res Vet Sci* (2017) 115:13–16. doi: 10.1016/j.rvsc.2017.01.018
161. Byrne AW, Graham J, Brown C, Donaghy A, Guelbenzu-Gonzalo M, Mcnair J, et al. Modelling the variation in skin-test tuberculin reactions, post-mortem lesion counts and case pathology in tuberculosis-exposed cattle: Effects of animal characteristics, histories and co-infection. *Transbound Emerg Dis* (2018) 65(3):844–58. doi: 10.1111/tbed.12814
162. Aranaz A, de Juan L, Bezos J, Álvarez J, Romero B, Lozano F, et al. Assessment of diagnostic tools for eradication of bovine tuberculosis in cattle co-infected with *Mycobacterium bovis* and *M. avium* subsp. *paratuberculosis*. *Vet Res* (2006) 37(4):593–606. doi: 10.1051/vetres:2006021
163. Broughan JM, Durr P, Clifton-Hadley R, Colloff A, Goodchild T, Sayers R et al "Bovine tuberculosis and Fasciola hepatica infection". In: *Society for Veterinary Epidemiology and Preventive Medicine (SVEPM)*. (2018).
164. Selemetas N, de Waal T. Detection of major climatic and environmental predictors of liver fluke exposure risk in Ireland using spatial cluster analysis. *Vet Parasitol* (2015) 209(3-4):242–53. doi: 10.1016/j.vetpar.2015.02.029
165. Salimi-Bejestani MR, Daniel RG, Felstead SM, Cripps PJ, Mahmoody H, Williams DJL. Prevalence of Fasciola hepatica in dairy herds in England and Wales measured with an ELISA applied to bulk-tank milk. *Vet Rec* (2005) 156(23):729–31. doi: 10.1136/vr.156.23.729
166. Byrne AW, Mcbride S, Lahuerta-Marin A, Guelbenzu M, Mcnair J, Skuce RA, et al. Liver fluke (Fasciola hepatica) infection in cattle in Northern Ireland: a large-scale epidemiological investigation utilising surveillance data. *Parasit Vectors* (2016) 9(1):209. doi: 10.1186/s13071-016-1489-2
167. Murphy TM, Fahy KN, Mcauliffe A, Forbes AB, Clegg TA, O'Brien DJ. A study of helminth parasites in culled cows from Ireland. *Prev Vet Med* (2006) 76(1-2):1–10. doi: 10.1016/j.prevetmed.2006.04.005
168. Garza-Cuartero L, O'Sullivan J, Blanco A, Mcnair J, Welsh M, Flynn RJ, et al. *Fasciola hepatica* infection reduces *Mycobacterium bovis* burden and mycobacterial uptake and suppresses the pro-inflammatory response. *Parasite Immunol* (2016) 38(7):387–402. doi: 10.1111/pim.12326
169. Caminade C, van Dijk J, Baylis M, Williams D. Modelling recent and future climatic suitability for fasciolosis in Europe. *Geospat Health* (2015) 9(2):301–8. doi: 10.4081/gh.2015.352
170. Ducheyne E, Charlier J, Vercruysse J, Rinaldi L, Biggeri A, Demeler J, et al. Modelling the spatial distribution of Fasciola hepatica in dairy cattle in Europe. *Geospat Health* (2015) 9(2):261–70. doi: 10.4081/gh.2015.348
171. Rinaldi L, Biggeri A, Musella V, de Waal T, Hertzberg H, Mavrot F, et al. Sheep and Fasciola hepatica in Europe: the GLOWORM experience. *Geospat Health* (2015) 9(2):309–17. doi: 10.4081/gh.2015.353
172. Selemetas N, Phelan P, O'Kiely P, Waal T, Td W. Weather and soil type affect incidence of fasciolosis in dairy cow herds. *Vet Rec* (2014) 175(15):371. doi: 10.1136/vr.102437
173. Mccann CM, Baylis M, Williams DJL. The development of linear regression models using environmental variables to explain the spatial distribution of Fasciola hepatica infection in dairy herds in England and Wales. *Int J Parasitol* (2010) 40(9):1021–8. doi: 10.1016/j.ijpara.2010.02.009
174. Fox NJ, White PCL, Mcclean CJ, Marion G, Evans A, Hutchings MR. Predicting impacts of climate change on Fasciola hepatica risk. *PLoS One* (2011) 6(1):e16126. doi: 10.1371/journal.pone.0016126
175. Corner LAL. The role of wild animal populations in the epidemiology of tuberculosis in domestic animals: how to assess the risk. *Vet Microbiol* (2006) 112(2-4):303–12. doi: 10.1016/j.vetmic.2005.11.015
176. Böhm M, Hutchings MR, White PC. Contact networks in a wildlife-livestock host community: identifying high-risk individuals in the transmission of bovine TB among badgers and cattle. *PLoS One* (2009) 4(4):e5016. doi: 10.1371/journal.pone.0005016
177. Drewe JA, O'Connor HM, Weber N, Mcdonald RA, Delahay RJ. Patterns of direct and indirect contact between cattle and badgers naturally infected with tuberculosis. *Epidemiol Infect* (2013) 141(07):1467–75. doi: 10.1017/S0950268813000691
178. O'Mahony DT. Badger (Meles meles) contact metrics in a medium-density population. *Mammalian Biology - Zeitschrift für Säugetierkunde* (2015) 80(6):484–90. doi: 10.1016/j.mambio.2015.07.002
179. Woodroffe R, Donnelly CA, Ham C, Jackson SYB, Moyes K, Chapman K, et al. Badgers prefer cattle pasture but avoid cattle: implications for bovine tuberculosis control. *Ecol Lett* (2016) 19(10):1201–8. doi: 10.1111/ele.12654
180. Santos N, Almeida V, Gortázar C, Correia-Neves M. Patterns of Mycobacterium tuberculosis-complex excretion and characterization of super-shedders in naturally-infected wild boar and red deer. *Vet Res* (2015) 46(1):129. doi: 10.1186/s13567-015-0270-4
181. Payne A, Chappa S, Hars J, Dufour B, Gilot-Fromont E. Wildlife visits to farm facilities assessed by camera traps in a bovine tuberculosis-infected area in France. *European Journal of Wildlife Research* (2016) 62(1):33–42. doi: 10.1007/s10344-015-0970-0
182. Barbier E, Boschiroli ML, Gueneau E, Rochelet M, Payne A, de Cruz K, et al. First molecular detection of *Mycobacterium bovis* in environmental samples from a French region with endemic bovine tuberculosis. *J Appl Microbiol* (2016) 120(5):1193–207. doi: 10.1111/jam.13090
183. Gallagher J, Muirhead R, Burn K. Tuberculosis in wild badgers (Meles meles) in Gloucestershire: pathology. *Vet Rec* (1976) 98(1):9–14. doi: 10.1136/vr.98.1.9
184. Gallagher J, Nelson J. Cause of ill health and natural death in badgers in Gloucestershire. *Vet Rec* (1979) 105(24):546–51.
185. Jenkins HE, Morrison WI, Cox DR, Donnelly CA, Johnston WT, Bourne FJ, et al. The prevalence, distribution and severity of detectable pathological lesions in badgers naturally infected with Mycobacterium bovis. *Epidemiol Infect* (2008) 136(10):1350–61. doi: 10.1017/S0950268807009909
186. MAFF. *"Bovine TB in badgers. Third report by Ministry of Agriculture, Fisheries and Food"*. London: MAFF (1979).
187. Gallagher J. Doctoral Thesis - The natural history of spontaneous TB in wild badgers. Doctor of Veterinary Medicine Thesis. University of London (1988).
188. Hutchings MR, Service KM, Harris S. Defecation and urination patterns of badgers Meles meles at low density in south west England. *Acta Theriol* (2001) 46:87–96. doi: 10.4098/AT.arch.01-10
189. Angelakis E, Raoult D. Q fever. *Vet Microbiol* (2010) 140(3-4):297–309. doi: 10.1016/j.vetmic.2009.07.016
190. Eisenberg SWF, Nielen M, Santema W, Houwers DJ, Heederik D, Koets AP. Detection of spatial and temporal spread of Mycobacterium avium subsp. paratuberculosis in the environment of a cattle farm through bio-aerosols. *Vet Microbiol* (2010) 143(2-4):284–92. doi: 10.1016/j.vetmic.2009.11.033
191. Bouzid F, Brégeon F, Lepidi H, Donoghue HD, Minnikin DE, Drancourt M. Ready experimental translocation of mycobacterium canettii yields pulmonary tuberculosis. *Infect Immun* (2017) 85(12):e00507-17. doi: 10.1128/IAI.00507-17

192. Kaneene JB, Hattey JA, Bolin CA, Averill J, Miller R. Survivability of *Mycobacterium bovis* on salt and salt-mineral blocks fed to cattle. *Am J Vet Res* (2017) 78(1):57–62. doi: 10.2460/ajvr.78.1.57
193. Maddock EC. Studies on the survival time of the bovine tubercle bacillus in soil, soil and dung, in dung and on grass, with experiments on the preliminary treatment of infected organic matter and the cultivation of the organism. *J Hyg* (1933) 33(1):103–17. doi: 10.1017/S002217240001843X
194. Courtenay O, Reilly LA, Sweeney FP, Hibberd V, Bryan S, Ul-Hassan A, et al. Is Mycobacterium bovis in the environment important for the persistence of bovine tuberculosis? *Biol Lett* (2006) 2(3):460–2. doi: 10.1098/rsbl.2006.0468
195. Barbier E, Rochelet M, Gal L, Boschiroli ML, Hartmann A. Impact of temperature and soil type on Mycobacterium bovis survival in the environment. *PLoS One* (2017) 12(4):e0176315. doi: 10.1371/journal.pone.0176315
196. Winder CL, Gordon SV, Dale J, Hewinson RG, Goodacre R. Metabolic fingerprints of Mycobacterium bovis cluster with molecular type: implications for genotype-phenotype links. *Microbiology* (2006) 152(Pt 9):2757–65. doi: 10.1099/mic.0.28986-0
197. Jankute M, Nataraj V, Lee OY-C, Wu HHT, Ridell M, Garton NJ, et al. The role of hydrophobicity in tuberculosis evolution and pathogenicity. *Sci Rep* (2017) 7(1):1315. doi: 10.1038/s41598-017-01501-0
198. Peel MC, Finlayson BL, Mcmahon TA. Updated world map of the Köppen-Geiger climate classification. *Hydrol Earth Syst Sci* (2007) 11(5):1633–44. doi: 10.5194/hess-11-1633-2007
199. Dick RS. Frequency patterns of arid, semi arid and humid climates in Queensland. *Capricornia* (1964) 1:21–30.
200. Mayes J, Wheeler D. Regional weather and climates of the British Isles - Part 1: Introduction. *Weather* (2013) 68(1):3–8. doi: 10.1002/wea.2041
201. Met Office. National Meteorological Library and Archive Fact sheet 4 — Climate of the British Isles. UK Met Office (2011). Available at: https://www.metoffice.gov.uk/binaries/content/assets/mohippo/pdf/library/factsheets/metlib_13_001_factsheet_4.compressed.pdf (accessed 26 Nov 2017).
202. United Nations. UN sunshine statistics by country (2017). Available at: http://data.un.org/Data.aspx?d=CLINO&f=ElementCode%3a15#f_1 (Accessed November 26, 2017).
203. World Bank. Annual precipitation data by country (2017). Available at: https://data.worldbank.org/indicator/AG.LND.PRCP.MM?end=2014&start=2014&view=map (Accessed November 26, 2017).
204. Sweeney J, Albanito F, Brereton A, Caffarra A, Charlton R, Donnelly A, et al. *Climate Change - refining the impacts for Ireland.* Wexford: E.P. Agency (2008).
205. Murphy J, Sexton D, Jenkins G, Boorman P, Booth B, Brown K, et al. UK Climate Projections science report: Climate change projections. Exeter, UK: Meteorological Office Hadley Centre (2010). 192 p.
206. CLIMATE CHANGE –Refining the Impacts for Ireland. (2008). Available at: www.epa.ie (21st March 2017).
207. Wint GR, Robinson TP, Bourn DM, Durr PA, Hay SI, Randolph SE, et al. Mapping bovine tuberculosis in Great Britain using environmental data. *Trends Microbiol* (2002) 10(10):441–4. doi: 10.1016/S0966-842X(02)02444-7
208. Pfeiffer DU, Robinson TP, Stevenson M, Stevens KB, Rogers DJ, Clements ACA, et al. *Spatial analysis in epidemiology*. Oxford: Oxford University Press (2008).
209. Jin R, Good M, More SJ, Sweeney C, Mcgrath G, Kelly GE. An association between rainfall and bovine TB in Wicklow, Ireland. *Vet Rec* (2013) 173(18):452.1–452. doi: 10.1136/vr.101777
210. Macdonald DW, Newman C, Buesching CD, Nouvellet P. Are badgers '*Under The Weather*'? Direct and indirect impacts of climate variation on European badger (*Meles meles*) population dynamics. *Glob Chang Biol* (2010) 66:2913–22. doi: 10.1111/j.1365-2486.2010.02208.x
211. Matz C, Kjelleberg S. Off the hook – how bacteria survive protozoan grazing. *Trends Microbiol* (2005) 13(7):302–7. doi: 10.1016/j.tim.2005.05.009
212. Rhodes SG, de Leij FAAM, Dale JW. Protozoa as an environmental reservoir of bovine tuberculosis. *Trends Microbiol* (2007) 15(8):338–9. doi: 10.1016/j.tim.2007.06.001
213. Thomas V, Mcdonnell G. Relationship between mycobacteria and amoebae: ecological and epidemiological concerns. *Lett Appl Microbiol* (2007) 45(4):349–57. doi: 10.1111/j.1472-765X.2007.02206.x
214. Toft C, Andersson SGE. Evolutionary microbial genomics: insights into bacterial host adaptation. *Nat Rev Genet* (2010) 11(7):465–75. doi: 10.1038/nrg2798
215. Mardare C, Delahay RJ, Dale JW. Environmental amoebae do not support the long-term survival of virulent mycobacteria. *J Appl Microbiol* (2013) 114(5):1388–94. doi: 10.1111/jam.12166
216. Sanchez-Hidalgo A, Obregón-Henao A, Wheat WH, Jackson M, Gonzalez-Juarrero M. *Mycobacterium bovis* hosted by free-living-amoebae permits their long-term persistence survival outside of host mammalian cells and remain capable of transmitting disease to mice. *Environ Microbiol* (2017) 19(10):4010–21. doi: 10.1111/1462-2920.13810
217. Barbier E, Chantemesse B, Rochelet M, Fayolle L, Bollache L, Boschiroli ML, et al. Rapid dissemination of Mycobacterium bovis from cattle dung to soil by the earthworm Lumbricus terrestris. *Vet Microbiol* (2016) 186:1–7. doi: 10.1016/j.vetmic.2016.01.025
218. Rutgers M, Orgiazzi A, Gardi C, Römbke J, Jänsch S, Keith AM, et al. Mapping earthworm communities in Europe. *Appl Soil Ecol* (2016) 97:98–111. doi: 10.1016/j.apsoil.2015.08.015
219. Kruuk H, Parish T. Feeding specialization of the European badger Meles meles in Scotland. *J Anim Ecol* (1981) 50(3):773–88. doi: 10.2307/4136
220. Cleary GP, Corner LAL, O'Keeffe J, Marples NM. The diet of the badger Meles meles in the Republic of Ireland. *Mammalian Biology - Zeitschrift für Säugetierkunde* (2009) 74(6):438–47. doi: 10.1016/j.mambio.2009.07.003
221. Rainey E, Butler A, Bierman S, Roberts A. *Scottish badgers and Biomathematics and Statistics Scotland. "Scottish Badger Distribution Survey 2006-2009".* (2009).
222. Lara-Romero C, Virgós E, Revilla E. Sett density as an estimator of population density in the European badger Meles meles. *Mamm Rev* (2012) 42(1):78–84. doi: 10.1111/j.1365-2907.2011.00194.x
223. Delahay RJ, Walker N, Smith GS, Wilkinson D, Clifton-Hadley RS, Cheeseman CL, et al. Long-term temporal trends and estimated transmission rates for Mycobacterium bovis infection in an undisturbed high-density badger (Meles meles) population. *Epidemiol Infect* (2013) 141(07):1445–56. doi: 10.1017/S0950268813000721
224. Doyle LP, Gordon AW, Abernethy DA, Stevens K. Bovine tuberculosis in Northern Ireland: risk factors associated with time from post-outbreak test to subsequent herd breakdown. *Prev Vet Med* (2014) 116(1-2):47–55. doi: 10.1016/j.prevetmed.2014.06.010
225. Gates MC, Volkova VV, Woolhouse MEJ. Risk factors for bovine tuberculosis in low incidence regions related to the movements of cattle. *BMC Vet Res* (2013) 9(1):225. doi: 10.1186/1746-6148-9-225
226. Gates MC, Volkova VV, Woolhouse MEJ. Impact of changes in cattle movement regulations on the risks of bovine tuberculosis for Scottish farms. *Prev Vet Med* (2013) 108(2-3):125–36. doi: 10.1016/j.prevetmed.2012.07.016
227. Brunton LA, Nicholson R, Ashton A, Alexander N, Wint W, Enticott G, et al. A novel approach to mapping and calculating the rate of spread of endemic bovine tuberculosis in England and Wales. *Spat Spatiotemporal Epidemiol* (2015) 13:41–50. doi: 10.1016/j.sste.2015.04.002
228. Cox DR, Donnelly CA, Bourne FJ, Gettinby G, Mcinerney JP, Morrison WI, et al. Simple model for tuberculosis in cattle and badgers. *Proc Natl Acad Sci U S A* (2005) 102(49):17588–93. doi: 10.1073/pnas.0509003102

6

In silico Comparison of Test-and-Cull Protocols for Bovine Tuberculosis Control

Héléna Ladreyt[1], Mathilde Saccareau[2,3], Aurélie Courcoul[3†] and Benoit Durand[3*†]

[1] French School of Veterinary Services (ENSV), Lyon, France, [2] Mathematical Modelling of Infectious Diseases Unit, Institut Pasteur, Paris, France, [3] Epidemiology Unit, Paris-Est University, Laboratory for Animal Health, French Agency for Food, Environment and Occupational Health and Safety (ANSES), Maisons-Alfort, France

***Correspondence:** Benoit Durand benoit.durand@anses.fr

† These authors have contributed equally to this work

Whole depopulation of cattle herds (WHD) confirmed infected by bovine tuberculosis (bTB) has led since the 1950s to a drop of herd incidence in France below 0.1% in 2000, justifying the current officially bTB free (OTF) status of the country. However, this protocol is expensive, ethically questionable, and difficult for breeders to accept because the number of confirmed animals in an infected herd is often very low. A test-and-cull protocol combining at least three screening sessions of the entire herd followed by the slaughter of all the non-negative animals has been used for some years. The aim of this work was to evaluate *in silico* the epidemiological effectiveness, the public costs and the acceptability to farmers of this test-and-cull protocol as well as of several ones. A stochastic compartmental model of within-herd bTB spread was used. Six test-and-cull protocols were compared: two versions of the official protocol and four alternatives with varying delays between screenings, and varying tests used. Protocols were simulated for an average French beef herd, and compared to WHD. Three key indicators were computed: the failure probability of the protocol (a failure being defined as an herd recovering its OTF status recovery while still infected, indicator of epidemiological effectiveness), its overall public cost and the percentage of farmers who would have dropped it to switch to WHD (indicator of acceptability to farmers). Failure probability ranged from 1.4 to 12.4% and was null (by definition) for WHD. The median cost varied between 2.7 and 78 K€ for the test-and-cull protocols, vs. 120 K€ for WHD. The percentage of dropout ranged from 7.8 to 22%. The optimal tradeoff between epidemiological effectiveness, public costs, and acceptability to farmers was obtained for protocols with an increased delay (6 months instead of 2 in the currently used protocol) between the last two screening sessions, with either 3 or 2 screening sessions. This study may help improving the official test-and-cull protocol applied in France under European Union regulation, by suggesting alternative protocols, very effective, cheaper, and more acceptable than WHD.

Keywords: bovine tuberculosis, dynamic modeling, cattle herd, disease control, test-and-cull protocol

INTRODUCTION

The European Commission recognizes most of the European countries officially bTB free (OTF) but the infection remains endemic in cattle herds in several parts of Europe such as Spain, Ireland, some regions of United Kingdom, and some regions of Italy (1–5). France has been OTF since 2001 (Decision 2001/26/EC), but this status, which is essential for trade, is threatened by the upsurge of the disease in cattle farms since 2004 (6).The surveillance and control of bTB in Europe focus on animal screening (in slaughterhouses and farms) and the elimination of infection in detected infected herds. The surveillance and control protocols vary according to the local epidemiological situation. In France, in areas with recent outbreaks or where wildlife is involved in bTB transmission, surveillance consists in yearly screening tests, and disease control protocols tend to be drastic. In areas where *Mycobacterium bovis* has not been detected for a long time, surveillance can be reduced to animal screening every 4 years, or can only be based on meat inspection in slaughterhouses, although screening tests are still performed each year in specific herds considered at-risk (e.g., herds producing raw milk or those identified by contact-tracing from recent outbreaks). Disease elimination protocols implemented in outbreaks have also evolved in France since the very first mandatory measures defined in the 1950s. Protocols became progressively more drastic until 1999, when whole depopulation became mandatory in herds where the infection by *M. bovis* had been confirmed (Ministerial Decree of 4 May 1999). These measures allowed an almost complete eradication of bTB in France, reducing the prevalence of 25% of herds infected in 1955 to less than 0.1% in 2001, thus justifying obtaining the officially bTB free (OTF) status (6, 7).

In this context, whole depopulation remains the recommended method of disease elimination in infected herds. In practice, however, it becomes less and less adapted to the epidemiological situation in France, where bTB prevalence remains very low (around 100 herds reported as infected per year) despite a slight increase since 2004 (6). This measure first entails significant public costs, partly due to compensations paid to farmers for all the slaughtered animals, of which only a small number are infected: the average cost for an outbreak (compensations and disinfection) was 107 k€ in 2014 (6). More globally, in 2012, of the 193 million euros dedicated to surveillance and eradication plans by the EU, more than a third was attributed to tuberculosis (8), and more than 17 million euros were spent for bTB control in 2014 in France (6). Studies are then needed to reduce bTB control costs as it is done in other countries (9). A second drawback of whole herd depopulation is that this disease elimination protocol is difficult to accept for obvious ethical reasons for farmers and welfare reasons for animals. In addition, since the within-herd prevalence of the infection is low, very few of the slaughtered animals are confirmed to be infected. Although this does not imply that negative animals are uninfected, the breeders have the impression to have unnecessarily culled their animals. This low acceptability of the protocol can lead to a real lack of effectiveness of the control strategy, which is a source of concern for the animal health authorities (10). Finally, besides cost and acceptability problems, the effectiveness of whole herd depopulation can sometimes be questioned with the recurrence of bTB in some farms after restocking (11). These factors motivated the evolution of French regulations toward a gradual reintroduction of a test-and-cull protocol. This selective slaughter of only animals reacting to a combination of tests was thus authorized under certain conditions throughout France in 2014.

Only one test-and-cull protocol is currently authorized, which has not been evaluated yet. The question arises whether it may be improved in terms of epidemiological effectiveness, public costs and acceptability to the farmer. The current test-and-cull protocol provides for three screening tests with 2 months between each. All three controls have to be consecutively negative to allow the herd regaining its OTF status. The two first screening tests associate single intradermal tuberculin skin test (SIT), gamma-interferon assay (IFN-γ), and a serology test, whereas the third one uses the single intradermal comparative cervical skin test (SICCT). In practice, in areas where the infection by atypical mycobacteria is known to be frequent in cattle, SIT may be replaced by SICCT to increase the specificity of screenings.

The aim of this work was to compare, through modeling and simulation, several test-and-cull scenarios in a bTB-infected farm, to determine the most epidemiologically effective scenario, while evaluating its public costs and its acceptability to the farmer.

MATERIALS AND METHODS

Model

The model was a stochastic compartmental model operating in monthly time steps. Only females involved in reproduction were represented, as other animals were assumed to play only a minor role in the epidemiological system, either because of their short lifespan (calves, beef cattle), or because they are very few (bulls). Each heifer or cow was represented by its age (in years) and its health state, with S (susceptible) for non-infected animals, E (latent) for infected animals that do not excrete the bacteria yet and do not have lesions, and I (infectious) for infected animals having lesions and excreting the bacteria. The dynamics of bTB

TABLE 1 | Parameters of the demographic process included in the model of within-herd bTB dynamics.

Parameter	Value*	Source
Size of the herd	141 animals	(13–15)
Maximal age of cows	15 years	(12)
Stabling period	November to March	(12)
Yearly culling rate	35%	(16)
Age of culled animals	≥ 4 years	(12)
Culling period	January to March	(12)

Values characterizing of an average French beef cattle herd.

in a cattle herd, from the *M. bovis* introduction to the elimination of infection was represented by three processes:

- The demographic process: The age structure resulted from the cull of animals, the culling rate being assumed to vary according to the month and to the age class (null for heifers, >0 for cows). The size of the herd was assumed constant and the herd closed: slaughtered animals (because of routine slaughter or due to disease control) were replaced by young animals born in the same herd.
- The infectious process: animals were assumed to be grouped into batches according to their age class, distinct batches being kept in separate buildings or on distant pastures. The transmission of *M. bovis* was thus assumed to only occur between animals of the same batch. However, because of the aging of animals, the composition of batches changed every year, and animal transfers between batches allowed *M. bovis* to spread inside the herd. *M. bovis* transmission intensity was assumed to vary according to whether the animals are housed inside a stable (high intensity of within-batch transmission) or allowed to graze (low intensity of within-batch transmission), the transmission parameter was thus assumed to vary accordingly.
- The detection and control process: it combined ante mortem tests (SIT, SICCT, IFN-γ, and serology), post mortem and confirmation tests (routine or detailed carcass inspection, PCR, bacterial culture, and histology), as well as the culling of all (whole herd depopulation) or specific (test-and-cull) animals. At the individual level, it was assumed that ante-mortem tests may allow detecting animals in the E and I states (according to the sensitivities of these tests), whereas only animals in the I state could be detected by carcass inspection (again according to the sensitivity of routine or detailed inspection). The detection and control process was represented by a succession of steps, one or several tests being implemented at each step on one or several animals. Moves from one step to another depended on the results of these tests, and on those of routine carcass inspection. This representation allowed the model to simulate detection and control programs of arbitrary degree of complexity.

The model parameters were estimated from field data using Approximate Bayesian Computation (ABC) methods. The duration of the latent state was thus estimated 3.5 months (95% credible interval: 2–8 months), the transmission parameter was estimated 0.43 month^{-1} (95% CI: 0.16–0.84) inside buildings, and 0.08 month^{-1} (95% CI: 0.01–0.32) on pastures. Based on these estimates, the model was then validated using an independent dataset.

The model was implemented using the R software. A detailed description of its structure, parameterization and validation can be found in Bekara et al. (12).

Parameters

Demographic and Infection Process

As most of herds detected infected in France are beef herds, only this type of herd (i.e., breeding and suckling herds) was addressed in our study, and the values of the parameters of the demographic process (**Table 1**) were chosen to represent a typical French beef herd, in 2017. Three animal batches were considered, 1-, 2-, and 3-year old heifers, and cows with their calves.

At the beginning of each simulation, the values of the two transmission parameters (inside buildings and on pastures) and of the duration of the latent period were randomly drawn from the joint posterior distribution produced by the ABC estimation procedure (12). Moreover, the infection was assumed to be brought in the herd by the introduction of a single infected animal (I health state), at a randomly chosen month of the first simulated year.

Modeled Surveillance and Control Measures

Two sets of possible surveillance measures (feasible under present French field conditions) were represented in the model. Herds were assumed subjected to routine screening, based on skin tests of animals over 1 year of age. If at least one reactor was detected, the herd was placed under movement restriction until

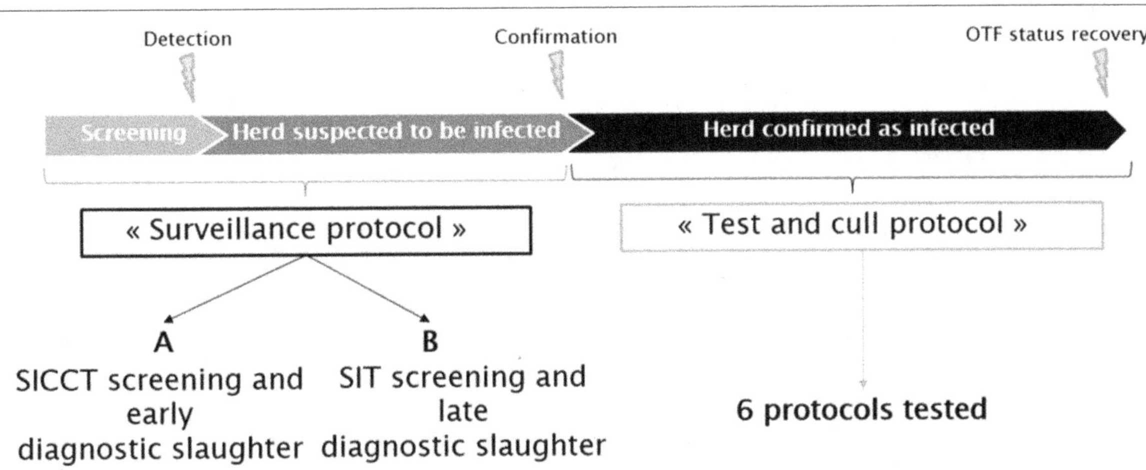

FIGURE 1 | Schematic representation of the bTB surveillance and control protocols applied in France in accordance with Council Directive 64/432/EEC.

confirmation (or not) of bTB infection. This phase (from the routine skin testing until the confirmation of infection) will be hereafter called the "surveillance protocol" (**Figure 1**). Two such surveillance protocols were distinguished. The first one, termed below "A," used a SICCT annual screening of the herds, followed by the slaughter of non-negative animals to infirm or confirm the suspicion. The second one, termed below "B," used a SIT annual screening of the herd. Reactors are retested in the following days with IFN-γ; the non-negative animals being then slaughtered for confirmatory purposes. When bTB infection is confirmed, the herd is kept under movement restriction during the implementation of the test-and-cull protocol, which ends when the herd is reported as free from bTB infection (the OTF status of the herd is recovered).

The current official test-and-cull protocol is based on three series of tests called "controls" (**Figure 2**) carried out on the entire herd (animals over 1 year of age) every 2 months. The first two controls combine a SIT ("SIT Official" protocol) or a SICCT ("SICCT Official" protocol, in the context of a surveillance of type A), an IFN-γ test, and a serological test. The third control consists of a SICCT. Moving from control X to control X+1 requires all the tested animals to be negative to all tests; otherwise the reactors are culled and the protocol moves back to the 1st control, 2 months later. The OTF status of the herd is recovered when the three controls are negative consecutively.

Based on these two reference protocols, several parameters were modified to specify alternative protocols: the inter-control time periods, the number of controls required and the type of tests used. Four new protocols were thus studied (**Figure 2**): a protocol where the time period between control 2 and control 3 was increased from 2 to 6 months (called "Increased delay" protocol), a protocol where a control was removed ("Two controls" protocol), a protocol where a control with SICCT, IFN-γ and serology was added ("Four protocols" protocol), and a protocol using only SICCT ("SICCT only" protocol).

TABLE 2 | Sensitivities and specificities of tests used for bTB surveillance and control in the model of within-herd bTB dynamics.

Test	Sensitivity (median [CI 95%])	Specificity (median [CI 95%])	References
SIT	0.81 [0.53; 0.94]	0.91 [0.63; 1.00]	(17)
SICCT	0.75 [0.61; 0.86]	1 [0.99; 1.00]	(17)
IFN bovine and avian PPD	0.70 [0.55; 0.92]	0.94 [0.88; 0.97]	(17)
IFN ESAT6	0.79 [0.64; 0.89]	0.99 [0.98; 1.00]	(17)
Serology	0.60 [0.31; 0.86]	0.93 [0.84; 0.97]	(17)
PCR	0.86 [0.65; 0.96]	1 [1.00; 1.00]	(17)
PCR NRL	1*	1	NRL
Histology	0.66 [0.41; 0.84]	1 [0.95; 1.00]	(17)
Culture	0.74 [0.46; 0.94]	1 [0.73; 1.00]	(17)
Routine necropsy (meat inspection)	0.71 [0.37; 0.92]	1 [0.99; 1.00]	(17)
Detailed necropsy (suspected animals)	0.96 [0.82; 1.00]	1 [0.99; 1.00]	(17)

**In the context of confirmation of positive PCR results obtained by local veterinary laboratories.*

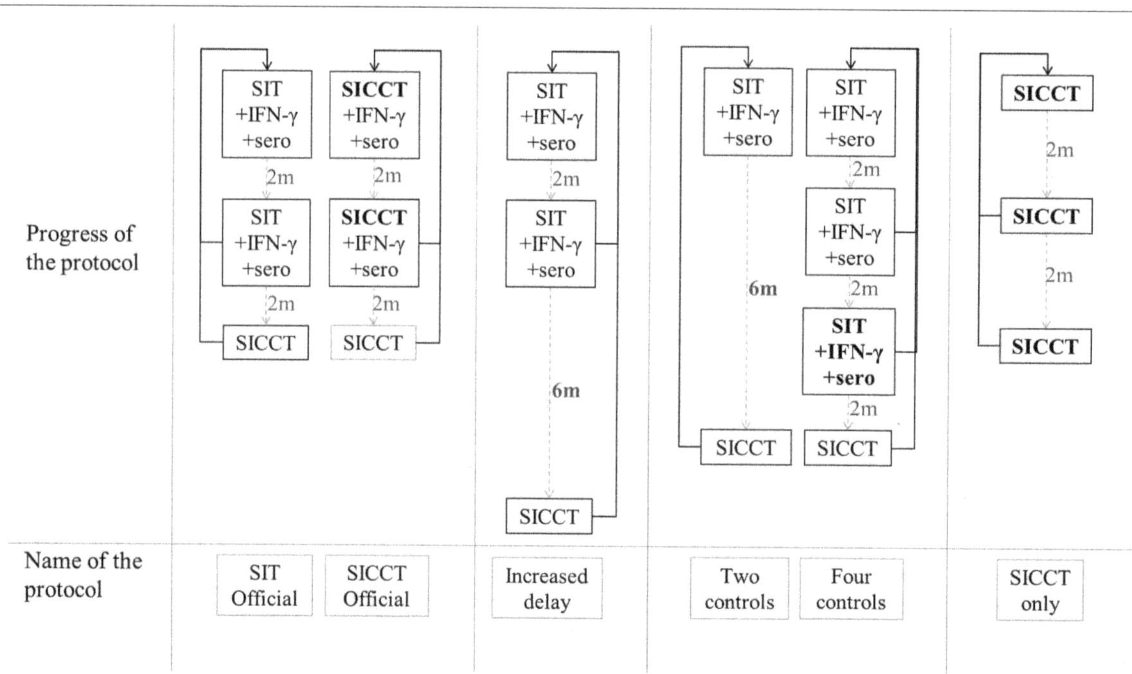

FIGURE 2 | Definition of the studied test-and-cull protocols for bTB control. SIT, single intradermal tuberculin skin tests; SICCT, single intradermal comparative cervical skin test; IFN-γ, gamma interferon test; sero, serology test; 2 m, time period of 2 months; 6 m, time period of 6 months, plain black arrows, non-negative control; dashed gray arrows, negative control.

These scenarios were compared to each other, and to whole depopulation protocol.

Tests sensitivities and specificities were fixed according to the literature and to the expertise of the French national reference laboratory (NRL) for bTB (**Table 2**).

Indicators

Epidemiological Effectiveness

The failure probability of the protocol was the probability that a herd would wrongly regain its OTF status while still infected (some infected animals, either latent E or infectious I, are still present but remain undetected). This corresponds to a failure of the system of detection of infected animals (e.g., lack of test sensitivity, animals not tested), and thus of the epidemiological effectiveness of the protocol. The number of infectious animals-months was considered a proxy for the risk of transmission of the infection to the neighboring farms and to the breeder or the farm staff. The number of infectious animals-months was computed as the sum across all infected animals of their total infectivity time (e.g., duration in months spent in I state).

Public Costs

The proportion of susceptible (S) animals among those culled during the test-and-cull protocol was an indicator of both cost and epidemiological effectiveness, as these false-positive animals are unnecessarily culled and compensated. It was computed as the number of susceptible animals culled during the test-and-cull protocol over the number of culled animals during the test-and-cull protocol (i.e., the number of animals to be compensated).

The overall public costs combined compensations paid to the farmer (for slaughtered animals, calculated based on expert opinions, data provided by French veterinary services (French Ministry of agriculture) of departments Dordogne and Cote d'Or and presented in **Table 3**) and the laboratory and veterinary costs (prices of analyses, veterinary visits and acts, presented in **Table 4**). The total farmer compensation costs were calculated for each simulation by summing the average compensation costs of each slaughtered animal, according to its age group. The total laboratory and veterinary costs were calculated by multiplying the number of tests and veterinary visits by their respective unitary costs.

Acceptability

Seven acceptability indicators were defined. First, the total number of culled animals (during surveillance protocol and test-and-cull protocol) was calculated (**Table 7A**, indicator 1 on **Figure 3**). Besides, the number of culled animal confirmed infected with *M. bovis* by culture (**Table 7A**) was computed as a proxy for acceptability: indeed, the animals culled but not confirmed infected by culture (even if they are infected) are most often seen by breeders as animals "slaughtered for nothing," which is one of their biggest sources of frustration. The total time needed for disease elimination and OTF status recovery (**Table 7B**, indicator 2 on **Figure 3**) represented the total time needed for the herd to actually get rid of the infection and correctly regain its OTF status. It could include periods when the herd had temporarily recovered its OTF status but was still infected (see "requalified herd" period while still I animals on **Figure 3**). The delay between a confirmation and an OTF status recovery represented the duration of strict movement restriction of the herd (**Table 7B**, indicator 3 on **Figure 3**), which is source of non-acceptability. Modeling allowed computing the duration of the wrongly movement restriction of the herd (**Table 7B**, indicator 4 on **Figure 3**) by measuring the delay between the slaughter of the last infected animal (E or I) (i.e., the "real elimination of the infection" moment on **Figure 3**) and the OTF status recovery (**Figure 3**). The number of veterinary visits (**Table 7A**) corresponded to the number of controls needed to eliminate the infection and recover the OTF status. This number of visits could be greater than the number of controls provided for by the protocol, when one or more controls had been unfavorable, leading to restart the protocol.

The global acceptability was finally evaluated by a synthetic indicator corresponding to the percentage of simulations for which the farmer would have dropped out the test-and-cull protocol before its end (percentage of drop out). The acceptability of the measures by the breeders is a difficult notion to evaluate without sociological survey. It was assumed, according to personal communications from local representatives of veterinary services, that farmers would drop out the protocol if the number of animals confirmed infected exceeded 3, or if the duration of the protocol exceeded 26 months.

TABLE 3 | Average compensation paid to beef cattle farmers per slaughtered animal according to the age group, calculated from compensation reports of seven French herds having been subjected to a test-and-cull protocol between 2014 and 2017, for bTB control.

Age group	Average compensation cost (€)
0–1 year	507
1–2 years	712
2–3 years	1232
3–6 years	906
6–10 years	758
10–15 years	759

(Source: French Ministry of Agriculture).

TABLE 4 | Unit costs of veterinary acts and laboratory analyses used for bTB control in France.

Act/Analysis	Average price (€)	Source
Veterinary visit	27.7	(18)
Blood sample	2.77	(18)
SIT	2.77	(18)
SICCT	6.93	(18)
IFN	50	LDA 24, personal communication, 2017
Serology	12	LDA 24, personal communication, 2017; LDA 21, personal communication, 2017
PCR	50	LDA 24, personal communication, 2017
Culture	50	LDA 24, personal communication, 2017
Histology	50	Pricing grid LAPVSO, Vet diagnostics

For each scenario, 1,000 simulations were conducted, leading to proportions (for binary indicators) or to distributions of indicator values, reported below based on medians, 2.5 and 97.5% percentiles. Finally, three key indicators were represented graphically: the failure probability, the overall public costs, and the percentage of dropout. The six studied test-and-cull protocols were then separately ranked according to each of these three key indicators, and the global rank of each protocol was computed as the average value of these three ranks.

RESULTS

Epidemiological Effectiveness

Among the test-and-cull protocols (**Figure 2**), the "Increased delay" had the lowest failure probability: respectively 1.4 and 1.5% after an A (i.e., SICCT annual screening and early diagnostic slaughter) and a B (i.e., SIT annual screening and retesting with IFN-γ before diagnostic slaughter) surveillance protocols (**Table 5**). On the contrary, the official protocols presented the highest failure probability: 8.3% after an A surveillance protocol ("SICCT Official" protocol) and 12.4% after a B surveillance protocol ("SIT Official" protocol). In general, the failure probability was slightly higher after a B surveillance protocol. After an A surveillance protocol, the number of infectious animals-months remained low regardless of the test-and-cull protocol (median of 1 to 2 animal-months). This number was higher after a B surveillance protocol (median of 3 to 4 animal-months).

Public Costs

Although the difference was moderate, the B surveillance protocol always induced higher public costs than the A one (**Table 6B**). Whole herd depopulation was clearly the most expensive protocol with a median overall cost of 120 K€ per infected herd. The "Four controls" protocol was the most expensive of the test-and-cull protocols, with median values between 73.2 and 78 K€. However, the others were not much cheaper except the "Two controls" which costed more than 20 K€ less, and the "SICCT only" which was the cheapest protocol, costing between 2.7 and 4.8 K€. In this latter case, very few animals were culled during the protocol (between 0 and 1 in median **Table 6A**) leading to lower compensations. In addition, this protocol did not use IFN-γ at all, which is an expensive screening test.

The proportion of S animals among the animals culled during the protocol was high and reached 100% in median after an

TABLE 5 | Epidemiological effectiveness indicators of test-and-cull protocols to control bTB in an average French beef cattle herd, compared to whole herd depopulation.

Protocol	Failure probability (%)		Number of infectious animals-months[a]	
Surveillance	**A**	**B**	**A**	**B**
Test-and-cull				
SIT Official	7.3	12.4	2 [0–92]	4 [0–140]
SICCT Official	8.3	/[b]	2 [0–80]	/
Increased delay	1.4	1.5	1 [0–50]	4 [0–92]
Four controls	5.0	5.0	2 [0–52]	3 [0–77]
Two controls	4.4	6.5	1 [0–54]	3 [0–111]
SICCT only	7.5	5.4	2 [0–65]	3 [0–89]
Whole depopulation	0 by def.	0 by def.	0 by def.	0 by def.

[a]*Median, brackets: 2.5 and 97.5% percentiles.*
[b]*"SICCT Official" can only be implemented in the context of a surveillance of type A, which uses SICCT for annual screening.*

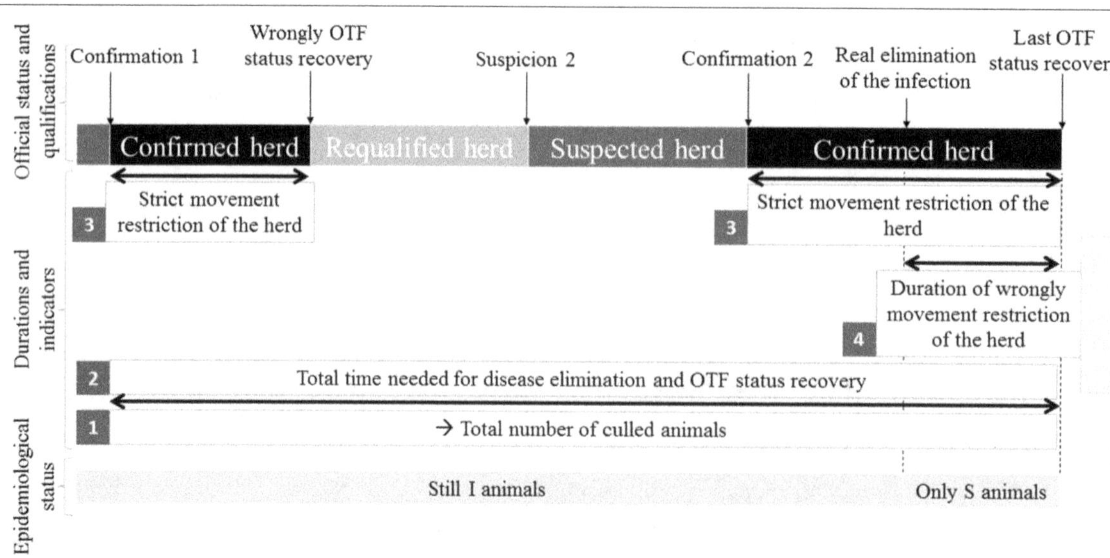

FIGURE 3 | Representation of four indicators [total number of culled animals (1), total time needed for disease elimination and OTF status recovery (2), strict movement restriction of the herd (3), duration of wrongly movement restriction of the herd (4)] in parallel with the evolution of the official and epidemiological status of the herd.

TABLE 6 | Public costs indicators of test-and-cull protocols to control bTB in an average French beef cattle herd, compared to whole herd depopulation.

Protocol	Number of culled animals during protocol[a]		Proportion of S among animals culled during protocol (%)[a]	
Surveillance	A	B	A	B
A				
Test-and-cull				
SIT Official	39 [25–107]	49 [28–131]	100 [83–100]	95.9 [66–100]
SICCT Official	20 [10–66]	/	100 [69–100]	/
Increased delay	40 [26–101]	49 [27–135]	100 [83–100]	95.9 [69–100]
Four controls	50 [37–127]	54 [34–131]	100 [88–100]	98.1 [82–100]
Two controls	22 [11–74]	29 [12–90]	100 [79–100]	96.4 [70–100]
SICCT only	0 [0–12]	1 [0–25]	0,0 [0–0]	0 [0–0]
Whole depopulation	141	141	100 [94–100]	99.3 [84–100]

Protocol	Lab/vet costs (K€)[a]		Compensation costs (K€)[a]		Overall cost (K€)[a]	
Surveillance	A	B	A	B	A	B
B						
Test-and-cull						
SIT Official	20.1 [18–55]	26.9 [18–69]	35.6 [23–102]	44.8 [25–130]	56 [41–158]	71.7 [43–201]
SICCT Official	20.3 [18–63]	/	18.4 [9–62]	/	40 [27–131]	/
Increased delay	20.2 [18–57]	27.1 [18–69]	36.0 [24–95]	44.2 [25–112]	56.9 [42–151]	71.3 [31–185]
Four controls	27.1 [23–68]	29.5 [22–69]	46.0 [34–115]	48.5 [31–120]	73.2 [58–182]	78 [54–187]
Two controls	11.2 [9–41]	17.7 [9–47]	20.3 [10–68]	26.4 [10–82]	31.6 [20–106]	44.8 [20–126]
SICCT only	2.7 [2–10]	3.6 [2–13]	0.0 [0–12]	0.9 [0–22]	2.7 [2–21]	4.8 [2–35]
Whole depopulation	0 [0–1]	0.2 [0–1.8]	120 [115–125]	120 [115–125]	120 [115–125]	120 [116–126]

[a]*Median, brackets: 2.5 and 97.5% percentiles.*

A surveillance, for all the protocols except the "SICCT only," meaning that all infected animals had been culled during the surveillance phase (**Table 6A**). Oppositely, for the "SICCT only," this percentage was null, due to the 100% specificity of SICCT. In the other protocols however, almost all culled animals were false positives. After a B surveillance, the percentage was smaller but remained very high (between 95.9 and 99.3% of culled animals in median were S).

Acceptability

After both A and B surveillances, the "Four control" protocol was the test-and-cull protocol leading to the highest number of culled animals (between 55 and 66 in median) (**Table 7A**). The "SICCT only" protocol only induced the culling of 6 and 14 animals in median. Whatever the protocol, an A surveillance induced fewer culling (between 13 and 8 animals). After an A surveillance, medians of the number of culture-confirmed animals were null regardless the test-and-cull protocol (**Table 7A**). Indeed, almost all animals culled were S (**Table 6A**). The median reached one confirmed animal after a B surveillance, regardless the test-and-cull protocol.

The median number of veterinary visits (or control sessions) needed to eliminate the infection and recover the OTF status showed that in most cases, after an A surveillance, the minimal number of controls was performed (i.e., the number of controls provided for by the protocol), although in some cases, the number of required visits was important (97.5% percentile between 6 and 10 visits). After a B surveillance however, an additional control, in median, was necessary to eliminate the infection and recover the OTF status (**Table 7A**). After an A surveillance, the total time needed for disease elimination and OTF status recovery varied in median between 6 months for the "SIT Official" protocol and 10 months for the "Increased delay" one (**Table 7B**). After a B surveillance, this duration was always about two months longer in median, varying from 8 months for the "SIT Official" and "SICCT only" protocols to 12 months for the "Increased delay" protocol. In whole depopulation, the regulatory depopulation duration is 30 days. However, it is necessary to add the time needed for the cleaning-disinfection operations, the repopulation, and the realization of the tests on the new animals to recover the OTF status. This duration is therefore hardly comparable to that of test-and-cull protocols.

Regardless the surveillance protocol, the median duration of strict movement restriction was similar to the total time needed for disease elimination and OTF status recovery (**Table 7B**). This shows that in most cases, there were no periods of herd

TABLE 7 | Acceptability indicators of test-and-cull protocols to control bTB in an average French beef cattle herd, compared to whole herd depopulation.

Protocol	Total number of culled animals[a]		Number of culled animal confirmed infected with *M. bovis* by culture[a]		Number of veterinary visits[a]	
Surveillance	**A**	**B**	**A**	**B**	**A**	**B**
A						
Test-and-cull						
SIT Official	39 [25–119]	49 [28–138]	0 [0–6]	1 [0–20]	3 [3–9]	4 [3–10]
SICCT Official	20 [10–74]	/	0 [0–7]	/	3 [3–9]	/
Increased delay	40 [26–111]	49 [27–135]	0 [0–6]	1 [0–22]	3 [3–8]	4 [3–10]
Four controls	55 [42–138]	66 [47–159]	0 [0–6]	1 [0–12]	4 [4–10]	5 [4–11]
Two controls	27 [16–89]	40 [22–123]	0 [0–6]	1 [0–15]	2 [2–6]	3 [2–7]
SICCT only	6 [3–29]	14 [4–49]	0 [0–6]	1 [0–17]	3 [3–10]	4 [3–11]
Whole depopulation	141 (by definition)	141 (by definition)	0 [0–4]	1 [0–9]	/	/

Protocol	Total time needed for disease elimination and OTF status recovery (months)[a]		Duration of strict movement restriction (months) [a]		Duration of wrongly movement restriction (months)[a]		Percentage of drop out (%)	
Surveillance	**A**	**B**	**A**	**B**	**A**	**B**	**A**	**B**
B								
Test-and-cull								
SIT Official	6 [6–32]	8 [6–34]	6 [6–11]	8 [6–17]	6 [4–7]	6 [4–7]	10.7	22
SICCT Official	7 [6–32]	/	7 [6–11]	/	6 [5–7]	/	11.3	/
Increased delay	10 [10–26]	12 [10–28]	10 [10–25]	12 [10–27]	10 [8–11]	10 [8–11]	8.5	20.1
Four controls	8 [8–33]	10 [8–34]	8 [8–20]	10 [8–21]	8 [6–9]	8 [6–9]	9.6	16
Two controls	8 [8–33]	10 [8–34]	8 [8–20]	10 [8–21]	8 [6–9]	8 [6–9]	7.8	21.1
SICCT only	7 [6–33]	8 [6–34]	6 [6–18]	8 [6–21]	6 [6–6]	6 [6–7]	12.8	22

[a]*Median, brackets: 2.5 and 97.5% percentiles.*

infection with false OTF status. However, the 97.5% percentiles showed that these two durations could differ up to 21 months. Thus, these situations were rare, but when they occurred, they lasted a long time (between 6 and 21 months), except for the "Increased delay" protocol where the difference was only 1 month. Duration of the wrongly movement restriction was also most of the time equal to the total time needed for disease elimination and OTF status recovery after an A surveillance (**Table 7B**). This means the infection was eliminated from the herd when the last infected animals were culled, during the surveillance period. The necropsy confirming the infection, the herd was declared infected and the test-and-cull protocol started although there was no more infected animal. Only the "SICCT Official" and "SICCT only" scenarios had differences of 1 month. However, after a B surveillance, the median durations of wrongly movement restriction were shorter than the total time needed for disease elimination and OTF status recovery. Infection was eliminated from the farm 2 months in median after the confirmation and the implementation of the test-and-cull protocol.

After an A surveillance, the "Two controls" protocol had the lowest percentage of drop out: 7.8% (**Table 7B**). After a B surveillance however, the "Four control" protocol was the one with the lowest but still quite high percentage of drop out of 16%. The "Two controls" implied 21.1% of drop out. "SICCT only" had the higher percentage of drop out in both A and B cases, but implied 12.8% of drop out after an A surveillance while it reached 22% of drop out after a B surveillance, like the "SIT Official" protocol.

Indeed, considering the percentage of drop out as the main indicator for acceptability, we can note that acceptability was better after an A surveillance, regardless the test-and-cull protocols.

Global Analysis and Ranking of the Protocols

The failure probability of the protocols function on their overall public cost is plotted in **Figure 4**. The percentage of drop out is indicated as a label for each protocol. In this representation, the optimal protocols should be located in the lowest left part of the graph, (attention needs also to be paid to the acceptability). **Figure 4** confirms that B surveillance (blue markers) induced increased public costs (blue markers being always on the right of red markers) and decreased acceptability (superscripts of blue markers being always higher than superscripts of red ones) and effectiveness (blue markers being higher than red ones except for the "SICCT only" protocol). These considerations should lead to prefer the A surveillance protocol. Each scenario was

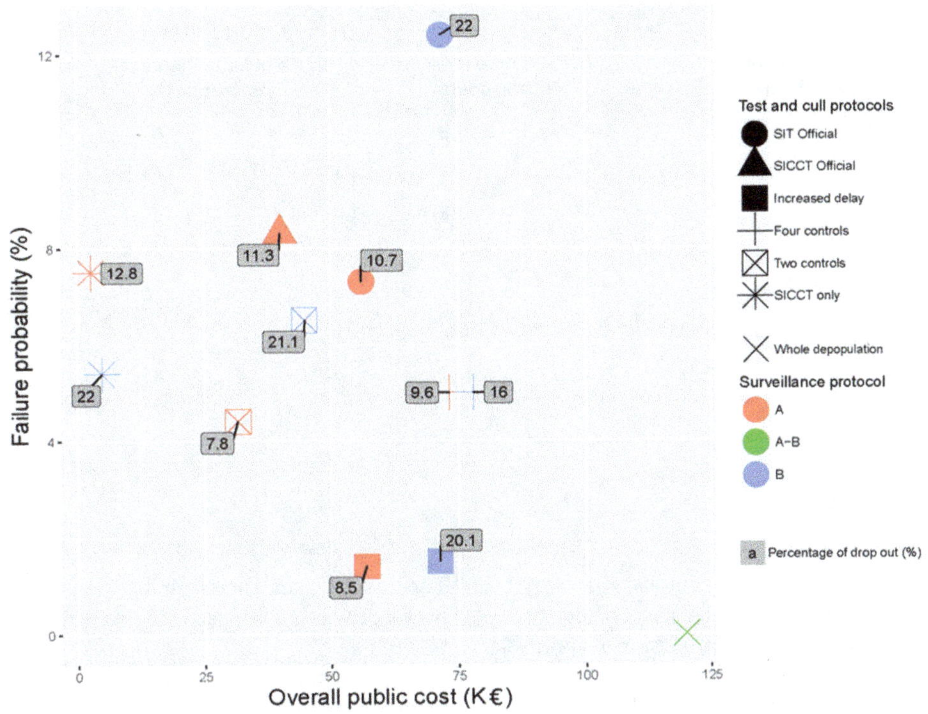

FIGURE 4 | Failure probability of the test-and-cull protocols for bTB control after both A and B surveillances schemes, according to their overall public cost and their percentage of drop out (labels) compared to whole depopulation.

then ranked for each indicator separately (**Table 8**). **Figure 4** and **Table 8** show that in both A and B cases, the "SICCT only" protocol was very economical. However, after an A surveillance its failure probability was the second highest (ranked 6th out of 7 protocols, see **Table 8**) and its percentage of drop out was the highest (ranked 7th out of 7). After a B surveillance, although its failure probability was enhanced (ranked 4th out of 6), its percentage of drop out was the second highest (ranked 4th out of 6, placed equal with "SIT Official"). Therefore, in both cases, the "SICCT only" protocol does not appear to be appropriate for bTB control. The "SIT Official" protocol was among the less effective and most expensive ones, especially after a B surveillance. Its percentage of drop out was the highest after a B surveillance (placed equal with the "SICCT only") and the 4th highest after an A surveillance. Similarly, the "SICCT Official" protocol was poorly ranked for each of the three indicators.

After an A surveillance (red markers), the "Two controls" and "Increased delay" protocols appeared to be the two best protocols. Both had a reasonable acceptability (<9% of drop out, 1st and 2nd rank), a reasonable failure probability (<5% of failure, 2nd and 3rd rank) and induced reasonable public costs (<60 K€TF and 2nd and 5th rank). The "Two controls" protocol was cheaper but had a higher failure probability whereas the "Increased delay" one was almost twice more expensive but with a much lower failure probability.

The average of the three ranks (failure probability, public costs and drop out percentage) allowed obtaining a global ranking of these protocols, while attributing the same importance to each of the three criteria (**Table 8**). The "Two controls" protocol was the best tradeoff (average rank of 2) after an A surveillance. After a B surveillance, the best tradeoff was obtained by the "Increased delay" protocol with an average rank of 2.3, closely followed by the "Four controls" and "SICCT only" protocols (average rank of 3) (**Table 8**).

DISCUSSION

In this study, we evaluated the official test-and-cull protocols implemented in France, in accordance with Council Directive 64/432/EEC as well as four alternative protocols. Their epidemiological effectiveness, the public costs they induce and their acceptability to farmers were compared.

For that purpose, a previously published and validated model was used (12), model that allowed representing the "true" health state of the animals and the detection and control events, in order to quantify events such as incorrectly assigning a bTB free status to the farm (19, 20). This model was chosen because it allowed parameterizing easily alternative surveillance and control protocols, and because its parameters were estimated from field data collected in France, and validated independently: Bekara et al. (12) performed both an internal validation using a leave-one-out cross-validation procedure, and an external validation to demonstrate the ability of the model to reproduce observational bTB data collected in France between 1980 and 2010, that were not used for parameter estimation. The model was parameterized based on French

TABLE 8 | Ranking of test-and-cull protocols to control bTB in an average French beef cattle herd, compared to whole herd depopulation, according to three key indicators, and average rank considering the three indicators being at the same level of importance.

Protocol	Rank for failure probability*		Rank for overall public cost*		Rank for percentage of drop out*		Mean rank**	
Surveillance	**A**	**B**	**A**	**B**	**A**	**B**	**A**	**B**
Test-and-cull								
SIT Official	5	6	4	4	4	4	4.3	4.7
SICCT Official	7	/	3	/	5	/	5	/
Increased delay	2	2	5	3	2	2	4	2.3
Four controls	4	3	6	5	3	1	4.3	3
Two controls	3	5	2	2	1	3	2	3.3
SICCT only	6	4	1	1	6	4	4.3	3
Whole depopulation	1	1	7	6	7	6	5	4.3
Total number of protocols	7	6	7	6	7	6	7	6

**1is the protocol with the lowest value, 6 or 7 is the one with the highest one.*
***The smaller the rank, the better the scenario.*

data with an average beef herd size (141 animals) that may be greater than in most of European countries. According to the Directorate General of the European Commission responsible for statistical information at Community level (Eurostat), the last calculated average size of beef herds would be 70 animals (21). The model could easily be adapted to different breeding contexts.

Results suggest that the official protocol could probably be improved, as alternative protocols appeared more effective, acceptable while inducing lower public costs.

The proportion of non-infected animals among the slaughtered animals appeared high, except with the "SICCT only" protocol. Following an A surveillance (based on SICCT annual screening and slaughter of positive animals to confirm suspicions), *M. bovis* was often very quickly eliminated from the infected farms (i.e., either at the time of the confirmation of infection, or in the first months following this confirmation). Moreover, the low specificity of the SIT and IFN-γ tests (17) led to the cull of many susceptible animals. This phenomenon was mitigated when using surveillance protocol B (based on SIT annual screening, IFN-γ on positive animals and slaughter of non-negative animals to confirm suspicions), but the simulated proportion of non-infected animals among the culled animals remained high, with a minimum value of 95.9% for protocols other than the "SICCT only." Indeed, even though the simulated scenario rankings were relatively similar following an A or a B surveillance, the surveillance protocol had a strong impact on the epidemiological effectiveness, the public costs and the acceptability to farmers. After an A surveillance, and therefore a drastic management of the suspicion, most herds did not contain infected animals at the start of the test-and-cull protocol, unlike after a B surveillance. Epidemiological effectiveness, costs and acceptability of the test-and-cull protocols were then enhanced. For example and according to acceptability, herds managed under surveillance protocol A had a shorter duration of strict movement restriction (about 2 months in median) than those managed under surveillance protocol B. The farmer can therefore be prepared to the fact that the protocol will last longer if the surveillance protocol of his herd was B.

We investigated the balance between the costs that can be invested in test-and-cull protocols and the consequences of choosing a specific scheme. It all depends on the goal: if it is to eradicate the infection, the most effective and acceptable protocols will have to be chosen, regardless of their cost. Indeed, without good acceptability, the actors will not follow the measures and the strategy will lose of power. In this case, "Increased delay" protocol is to be implemented. If, however, one is willing to accept a small percentage of outbreaks wrongly regaining their bTB free-status, then less effective but less expensive scenarios may be chosen, such as the "Two controls" protocol in the context of reducing public expenditure. In both cases, the good effectiveness of the "Increases delay" and "Two controls" protocols highlights the importance of long inter-control delays for the epidemiological effectiveness of the scenarios. This appears to be valid even when very few animals are actually infected.

Field observations bring support to the results we obtained. According to a study on the typology of French farms that were subjected to the test-and-cull official protocol between 2014 and 2017 (22), infection was laboratory-confirmed in <4 animals in 95% of the farms. In our simulations, we obtained a very low number of laboratory-confirmed infected animals (between 0 and 1 in median) for the official scenarios, which is thus consistent with field observations. In the same way, the number of control sessions observed in the field (on average 3.3 visits) was close to the figure we obtained (median of 3 to 4 visits for the official protocols).

In the model, births were assumed to compensate for animal culls, herd size thus remaining constant. This simplifying assumption may not accurately represent reality. First, some breeders decide to reduce the size of their herd when starting the test-and-cull protocol, for reasons of biosecurity and easier management of the batches (personal communication 2017: F.

Chevalier, French national referent for bTB). Then, if many animals are slaughtered (rightly or wrongly), it can surpass the amount of births and prevent renewal. Thus, the number of young cattle in the model could be over-estimated. However, these young cattle probably play a minor role in infectious dynamics and are, in practice, not tested because they are too young. The impact of this simplification on our results is therefore assumed to be low.

The overall indicator of acceptability (percentage of drop out) was calculated taking into account the number of confirmed animals and the duration of the test-and-cull protocol. The number of animal reacting to tests may also have been a relevant parameter, but it was too difficult to determine an adequate threshold. In the field, when the number of reactors is high, veterinary services can advise or even force the breeder to shift from the test-and-cull protocol to whole herd depopulation. However, no official or empirical value exists to support that. This is why we decided not to take into account this parameter for the definition of acceptability.

The six studied test-and-cull protocols have been compared and ranked according to 3 key indicators, and according to an overall rank that gave the same level of importance to each. However, in real life, the choice of a control strategy does not always obey a pure epidemiological, economic or social rationality (23). Using a multicriteria decision analysis method (MCDA) would allow investigating more precisely the overall ranking of the protocols according to the expectations of the decision-makers (24).

Even though we focused on test-and-cull protocols applied or feasible in France, some of the protocols we analyzed are also relevant at the European level. The bTB surveillance and control protocols used in EU countries are indeed not country-specific, as these protocols and the tests they include stem from the European legislation (especially the Council Directive 64/432/ECC). As an example, test and cull is very common in the United Kingdom, where bTB can reach in some areas the highest prevalence of the EU (except in Scotland which is OTF), or in Spain (1, 4). For example, England and Northern Ireland eradication program incorporate the surveillance protocol we called "A" (13, 25, 26). A SICCT is performed on the whole herd and reactors are immediately removed for slaughter. If postmortem evidence of *M. bovis* infection cannot be demonstrated in any of the slaughtered reactors, OTF herd status that was suspended may be restored after one single skin test of all the animals with negative results, minimum 60 days later. However, if the infection is confirmed or if more than two animals had reacted to the SICCT, the herd loses its OTF status and enters in a "test and cull protocol" close to one of those we tested: the "SICCT only." Indeed, two consecutively negative SICCT on the whole herd are required to restore the OTF herd status while we modeled a three control protocol. Although other protocols used in EU countries could easily be implemented and compared using the model we used (which was designed for that purpose), it can be expected that the main results would remain valid, such as the reduced failure probability when inter-control delays are lengthened, or the positive effect of type A surveillance on epidemiological effectiveness, on cost and acceptability.

In conclusion, this study aimed at contributing to the identification of points on which decision-makers should act to improve the detection and control of bTB. It appears that there is room for an improvement of the present official test-and-cull protocol implemented in France in line with Council Directive 64/432/EEC, in particular by allowing an increase in the time interval between controls. Decision-makers may use this study to communicate with field actors and justify the needed modification of the French regulations concerning the bTB control. As tests and protocols are close between European countries it could be interesting to extend this study to other regions facing bTB taking into account their specificities in terms of epidemiological situation and cattle breeding.

AUTHOR CONTRIBUTIONS

HL, MS, AC, and BD conceived and designed the study. HL, MS, and BD encoded the model and indicators. HL, MS, AC, and BD performed the analysis. HL wrote the manuscript. HL, MS, AC, and BD revised the manuscript. All the authors approved the submitted version of the manuscript.

ACKNOWLEDGMENTS

The authors thank the French Ministry of Food and Agriculture, Directorate General for Food (DGAl) and the School of French Veterinary Services (ENSV) which funded Helena Ladreyt's internship grant. The authors also warmly thank Fabrice Chevalier (DGAl), Maria-Laura Boschiroli (NRL), Taeb Slassi and Christophe Constant (French Veterinary Services) for their expertise on bTBmanagement in France and the communication of the data, and Valentine Poirier and Adrien Bouveret (interns) for communicating the field data. This work was supported by the Laboratoire d'Excellence Integrative Biology of Emerging Infectious Diseases program (grant ANR-10-LABX-62-IBEID).

REFERENCES

1. Ciaravino G, García-Saenz A, Cabras S, Allepuz A, Casal J, García-Bocanegra I, et al. Assessing the variability in transmission of bovine tuberculosis within Spanish cattle herds. *Epidemics* (2018) 23:110–20. doi: 10.1016/j.epidem.2018.01.003
2. Allen AR, Skuce RA, Byrne AW. Bovine Tuberculosis in Britain and Ireland - A Perfect Storm? The confluence of potential ecological and epidemiological impediments to controlling a chronic infectious disease. *Front Vet Sci.* (2018) 5:109. doi: 10.3389/fvets.2018.00109
3. Caminiti A, Pelone F, Battisti S, Gamberale F, Colafrancesco R, Sala M, et al. Tuberculosis, brucellosis and leucosis in cattle: a cost description of eradication programmes in the Region of Lazio, Italy. *Transbound Emerg Dis.* (2017) 64:1493–504. doi: 10.1111/tbed.12540
4. Schiller I, Waters WR, RayWaters W, Vordermeier HM, Jemmi T, Welsh M, et al. Bovine tuberculosis in Europe from the perspective of an officially

tuberculosis free country: trade, surveillance and diagnostics. *Vet Microbiol.* (2011) 151:153–9. doi: 10.1016/j.vetmic.2011.02.039

5. *Animal Health-Regulatory Committee-Presentations Food Safety-European Commission* (2018). Available online at: /food/animals/health/regulatory_committee/presentations_en
6. Cavalerie L, Courcoul A, Boschiroli ML, Réveillaud E, Gay P. Tuberculose bovine en France en 2014: une situation stable. *Bull Épidémiol Santé Animale et Alimentation* (2014) 71:4–11. Available online at: https://be.anses.fr/sites/default/files/BEP-mg-BE71-art1.pdf
7. Bénet J-J, Boschiroli M-L, Dufour B, Garin-Bastuji B. Lutte contre la tuberculose bovine en France de 1954 à 2004: analyse de la pertinence épidémiologique de l'évolution de la réglementation. *Epidémiol Santé Anim.* (2006) 50:127–43. Available online at: http://aeema.vet-alfort.fr/images/2006-50/50.14.pdf
8. Delmotte D, Lecomte S. *Tuberculose: Il Faut Soutenir Davantage les Éleveurs. Arsia infos (113)* (2013) Available online at: http://www.arsia.be/wp-content/uploads/2013/10/AI-octobre-2013.pdf
9. Smith RL, Tauer LW, Schukken YH, Lu Z, Grohn YT. Minimization of bovine tuberculosis control costs in US dairy herds. *Prevent Vet Med.* (2013) 112:266–75. doi: 10.1016/j.prevetmed.2013.07.014
10. Ciaravino G, Ibarra P, Casal E, Lopez S, Espluga J, Casal J, et al. Farmer and Veterinarian Attitudes towards the Bovine Tuberculosis Eradication Programme in Spain: what is going on in the field? *Front Vet Sci.* (2017) 4:202. doi: 10.3389/fvets.2017.00202
11. Good M, Clegg TA, Duignan A, More SJ. Impact of the national full herd depopulation policy on the recurrence of bovine tuberculosis in Irish herds, 2003 to 2005. *Vet Rec.* (2011) 169:581. doi: 10.1136/vr.d4571
12. Bekara MEA, Courcoul A, Bénet J-J, Durand B. Modeling tuberculosis dynamics, detection and control in cattle herds. *PLoS ONE* (2014) 9:e108584. doi: 10.1371/journal.pone.0108584
13. Defra. *European Commission, SANCO.* UK bTB eradication plan 2013. 2012/761/EU. (2013).
14. *Agreste, Statistique Agricole Annuelle.* Effectif des animaux en fin d'année 2015 (2017). Available online at: http://agreste.agriculture.gouv.fr/IMG/pdf/saa2017T10bspca.pdf
15. Institut de l'élevage, CNE. *Chiffres clé 2015, Productions Bovines Lait et Viande* (2015). Available online at: http://idele.fr/presse/publication/idelesolr/recommends/chiffres-cles-des-filieres-bovine445-ovine-et-caprine-2016.html
16. Roche B, Dedieu B, Ingrand S. Taux de renouvellement et pratiques de réforme et de recrutement en élevage bovin allaitant du Limousin. *INRA Prod Anim.* (2001) 14:255–63. Available online at: https://www6.inra.fr/productions-animales/2001-Volume-14/Numero-4-2001/Taux-de-renouvellement-et-pratiques-de-reforme
17. Nuñez-Garcia J, Downs SH, Parry JE, Abernethy DA, Broughan JM, Cameron AR, et al. Meta-analyses of the sensitivity and specificity of ante-mortem and post-mortem diagnostic tests for bovine tuberculosis in the UK and Ireland. *Prev Vet Med.* (2017) 153:94–107 doi: 10.1016/j.prevetmed.2017.02.017
18. *CGAAER Modalités De Fixation Des Tarifs des Prophylaxies Animales.* (2015) Available online at: http://agriculture.gouv.fr/modalites-de-fixation-des-tarifs-des-prophylaxies-animales-0
19. Vynnycky E, White RG. *An Introduction to Infectious Disease Modelling* Oxford: Oxford University Press Inc. (2010).
20. Sabatier P, Bicout DJ, Durand B, Dubois MA. Le recours à la modélisation en épidémiologie animale. *Epidémiol Santé Anim.* (2005) 47:15–33. Available online at: http://aeema.vet-alfort.fr/images/2005-47/47.03.pdf
21. European Commission. *Agriculture and Rural Development.* EU beef farms report 2012. (2013).
22. Poirier V. *Elevages Foyers de Tuberculose Bovine Ayant fait l'objet d'un Assainissement par Abattage Partiel Depuis son Autorisation sur Tout le Territoire National en 2014: Typologie des Élevages Concernés, Étude de L'efficacité du Dispositif.* Master's thesis, Université Paris Saclay (2017) Available online at: http://theses.vet-alfort.fr/telecharger.php?id=2235
23. Marsot M, Rautureau S, Dufour B, Durand B. Impact of stakeholders influence, geographic level and risk perception on strategic decisions in simulated foot and mouth disease epizootics in France. *PLoS ONE* (2014) 9:e86323. doi: 10.1371/journal.pone.0086323
24. Thokala P, Devlin N, Marsh K, Baltussen R, Boysen M, Kalo Z, et al. Multiple criteria decision analysis for health care decision making—an introduction: report 1 of the ISPOR MCDA Emerging Good Practices Task Force. *Value Health* (2016) 19:1–13. doi: 10.1016/j.jval.2015.12.003
25. O'Hagan MJH, Stegeman JA, Doyle LP, Stringer LA, Courcier EA, Menzies FD. The impact of the number of tuberculin skin test reactors and infection confirmation on the risk of future bovine tuberculosis incidents; a Northern Ireland perspective. *Epidemiol Infect.* (2018) 146:1495–502. doi: 10.1017/S0950268818001310
26. *Animal Health and Veterinary Laboratories Agency.* Dealing with TB in your herd - What happens if TB is identified in your herd? (2014).

7

Use of the Human Vaccine, *Mycobacterium bovis* Bacillus Calmette Guérin in Deer

Mitchell V. Palmer and Tyler C. Thacker*

Infectious Bacterial Diseases of Livestock Research Unit, National Animal Disease Center, Agricultural Research Service, United States Department of Agriculture, Ames, IA, United States

***Correspondence:**
Mitchell V. Palmer
mitchell.palmer@ars.usda.gov

The only vaccine ever approved for human tuberculosis was developed a century ago from an isolate of *Mycobacterium bovis* derived from a tuberculous cow. Initial safety and efficacy studies of an attenuated version of this isolate were conducted in cattle and other animals. In 1921 the first human, an infant, was orally dosed with this attenuated strain that came to be known as *M. bovis* bacillus Calmette-Guérin (BCG); named for Albert Calmette and Camille Guérin, the two French scientists that developed the strain. Since 1921, billions of people have been vaccinated with BCG making it the oldest, most widely used, and safest vaccine in use today. It is also the tuberculosis vaccine most studied for use in wildlife, including deer. While BCG vaccination of deer may not reliably prevent infection, it consistently decreases lesion severity, minimizing large, necrotic lesions, which often contain large numbers of bacilli. It is believed that decreased lesion severity correlates with decreased disease transmission; however, this hypothesis remains to be proven. Safety studies in white-tailed deer show BCG may persist in lymphoid tissues for up to 12 months; a factor to be considered in deer used for food. Beyond efficacy and safety, methods of vaccine delivery to free-ranging deer are also under investigation, both in the laboratory and in the field. The ideal delivery method is effective, efficient and safe for non-target species, including livestock. Ingestion of BCG by cattle is of special concern as such cattle may present as "false positives" using currently approved diagnostic methods, thus interfering with efforts by animal health agencies to monitor cattle for tuberculosis. An effective BCG vaccine for deer would be of value in regions where free-ranging deer represent a potential source of *M. bovis* for livestock. Such a vaccine would also be beneficial to farmed deer where *M. bovis* represents a serious threat to trade and productivity.

Keywords: BCG, deer, mycobacterium, tuberculosis, vaccine, wildlife

INTRODUCTION

Mycobacterium bovis is the cause of tuberculosis in most animal species, including man. Clinical signs and pathological manifestations of *M. bovis* in humans can be identical to infection with the more common cause of human tuberculosis, *Mycobacterium tuberculosis*. The range of susceptible hosts to *M. bovis* is broad and includes most species of both livestock and wildlife. For decades, most developed countries have conducted costly campaigns to eradicate tuberculosis from cattle with varying success (1). In cases where a wildlife reservoir of *M. bovis* infection exists, eradication has been difficult, if not impossible (2) due to transmission of *M. bovis* from livestock to wildlife (spillover) and subsequent transmission from wildlife back to livestock (spillback). In northeast Michigan, USA there is a focus of *M. bovis* infection in free-ranging white-tailed deer (*Odocoileus virginianus*) where infected deer have been implicated as the source of infection in 69 cattle herds from 1995 through 2017. Control efforts, including increased hunting have been effective in decreasing disease prevalence from 4.9% in 1995 to 1.7% in 2004, but prevalence continues to remain at approximately 2% (3, 4).

In addition to white-tailed deer in the US, there is general consensus that the European badger (*Meles meles*) in the United Kingdom and the Republic of Ireland, the brushtail possum (*Trichosurus vulpecula*) in New Zealand, and the European wild boar (*Sus scrofa*) in the Iberian Peninsula represent wildlife reservoirs of *M. bovis* and can be a persistent source of re-infection of cattle (5–12). Attempts to control or eliminate these reservoirs of infection have involved population reductions through hunting, trapping or poisoning, as well as physical exclusion of wildlife from cattle feeding areas through barrier fencing. In all cases, vaccination of wildlife to reduce wildlife-to-cattle transmission has been investigated, with some vaccines progressing to field trials (13, 14). The goal of vaccination is to induce an immune response such that the animal is resistant to infection or if infection occurs, disease severity is lessened and transmission is reduced or eliminated. Thus, a successful wildlife vaccine need not provide complete protection from infection (15, 16).

Vaccines other than BCG have been successfully used in wildlife to control rabies in raccoons (*Procyon lotor*), foxes (*Vulpes vulpes*), skunks (*Mephitis mephitis*) and coyotes (*Canis latrans*) in Europe and North America (17–19); plague in North American black-tailed prairie dogs (*Cynomys ludovicianus*) (20–23); and classical swine fever in wild boar (*Sus scrofa*) in Europe (24). There have been no widespread efforts to vaccinate wildlife to control tuberculosis, although there is currently one approved vaccine for use in European badgers (25) and field trials are progressing (14).

HISTORY OF BCG

The most studied tuberculosis vaccine in deer, as well as other wildlife is the attenuated strain of *M. bovis* known as bacillus Calmette-Guérin (BCG), named for Albert Calmette and Camille Guérin, two French scientists at the Pasteur Institute that developed the strain (26). BCG vaccines are the oldest vaccines still in use today; moreover, with over four billion people vaccinated in over 180 countries it is history's safest and most widely used vaccine (27) and it remains the only approved tuberculosis vaccine for humans. Protective immunity in adults is highly variable, ranging from 0 to 80% depending on the study (28). In adults, BCG vaccination does not reliably prevent infection, development of latent tuberculosis, or reactivation of latent disease (29). However, in infants BCG has proven beneficial and highly cost-effective in protecting children from tuberculous meningitis (30, 31).

In 1901, French veterinarian and microbiologist, Edmond Nocard transferred to Calmette and Guérin a virulent isolate of *M. bovis* he had recovered from a cow with tuberculous mastitis (32). From this isolate, BCG was developed through continuous subculture on a media composed of ox bile, glycerin and potatoes. In 1919, after 13 years and 231 subculture passages, virulence in various animal models was lost (i.e., rabbits, guinea pigs, cows, horses, hamsters, mice, dogs, chickens, non-human primates) (33–35). The attenuation of BCG was shown to be irreversible upon further cultivation on bile-potato medium (36) and passage through various animal species (33). The first human was vaccinated in 1921 when an infant was orally dosed with live BCG. The infant's mother had died of tuberculosis and the infant's caregiver, the grandmother, had clinical tuberculosis. In spite of what must have been significant exposure to virulent *M. tuberculosis*, the child developed normally with no signs of tuberculosis (33). In the following 3 months after this first vaccination, 317 infants were vaccinated and by 1924 more than 660 infants had been orally vaccinated (26). Oral, subcutaneous, intraperitoneal and intravenous routes of administration all proved safe. Although originally given orally, the current recommendation for BCG vaccination is intradermal injection (37). The original BCG was not cloned, but was distributed to many laboratories worldwide, where the vaccine was propagated, such that today there are many genetically variant BCG strains, none of which are identical to each other or to the original vaccine (26, 32, 38). The various substrains differ in immunogenicity and potency; a possible reason for historically large ranges of observed efficacy in human studies around the world (26, 32, 39). Currently, five strains account for >90% of the BCG used worldwide; Pasteur 1173 P2, Danish 1331, Glaxo 1077, Tokyo 172-1, Russian BCG-I and Moreau RDJ (40). The two strains most commonly used in deer studies are strains Danish 1331 and Pasteur 1173 P2. The isolate that would later become BCG Danish was received directly from Calmette in 1931 by Statens Serum Institut. In 1960, batch 1331 was freeze-dried and eventually adopted as the primary Danish 1331 seed-lot in 1966 (32). The strain Pasteur 1173 P2 originated in 1961; produced from a colony closely resembling the original descriptions of BCG by Calmette (32). In white-tailed deer studies, both strains have demonstrated some degree of protection (41).

Calmette and Guérin recognized in animal studies that vaccination prevented disease, but did not always prevent infection (36), a finding consistent with most modern BCG studies in animals (42–45). Although developed as a vaccine for humans, it was first proven efficacious in cattle circa 1911. Calmette and Guérin recommended widespread oral BCG vaccination of neonatal calves, since older calves may have already been infected with virulent *M. bovis* (36). Safety studies in other mammals including horses, sheep, dogs, rabbits, guinea pigs, non-human primates, rats, mice, chickens, and pigeons showed no untoward effects (33).

MODEL OF INFECTION

To study vaccine-induced protection, a reliable model of infection is of paramount importance. The ideal model is repeatable, technically feasible, and produces disease similar to that seen in natural infection. The best and most widely used model of tuberculosis in deer was developed in New Zealand using red deer (*Cervus elaphus*) and a low dose (200–500 colony forming units, CFU) intratonsilar inoculation (46); where virulent *M. bovis* is deposited into one or both palatine tonsillar crypts. Using this model, many experiments were carried out to identify critical variables in BCG studies, such as dose, route, boosting and detailed immune responses (47–52). The red deer model has been extended for use in white-tailed deer (53). In both deer species, the intratonsilar model results in primary involvement of the medial retropharyngeal lymph node (46, 53), the most commonly affected tissue in naturally infected deer (54–56). The frequent involvement of the medial retropharyngeal lymph node suggests that the primary route of infection in deer is oral; although contribution by aerosol cannot be excluded (57–59). Further supporting a primary oral route of infection is the finding that experimental infection of white-tailed deer via an aerosol did not result in lesion distribution similar to natural infection, but rather resulted in disease focused on the lungs and pulmonary lymph nodes (60).

VACCINE EFFICACY

Vaccine doses of 10^4-10^7 CFU of BCG provided significant levels of protection against infection and disease (lesion development) in red deer (51), while 10^7 CFU (parenteral) and 10^8 CFU (oral) demonstrated similar efficacy in white-tailed deer (41, 61, 62).

There are no known antemortem immune responses that correlate to BCG-induced protection. Measurements of immune responses to vaccination such as intradermal skin testing or cytokine production do not predict protection in any species. Rather, BCG efficacy is measured through postmortem quantitative or semi quantitative assessments of disease severity, as well as measuring the level of tissue colonization (63, 64). Disease severity assessments include subjective scoring of gross lesions based on size, number, presence of liquefactive or caseous necrosis or fibrous encapsulation, and the number of tissues with lesions and from which virulent *M. bovis* can be isolated. Protection has also been evaluated by considering the extent and distribution of lesions, that is, animals with lesions limited to a single body region are considered more protected than those with lesions in multiple anatomic locations such as cranial lymph nodes, thoracic lymph nodes and abdominal organs (41, 43, 61, 62, 65).

In white-tailed deer and red deer, oral (43, 51, 62) or subcutaneous (41, 43, 51, 61) BCG vaccination results in fewer lesions, as well as fewer tissues from which virulent *M. bovis* may be isolated. Using subjective gross lesion scoring, BCG vaccination of deer decreases lesion severity and limits disease dissemination. Microscopic examination of tissues reveals that vaccinated deer have fewer large necrotic lesions that contain large numbers of acid-fast bacilli compared to non-vaccinated animals (41, 43, 61, 62). Both live and inactivated BCG in saline and oil adjuvant, as well as a recombinant BCG expressing the inflammatory cytokine IL-2 have been evaluated in red deer (66, 67). Detailed studies show significant immune responses to some of these preparations; however, necropsy and pathology results are not always available from these studies making vaccine efficacy determination difficult. Studies in red deer have also shown that a homologous prime boost regime (i.e., two doses 4-8-weeks apart), further reduces infection and disease (48, 68, 69). A single study in white-tailed deer demonstrated no significant difference between a single vaccination and a homologous prime-boost approach (61). Reduction of disease transmission through BCG vaccination remains to be demonstrated in deer.

In other wildlife species, the time to seroconversion, and transmission from adults to offspring have been used to demonstrate BCG-induced protection in European badgers (13, 14). The median time to seroconversion was significantly longer for vaccinated badgers (413 days), compared to non-vaccinates (230 days) (14). In addition to a direct protective effect of badger vaccination, there was a positive indirect effect on unvaccinated badger cubs. When at least one third of a badger social group was BCG vaccinated, the probability of an unvaccinated badger cub testing positive for *M. bovis* infection was reduced by 79% (13). The use of such metrics in deer would be difficult due to differing social structures, fecundity and biology.

VACCINE DELIVERY

The most efficacious vaccine is of little use if it cannot be delivered to the target population. An effective means of delivery requires knowledge of host feeding behavior, climatic effects on bait matrix composition, environmental survivability of the vaccine, and bait attractiveness and palatability to the target host. In most cases the only effective means to vaccinate wildlife is through an oral bait. Oral vaccines have been used experimentally to protect white-tailed deer from the prion-based, chronic wasting disease (70, 71), as well as brucellosis (72).

A variety of oral baits have been evaluated in wildlife. Dried shell corn has been used to deliver an acaricide to free-ranging white-tailed deer (73, 74) while Hakim, et al showed that free-ranging white-tailed deer found a liquid bait composed of apple juice, water and glycerin palatable; thus a plausible means of delivering pharmaceutical agents (75). A molasses-based bait for potential BCG delivery was evaluated for palatability, attractiveness and stability under various environmental conditions (76). Although environmentally stable and attractive for captive deer, field testing demonstrated a lack of palatability to free-ranging deer. A lipid formulation of BCG has been used as an oral vaccine for brushtail possums (77, 78), and European badgers (45, 79). The same BCG lipid-formulated bait has been used in white-tailed deer, and although vaccination was achievable (43, 80), deer found the lipid formulation unpalatable. In Spain, baits prepared from feed mixed with paraffin, sucrose and cinnamon-truffle powder worked well to deliver BCG to wild boar (81, 82), but have not been evaluated in deer.

A potential hazard of oral bait vaccines, is the difficulty of preventing non-target species from consuming the vaccine bait. Cattle are a non-target species of special interest as it is possible that BCG ingestion could result in sensitization to the tuberculin used in intradermal skin testing resulting in false positive results; thus, confounding accurate identification of infected cattle (83). Alternative diagnostic tests, able to differentiate infected from vaccinated (DIVA) cattle would be needed to avoid this confounding problem (84–86). In addition to exposure of non-target species to vaccine, dosage is difficult to control using oral baits. The effect of higher than recommended doses of vaccine should be evaluated in the target population. In red deer, no untoward effects have been seen using subcutaneous doses of BCG up to 1×10^8 CFU (68); 10–100 times the regular dose, or in white-tailed deer using oral doses of 1×10^9 (80, 87) to 1×10^{10} CFU; 10–100 times the regular dose.

Studies in red deer did not demonstrate shedding of BCG from vaccinates to non-vaccinates (66); however, evidence shows that BCG-vaccinated white-tailed deer shed vaccine and cohorts can become "secondarily vaccinated" (88, 89). It remains to be evaluated whether deer vaccinated secondarily through shed BCG possess any protection against infection with virulent *M. bovis*. If secondary vaccination were to provide protection, this self-disseminating feature could serve to increase vaccine coverage without additional labor or cost. However, the shedding of BCG by deer increases the possibility that non-target species such as cattle could be exposed to BCG. Thus far, indirect contact of calves with BCG-vaccinated white-tailed deer has not resulted in deer-to-cattle transfer of BCG (88, 89).

By comparison, orally vaccinated possums and badgers were shown to shed BCG in feces for up to 7 and 17 days, respectively, after vaccination (44, 90), while excretion could not be detected in orally vaccinated wild boar (82).

SAFETY

Vaccine safety may be viewed from both the perspective of either the vaccinated animal or humans that may come into contact with vaccinated animals. No untoward effects have been reported in BCG-vaccinated deer, possums or badgers (66, 91, 92). In white-tailed deer vaccinated subcutaneously with BCG, but not challenged with virulent *M. bovis*, microscopic, but not gross lesions due to BCG were reported in various lymph nodes (superficial cervical, tracheobronchial, hepatic) as late as 250 days after vaccination (41).

Although BCG has proven safe in humans with uncompromised immune systems, use of BCG in immunocompromised individuals can result in disseminated disease, with infection in various organs and body systems (93, 94). Because BCG may persist in tissues of vaccinated deer, hunters could potentially be exposed to BCG while field dressing vaccinated deer and unlike many other wildlife hosts of *M. bovis*, deer may be consumed as food by humans. In BCG-vaccinated white-tailed deer, vaccine was recovered from lymphoid tissues up to 12 months after oral dosing of 10^9 CFU. Lowering the dose to 10^8 CFU decreased persistence to 9 months. Persistent and viable BCG were limited to lymphoid tissues such as cranial lymph nodes, tracheobronchial, hepatic and mesenteric lymph nodes. Importantly, samples of muscles commonly consumed by hunters (epaxial, sublumbar, supraspinatus, triceps, semimembranosus, semitendinosus and biceps femoris) did not yield viable BCG at any time point (80, 87). In BCG-vaccinated red deer, viable vaccine could be recovered from various lymph nodes and the site of vaccination 14 weeks after vaccination, although the numbers of recoverable CFU were extremely low, 32–57 CFU/node and 150–190 CFU/vaccination site, representing 0.007–0.009% and 0.002–0.003%, respectively, of the original inoculum dose (2×10^6 CFU) (67). It has been shown that thoroughly heating meat products to 60°C (140^0 F) for 6 min kills virulent *M. bovis* (95) and *M. avium* (96). It is assumed the same would be true for *M. bovis* BCG. As humans generally avoid consumption of lymphoid organs and usually cook meat before consumption (97), the potential exposure of humans to BCG from vaccinated deer is very low.

By comparison, BCG has been found in the tissues of orally vaccinated badgers 30 weeks after vaccination (44) and in possums 8 weeks after oral vaccination (90). In contrast, BCG could not be found in the tissues of orally vaccinated wild boar (82) even when examined 30 days after vaccination (98), an important finding as wild boar, similar to deer, are often used for food.

NON-TUBERCULOUS MYCOBACTERIA

Many saprophytic, non-pathogenic species of mycobacteria exist in soil and water. These mycobacteria may be collectively described as non-tuberculous mycobacteria (NTM). Numerous NTM have been isolated from deer (41, 61, 62, 80, 99–101), some of which were found within lesions consistent with tuberculosis. Although some studies have suggested that preexisting sensitivities to *M.avium*, or other NTM, has no effect or confers some degree of protection against virulent challenge (102–106), others show interference with BCG efficacy by NTM exposure in humans, laboratory animals and cattle (102, 104, 107, 108). One proposed mechanism for this reduced efficacy is that pre-existing immune sensitivity to NTM restricts BCG multiplication following vaccination, resulting in dampening of critical cytokine responses, such as that of interferon-gamma (108). For this reason, it is recommended that humans and calves be vaccinated as neonates prior to NTM exposure. It is, as yet unclear how exposure to NTM affects BCG efficacy in deer. Vaccination of neonates, although possible in farmed deer, would prove very difficult in free ranging deer.

FUTURE DIRECTIONS

Self-disseminating Virus-Based Vaccines

One limitation of traditional oral or parenteral vaccination is the need to administer vaccine to every animal individually. Furthermore, with many inactivated vaccines, adequate protection requires subsequent booster vaccinations. In contrast, self-disseminating vaccines are designed to exploit replicating virus-based vectors to spread within the target animal population without the need for individual animal inoculation (109). Vaccination of a limited number of animals introduces the vaccine into the target population and the vaccine is spread naturally as it is shed by vaccinates. Ideal self-disseminating vaccines are viruses with high immunogenicity and high horizontal transmission levels, but with a robust species barrier to minimize infection of non-target species.

Examples of self-disseminating virus-based vaccines include a cytomegalovirus-based vaccine targeting deer mice (*Peromyscus maniculatus*) to interrupt transmission of Sin Nombre hantavirus, and a myxoma virus-based vaccine targeting European hares (*Oryctolagus cuniculus*) to prevent myxomatosis and rabbit hemorrhagic disease [reviewed in Murphy et al. (109)]. A similar self-disseminating viral vectored vaccine targeting white-tailed deer to prevent deer-to-deer and deer-to-cattle transmission of *M. bovis* may one day be possible.

Plant-Based Vaccines

Another alternative to traditional vaccination is the use of plant-based vaccines (110). Selected immunogenic antigens of the pathogen are introduced into a plant, creating a recombinant edible vaccine. Ingestion of the plant material induces a protective immune response against that particular pathogen. Plant-based vaccines are cost-effective and amenable to large scale production (110); moreover, using plants that are part of the normal diet of the target population minimizes issues of palatability and acceptance. Edible vaccines have been produced in tobacco, cereal grains, fruits (banana, tomato), leaves (lettuce, alfalfa), tubers (potato, carrot), and legumes (cow pea, soybean) (111). When produced in plants, antigenic proteins of the vaccine are bioencapsulated in plant cells, to be released when plant cells are digested by microbes of the gut (112). This may be particularly advantageous with diseases such as tuberculosis where mucosal immune responses are critical. Transgenic carrots, tobacco, lettuce and arabidopsis expressing *M. tuberculosis* proteins have been tested in mice and piglets and shown to induce both humoral and cell-mediated immunity (112–115).

Inactivated Vaccines

Attenuated live vaccines, like BCG have some drawbacks. The possibility exists that vaccine shed by vaccinates, may contaminate not only the environment, but also potentially expose various non-target species. Use of genetically altered subunit vaccines may be an alternative; however, there could be public resistance to the use of genetically altered microbes. Heat-inactivated *M. bovis* (oral and parenteral) has been shown to reduce disease severity in wild boar (82, 116) similar to protection provided through vaccination with BCG (117), without risk of environmental contamination or spread to non-target species. Similarly, heat-inactivated *M. bovis* has been shown to decrease disease severity in experimentally infected red deer (118). Another noted advantage to heat-inactivated *M. bovis* is that vaccinated calves did not have false positive responses in either antibody-based assays or interferon gamma release assays measuring cell-mediated immune responses (118) reducing concern that vaccine exposed cattle would be falsely identified as *M. bovis* infected during routine surveillance.

CONCLUSIONS

Between 1940 and 2004, more than 335 emerging infectious disease events were reported in the scientific literature. The majority (60%) of those events involved zoonoses, most of which (72–80%) had an epidemiologically important wildlife host (119, 120). Controlling or eliminating disease, which has become established in wildlife is extremely difficult, with seemingly few solutions, such as population reduction, separation of wildlife from livestock and disease control through vaccination. Varying degrees of success have been achieved with rabies, plague and classical swine fever. In the case of tuberculosis in deer and other wildlife, the challenge is indeed monumental. In spite of millions of research dollars and countless hours of research effort toward a new human vaccine, the only approved vaccine remains one that is 100 years old and provides questionable protection in some settings. Far less money and effort have been expended exploring a vaccine for animal tuberculosis. Nevertheless, there is reason to be optimistic. Regardless of the species, research to date on BCG vaccination consistently demonstrates a decrease in disease severity, which likely results in decreased disease transmission, and progress is being made in the development of oral baits as vaccine delivery devices. Moreover, advances are being made in the next-generation of human vaccines based on BCG (79), some of which may prove useful for vaccination of deer or other wildlife.

AUTHOR CONTRIBUTIONS

All authors listed have made a substantial, direct and intellectual contribution to the work, and approved it for publication.

REFERENCES

1. Palmer MV, Waters WR. Bovine tuberculosis and the establishment of an eradication program in the United States: role of veterinarians. *Vet Med Int.* (2011) 2011:816345. doi: 10.4061/2011/816345
2. Palmer MV, Thacker TC, Waters WR, Gortazar C, Corner LA. *Mycobacterium bovis*: a model pathogen at the interface of livestock, wildlife, and humans. *Vet Med Int.* (2012) 2012:236205. doi: 10.1155/2012/236205
3. O'Brien DJ, Schmitt SM, Fitzgerald SD, Berry DE. Management of bovine tuberculosis in Michigan wildlife: current status and near term prospects. *Vet Microbiol.* (2011) 151:179–87. doi: 10.1016/j.vetmic.2011.02.042
4. O'Brien DJ, Schmitt SM, Rudolph BA, Nugent G. Recent advances in the management of bovine tuberculosis in free-ranging wildlife. *Vet Microbiol.* (2011) 151:23–33. doi: 10.1016/j.vetmic.2011.02.022
5. Ekdahl MO, Smith BL, Money DFL. Tuberculosis in some wild and feral animals in New Zealand. *NZ Vet J.* (1969) 18:44–5. doi: 10.1080/00480169.1970.33860
6. Muirhead RH, Gallagher J, Burn KJ. Tuberculosis in wild badgers in gloucestershire: epidemiology. *Vet Rec.* (1974) 95:552–5. doi: 10.1136/vr.95.24.552
7. Noonan NL, Sheane WD, Harper LR, Ryan PJ. Wildlife as a possible reservoir of bovine tuberculosis. *Ir Vet J.* (1975) 29:1.

8. Collins DM, Gabric DM, de Lisle GW. Typing of *Mycobacterium bovis* isolates from cattle and other animals in the same locality. *NZ Vet J.* (1988) 36:45–6. doi: 10.1080/00480169.1988.35476
9. Morris RS, Pfeiffer DU. Directions and issues in bovine tuberculosis epidemiology and control in New Zealand. *NZ Vet J.* (1995) 43:256–65. doi: 10.1080/00480169./1995.35904
10. Gortazar C, Vicente J, Gavier-Widen D. Pathology of bovine tuberculosis in the European wild boar (*Sus scrofa*). *Vet Rec.* (2003) 152:779–80. doi: 10.1136/vr.152.25.779
11. Vicente J, Hofle U, Garrido JM, Fernandez-De-Mera IG, Juste R, Barral M, et al. Wild boar and red deer display high prevalences of tuberculosis-like lesions in Spain. *Vet Res.* (2006) 37:107–19. doi: 10.1051/vetres:20 05044
12. Naranjo V, Gortazar C, Vicente J, de la Fuente J. Evidence of the role of European wild boar as a reservoir of *Mycobacterium tuberculosis* complex. *Vet Microbiol.* (2008) 127:1–9. doi: 10.1016/j.vetmic.2007.10.002
13. Carter SP, Chambers MA, Rushton SP, Shirley MD, Schuchert P, Pietravalle S, et al. BCG vaccination reduces risk of tuberculosis infection in vaccinated badgers and unvaccinated badger cubs. *PLoS ONE* (2012) 7:e49833. doi: 10.1371/journal.pone.0049833
14. Gormley E, Ni Bhuachalla D, O'Keeffe J, Murphy D, Aldwell FE, Fitzsimons T, et al. Oral vaccination of free-living badgers (*Meles meles*) with bacille Calmette Guerin (BCG) vaccine confers protection against tuberculosis. *PLoS ONE* (2017) 12:e0168851. doi: 10.1371/journal.pone.0168851
15. Buddle BM, Wedlock DN, Denis M. Progress in the development of tuberculosis vaccines for cattle and wildlife. *Vet Microbiol.* (2006) 112:191–200. doi: 10.1016/j.vetmic.2005.11.027
16. Beltran-Beck B, Ballesteros C, Vicente J, de la Fuente J, Gortazar C. Progress in oral vaccination against tuberculosis in its main wildlife reservoir in Iberia, the Eurasian wild boar. *Vet Med Int.* (2012) 2012:978501. doi: 10.1155/2012/978501
17. Rosatte R, MacDonald E, Sobey K, Donovan D, Bruce L, Allan M, et al. The elimination of raccoon rabies from Wolfe Island, Ontario: animal density and movements. *J Wildl Dis.* (2007) 43:242–50. doi: 10.7589/0090-3558-43.2.242
18. Slate D, Algeo TP, Nelson KM, Chipman RB, Donovan D, Blanton JD, et al. Oral rabies vaccination in north america: opportunities, complexities, and challenges. *PLoS Negl Trop Dis.* (2009) 3:e549. doi: 10.1371/journal.pntd.0000549
19. Maki J, Guiot AL, Aubert M, Brochier B, Cliquet F, Hanlon CA, et al. Oral vaccination of wildlife using a vaccinia-rabies-glycoprotein recombinant virus vaccine (RABORAL V-RG®): a global review. *Vet Res.* (2017) 48:57. doi: 10.1186/s13567-017-0459-9
20. Creekmore TE, Rocke TE, Hurley J. A baiting system for delivery of an oral plague vaccine to black-tailed prairie dogs. *J Wildl Dis.* (2002) 38:32–9. doi: 10.7589/0090-3558-38.1.32
21. Rocke TE, Smith SR, Stinchcomb DT, Osorio JE. Immunization of black-tailed prairie dog against plague through consumption of vaccine-laden baits. *J Wildl Dis.* (2008) 44:930–37. doi: 10.7589/0090-3558-44.4.930
22. Rocke TE, Tripp DW, Russell RE, Abbott RC, Richgels KLD, Matchett MR, et al. Sylvatic plague vaccine partially protects prairie dogs (*Cynomys* spp.) in field trials. *Ecohealth* (2017) 14:438–50. doi: 10.1007/s10393-017-1253-x
23. Tripp, DW, Rocke TE, Runge JP, Abbott RC, Miller MW. Burrow dusting or oral vaccination prevents plague-associated prairie dog colony collapse. *Ecohealth* (2017) 14:451–62. doi: 10.1007/s10393-017-1236-y
24. Rossi S, Pol F, Forot B, Masse-Provin N, Rigaux S, Bronner A, et al. Preventive vaccination contributes to control classical swine fever in wild boar (*Sus scrofa* sp.). *Vet Microbiol.* (2010) 142:99–107. doi: 10.1016/j.vetmic.2009.09.050
25. Chambers MA, Carter SP, Wilson GJ, Jones G, Brown E, Hewinson RG, et al. Vaccination against tuberculosis in badgers and cattle: an overview of the challenges, developments and current research priorities in Great Britain. *Vet Rec.* (2014) 175:90–6. doi: 10.1136/vr.102581
26. Abdallah AM, Behr MA. Evolution and strain variation in BCG. *Adv Exp Med Biol.* (2017) 1019:155–69. doi: 10.1007/978-3-319-64371-7_8
27. Fine PE. Bacille Calmette-Guerin vaccines: a rough guide. *Clin Infect Dis.* (1995) 20:11–4. doi: 10.1093/clinids/20.1.11
28. Andersen P, Doherty TM. The success and failure of BCG - implications for a novel tuberculosis vaccine. *Nat Rev Microbiol.* (2005) 3:656–62. doi: 10.1038/nrmicro1211
29. Andersen P. Tuberculosis vaccines- an update. *Nat Rev Microbiol.* (2007) 5:484–7. doi: 10.1038/nrmicro1713
30. Colditz GA, Berkey CS, Mosteller F, Brewer TF, Wilson ME, Burdick E, et al. The efficacy of bacillus Calmette-Guerin vaccination of newborns and infants in the prevention of tuberculosis: meta-analysis of the published literature. *Pediatrics* (1995) 96:29–35.
31. Trunz BB, Fine PEM, Dye C. Effect of BCG vaccination on childhood tuberculous meningitis and miliary tuberculosis worldwide: a meta-analysis and assessment of cost-effectiveness. *Lancet* (2006) 367:1173–80. doi: 10.1016/s0140-6736(06)68507-3
32. Oettinger T, Jorgensen M, Ladefoged A, Haslov K, Andersen P. Development of the *Mycobacterium bovis* BCG vaccine: review of the historical and biochemical evidence for a genealogical tree. *Tuber Lung Dis.* (1999) 79:243–50. doi: 10.1054/tuld.1999.0206
33. Calmette A. Preventive vaccination against tuberculos with BCG. *Proc R Soc Med.* (1931) 24:85–94.
34. Sakula A. BCG: who were Calmette and Guerin? *Thorax* (1983) 38:806–12. doi: 10.1136/thx.38.11.806
35. Corbel MJ, Fruth U, Griffiths E, Knezevic I. Report on a WHO consultation on the characterisation of BCG strains, Imperial College, London 15–16 December 2003. *Vaccine* (2004) 22:2675–80. doi: 10.1016/j.vaccine.2004.01.050
36. Locht, C. The history of BCG. In: Nor NM, Acosta A, Sarmiento, ME, editors. *The Art and Science of Tuberculosis Vaccine Development.* 2nd ed. Selanger Darul Etsun: Oxford University Press. (2010). p. 5 70–91.
37. WHO. BCG vaccine. World Health Organization position paper. *Wkly Epidemiol Rec.* (2004) 79:27–38. Available online at: http://www.who.int/wer
38. Fine PE. The BCG story: lessons from the past and implications for the future. *Rev Infect Dis.* (1989) 11(Suppl. 2):S353–59. doi: 10.1093/clinids/11.Supplement_2.S353
39. Gheorghiu M. The present and future role of BCG vaccine in tuberculosis control. *Biologicals* (1990) 18:135–41. doi: 10.1016/1045-1056(90)90025-U
40. WHO. *Infromation Sheet: observed Rate of Vaccine Reactions Bacille Calmette-Guerin (BCG) Vaccine.* Geneva: WHO (2012).
41. Palmer MV, Thacker TC, Waters WR. Vaccination with *Mycobacterium bovis* BCG strains Danish and Pasteur in white-tailed deer (*Odocoileus virginianus*) experimentally challenged with *Mycobacterium bovis*. *Zoonoses Public Health* (2009) 56:243–51. doi: 10.1111/j.1863-2378.2008.0 1198.x
42. Aldwell FE, Keen DL, Parlane NA, Skinner MA, de Lisle GW, Buddle BM. Oral vaccination with *Mycobacterium bovis* BCG in a lipid formulation induces resistance to pulmonary tuberculosis in brushtail possums. *Vaccine* (2003) 22:70–6. doi: 10.1016/S0264-410X(03)00539-5
43. Nol P, Palmer MV, Waters WR, Aldwell FE, Buddle BM, Triantis JM, et al. Efficacy of oral and parenteral routes of *Mycobacterium bovis* bacille Calmette-Guerin vaccination against experimental bovine tuberculosis in white-tailed deer (*Odocoileus virginianus*): a feasibility study. *J Wildl Dis.* (2008) 44:247–59. doi: 10.7589/0090-3558-44.2.247
44. Corner LA, Costello E, O'Meare D, Lesellier S, Aldwell FE, Singh M, et al. Oral vaccination of badgers (*Meles meles*) with BCG and protective immunity against endobronchial challenge with *Mycobacterium bovis*. *Vaccine* (2010) 28:6265–72. doi: 10.1016/j.vaccine.2010.06.120
45. Chambers MA, Aldwell F, Williams GA, Palmer S, Gowtage S, Ashford R, et al. The effect of oral vaccination with *Mycobacterium bovis* BCG on the development of tuberculosis in captive european badgers (*Meles meles*). *Front Cell Infect Microbiol.* (2017) 7:6. doi: 10.3389/fcimb.2017.00006
46. Mackintosh C, Waldrup K, Labes RE, Buchan G, Griffin F. Intratonsilar inoculation: an experimental model for tuberculosis in deer. In: Griffin F, DeLisle G, editors. *Tuberculosis in Wildlife and Domestic Animals.* Dunedin: Univeristy of Otago Press. 121–22.

47. Mackintosh CG, Griffin JFT. Epidemiological aspects of deer tuberculosis research. In: *Proceedings of the New Zealand Veterinary Association Deer Branch*. Palmerstown North: New Zealand Veterinary Association. (1994). p. 106–13.
48. Griffin JF, Mackintosh CG, Slobbe L, Thomson AJ, Buchan GS. Vaccine protocols to optimise the protective efficacy of BCG. *Tuber. Lung Dis.* (1999) 79:135–43. doi: 10.1054/tuld.1998.0202
49. Griffin JF, Mackintosh CG. Tuberculosis in deer: perceptions, problems and progress. *Vet J.* (2000) 160:202–19. doi: 10.1053/tvjl.200 0.0514
50. Mackintosh CG, Qureshi T, Waldrup K, Labes RE, Dodds KG, Griffin JFT. Genetic resistance to experimental infection with *Mycobacterium bovis* in red deer (*Cervus elaphus*). *Infect Immun.* (2000) 68:1620–25. doi: 10.1128/IAI.68.3.1620-1625.2000
51. Griffin JF, Chinn DN, Rodgers CR, Mackintosh CG. Optimal models to evaluate the protective efficacy of tuberculosis vaccines. *Tuberculosis* (2001) 81:133–9. doi: 10.1054/tube.2000.0271
52. Griffin JF, Rodgers CR, Liggett S, Mackintosh CG. Tuberculosis in ruminants: characteristics of intra-tonsilar *Mycobacterium bovis* infection models in cattle and deer. *Tuberculosis* (2006) 86:404–18. doi: 10.1016/j.tube.2005.10.003
53. Palmer MV, Whipple DL, Olsen SC. Development of a model of natural infection with *Mycobacterium bovis* in white-tailed deer. *J Wildl Dis.* (1999) 35:450–7. doi: 10.7589/0090-3558-35.3.450
54. Lugton IW, Wilson PR, Morris RS, Griffin JF, de Lisle GW. Natural infection of red deer with bovine tuberculosis. *NZ Vet J.* (1997) 45:19–26. doi: 10.1080/00480169.1997.35983
55. Schmitt SM, Fitzgerald SD, Cooley TM, Bruning-Fann CS, Sullivan L, Berry D, et al. Bovine tuberculosis in free-ranging white-tailed deer from Michigan. *J Wildl Dis.* (1997) 33:749–58. doi: 10.7589/0090-3558-3 3.749
56. Palmer MV, Whipple DL, Payeur JB, Alt DP, Esch KJ, Bruning-Fann CS, et al. Naturally occurring tuberculosis in white-tailed deer. *J Am Vet Med Assoc.* (2000) 216:1921–24. doi: 10.2460/javma.2000.2 16.1921
57. Lugton IW, Wilson PR, Morris RS, Nugent G. Epidemiology and pathogenesis of *Mycobacterium bovis* infection of red deer (*Cervus elaphus*) in New Zealand. *NZ Vet J.* (1998) 46:147–56. doi: 10.1080/00480169.1998.36079
58. Lugton I. Mucosa-associated lymphoid tissues as sites for uptake, carriage and excretion of tubercle bacilli and other pathogenic mycobacteria. *Immunol Cell Biol.* (1999) 77:364–72. doi: 10.1046/j.1440-1711.1999.0 0836.x
59. Palmer MV, Waters WR, Whipple DL. Shared feed as a means of deer-to-deer transmission of *Mycobacterium bovis*. *J Wildl Dis.* (2004) 40:87–91. doi: 10.7589/0090-3558-40.1.87
60. Palmer MV, Waters WR, Whipple DL. Aerosol exposure of white-tailed deer (*Odocoileus virginianus*) to *Mycobacterium bovis*. *J Wildl Dis.* (2003) 39:817–23. doi: 10.7589/0090-3558-39.4.817
61. Palmer MV, Thacker TC, Waters WR. Vaccination of white-tailed deer (*Odocoileus virginianus*) with *Mycobacterium bovis* bacillus Calmette Guerin. *Vaccine* (2007) 25:6589–97. doi: 10.1016/j.vaccine.2007.0 6.056
62. Palmer MV, Thacker TC, Waters WR, Robbe-Austerman S. Oral vaccination of white-tailed deer (*Odocoileus virginianus*) with *Mycobacterium bovis* Bacillus Calmette-Guerin (BCG). *PLoS ONE* (2014) 9:e97031. doi: 10.1371/journal.pone.0097031
63. Buddle BM, Parlane NA, Wedlock DN, Heiser A. Overview of vaccination trials for control of tuberculosis in cattle, wildlife and humans. *Transbound Emerg Dis.* (2013) 60(Suppl. 1):136–46. doi: 10.1111/tbed.12092
64. Vordermeier HM, Perez de Val B, Buddle BM, Villarreal-Ramos B, Jones GJ, Hewinson RG, et al. Vaccination of domestic animals against tuberculosis: review of progress and contributions to the field of the TBSTEP project. *Res Vet Sci.* (2014) 97(Suppl):S53–60. doi: 10.1016/j.rvsc.2014.0 4.015
65. Griffin JF, Mackintosh CG, Buchan GS. Animal models of protective immunity in tuberculosis to evaluate candidate vaccines. *Trends Microbiol.* (1995) 3:418–24. doi: 10.1016/S0966-842X(00)88994-5
66. Griffin JF, Hesketh JB, Mackintosh CG, Shi YE, Buchan GS. BCG vaccination in deer: distinctions between delayed type hypersensitivity and laboratory parameters of immunity. *Immunol Cell Biol.* (1993) 71:559–70. doi: 10.1038/icb.1993.62
67. Slobbe L, Lockhart E, O'Donnell MA, MacKintosh C, De Lisle G, Buchan, G. An *in vivo* comparison of bacillus Calmette-Guerin (BCG) and cytokine-secreting BCG vaccines. *Immunology* (1999) 96:517–23. doi: 10.1046/j.1365-2567.1999.00702.x
68. Griffin JF. Veterinary tuberculosis vaccine development. *Clin Infect Dis.* (2000) 30 (Suppl. 3):S223–8. doi: 10.1086/313865
69. Griffin JFT, Mackintosh CG, Rodgers CR. Factors influencing the protective efficacy of a BCG homologous prime-boost vaccination regime against tuberculosis. *Vaccine* (2006) 24:835–45. doi: 10.1016/j.vaccine.2005.0 7.033
70. Goni F, Mathiason CK, Yim L, Wong K, Hayes-Klug J, Nalls A, et al. Mucosal immunization with an attenuated Salmonella vaccine partially protects white-tailed deer from chronic wasting disease. *Vaccine* (2015) 33:726–33. doi: 10.1016/j.vaccine.2014.11.035
71. Taschuk R, Scruten E, Woodbury M, Cashman N, Potter A, Griebel P, et al. Induction of PrP(Sc)-specific systemic and mucosal immune responses in white-tailed deer with an oral vaccine for chronic wasting disease. *Prion* (2017) 11:368–80. doi: 10.1080/19336896.2017.13 67083
72. Arenas-Gamboa AM, Ficht TA, Davis DS, Elzer PH, Wong-Gonzalez A, Rice-Ficht AC. Enhanced immune response of red deer (*Cervus elaphus*) to live RB51 vaccine strain using composite microspheres. *J Wildl Dis.* (2009) 45:165–73. doi: 10.7589/0090-3558-45.1.165
73. Pound JM, Miller JA, George JE, Lemeilleur CA. The "4-poster" passive topical treatment device to apply acaracide for controlling ticks (Acari: *Ixodidae*) feeding on white-tailed deer. *J Med Entomol.* (2000) 37:588–94. doi: 10.1603/0022-2585-37.4.588
74. Grear JS, Koethe R, Hoskins B, Hillger R, Dapsis L, Pongsiri M. The effectiveness of permethrin-treated deer stations for control of the Lyme disease vector *Ixodes scapularis* on Cape Cod and the islands: a five-year experiment. *Parasit Vectors* (2014) 7:292–30. doi: 10.1186/1756-330 5-7-292
75. Hakim S, McShea WJ, Mason JR. The attractiveness of a liquid bait ot white-tailed deer in central Appalachian mountains, Virginia, USA. *J Wildl Dis.* (1996) 32:395–8. doi: 10.7589/0090-3558-32.2.395
76. Palmer MV, Stafne MR, Waters WR, Thacker TC, Phillips GE. Testing a molasses-based bait for oral vaccination of white-tailed deer (*Odocoileus virginianus*) against *Mycobacterium bovis*. *Er J Wildl Res.* (2014) 60:265–70. doi: 10.1007/s10344-013-0777-9
77. Cross ML, Henderson RJ, Lambeth MR, Buddle BM, Aldwell FE. Lipid-formulated bcg as an oral-bait vaccine for tuberculosis: vaccine stability, efficacy, and palatability to brushtail possums (*Trichosurus vulpecula*) in New Zealand. *J Wildl Dis.* (2009) 45:754–65. doi: 10.7589/0090-3558-4 5.3.754
78. Ramsey DS, Aldwell FE, Cross ML, de Lisle GW, Buddle BM. Protection of free-living and captive possums against pulmonary challenge with *Mycobacterium bovis* following oral BCG vaccination. *Tuberculosis* (2009) 89:163–8. doi: 10.1016/j.tube.2008.11.002
79. Neiuwenhuizen NE, Kaufmann SHE. Next generation vaccines based on Bacille Calmette Guerin. *Front Immunol.* (2018) 9:121. doi: 10.3389/fimmu.2018.00121
80. Palmer MV, Thacker TC, Waters WR, Robbe-Austerman S, Aldwell FE. Persistence of *Mycobacterium bovis* bacillus Calmette-Guerin (BCG) Danish in white-tailed deer (*Odocoileus virginianus*) vaccinated with a lipid-formulated oral vaccine. *Transboundary Emerg Dis.* (2012) 61:266–72. doi: 10.1111/tbed.12032
81. Ballesteros C, Gortazar C, Canales M, Vicente J, Lasagna A, Gamarra JA, et al. Evaluation of baits for oral vaccination of European wild boar piglets. *Res Vet Sci.* (2009) 86:388–93. doi: 10.1016/j.rvsc.2008.0 9.003
82. Beltran-Beck B, de la Fuente J, Garrido JM, Aranaz A, Sevilla I, Villar M, et al. Oral vaccination with heat inactivated *Mycobacterium bovis* activates the complement system to protect against tuberculosis. *PLoS ONE* (2014) 9:e98048. doi: 10.1371/journal.pone.0098048

83. Buddle BM, Hewinson RG, Vordermeier HM, Wedlock DN. Subcutaneous administration of a 10-fold-lower dose of a commercial human tuberculosis vaccine, *Mycobacterium bovis* bacillus Calmette-Guerin Danish, induced levels of protection against bovine tuberculosis and responses in the tuberculin intradermal test similar to those induced by a standard cattle dose. *Clin Vaccine Immunol.* (2013) 20:1559–62. doi: 10.1128/CVI.00435-13
84. Whelan C, Whelan AO, Shuralev E, Kwok HF, Hewinson G, Clarke J, et al. Performance of the Enferplex TB assay with cattle in Great Britain and assessment of its suitability as a test to distinguish infected and vaccinated animals. *Clin Vaccine Immunol.* (2010) 17:813–7. doi: 10.1128/CVI.00489-09
85. Vordermeier M, Jones GJ, Whelan AO. DIVA reagents for bovine tuberculosis vaccines in cattle. *Expert Rev Vaccines* (2011) 10:1083–91. doi: 10.1586.erv.11.22
86. Rhodes SG, McKinna LC, Steinbach S, Dean GS, Villarreal-Ramos B, Whelan AO, et al. Use of antigen-specific interleukin-2 to differentiate between cattle vaccinated with *Mycobacterium bovis* BCG and cattle infected with *M. bovis. Clin Vaccine Immunol.* (2014) 21:39–45. doi: 10.1128/CVI.00522-13
87. Palmer MV, Thacker TC, Waters WR, Robbe-Austerman S, Lebepe-Mazur SM, Harris NB. Persistence of *Mycobacterium bovis* Bacillus Calmette-Geurin (BCG) in white-tailed deer (*Odocoileus virginianus*) after oral or parenteral vaccination. *Zoonoses Public Health* (2010) 57:e206–12. doi: 10.1111/j.1863-2378.2010.01329.x
88. Palmer MV, Thacker TC, Waters WR, Robbe-Austerman S,Harris B. Investigations on deer to deer and deer to cattle transmission of the vaccine *Mycobacterium bovis* Bacillus Calmette-Guerin (BCG). *J Vaccines Vaccinat.* (2010) 1:1–6. doi: 10.4172/2157-7560.1000104
89. Nol P, Rhyan JC, Robbe-Austerman S, McCollum MP, Rigg TD, Saklou NT, et al. The potential for transmission of BCG from orally vaccinated white-tailed deer (*Odocoileus virginianus*) to cattle (*Bos taurus*) through a contaminated environment: experimental findings. *PLoS ONE* (2013) 8:e60257. doi: 10.1371/journal.pone.0060257
90. Wedlock DN, Aldwell FE, Keen D, Skinner MA, Buddle BM. Oral vaccination of brushtail possums (*Tichosurus vulpecula*) with BCG: immune responses, persistence of BCG in lymphoid organs and excretion in faeces. *NZ Vet J.* (2005) 53:301–6. doi: 10.1080/00480169.2005.36564
91. Aldwell FE, Pfeffer A, DeLisle GW, Jowett G, Heslop J, Keen D, et al. Effectiveness of BCG vaccination in protecting possums against bovine tuberculosis. *Res. Vet. Sci.* (1995) 58:90–5. doi: 10.1016/0034-5288(95)90095-0
92. Corner LA, Costello E, Lesellier S, O'Meara D, Gormley E. Vaccination of European badgers (*Meles meles*) with BCG by the subcutaneous and mucosal routes induces protective immunity against endobronchial challenge with *Mycobacterium bovis*. *Tuberculosis* (2008) 88:601–9. doi: 10.1016/j.tube.2008.03.002
93. Talbot EA, Perkins MD, Silva SF, Frothingham R. Disseminated bacille Calmette-Guerin disease after vaccination: case report and review. *Clin Infect Dis.* (1997) 24:1139–46. doi: 10.1086/513642
94. Norouzi S, Aghamohammadi A, Mamishi S, Rosenzweig SD, Rezaei N. Bacillus Calmette-Guerin (BCG) complications associated with primary immunodeficiency diseases. *J Infect.* (2012) 64:543–54. doi: 10.1016/j.jinf.2012.03.012
95. Merkal RS, Whipple DL. Inactivation of *Mycobacterium bovis* in meat products. *Appl Environ Microbiol.* (1980) 40:282–4.
96. Merkal RS, Lyle PS, Whipple DL. Heat inactivation of *in vivo*- and *in vitro*-grown mycobacteria in meat products. *Appl Environ Microbiol.* (1981) 41:1484–5.
97. Wilkins MJ, Bartlett PC, Frawley B, O'Brien DJ, Miller CE, Boulton ML. *Mycobacterium bovis* (bovine TB) exposure as a recreational risk for hunters: results of a Michigan Hunter Survey, 2001. *Int J Tuberc Lung Dis.* (2003) 7:1001–9. Available online at: https://www.theunion.org/what-we-do/journals/ijtld
98. Nol P, Robbe-Austerman S, Rhyan JC, McCollum MP, Triantis JM, Beltran-Beck B, et al. Determining the persistence of *Mycobacterium bovis* bacille Calmette-Guerin Danish in select tissues of orally vaccinated feral swine (*Sus scrofa* ssp.). *Res Vet Sci.* (2016) 104:50–2. doi: 10.1016/j.rvsc.2015.11.007
99. Pate M, Zolnir-Dovc M, Kusar D, Krt B, Spicic S, Cvetnic Z, et al. The first report of *Mycobacterium celatum* isolation from domestic pig (*Sus scrofa domestica*) and Roe deer (*Capreolus capreolus*) and an overview of human infections in Slovenia. *Vet Med Int.* (2011) 2011:432954. doi: 10.4061/2011/432954
100. Thacker TC, Robbe-Austerman S, Harris B, Palmer MV, Waters WR. Isolation of mycobacteria from clinical samples collected in the United States from 2004 to 2011. *BMC Vet Res.* (2013) 9:100. doi: 10.1186/1746-6148-9-100
101. Ronai Z, Eszterbauer E, Csivincsik A, Gutl CF, Dencso L, Janosi S, et al. Detection of wide genetic diversity and several novel strains among non-avium nontuberculous mycobacteria isolated from farmed and wild animals in Hungary. *J Appl Microbiol.* (2016) 121:41–54. doi: 10.1111/jam.13152
102. Palmer CE, Long MW. Effects of infection with atypical mycobacteria on BCG vaccination and tuberculosis. *Am Rev Respir Dis.* (1966) 94:553–68. doi: 10.1164/arrd.1966.94.4.553
103. Edwards ML, Goodrich JM, Muller D, Pollack A, Ziegler JE, Smith DW. Infection with *Mycobacterium avium*-intracellulare and the protective effects of Bacille Calmette-Guerin. *J Infect Dis.* (1982) 145:733–41. doi: 10.1093/infdis/145.2.733
104. Orme IM, Collins FM. Efficacy of *Mycobacterium bovis* BCG vaccination in mice undergoing prior pulmonary infection with atypical mycobacteria. *Infect Immun.* (1984) 44:28–32.
105. Orme IA, Roberts AR, Collins FM. Lack of evidence for a reduction in the efficacy of subcutaneous BCG vaccination in mice infected with nontuberculous mycobacteria. *Tubercle* (1986) 67:41–6. doi: 10.1016/0041-3879(86)90030-9
106. Hope JC, Thom ML, Villarreal-Ramos B, Vordermeier HM, Hewinson RG, Howard CJ. Exposure to *Mycobacterium avium* induces low-level protection from *Mycobacterium bovis* infection but compromises diagnosis of disease in cattle. *Clin Exp Immunol.* (2005) 141:432–9. doi: 10.1111/j.1365-2249.2005.02882.x
107. Black GF, Dockrell HM, Crampin AC, Floyd S, Weir RE, Bliss L, et al. Patterns and implications of naturally acquired immune responses to environmental and tuberculous mycobacterial antigens in Northern Malawi. *J Infect Dis.* (2001) 184:322–9. doi: 10.1086/322042
108. Buddle BM, Wards BJ, Aldwell FE, Collins DM, de Lisle GW. Influence of sensitisation to environmental mycobacteria on subsequent vaccination against bovine tuberculosis. *Vaccine* (2002) 20:1126–33. doi: 10.1016/S0264-410X(01)00436-4
109. Murphy AA, Redwood AJ, Jarvis MA. Self-disseminating vaccines for emerging infectious diseases. *Expert Rev Vaccines* (2016) 15:31–9. doi: 10.1586/14760584.2016.1106942
110. Shahid N, Daniell H. Plant-based oral vaccines against zoonotic and non-zoonotic diseases. *Plant Biotechnol J.* (2016) 14:2079–99. doi: 10.1111/pbi.12604
111. Aswathi PB. Plant based edible vaccines against poultry diseases: a review. *Adv Anim Vet Sci.* (2014) 2:305–11. doi: 10.14737/journal.aavs/2014/2.5.305.311
112. Permyakova NV, Zagorskaya AA, Belavin PA, Uvarova EA, Nosareva OV, Nesterov AE, et al. Transgenic carrot expressing fusion protein comprising *M.* tuberculosis antigens induces immune response in mice. *Biomed Res Int.* (2015) 2015:417565. doi: 10.1155/2015/417565
113. Rigano MM, Dreitz S, Kipnis AP, Izzo AA, Walmsley AM. Oral immunogenicity of a plant-made, subunit, tuberculosis vaccine. *Vaccine* (2006) 24:691–95. doi: 10.1016/j.vaccine.2005.08.009
114. Floss DM, Mockey M, Zanello G, Brosson D, Diogon M, Frutos R, et al. Expression and immunogenicity of the mycobacterial Ag85B/ESAT-6 antigens produced in transgenic plants by elastin-like peptide fusion strategy. *J Biomed Biotechnol.* (2010) 2010:274346. doi: 10.1155/2010/274346

115. Lakshmi PS, Verma D, Yang X, Lloyd B, Daniell H. Low cost tuberculosis vaccine antigens in capsules: expression in chloroplasts, bio-encapsulation, stability and functional evaluation *in vitro*. *PLoS ONE* (2013) 8:e54708. doi: 10.1371/journal.pone.0054708
116. Diez-Delgado I, Rodriguez O, Boadella M, Garrido JM, Sevilla IA, Bezos J, et al. Parenteral vaccination with heat-inactivated *Mycobacterium bovis* reduces the prevalence of tuberculosis-compatible lesions in farmed wild boar. *Transbound Emerg Dis*. (2017) 64:e18–21. doi: 10.1111/tbed.12526
117. Garrido JM, Sevilla IA, Beltran-Beck B, Minguijon E, Ballesteros C, Galindo RC, et al. Protection against tuberculosis in Eurasian wild boar vaccinated with heat-inactivated *Mycobacterium bovis*. *PLoS ONE* (2011) 6:e24905. doi: 10.1371/journal.pone.0024905
118. Thomas J, Risalde MA, Serrano M, Sevilla I, Geijo M, Ortiz JA, et al. The response of red deer to oral administration of heat-inactivated *Mycobacterium bovis* and challenge with a field strain. *Vet Microbiol.* (2017) 208:195–202. doi: 10.1016/j.vetmic.2017.08.007
119. Jones KE, Patel NG, Levy MA, Storeygard A, Balk D, Gittleman JL, et al. Global trends in emerging infectious diseases. *Nature* (2008) 451:990–3. doi: 10.1038/nature06536
120. Gortazar C, Diez-Delgado I, Barasona JA, Vicente J, De La Fuente J, Boadella M. The wild side of disease control at the wildlife-livestock-human interface: a review. *Front Vet Sci.* (2014) 1:27. doi: 10.3389/fvets.2014.00027

8

Risk Perceptions and Protective Behaviors toward Bovine Tuberculosis among Abattoir and Butcher Workers

Fikre Fekadu[1], *Tariku Jibat Beyene*[1,2], *Ashenafi Feyisa Beyi*[1,3], *Bedaso Mammo Edao*[1,4], *Takele Beyene Tufa*[1], *Fanos Tadesse Woldemariyam*[1,5] *and Fanta Desissa Gutema*[1,6]*

[1] College of Veterinary Medicine and Agriculture, Addis Ababa University, Bishoftu, Ethiopia, [2] Centre for Outcomes Research and Epidemiology, Department of Diagnostic Medicine, Pathobiology, College of Veterinary Medicine, Kansas State University, Manhattan, KS, United States, [3] Department of Veterinary Microbiology and Preventive Medicine, College of Veterinary Medicine, Iowa State University, Ames, IA, United States, [4] Department of Veterinary Medicine, University of Cambridge, Cambridge, United Kingdom, [5] Faculty of Bioscience Engineering, KU Leuven, Leuven, Belgium, [6] Faculty of Veterinary Medicine, Ghent University, Ghent, Belgium

Correspondence:
Fanta Desissa Gutema
fantadesissa@gmail.com

Bovine Tuberculosis (BTB) is a serious cause of economic losses and public health threat, especially in developing countries. Humans acquire BTB through consumption of raw or undercooked meat, inhalation of aerosol and occupational exposure. A cross-disciplinary approach to study diseases connecting society and biology helps to understand the ways in which social, cultural, behavioral, and economic circumstances influence a healthy life. The objective of this study was to assess the risk perceptions and protective behaviors toward BTB among abattoir and butcher workers in central Ethiopia. A health belief model was used to generate the desired data following health belief model constructs. A total of 300 meat handlers working in local abattoirs, export abattoirs and butcher houses in Bishoftu, Modjo, Dukem, and Akaki towns of central Ethiopia were selected using a systematic random sampling method. Univariate and multivariable logistic regression analysis were used to assess factors associated with risk of exposure to BTB through the consumption of raw meat. The results showed that among the study participants, 95% heard about BTB and 93% knew that eating raw meat could be a source of BTB for humans. More than 62.7% of the respondents in the high risk group strongly agreed that contracting BTB would prevent them from coming to work, keep them in bed for an extended period of time and cause death. The majority of the respondents believed that free provision of personal protective clothing, compensation with test and slaughter campaigns, television and radio advertisements, educational programs and government-imposed penalties would help in prevention of BTB. Despite the high perceived severity and risk perception, the multivarable logistic regression model showed low-risk protective behavior among male (OR: 2.3, 95% CI: 1.2–4.3) and older age (>30) individuals (OR: 14.4 95% CI: 2.1–125.8). The study also noted the importance of media for health education as means for prevention of BTB. The authors strongly recommended the need of promotion of behavioral change toward the consumption of raw meat wich would have potential implications for the public health impacts of zoonotic tuberculosis and ultimately help national and global efforts toward prevention and control of tuberculosis.

Keywords: bovine tuberculosis, health belief model, protective behavior, raw meat, risk perception, Ethiopia

INTRODUCTION

Bovine Tuberculosis (BTB) is a zoonotic Tuberculosis disease (TB) caused by *Mycobacterium bovis (M. bovis)* with cattle being serving as a primary host. In 2016, an estimated 147,000 new human cases of zoonotic TB and 12,500 deaths due to the disease occurred globally. The African region carries the heaviest burden, followed by the South-East Asian region (1–3). In Africa, zoonotic TB due to *M. bovis* is transmitted through inhalation of aerosols, leading to pulmonary TB, and through ingestion of contaminated animal products such as milk and meat, leading primarily to extrapulmonary TB (4). In most developed countries, it was eliminated or controlled in the domestic animal population through strict control and eradication measures including test-and-slaughter strategies and compulsory pasteurization of milk. As a result, human infection is reduced, even though the potential risk remains in place (5, 6).

In Ethiopia, the average prevalence of bovine tuberculosis based on studies done between 2000 and 2016 showed to be 6% in cattle. The prevalence also varied based on the breeds of cattle and the production systems (7). The fact that *M. bovis* is frequently isolated from various animal organs/tissues such as lesions in the lungs and lymph nodes at slaughterhouses gestures that the disease can spread through both direct and indirect modes to human (8). Out of all human TB cases, the contribution of *M. bovis* was estimated to be 17.0% (9). This is of great importance, especially for livestock traders, farmers and animal product handlers.

Occupational exposures to *M. bovis* have been reported in many countries including Australia (10). In Nigeria, 10% prevalence of TB was diagnosed among livestock traders; and about one-quarter of the identified TB cases were caused by *M. bovis* strains. This study indicated that several factors including poor living conditions contributed to exposure of the people to *M. bovis* infections (11). In addition to the health effects, the economic loss in livestock caused by TB is enormous. Direct economic losses due to the infection become evident by 10 to 18% and 15% reduction in milk and meat production, respectively (12).

Collecting data on the status of BTB can enhance the understanding of the effects and patterns of transmission of the diseases and the associated determinant factors in population (13). To communicate the potential risks and protective measures effectively, health authorities need to understand the determinants of a particular behavior such as the role of beliefs, the perception of risk, benefits, and barriers to change to protect oneself (14, 15).

The Health Belief Model (HBM), a theory that is used to incorporate each of these factors, allows researchers to assess what might constitute one's protective behavior which is influenced by constructs of knowledge, perceived benefits, perceived susceptibility and severity, perceived barrier, self-efficacy, and cue to action (16). Addressing the occupational risks related to such infectious diseases is necessary by exploring the risk perception and protective behavior against the disease. According to this model, meat handlers at abattoirs and butcher shops are likely to overlook health-related precautionary measures including avoiding eating raw meat and refrain from contacting contaminated meat, if the meat handlers consider BTB to be a threat to their health and believe to be susceptible to the disease BTB. In other words, a meat handler and trader are less likely to eat the visibly infected parts of the meat when they feel they are at a heightened risk of BTB owing to their general work conditions such as working in the abattoirs and habits of processing raw meat with inadequate protective wear and not washing their hands before and after processing meat. A meat handler is also likely to read messages related to health if they believe that the benefits of the measures taken as a precaution to avert BTB outweigh the costs and if factors have synergistic rather than hindering contributions. The meat handlers will also need to feel that they are capable of undertaking the required actions to avoid risky behaviors which are called here self-efficacy. The cues or readiness to action component of the model is the least systematically studied or understood of all constructs (16).

However, such information is limited in Ethiopia. To this end, addressing the occupational risks related to such infectious diseases is needed by exploring the risk perception and protective behaviors against the disease. Therefore, the objective of this study was to assess the occupational exposure risk perceptions and protective behaviors toward BTB among abattoir and butcher house workers in four selected towns of central Ethiopia.

MATERIALS AND METHODS

Study Site and Population

The study was conducted in four selected towns in central Ethiopia (Bishoftu, Modjo, Dukem, and Akaki towns) on randomly selected people working in local and export abattoirs as well as butcher houses (**Figure 1**). The study population consists of people living in the towns working in abattoirs and butcher houses. The eligibility criteria were meat handlers who were 15 years old or above, working in local or export abattoirs and butcher houses.

Study Design and Theoretical Framework

The study employed a cross-sectional study design following the HBM. The model is commonly used to explain a wide variety of health behaviors and can be successfully used to guide public health interventions (16). It emphasizes the subjective perceptions of the individuals in understanding behaviors. Perceived susceptibility and severity of a health hazard as well as perceived benefits and barriers of preventive health behaviors are key components of the HBM. They are theorized to underline the cognitive processes involved in health-related decision making (17). The current study followed similar protocol used by Hambolu et al. (18) in adopting the HBM.

The main study outcome was whether respondents did or did not eat raw meat. Those who ate raw meat were classified as "high risk" and otherwise "low risk." The independent variables were related to socio-demographic variables, knowledge

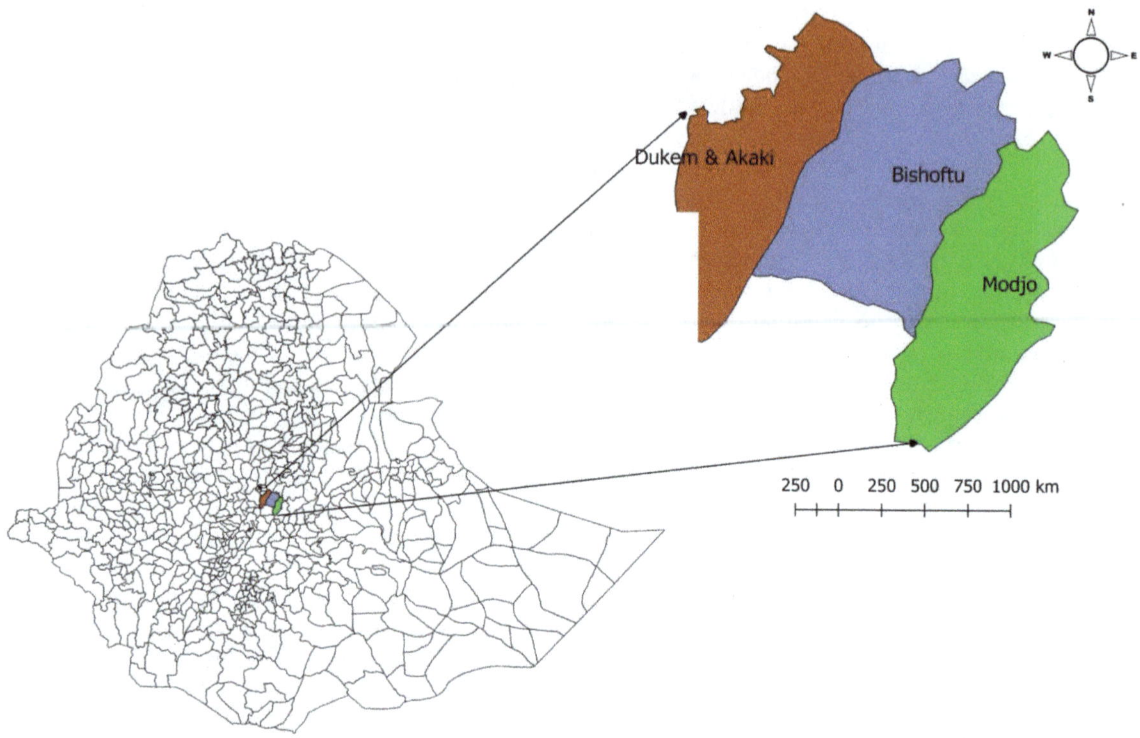

FIGURE 1 | Map of the study sites.

indicators related to TB and BTB, other risky behaviors related to BTB, participants' perceived susceptibility, perceived severity, perceived barriers, self-efficacy, and cues to action to BTB.

Sample Size and Sampling

The sample size was calculated by considering 74.4% expected prevalence of raw meat eating habit (16), 95% confidence interval and 5% required precision. Accordingly, the minimum target sample size was 289 and we collected data from 300 study people working the abattoirs in the study area.

Data Collection Tool and Eligibility

Data were collected through face-to-face interview using a pre-tested and structured questionnaire. The questionnaire format consisted of four sections. The first part included questions about participants' socio-demographic characteristics such as age, gender, level of education, monthly income, and religion. The second part comprised of questions examining the knowledge on BTB, with response options of "yes," "no" or "I don't know." The third part had items asking about risk-taking behavior, including whether participants eating raw meat with response options of either "yes" or "no." The final part consists of questions relating to each of the health belief model constructs: perceived susceptibility, severity, barriers, self-efficacy, and readiness or cues to action. For the items in the health belief model constructs, participants were asked to indicate their level of agreement to the given statements eliciting their own views on a five-point Likert scale:(1) Strongly disagree, (2) Disagree, (3) Neither agree nor disagree, (4) Agree, and (5) Strongly Agree.

Statistical Analysis

The collected data were entered into excel spreadsheet and analyzed using SPSS version 20. As all the variables were categorical, the values in each category were presented together with their corresponding percentages. Univariate and multivariate logistic regression analyses were conducted to examine the effects of the independent variables on the dependent variable (eating raw meat). Correlation between responses to items within a construct was tested using Cronbach alpha. If the correlation was high (> 0.7), then the average of the Likert scale was considered. Candidate variables having a *P*-value less than 0.05 during the univariate analysis were further included in the multivariate logistic regression model to see their association with risk of consuming raw meat. The significance level was set at $\alpha < 0.05$ (19).

RESULTS

Socio-Demographic Characteristics

A total of 300 people were interviewed and all responded to the questionnaires. Of these, 75% (225) of the respondents had eaten/consumed raw meat and categorized as having high-risk behavior whereas the remaining who did not consume raw meat (25%) were referred as "the low-risk group."

Eighty percent (241/300) of the respondents were male, and more than half of them (165/300) were in the age category of 21–30 years. The univariate analysis showed that among the socio-demographic variables, only the gender variable was shown to have a significant difference across proportions of categories of a variable as compared between low and high risk groups ($P < 0.01$). Irrespective of the risk category, people in the categories of male gender, 21–30 age range, Orthodox religion followers, those who work in abattoirs, and those with income range of 1–5 USD per day where found to make 80.3, 55, 83.3, 69.3, and 97% of the participants having the habit of consuming raw meat, respectively (**Table 1**).

Knowledge

Among the respondents, about 95.3% of the respondents had awareness about TB. In spite of this fact, 97.3% of them were found to consume raw meat becoming a high-risk group. Ninety-three percent of all the interviewed people knew about the transmission mode of TB from animals to humans. More than 70% of them were aware about that the healthy-looking meat could be contaminated. On the other hand, about 90% of respondents knew that consumption of contaminated meat could be a source of BTB in humans (**Table 2**). Based on the univariate analysis, all the variables related to knowledge about BTB: heard of TB, spread of TB from animals to humans, healthy-looking meat contains TB causing pathogen and consumption of contaminated meat can be a source of infection in humans were found statistically associated with the high-risk behavior of the habit of consuming raw meat ($P < 0.05$).

Perceived Susceptibility

The univarate logistic regression analysis showed statistically significant association of all the considered evidence for the respondents' perceived susceptibility with the high risk behavior for contracting BTB ($P < 0.05$). Most of respondents perceived that they had a probability of increased chance of contracting BTB because of their work, when they use bare hands, when they would eat in the slaughterhouses and perceived that contaminated (unwashed) hands and eating raw meat (**Table 3**).

Perceived Barriers to Prevention

Contrary to the perceived susceptibility all the attributes of the perceived barriers to prevention of BTB were not statistically associated with the high-risk behavior ($P > 0.05$) (**Table 4**).

Perceived Severity

More than 62.7% of the respondents in the high risk group strongly agreed that contracting BTB would prevent them from coming to work, keep them in bed for an extended period of time and cause death. These were statistically significant ($p < 0.05$). There were no significant difference between high risk and low-risk groups based on contacting BTB is scaring and treatable or not ($P > 0.05$) (**Table 5**).

TABLE 1 | Univariate analysis of demographic characteristics and their association with raw meat eating habit of abattoir and butcher house workers.

Variables	Number (%) $n = 300$	High risk (%) $n = 225$	Low risk (%) $n = 75$	*p*-value
GENDER				
Male	241(80.3)	153 (68.0)	63(84.4)	<0.01
Female	59 (19.7)	72(32.0)	12(15.6)	
AGE				
15–20	18 (6.0)	21(9.3)	4(4.9)	0.06
21–30	165 (55.0)	135(60.0)	40(53.3)	
31–40	68 (22.7)	42(18.7)	18(24.1)	
>40	49 (14.3)	27(12.0)	13(17.7)	
LEVEL OF EDUCATION				
Illiterate	11 (3.7)	12(5.4)	4(4.9)	0.66
At school	274 (91.3)	200(89.3)	69(92.0)	
Graduate	15 (5.0)	12(5.3)	2(3.1)	
RELIGION				
Orthodox	250 (83.3)	198(88.0)	61(81.8)	0.46
Muslim	18 (6.0)	12(5.3)	5(6.2)	
Protestant	27 (9.0)	15(6.7)	7(9.8)	
Traditional	5 (1.7)	0(0.0)	2(2.2)	
OCCUPATION				
Abattoir worker	208 (69.3)	171 (76.0)	50 (67.1)	0.19
Butcher man	92 (30.7)	54 (24.0)	25 (32.9)	
INCOME PER DAY				
<1 USD	6 (2.0)	3 (1.3)	2 (2.2)	0.85
1–5 USD	291 (97.0)	219 (97.3)	73 (96.9)	
>6 USD	3 (1.0)	3 (1.3)	1 (0.9)	

TABLE 2 | Univariate analysis of knowledge about bovine tuberculosis (BTB) by risk categories among workers of abattoirs and butcher shops.

Knowledge related variables	Number (%)	High risk (%) $N = 225$	Low risk (%) $N = 75$	*p*-value
HAVE YOU HEARD OF TB?				
Yes	286 (95.3)	201 (89.3)	73 (97.3)	0.02
No	2 (0.7)	3 (1.3)	3 (0.4)	
Don't Know	12 (4.0)	33 (14.7)	33 (3.6)	
CAN TB SPREAD FROM ANIMALS TO HUMANS?				
Yes	279 (93.0)	192 (85.3)	72 (95.6)	<0.01
No	2 (3.3)	0 (0)	1 (0.9)	
Don't know	19 (4.0)	33 (14.7)	3 (3.6)	
CAN HEALTHY LOOKING MEAT CONTAIN TB CAUSING PATHOGENS?				
Yes	221 (73.7)	138 (61.3)	58 (77.8)	0.02
No	25 (8.3)	24 (10.7)	6 (7.6)	
Don't know	54 (18.0)	63 (28)	11 (14.7)	
IS CONSUMPTION OF CONTAMINATED MEAT A SOURCE OF BTB INFECTION IN HUMANS?				
Yes	267 (89.0)	186 (82.7)	68 (91.1)	<0.01
No	6 (2.0)	0 (0)	2 (2.7)	
Don't know	27 (9.00)	39 (17.3)	5 (6.2)	

TABLE 3 | Univariate analysis of perceived susceptibility to bovine tuberculosis (BTB) by risk groups (Percent sum up to 100 for each risk group across the levels of Likert scales.

Questions	Strongly disagree (%)	Disagree (%)	Neither agree nor disagree (%)	Agree (%)	Strongly agree (%)	p-value
DO YOU THINK THAT YOU HAVE AN INCREASED CHANCE OF CONTRACTING BTB BECAUSE OF YOUR WORK?						
Low risk	26.7	2.7	6.7	30.7	33.3	0.02
High risk	19.1	2.2	2.2	22.2	53.3	
DO YOU THINK THAT YOU ARE AT INCREASED RISK OF CONTRACTING BTB WHEN YOU USE A BARE HAND?						
Low risk	26.7	1.3	6.7	36.0	29.3	<0.01
High risk	17.3	1.3	2.2	27.1	52.0	
DO YOU THINK THAT YOU ARE AT INCREASED RISK OF CONTRACTING BTB WHEN YOU EAT IN THE SLAUGHTER SLAB?						
Low risk	24.0	1.3	6.7	41.3	26.7	<0.01
High risk	10.7	0.4	8.5	27.2	52.7	
DO YOU THINK THAT YOU ARE AT INCREASED RISK OF CONTRACTING BTB WHEN YOU DON'T WASH YOUR HANDS AFTER HANDLING CARCASSES?						
Low risk	24.3	1.4	4.1	36.5	33.8	0.01
High risk	14.2	0.4	2.7	25.2	57.1	
DO YOU THINK THAT YOU ARE AT INCREASED RISK OF CONTRACTING BTB WHEN YOU EAT RAW MEAT?						
Low risk	69.3	1.3	4.0	14.7	10.7	<0.01
High risk	15.5	0.9	2.7	45.1	35.4	

TABLE 4 | Univariate analysis of perceived barriers to prevent bovine tuberculosis (BTB) among workers of abattoirs and butcher shops.

Questions	Strongly disagree (%)	Disagree (%)	Neither agree nor disagree (%)	Agree (%)	Strongly agree (%)	p-value
DO YOU NEED TO TASTE MEAT BEFORE SELLING TO SHOW THAT IT IS SAFE?						
Low risk	80.0	0.0	0.0	1.3	18.7	0.36
High risk	72.0	0.0	0.0	0.9	26.8	
CANNOT WEAR PROTECTIVE CLOTHING BECAUSE THEY ARE NOT CONDUCIVE TO WORK?						
Low risk	94.7	0.0	0.0	4.0	1.3	0.11
High risk	98.2	0.9	0.9	0.4	0.9	
CANNOT WEAR PROTECTIVE CLOTHING BECAUSE THEY ARE EXPENSIVE?						
Low risk	98.7	0.0	0.0	1.3	0.0	0.30
High risk	99.6	0.4	0.0	0.0	0.4	
DO NOT WEAR PROTECTIVE CLOTHING BECAUSE MY COLLEAGUES DO NOT?						
Low risk	98.7	0.0	0.0	1.3	0.0	0.26
High risk	99.1	0.4	0.0	0.0	0.9	

Self-Efficacy

Only 25% of the respondents in the high risk group agreed or strongly agreed that they were able to tell if carcasses were infected with TB or not ($P < 0.05$). There were no significant difference between high risk and low-risk groups based on the capacity to buy protective wear and wearing of protective wear when their colleagues are not wearing $P > 0.05$ (**Table 6**).

Cue to Action

Over 65% of respondents in the high risk group agreed or strongly agreed that free provision of protective clothing and compensation with test and slaughter campaigns would help to protect BTB ($P < 0.05$). Even though, not statically significant ($P > 0.05$), the majority of the respondents agreed or strongly agreed that both television and radio advertisements, educational programs, and government-imposed penalties would help to protect BTB (**Table 7**).

Evaluation of the way the public protection could be prompted shows that the majority of respondents agreed or strongly agreed that radio advertisements and adequate compensation would help (**Figure 2**). In addition, about 65% of respondents felt that they would need educational programs and free provision of protective clothing in order to comply with the procedures and 60% felt that government-imposed penalties for those who do not practice safe measures would work.

All the potential predictors of the high-risk behavior for contacting BTB under each construct of HBM based the univariate analysis having statistically significant association at a p-value less than 0.05 and high correlation (>0.7) between significant variables with in each construct were further analyzed using multivariate logistic regression to determine the predictors of the high risk behavior. The analyses were done using the

TABLE 5 | Univariate analysis of perceived severity to prevent bovine tuberculosis (BTB) among workers of abattoirs and butcher shops.

Questions	Strongly disagree	Disagree	Neither agree nor disagree	Agree	Strongly agree	*P*-value
DO YOU THINK THAT CONTRACTING BTB WILL PREVENT YOU COMING TO WORK?						
Low risk	6.7	0.0	5.3	29.3	57.3	<0.01
High risk	2.7	0.0	1.3	17.3	78.7	
DO YOU THINK THAT CONTRACTING BTB WILL KEEP YOU IN BED FOR AN EXTENDED PERIOD OF TIME?						
Low risk	10.7	0.0	4.0	28.0	56.0	0.02
High risk	4.4	0.0	1.3	20.0	74.2	
DO YOU THINK THAT CONTRACTING BTB SCARES YOU?						
Low risk	29.3	4.0	4.0	14.7	46.7	0.12
High risk	21.7	1.8	1.3	12.4	62.7	
DO YOU THINK THAT BTB CAN CAUSE DEATH						
Low risk	5.3	2.7	2.7	22.7	65.3	0.01
High risk	2.7	0.4	1.8	10.7	84.4	
DO YOU THINK THAT TB IS TREATABLE?						
Low risk	5.33	2.7	4.0	12.0	74.7	0.53
High risk	3.6	0.9	2.2	10.2	83.1	

TABLE 6 | Univariate analysis of self- efficacy to prevent bovine tuberculosis (BTB) among workers of abattoirs and butcher shops in Central Ethiopia.

Questions	Strongly disagree	Disagree	Neither agree nor disagree	Agree	Strongly agree	*P*-value
CAN YOU BUY PROTECTIVE WEAR?						
Low risk	85.3	2.7	1.3	1.3	9.3	0.25
High risk	78.7	0.9	0.4	4.4	15.6	
CAN YOU WEAR PROTECTIVE WEAR EVEN IF YOUR COLLEAGUES ARE NOT?						
Low risk	1.3	0.0	1.3	1.3	96.0	0.39
High risk	1.3	0.0	0.0	1.3	97.3	
ARE YOU ABLE TO TELL IF CARCASSES ARE INFECTED WITH TB OR NOT?						
Low risk	76.0	6.7	2.7	2.7	12.0	<0.01
High risk	63.1	2.2	0.9	25.3	8.4	

TABLE 7 | Univariate analysis of Cues to action to prevent bovine tuberculosis (BTB) among workers of abattoirs and butcher shops in Central Ethiopia.

Questions	Strongly disagree	Disagree	Neither agree nor disagree	Agree	Strongly agree	*P*-value
DO YOU THINK THAT EDUCATIONAL PROGRAMS WOULD HELP TO PROTECT BTB?						
Low risk	5.3		5.3	32.0	56.0	0.29
High risk	4.4		2.2	26.2	67.1	
DO YOU THINK THAT SUPPLY OF FREE CLOTHING WOULD HELP TO PROTECT BTB?						
Low risk	4.0	0.0	9.3	34.6	52.0	0.01
High risk	1.3	0.4	2.2	27.1	68.8	
DO YOU THINK THAT ADEQUATE COMPENSATION FOR COOPERATING WITH TEST AND SLAUGHTER CAMPAIGNS WOULD HELP TO PROTECT BTB?						
Low risk	5.3		13.3	34.6	44.0	<0.01
High risk	1.7		4. %	28.4	65.3	
DO YOU THINK THAT GOVERNMENT IMPOSED PENALTIES WOULD HELP TO PROTECT BTB?						
Low risk	2.6	2.6	6.6	22.6	64.0	0.06
High risk	2.2	0.0	2.6	25.3	69.7	
DO YOU THINK THAT TELEVISION ADVERTISEMENT WOULD HELP TO PROTECT BTB?						
Low risk	1.3		5.3	20.0	72.0	0.66
High risk	0.8		2.6	18.6	77.7	
DO YOU THINK THAT RADIO ADVERTISEMENT WOULD HELP TO PROTECT BTB?						
Low risk	1.3		5.3	18.6	73.3	0.39
High risk	0.8		1.7	18.6	78.6	

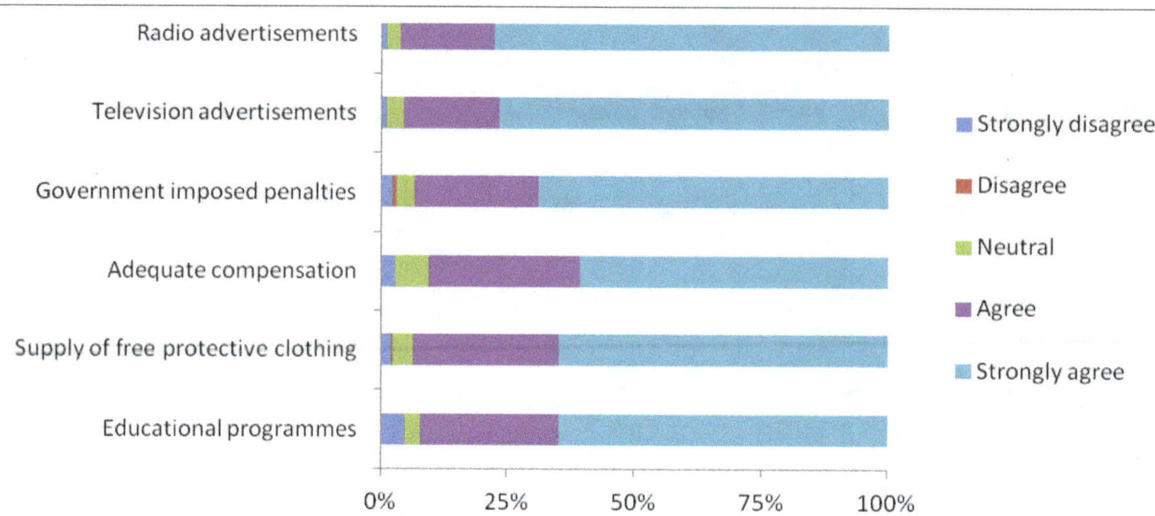

FIGURE 2 | Major interventions for facilitating the adoption of protective behaviors and practices.

TABLE 8 | Multivariate logistic regression analysis of HBM constructs to prevent bovine tuberculosis (BTB) among workers of abattoirs and butcher shops.

Risk factors identified	Adjusted odds ratio (95% CI)	*P*-value
PERCEIVED SUSCEPTIBILITY		
High susceptibility	1	
Low susceptibility	1.6 (1.2–2.1)	<0.01
GENDER		
Female	1	
Male	2.3 (1.2–4.3)	0.01
AGE CATEGORY		
<15	1	
15–20	4.6 (0.6–44.2)	0.15
21–30	6.4 (0.9–51.5)	0.15
31–40	14.4 (2.1–125.8)	<0.01
>40	9.6 (1.3–89.9)	0.03

significant variables and averaged Likert scale of the significant variables under each construct. Accordingly, only the male gender, those who claim to be older and those who perceive that are not susceptible to BTB were associated with the risk of high risk behavior of consuming raw meat (**Table 8**).

DISCUSSION

This study attempted to assess the risk perceptions and protective behaviors on BTB and identify the determinants of the high-risk behavior, eating raw meat, among workers of abattoirs and butcher shops in central Ethiopia using the health belief model. The present study showed the high prevalence of the risky behavior of eating raw meat for BTB (75%, 225/300), which was in agreement with the findings of Biru et al. (20) in which 79.3% people were found to consume raw meat in and around Sululta, central Ethiopia. About 95% of the respondents were aware of TB, and 93% of them were aware that TB can spread from animals to humans and the was relatively higher as compared to a previous study (21), which reported that about 82% of the respondents in western highland regions of Cameroon aware of TB. The high-risk group was found to exhibit better knowledge (95.3%) about TB, despite that, they were found to consume raw meat becoming a high-risk group. This is not in line with theories of the health belief model as well as other health behavior models, which might be due to the longtime and deep entrenched cultural habit of eating raw meat in Ethiopia, particularly eating "*kurt*" (raw beef) and "*kitfo*" (raw or undercooked minced beef mixed with blend of several spices) in many social groups including educated people such as animal and human health professionals in the country (22).

The health belief model recognizes the importance of raising awareness in the populations for the promotion of health and disease protective life strategy. Our finding was in contrary to other findings that concluded as "patchy awareness" and lack of knowledge of zoonosis combined with raw meat eating habits and poor livestock keeping systems are likely to expose respondents to an increased risk of contracting zoonosis (18, 23).

Out of the demographic factors male gender and age (above30 years) were found to associate with the high-risk behavior, consumption of raw meat. This might be due to the fact that most of the workers in the abattoir were male individuals (80.3%). The finding of risky behavior related to the age was not in agreement with another finding, this might be due to the raw meat eating culture of adult people as compared to young ones in Ethiopia (22). In this study, the male respondents were found to be more in a high-risk group compared to the female counterpart. This finding is in agreement with the reports of Hambolu et al. (18) who reported 78.2% of males were in the high group in Nigeria. As the matter of the fact and the high probability of the exposure, older groups and male individuals working in abattoirs in Ethiopia will be at greater risk of contracting BTB. Behavioral sciences explain that the observed predominance of risk-bearing behavior among males as inherently linked to the social construction of masculinity in many African countries. Given that, further in depth studies might be required to get insight into the Ethiopian context (23).

In our study, even though they were not statistically significant, free provision of personal protective clothing, compensation with test and slaughter campaigns wherever economic benefits allow, television and radio advertisements, educational programs and government-imposed penalties found to help to protect BTB. These findings are comparable with a study conducted in Nigeria (18).

The respondents perceived susceptibility to contracting BTB showed that there was increased chance of contracting BTB because of handling meat using a bare and contaminated hand, their work, eating at slaughter slab and eating raw meat. In terms of perceived barrier namely the perception that one cannot wear personal protective clothing because they are not conducive for work, and the perception that one cannot sell meat without tasting were not found to be predictors of the high-risk behavior. However, according to Janz et al. (24) the perceived barriers were the most important predictors of behavior while perceived susceptibility was the most important amongst predictors of preventative behavior.

The main limitation of this study was the use of cross-sectional study design, which is unable to verify causal relationships between the dependent and independent variables. It is documented that other methods such as longitudinal designs have a clear superiority in studies of belief-behavior relationships (25). The face to face semi-structured interviews which were used in this study might have increased the likelihood of respondents' inclination to give socially acceptable answers as also hypothesized by Hambolu et al. (18). Despite the limitation, there was a high response rate (100%), making the results likely to be the beliefs of the study population.

In conclusion, the study revealed low-risk protective behavior among male and older age (>30) individuals despite the high-risk perception and the importance of media for health education as means for prevention of BTB. We believe that the findings of the study would help and serve as a baseline data for policy and decision makers to take appropriate actions aimed at mitigating the risk of tuberculosis transmission to humans from animals following consumption of raw meat. Avoiding eating raw meat, avoiding handling of meat using bare and contaminated hands, creation of awareness for workers in abattoirs and butcher houses in particular and the general population in general about zoonotic importance of BTB using radio and television streaming and a national level study to assess the public perception regarding zoonotic importance of BTB were recommended.

ETHICS APPROVAL AND CONSENT TO PARTICIPATE

This research was approved by the Academic Commission of College of Veterinary Medicine and Agriculture, Addis Ababa University. As the research was not involving invasive procedures and collection of biological samples, separate ethical clearance was not solicited. The study purpose was explained to participants and verbal agreement was obtained before proceeding to the study. Due to the low literacy rate and lack of interest of the participants to put their signature on consent form, the researchers opt to collect the desired data merely based on oral consent.

AUTHOR CONTRIBUTIONS

FF collected field data. TB, FG, AB, FW conceived the idea of the study, participated in the study and questionnaire design, organized the data collection, wrote the draft of the manuscript, and completed the final version for submission. TB analyzed the data and interpreted the results. TT participated in developing the research idea and study design. BE participated in the development of the idea, supervised the work, and edited the final version of the manuscript before submission.

ACKNOWLEDGMENTS

The authors would like to thank all study participants and Addis Ababa University, College of Veterinary Medicine and Agriculture for supporting this study. The authors acknowledge Dr. Samson Leta for developing the map of the study sites.

REFERENCES

1. WHO. *Zoonotic tuberculosis.* World Health Organization (Accessed May 18, 2018). Available online at http://www.who.int/tb/zoonoticTB.pdf (2017).
2. Amanfu W. The situation of tuberculosis and tuberculosis control in animals of economic interest. *Tuberculosis* (2006) 86:330–5. doi: 10.1016/j.tube.2006.01.007
3. Zinsstag J, Esther S, Roth F, Rudovick K. Economics of bovine tuberculosis. In: Thoen COS, JH, Gilsdorf MJ, editors. *Mycobacterium Bovis Infection in Animals and Humans. 2nd Edn.* Oxford: Blackwell Publishing Ltd. (2006). pp 70–79.
4. Oliver SP, Boor KJ, Murphy SC, Murinda SE. Food safety hazards associated with consumption of raw milk. *Foodborne Pathog Dis.* (2009) 6:793–806. doi: 10.1089/fpd.2009.0302
5. Ayele W, Neill S, Zinsstag J, Weiss M, Pavlik I. Bovine tuberculosis: an old disease but a new threat to Africa. *Int J Tuberc Lung Dis.* (2004) 8:924–37.
6. Moda G, Daborn C, Grange J, Cosivi O. The zoonotic importance of *Mycobacterium bovis. Tuberc Lung Dis.* (1996) 77:103–8. doi: 10.1016/S0962-8479(96)90022-2
7. Sibhat B, Asmare K, Demissie K, Ayelet G, Mamo G, Ameni G. Bovine tuberculosis in Ethiopia: a systematic review and meta-analysis. *Prev Vet Med.* (2017) 147:149–57. doi: 10.1016/j.prevetmed.2017.09.006
8. Cadmus S, Palmer S, Okker M, Dale J, Gover K, Smith N, et al. Molecular analysis of human and bovine tubercle bacilli from a local setting in Nigeria. *J Clin Microbiol.* (2006) 44:29–34. doi: 10.1128/JCM.44.1.29-34.2006
9. Regassa A, Medhin G, Ameni G. Bovine tuberculosis is more prevalent in cattle owned by farmers with active tuberculosis in central Ethiopia. *Vet J.* (2008) 178:119–25. doi: 10.1016/j.tvjl.2007.06.019

10. Robinson P, Morris D, Antic R. *Mycobacterium bovis* as an occupational hazard in abattoir workers. *Int Med J.* (1988) 18:701–3. doi: 10.1111/j.1445-5994.1988.tb00156.x
11. Adesokan H, Jenkins A, van Soolingen D, Cadmus S. *Mycobacterium bovis* infection in livestock workers in Ibadan, Nigeria: evidence of occupational exposure. *Int J Tuberc Lung Dis.* (2012) 16:1388–92. doi: 10.5588/ijtld.12.0109
12. Radostits O, Blood D. Disease caused by mycobacteria IV. In: Bailliere T, Editor. *Veterinary Medicine, 7th Edn.* London: Elsevier Health Sciences (1994). p. 710–40.
13. Nega M, Mazengia H, Mekonen G. Prevalence and zoonotic implications of bovine tuberculosis in Northwest Ethiopia. *Int J Med Sci.* (2012) 2:188–92.
14. Champion VL, Skinner CSi, Rimer BK, Viswanath K. *Health Behavior and Health Education: Theory, Research, and Practice.* Hoboken, NJ: John Wiley and Sons (2008).
15. Shillitoe R, Christie M. Determinants of self-care: the health belief model. *Holistic Med.* (1989) 4:3–17. doi: 10.3109/13561828909043602
16. Baum A. *Cambridge Handbook of Psychology, Health and Medicine.* Cambridge: Cambridge University Press (1997).
17. Rosenstock IM, Strecher VJ, Becker MH. Social learning theory and the health belief model. *Health Educ Behav.* (1988) 15:175–83. doi: 10.1177/109019818801500203
18. Hambolu D, Freeman J, Taddese HB. Predictors of bovine TB risk behaviour amongst meat handlers in Nigeria: a cross-sectional study guided by the health belief model. *PLoS ONE* (2013) 8:e56091. doi: 10.1371/journal.pone.0056091
19. Dohoo I, Martin W, Henrik. S. *Veterinary Epidemiologic Research, 2nd Edn.* Charlottetown, PE:AVC (2009).
20. Biru A, Ameni G, Sori T, Desissa F, Teklu A, Tafess K. Epidemiology and public health significance of bovine tuberculosis in and around Sululta District, Central Ethiopia. *Afr J Microbiol Res.* (2014) 8:2352–8. doi: 10.5897/AJMR2013.6325
21. Awah Ndukum J, Kudi AC, Bradley G, Ane-Anyangwe I, Fon-Tebug S, Tchoumboue J. Prevalence of bovine tuberculosis in abattoirs of the littoral and Western highland regions of cameroon: a cause for public health concern. *Vet Med Int.* (2010) 2010:495015. doi: 10.4061/2010/495015
22. Gebremedhin EZ, Abebe AH, Tessema TS, Tullu KD, Medhin G, Vitale M, et al. Seroepidemiology of *Toxoplasma gondii* infection in women of child-bearing age in central Ethiopia. *BMC Infect. Dis.* (2013) 13:101. doi: 10.1186/1471-2334-13-101
23. Davidson KW, Trudeau KJ, Van Roosmalen E, Stewart M, Kirkland S. Perspective: gender as a health determinant and implications for health education. *Health Educ Behav.* (2006) 33:731–43. doi: 10.1177/1090198106288043
24. Janz NK, Becker MH. The health belief model: a decade later. *Health Educ Q.* (1984) 11:1–47. doi: 10.1177/109019818401100101
25. Rosenstock IM, Strecher VJ, Becker MH. The health belief model and HIV risk behavior change. *In Preventing AIDS.* Boston, MA: Springer (1994). p. 5–24.

9

Infection of Wildlife by *Mycobacterium bovis* in France Assessment through a National Surveillance System, Sylvatub

Édouard Réveillaud[1†], Stéphanie Desvaux[2], Maria-Laura Boschiroli[3], Jean Hars[2], Éva Faure[4], Alexandre Fediaevsky[5†], Lisa Cavalerie[5], Fabrice Chevalier[5], Pierre Jabert[5], Sylvie Poliak[6], Isabelle Tourette[7], Pascal Hendrikx[1†] and Céline Richomme[8]*

[1] Anses, Unit of Coordination and Support to Surveillance, Maisons-Alfort, France, [2] French Hunting and Wildlife Agency (ONCFS), Studies and Research Department, Auffargis, France, [3] University Paris-Est–Anses, French Reference Laboratory for Tuberculosis, Maisons-Alfort, France, [4] National Hunters Federation (FNC), Issy-les-Moulineaux, France, [5] French General Directorate for Food (DGAL), Animal Health Unit, Paris, France, [6] French Association of Directors and Managers of Public Veterinary Laboratories of Analyses (Adilva), Paris, France, [7] French National Federation of Animal Health Defense Associations (GDS France), Paris, France, [8] Anses, Nancy Laboratory for Rabies and Wildlife, Malzéville, France

***Correspondence:**
Stéphanie Desvaux
stephanie.desvaux@oncfs.gouv.fr

Mycobacterium bovis infection was first described in free-ranging wildlife in France in 2001, with subsequent detection in hunter-harvested ungulates and badgers in areas where outbreaks of bovine tuberculosis (TB) were also detected in cattle. Increasing concerns regarding TB in wildlife led the French General Directorate for Food (DGAL) and the main institutions involved in animal health and wildlife management, to establish a national surveillance system for TB in free-ranging wildlife. This surveillance system is known as "Sylvatub." The system coordinates the activities of various national and local partners. The main goal of Sylvatub is to detect and monitor *M. bovis* infection in wildlife through a combination of passive and active surveillance protocols adapted to the estimated risk level in each area of the country. Event-base surveillance relies on *M. bovis* identification (molecular detection) (*i*) in gross lesions detected in hunter-harvested ungulates, (*ii*) in ungulates that are found dead or dying, and (*iii*) in road-killed badgers. Additional targeted surveillance in badgers, wild boars and red deer is implemented on samples from trapped or hunted animals in at-risk areas. With the exception of one unexplained case in a wild boar, *M. bovis* infection in free-living wildlife has always been detected in the vicinity of cattle TB outbreaks with the same genotype of the infectious *M. bovis* strains. Since 2012, *M. bovis* was actively monitored in these infected areas and detected mainly in badgers and wild boars with apparent infection rates of 4.57–5.14% and 2.37–3.04%, respectively depending of the diagnostic test used (culture or PCR), the period and according to areas. Sporadic infection has also been detected in red deer and roe deer. This surveillance has demonstrated that *M. bovis* infection, in different areas of France, involves a multi-host system including cattle and wildlife. However, infection rates are lower than those observed in badgers in the United Kingdom or in wild boars in Spain.

Keywords: bovine tuberculosis, *Mycobacterium bovis*, surveillance, wildlife, badger, wild boar, France

INTRODUCTION

Wildlife can serve as a reservoir for multiple pathogens and may serve as a sentinel of the disease risk to humans and domestic animals. As a result, disease surveillance in wildlife is strongly recommended to provide data on the epidemiological role of wild animals and for the development of adapted disease control measures (1).

Bovine tuberculosis (TB) is a contagious and zoonotic disease caused by *Mycobacterium bovis*, and occasionally by *M. caprae* or *M. tuberculosis* (hereafter referred to as MTBC). This pathogen primarily infects cattle but can be transmitted to a wide range of host mammals, especially numerous wild animals such as Eurasian badgers (*Meles meles*), wild boars (*Sus scrofa*), red deer (*Cervus elaphus*), and roe deer (*Capreolus capreolus*) (2). In the United Kingdom (UK) and in Ireland, the Eurasian badger is considered as TB reservoir, as is the wild boar in Spain. These species are involved in the transmission of *M. bovis* to cattle (3–6).

France is officially declared TB-free since 2001 in the bovine population, because <0.1% of cattle herds being infected annually. However, outbreaks still occur and the number of infected herds has increased since 2004 in certain parts of the country, especially in the South-West: Dordogne, Charente and Pyrénées-Atlantiques (French administrative division called departments) and in the East of France (Côte-d'Or) (7).

In France, TB in wild animals was first detected in 2001 in the Brotonne forest (Normandy) in hunter-harvested red deer exhibiting gross lesions. In 2006, despite control measures (culling), apparent prevalence rates in this forest reached 24% in red deer and 42% in wild boars, the closed environment and high density of wild ungulates were considered major risk factors to explain such high prevalence rates (8). Elsewhere in France, sporadic cases of TB infection have been detected in red deer and/or wild boar in several areas: Côte-d'Or (Burgundy region), Corsica, Pyrénées-Atlantiques, Dordogne, and Ariège in 2002, 2003, 2005, and 2010, respectively. The first cases in wild ungulates were systematically detected by carcass examination in hunter-harvested animals. Since then, event-based surveillance programs (also called passive surveillance) and targeted (or active) surveillance programs for the disease including the badger have been implemented in these areas. TB infection in badgers was initially detected in 2009 in Côte-d'Or (5.7%, $n = 918$ in the 2009–2011 period), then in 2010 in Dordogne and Charente (4.8%, $n = 417$ in 2010–2011). In wild boars, prevalence rates observed in 2008 reached locally 16.5% in Côte-d'Or and 4.4% in 2010–2011 in Dordogne (9). All these cases were detected in the vicinity of cattle outbreaks (10–12).

Increasing concern regarding the status of TB infections in wildlife led the French General Directorate for Food (DGAL) and the main institutions involved in animal health and wildlife management to establish a national surveillance system for TB in free-ranging wildlife: the "Sylvatub" system. This system coordinated by the French platform for epidemiological surveillance in animal health (ESA-Platform), was launched in September 2011. The main aims of Sylvatub are to detect TB in wildlife, to estimate and monitor infection levels in infected areas, to characterize *M. bovis* strains isolated from wildlife and to harmonize surveillance at the national level.

This article summarizes the key data collected on TB infection in France between 2011 and 2017 in badgers, wild boars, red deer, and roe deer. We describe the organization of the Sylvatub system and the findings in terms of TB prevalence in wild boars and badgers, and necropsy data gathered during event-based and targeted surveillance in the four species.

MATERIALS AND METHODS

Stakeholders and Organization of Sylvatub

The organizational structure of the system is shown in **Figure 1** and was described by Rivière et al. (12). Briefly, the DGAL is in charge of the Sylvatub system. Coordination and technical operations are performed by the ESA-Platform (www.plateforme-esa.fr). National governance is ensured by a steering committee and a technical subcommittee, where the different institutions or organizations involved in Sylvatub are represented (**Figure 1**).

The implementation of Sylvatub is based on the regular involvement of national stakeholders [national reference laboratory (NRL) for TB and the national coordinator of Sylvatub] and local stakeholders: veterinary services in charge of Sylvatub coordination, public administration in charge of the environment, hunting federations, associations of "*lieutenants de louveterie*" (historically called wolf-hunter, nowadays being state but volunteer officers in charge of pest control and who supervised badger trapping), trappers associations (volunteers who are duly trained and authorized), French hunting and wildlife agency services, local veterinary laboratories for animal health, cattle breeders, and finally veterinary associations.

Sylvatub: A Risk-Based Surveillance System

Sylvatub targets the wildlife species considered in 2011 to be the most relevant in the TB multi-host system: badgers, wild boars, red deer, and roe deer. Sylvatub's surveillance system components are based on event-based and targeted surveillance. These components are applied according to a risk-based surveillance approach, with three different levels of surveillance, applied at the level of French department (**Table 1**) and defined as follows:

- Level 3, for areas with several outbreaks in cattle and cases in wildlife. This level is applied for at least 4 years, to monitor infection levels in wildlife and to assess the efficacy of control measures;
- Level 2, for areas with sporadic at-risk outbreaks in cattle and/or areas in geographic proximity to high-risk areas. This level is applied for at least 1 year or for as long as necessary to develop a clear understanding of the epidemiological situation. A lower or higher surveillance level is subsequently applied, depending on the results obtained;
- Level 1, elsewhere in the country where no domestic and wild animal has been found infected for a long period of time.

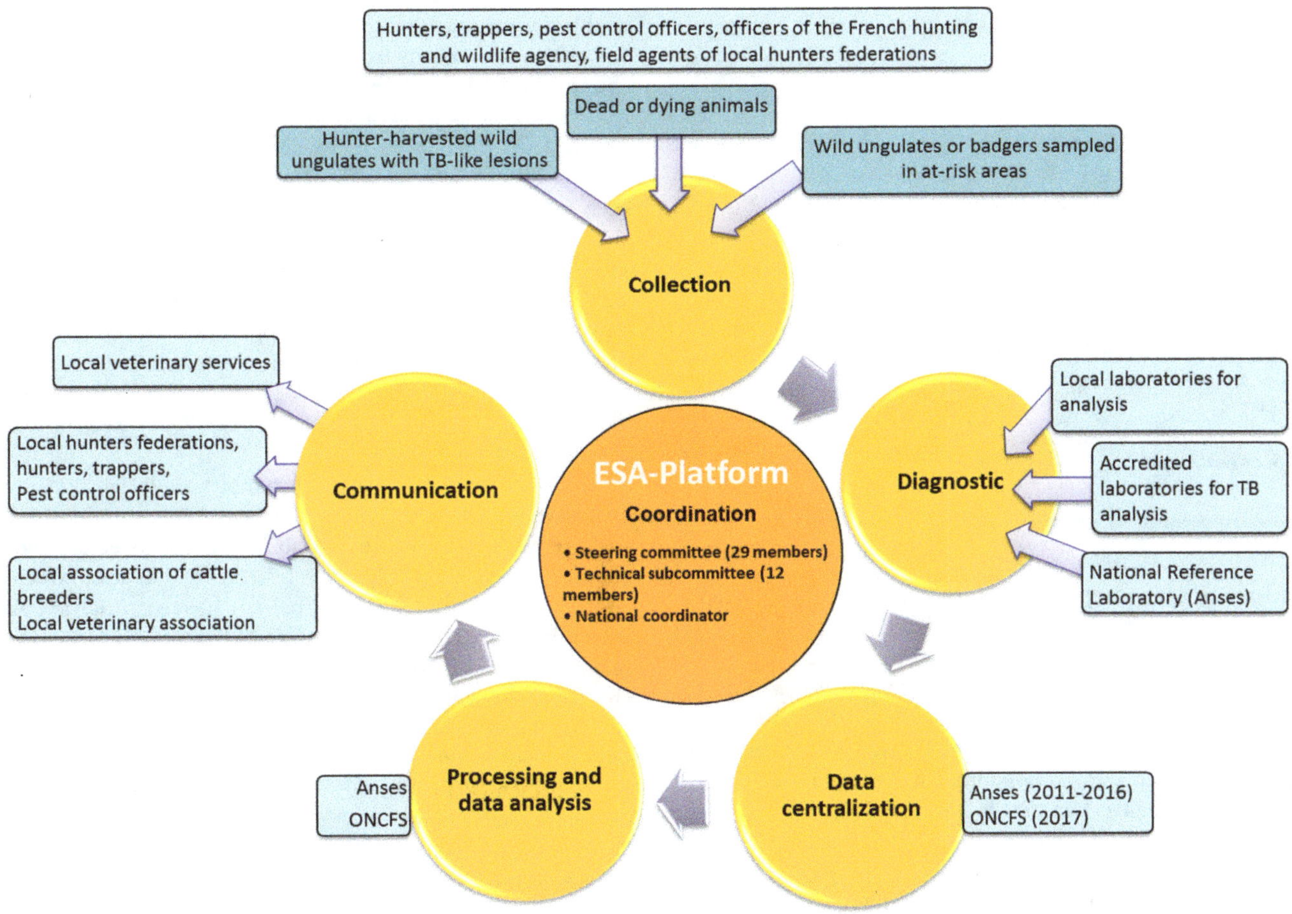

FIGURE 1 | Simplified organization of Sylvatub. *Steering committee members*: French General Directorate for Food (DGAL), Ministry of the Environment (MEDDE), Regional Directorates for Food (DRAAF), Anses, French hunting and wildlife agency (ONCFS), National Hunters Federation (FNC), French association of pest control officers, French association of approved trappers, the French National Federation of Animal Health Defense Associations (GDS France), National veterinary association (SNGTV), Coop de France and French Association of Directors and Managers of Public Veterinary Laboratories of Analyzes (Adilva), Regional veterinary epidemiologists. *Technical subcommittee members*: DGAL, Anses, ONCFS, DRAAF, FNC, GDS France, Adilva.

The local surveillance level is re-evaluated twice a year, to align with the epidemiological situation in cattle and wildlife populations.

Event-Based Surveillance Through Detailed Game Carcass Examination

This surveillance component is applied to all geographic areas, i.e., regardless of the local risk, to hunted wild boars, red deer, and roe deer. It is based on the analysis of animals with macroscopic TB-like lesions detected by hunters during post-mortem examination of all hunted games. The detection of gross lesions is supported by a national network of more than 55,000 hunters trained by the National Hunters Federation (FNC) for food safety purpose. Additionally to this framework, voluntary training courses were organized in the field to train hunters for recognition and reporting of TB-like lesions (internal abscesses or gross lymph nodes) and sampling of affected organs.

Event-Based Surveillance Through the SAGIR Network: Wild Animals Found Dead, Moribund or With Abnormal Behavior

Event-based surveillance on dead and dying wild animals, through the SAGIR network (French hunting and wildlife agency/local hunters federations/FNC), has been implemented in France since 1986 (13). Within the Sylvatub system, dead animals belonging to TB-receptive species (badgers, wild boars, red, and roe deer) collected as part of the SAGIR network are tested for TB (*i*) in the presence of TB-like lesions for level 1 departments, and (*ii*) systematically for level 2 and 3 departments. Moreover, efforts are made to collect and test road-kill badgers in all the level 2 and 3 departments.

Targeted Surveillance

Targeted surveillance may concern badgers, wild boars and/or red deer in level 3 departments depending on the population abundance and distribution, and badgers only in level 2

TABLE 1 | Surveillance methods implemented depending on the estimated risk level.

Surveillance methods	Level 1	Level 2	Level 3
Event-based surveillance: - Detailed game carcass examination (wild ungulates) - SAGIR[(1)] network (wild ungulates, badgers)	X	X	X
Strengthened event-based surveillance: - SAGIR network strengthened (red deer, wild boars, badgers) - Road-killed animals (badgers, wild ungulates)		X	X
Targeted surveillance in badgers in at-risk areas or around sporadic bovine outbreaks		X	X
Targeted surveillance in wild boars and red deer in at-risk areas			X

[(1)] *Monitoring of dead or dying animals.*

departments. This component of surveillance is implemented in "at-risk areas" determined as areas of about seven kilometers in radius around pastures of cattle outbreaks detected in the previous 4 years, and hunting or trapping locations of all infected wild animals. For badgers, at-risk areas are divided in two sub-areas: "infected area" (2 km radius) and "buffer area" (5 km radius around the infected area) to take into consideration badger home range which is smaller than in wild ungulates.

Sample sizes are determined to detect TB infection in at-risk areas, assuming a prevalence of 3%, with a 95% confidence interval. For wild boar and red deer, samples are defined for the whole at-risk area, whereas for badgers, one sample is for the infected area and one is for the buffer area. In large areas where wild populations could be considered as infinite, a sample of 130 animals per species is required. This sample size takes into account diagnostic test sensitivity (estimated at ~75% for PCR; see below). However, sample sizes are adjusted based on the surface of the area. In practice, samples between 60 and 260 red deer, wild boars, and badgers are programmed annually in each area. These are samples of hunted wild boars and deer or trapped badgers for control measures in infected areas.

Additionally, around sporadic cattle outbreaks outside at-risk areas (in level 2 and 3 departments), systematic TB analysis is conducted on a sample of about 15 badgers trapped within a radius of one or two kilometers depending on the number and localization of badger's setts. These small areas are called "prospecting areas."

Animals are collected even if no macroscopic TB lesions are detected by field stakeholders.

Tissue Collection and Laboratory Investigations

Sample Collection

Wild boars and red deer are collected by hunters, under the supervision of the local hunting federations during the hunting season (generally from August to March each year), and badgers are collected by trappers (accreditation required), under the supervision of pest control officers. In infected areas, where one of the control measures is to reduce badger populations, badger can be trapped, mostly from March to August. Field stakeholders (hunters, trappers, pest control officers) submit animals, organs, or tissues (from a standardized list of samples described in **Tables 2, 3**) directly to the local laboratory or store them in cooling rooms or freezers for later analysis. Data is collected for each animal on the species, estimated age (juvenile or adult), sex, date, location of collection and body condition (degradation, presence of lesions in the carcass, etc.). Age determination is based on animal size for badgers and/or weight and hunters' knowledge for wild ungulates. Trappers and pest control officers are volunteers but a financial compensation is provided for them.

Tissue samples are taken in local laboratories even if no TB-like lesions are detected except for SAGIR network animals in level 1 department.

Tables 2, 3 shows the field samples collected for testing and changes over time. For wild boars, from mid-2013 until the present time, only the head has been collected and the submaxillary lymph nodes are tested. For badgers, which are relatively small, the entire animal is collected. Analyses at the local laboratory consist of post-mortem necropsy to detect TB-like lesions (caseo-granulomas, mineralized nodules, or purulent abscesses), polymerase chain reaction (PCR) and/or bacterial culture on pooled lymph node samples and on pooled samples with TB-like lesions.

As presented previously, diagnostic schemes differ between surveillance components: either TB testing is performed only if TB lesions are detected (SAGIR event-based surveillance in level 1 departments), or TB testing is performed systematically (for all suspect hunted carcasses and all SAGIR animals in level 2 and 3 departments, as well as for targeted surveillance in level 2 and 3 departments).

Analyses are performed as indicated in **Tables 2, 3**. The year 2015 marked a diagnostic-methodological transition for badger surveillance as these two diagnostic schemes were used depending on the local laboratory and the time of year. Changing from culture to PCR as a first line test was decided after having demonstrated that in cattle PCR provides a better sensitivity for TB detection without losing specificity (14).

Microbiological Culture

Bacterial culture is performed following the protocol established by the French NRL (NF U 47-104) for isolation of *M. bovis*. Two to 5 g of sampled tissues were crushed with a 4% sulfuric acid solution to decontaminate the tissue. After 10 min, the acid was neutralized by adding a 6% sodium hydroxide solution. After decontamination, the supernatant was seeded on two different media: Löwenstein-Jensen and Coletsos. All seeded media were incubated at 37°C +/- 3°C for three months and exanimated every 2 weeks. If contamination is observed during the first month, samples are decontaminated a second time with 4% sodium hydroxide and then neutralized with 10% sulfuric acid solution.

The isolated *M. tuberculosis* complex (MTBC) colonies are confirmed by DNA amplification (15) targeting the IS*6110*

TABLE 2 | Diagnostic methods used in badgers from 2012 to 2017.

		2012	2013	2014	2015	2016	2017
	Field samples	**Entire carcass**					
Badgers	Pooled samples at local laboratory	- Retropharyngeal, tracheobronchial, mediastinal, hepatic lymph nodes and salivary glands; - Pool of lesions (if present)		- Retropharyngeal, tracheobronchial, mediastinal and hepatic lymph nodes - Pool of lesions (if present)			
	Analysis at local laboratory	Culture; PCR on pool of lesions			Culture; PCR on pool of lesions or PCR, culture on positive PCR pools	PCR; Culture on positive PCR pools	

TABLE 3 | Diagnostic methods used in wild boars and deer for the hunting seasons from 2011 to 2017.

		2011–2012	2012–2013	2013–2014	2014–2015	2015–2016	2016–2017
Wild boars	Field samples	Head, pulmonary system, organs with lesions if present		Head, organs with lesions if present			
	Pooled samples at local laboratory	Cephalic and pulmonary lymph nodes; Pool of lesions (if present)		Submandibular lymph nodes; Pool of lesions (if present)			
	Analysis at local laboratory	Culture; PCR on pool of lesions				PCR; Culture on positive PCR pools	
Deer	Field samples	Head, pulmonary and digestive systems, organs with lesions if present					
	Pooled samples at laboratory	- Retropharyngeal, tracheobronchial, mediastinal and mesenteric lymph nodes; - Pool of lesions (if present)					
	Analysis at local laboratory	Culture; PCR on pool of lesions				PCR; Culture on positive PCR pools	

sequence present in all species of MTBC (16), and *M. bovis* is confirmed by spoligotyping (see below).

Tissue PCRs

DNA extraction is performed on a pool of lymph nodes (retropharyngeal, pulmonary and mesenteric) and on organs with gross lesions when present, after mechanical lysis using an LSI MagVet^{TM} Universal Isolation Kit (Life Technologies) with a KingFisher^{TM} Flex automate (Thermo Scientific), following the manufacturer's instructions. The LSIV and MAX^{TM} MTBC Real-Time PCR kit (Life Technologies), which targets IS*6110*, is used. A volume of 5 μL of the extracted DNA is mixed with 20 μL of reaction mix, and the reaction is carried out at 50°C for two min (1 cycle), followed by one cycle of 10 min at 95°C and 45 cycles of 15 s at 95°C, and one min at 60°C. Results are interpreted following the manufacturer's recommendations and by comParison with negative and positive controls. If DNA amplification is positive, *M. bovis* or any other MTBC species is confirmed by spoligotyping (see below).

Spoligotyping

Spoligotyping is performed as described by Zhang et al. (17), using TB-SPOL kits purchased from Beamedex® (Beamedex SAS, Orsay, France) on Bio-PLex 200/Luminex 200®. Molecular typing is performed either on MTBC isolates or directly on PCR-positive sample DNA. The presence or absence of the 43 spacer sequences contained in the DR locus is represented in a binary code of 43 entries. Spoligotypes are named according to an agreed international convention (www.mbovis.org).

Data Analysis

An infected animal is defined as an animal with an analytical result demonstrating *M. bovis* (or if it had been found *M. tuberculosis* or *M. caprae)* by molecular diagnosis or by bacterial culture.

All results presented in this article come from the Sylvatub national database.

Results are presented by calendar year for badgers and by 12 month period starting with the beginning of the wild boar hunt (August to the end of July). The Sylvatub system was set up in September 2011; as a result surveillance findings for wild ungulates are presented from the 2011–2012 hunting season to the 2016–2017 hunting season and from 2012 to 2017 for badgers.

To simplify, at-risk areas are renamed with numbers as follows, by chronological order of detection of TB in wildlife: 1: Brotonne-Mauny forest (Seine-Maritime); 2: Côte-d'Or; 3: Dordogne/Charente/Charente-Maritime/Haute-Vienne/Corrèze/Gironde; 4: Dordogne/Lot; 5: Béarn (Pyrénées-Atlantiques/Landes/Gers); 6: Ardennes/Marne; 7: Marne (Reims mountain); 8: Loir-et-Cher (Sologne); 9: Lot-et-Garonne; 10: Pays Basque; and 11: Ariège/Haute-Garonne (**Figure 2**).

In this paper, apparent prevalence rates are indicated based on the diagnostic test used (culture or PCR). Furthermore, results were aggregated into two periods of 2 years each to calculate prevalence rates with more precision: P1 (2013 and 2014 for badger surveillance; the 2012-2013 and 2013-2014 hunting seasons for wild ungulate surveillance) and P2 (2016 and 2017 for badger surveillance; the 2015-2016 and 2016-2017 hunting seasons for wild ungulate surveillance). In P1, the

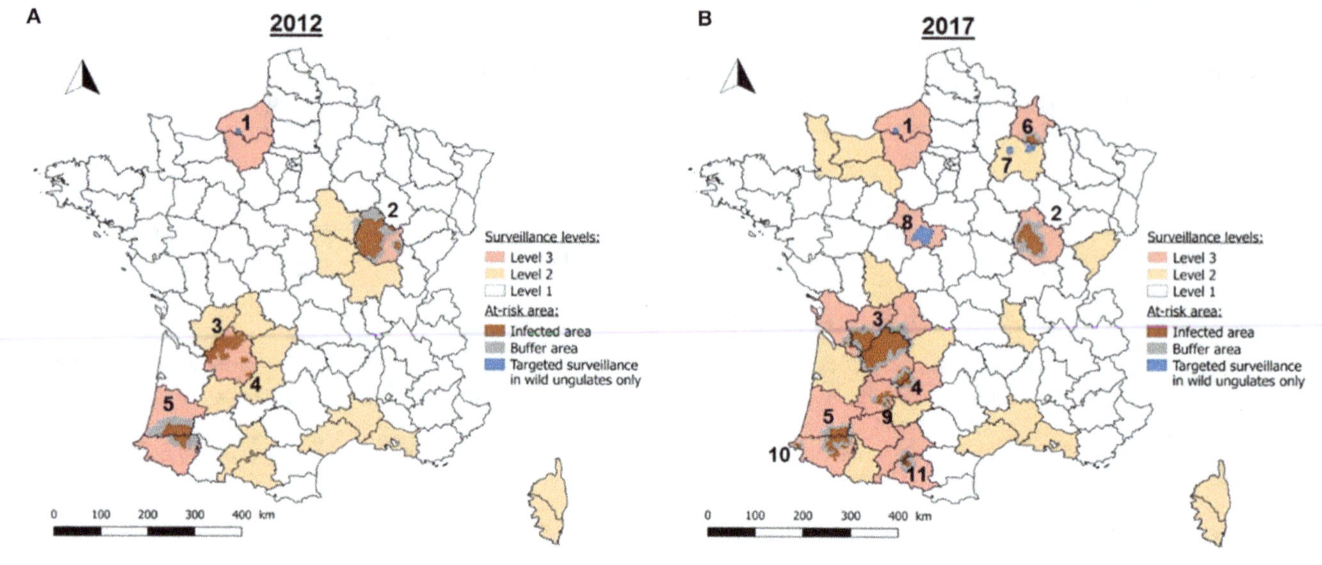

FIGURE 2 | Changes in surveillance levels and at-risk areas between 2012 **(A)** and 2017 **(B)** (*1*: Brotonne-Mauny forest; *2*: Côte-d'Or; *3*: Dordogne/Charente/Charente-Maritime/Haute-Vienne/Corrèze/Gironde; *4*: Dordogne/Lot; *5*: Béarn; *6*: Ardennes/Marne; *7*: Marne (Reims Mountain); *8*: Loir-et-Cher (Sologne); *9*: Lot-et-Garonne; *10*: Pays Basque; *11*: Ariège/Haute-Garonne).

diagnostic test used was sample culture, whereas in P2, PCR was used. We focused on areas where sampled animals were most numerous and where infection was confirmed to present and compare these results. To compare results in badgers between event-based and targeted surveillances, we focused in the at-risk area 3 because it is the only area where the number of analyzed badgers was sufficient for each of these surveillance components.

Regarding the number of analyzed animals, we counted only those with an interpretable analysis result (positive or negative). Apparent prevalence and 95% confidence intervals were calculated using exact binomial tests and *p*-values using the Fisher's exact test. Data analysis was performed using LibreOffice Calc (version 5.2) and R Studio software (version 3.3.1). Maps were generated using QGIS software (version 2.16.3).

RESULTS

Functioning Results

Since its implementation in 2012, Sylvatub has been gradually strengthened due to the larger number of areas where wild animals have been found infected, the enlargement of infected areas affecting cattle, and the detection of sporadic cattle outbreaks in new areas. This is reflected in the increase of number of departments at level 2 and 3 (from 21 in 2012 to 32 in 2017) (**Figure 2**). The surveillance levels for the departments were re-evaluated by the steering committee 10 times between 2011 and the end of 2017.

In 2012, there were five distinct at-risk areas. Since then, six other at-risk areas have been defined, with a total of 11 areas in 2017. Targeted surveillance was implemented for wild boars and red deer in three at-risk areas (numbered 1, 7, and 8), for wild boars and badgers in four at-risk areas (numbered 9, 5, 10, and 11) and for the three species in four at-risk areas (numbered 2, 3, 4, and 6) depending on the populations abundance and distribution.

In the meantime, size of these at-risk areas was expanded for five areas (3, 4, 6, 10, and 11), reduced for two areas (2 and 5) and remained approximately stable for the others (see details in **Supplementary Table 1**). The surface area of mainland France classified as at-risk was 14,397 km^2 in 2012 and 20,434 km^2 in 2017.

Event-Based Surveillance

The number of wild boars, red and roe deer collected by event-based surveillance increased from 77 in 2011–2012 to 134 in 2015–2016. In total, 316 wild boars, 197 roe deer, and 98 red deer have been collected since 2011. The number of dead or dying badgers collected per year (SAGIR and road-killed badgers) has increased from 70 badgers in 2012 to 582 in 2015. This number has been stable since 2015 with about 580 badgers collected per year, most of them being road-killed badgers.

Targeted Surveillance

An average of 296 red deer (min: 226; max: 380), 1,420 wild boars (min: 1,078; max: 2,175) and 1,881 badgers (min: 1,447; max: 2,239) were analyzed per year between 2011 and 2017.

TB Infection in Wildlife

TB Infection in Badgers

Event-based surveillance

Among the 2,491 badgers collected by event-based surveillance in 45 departments, 2,397 were analyzed (2,372 with an interpretable analysis result), and 89 were found infected with *M. bovis* (**Figure 3**). In all, 84 of these infected animals were found in the vicinity of cattle outbreaks (75 infected badgers in infected areas, five in buffer areas and four in prospecting areas). Five infected badgers ($n = 716$) were from outside but very close (<3.5 km) to at-risk areas (areas 3 and 9). In infected area 3, where badgers collected by event-based surveillance are numerous, apparent prevalence rates seems to be stable between P1 (8.2%; 95% CI: 4.2–14.2%) and P2 (9.6%; 95% CI: 6.8–13.1%).

Targeted surveillance

From 2012 to 2017, 378 badgers ($n = 10{,}184$) were found infected with *M. bovis* by targeted surveillance in at-risk areas 2, 3, 4, 5, 6, 9, 10, and 11. In all, 340 of these badgers ($n = 6{,}870$) originated from infected areas and 27 ($n = 3{,}314$) from buffer areas (**Figure 4**). Targeted surveillance has not been implemented in at-risk areas 1, 7 and 8, where badger populations are very small.

In infected areas, apparent prevalence rate observed with culture (from 2012 to 2014) was on average 4.57% ($n = 3{,}198$) and with PCR (2016-2017) on average 5.14% ($n = 2{,}412$) (**Supplementary Table 2**). In buffer areas, apparent prevalence rate observed with culture was on average 1.33% ($n = 1{,}508$) and with PCR on average 0.41% ($n = 1{,}217$) (**Supplementary Table 2**). Regarding results in the four main infected areas (areas 2, 3, 5 and 6) for the two periods (P1 and P2), prevalence in badgers was significantly lower in P1 in infected area 3 than in the three other areas ($p < 0.001$; $p = 0.009$; $p = 0.0351$, respectively). In P2, prevalence was higher in infected area 5 than in areas 2 and 3 ($p = 0.02$; $p = 0.013$, respectively) (**Table 4**).

In area 2, apparent prevalence was higher in P1 than in P2 ($p = 0.008$) (**Table 4**).

The targeted surveillance in prospecting areas has detected two sites of infection: in Ardennes in 2013, five infected badgers were detected from a total sample of 37 badgers collected close to four bovine TB outbreaks and, in 2015, in the Pays Basque (Pyrénées-Atlantiques), two infected badgers were detected from a sample of nine badgers, also sampled on the outskirts of four bovine TB outbreaks. As a result of these findings, infected and buffer areas were defined in these two departments and other cattle outbreaks were discovered nearby.

Males were found to have significantly higher infection rates (4.95%, $n = 3{,}394$) than females (2.02%, $n = 4{,}213$) ($p < 0.001$).

In infected area 3, prevalence were significantly higher (in P1 and P2) in badgers collected by event-based surveillance (mainly road-killed badgers) than by targeted surveillance (mainly trapped badgers) ($p = 0.006$ and $p = 0.01$, respectively) (**Table 5**).

TB Infection in Wild Boars and Deer

Event-based surveillance

Among the 323 free ranging wild boars collected from 2011–2012 to 2016–2017 in 53 departments, 258 were analyzed, 241 had an

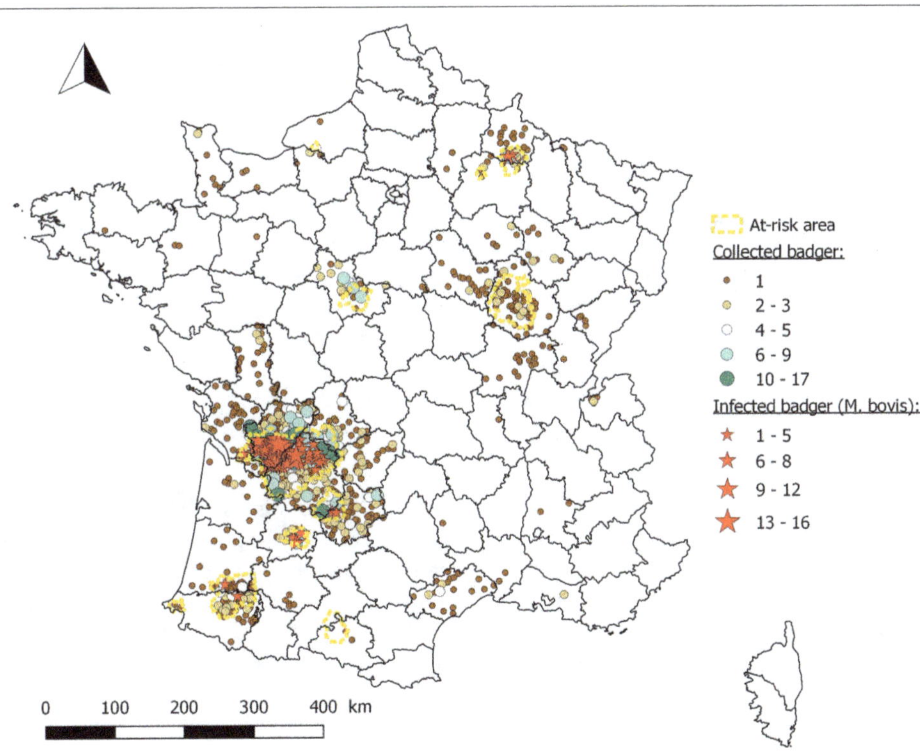

FIGURE 3 | Location of badgers collected and found infected by event-based surveillance from 2012 to 2017.

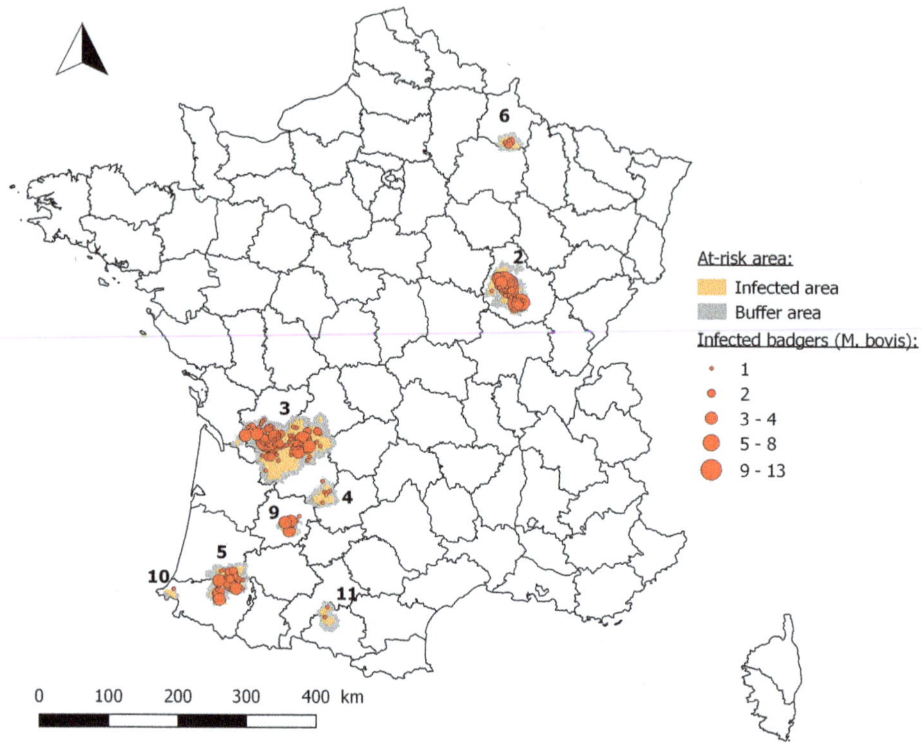

FIGURE 4 | Location of infected badgers collected by targeted surveillance from 2012 to 2017 (*2*: Côte-d'Or; *3*: Dordogne/Charente/Charente-Maritime/Haute-Vienne/Corrèze/Gironde; *4*: Dordogne/Lot; *5*: Béarn; *6*: Ardennes/Marne; *9*: Lot-et-Garonne; *10*: Pays Basque; *11*: Ariège/Haute-Garonne).

TABLE 4 | Apparent prevalence rates in badgers collected by targeted surveillance in the four main infected areas of France between 2013-2014 (Period 1: P1) and 2016-2017 (Period 2: P2) [percentages are given with 95% confidence intervals (CI); in brackets number of infected/analyzed animals].

No. of the infected area (full name of the area)	P1 (2013–2014) *Culture*	P2 (2016–2017) *PCR*
	Apparent prevalence rates [95% CI] (No. of infected badgers/no. analyzed)	
2 (Côte-d'Or)	8.1% [6.3–10.3%] (61/751)	4.2% [2.6–6.2%] (22/528)
3 (Dordogne/Charente/Charente-Maritime/Haute-Vienne/Corrèze/Gironde)	2.7% [1.7–4.1%] (22/805)	5.3% [4.1–6.8%] (61/1143)
5 (Béarn)	5.9% [3.9–6.8%] (26/439)	7.9% [5.2–11.2%] (27/344)
6 (Ardennes/Marne)	6.7% [3.1–12.4%] (9/134)	3.1% [0.4–10.7%] (2/65)

TABLE 5 | Comparison of apparent prevalence rates in badgers obtained by event-based surveillance and by targeted surveillance for two periods in infected area 3 [percentages are given with 95% confidence intervals (CI); in brackets number of infected/analyzed animals].

Type of surveillance component	P1 (2013–2014) *Culture*	P2 (2016–2017) *PCR*
	Apparent prevalence rates [95% CI] (No. of infected badgers/no. analyzed)	
Event-based surveillance	8.2% [4.2–14.2%] (11/134)	9.6% [6.8–13.1%] (35/365)
Targeted surveillance	2.7% [1.7–4.1%] (22/805)	5.3% [4.1–6.8%] (61/1143)

interpretable analysis result and 29 were found to be infected in six departments (Dordogne, Charente, Côte-d'Or, Haute-Corse, Corse-du-Sud, and Loir-et-Cher). Ten came from at-risk areas (level 2 and 3 departments), 18 came from Corsica and one wild boar found infected in January 2015 in Loir-et-Cher, a livestock TB-free area since 1986 (**Figure 5**). This wild boar was found in open forest, although the area is surrounded by private game parks. *M. bovis* was also isolated from a wild boar in a closed game park in the Reims Mountain (Marne) in 2012 (18). Data for this case were not integrated in Sylvatub database because it was not a free ranging wildlife animal.

A total of 107 red deer and 190 roe deer have been collected through event-based surveillance since 2011 from 35 and 48 departments, respectively. Two red deer submitted by hunters both in 2016 were found to be infected in areas 2 and 3, and five infected roe deer were detected in area 3 in 2012, 2013, 2015, and 2016. For more details on roe deer surveillance in France see Lambert et al. (19) (**Figure 5**).

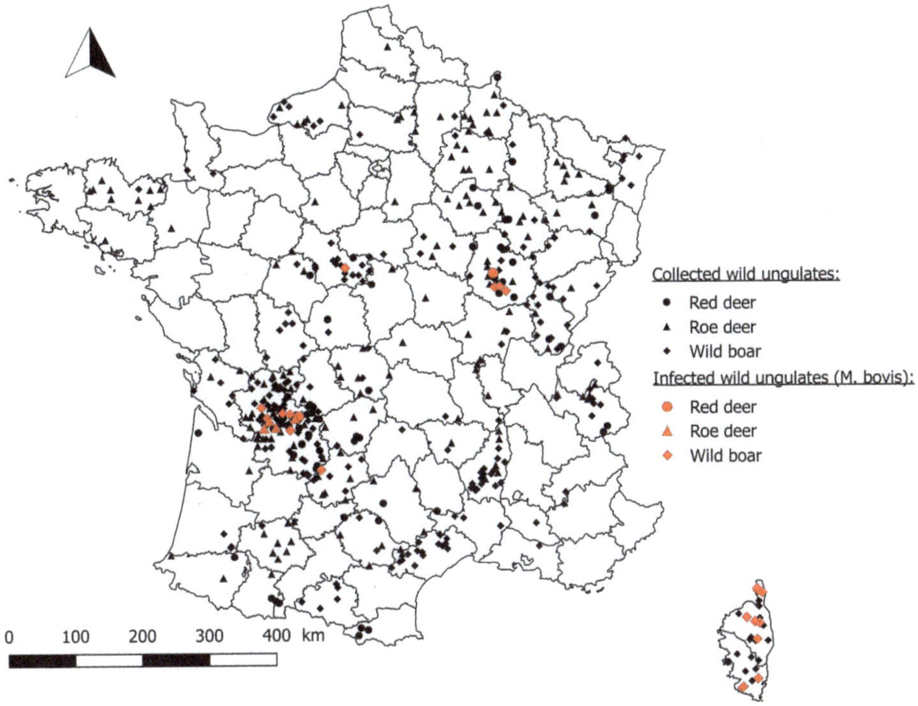

FIGURE 5 | Location of wild ungulates collected by event-based surveillance from 2011 to 2017.

Targeted surveillance

Targeted surveillance on wild boars was implemented in 11 at-risk areas with 7,634 wild boars analyzed since 2011. In total, 180 wild boars were found infected with *M. bovis* in seven at-risk areas. In at-risk areas where infection in wild boars was known, apparent prevalence rate observed with culture (from 2011 to 2015) was on average 3.04% ($n = 3{,}786$), and with PCR (2015–2017) on average 2.37% ($n = 2{,}536$) (**Supplementary Table 3**). Prevalence in the main at-risk areas was between 1.5 and 4.3% in P1, and between 0.5 and 4.4% in P2 (**Table 6**). No infected wild boar has been found in areas 6, 7, 8, and 10 (**Supplementary Table 3**). In the Brotonne-Mauny forest (area 1) surveillance in wild boars has been implemented since 2001 due to the detection of infection at high prevalence rates in deer and wild boars (20). From that time point onwards, one to five additional infected wild boars were found each year between 2011 and 2017 (among about 200 wild boars analyzed/year) (**Supplementary Table 3**). Furthermore, following the discovery of one infected wild boar in Loir-et-Cher (Sologne), 986 wild boars were analyzed from 2015 to 2017 in open forest and in 12 game parks, but no additional wild boar was found to be infected.

Infection in males and in females was similar (2.4%, $n = 2{,}947$ and 2.5%, $n = 2{,}753$, respectively) ($p = 0.80$).

Targeted surveillance on red deer was implemented in seven at-risk areas, where 1,817 red deer carcasses have been examined including 1,491 analyzed since 2011. Six red deer were found infected in area 2. Results by year and by area are detailed in **Supplementary Table 4**.

M. bovis Strains Isolated in Wildlife

In total, nine genotypes of *M. bovis* have been identified in wildlife in France (**Figure 6**). Some of these genotypes are found in different at-risk areas (SB0120 in areas 2, 3, and 6 and in the Corsica region, SB134 in areas 1, 2, and 11), but their variable number tandem repeat (VNTR) profiles are different (**Table 7**). We should note the presence of two different genotypes in two areas: SB0120 and SB0134 in area 2, and SB0120 and SB0840 in Corsica. In area 5, the two genotypes SB0821 and SB0832 are in geographic proximity, but nevertheless in different sectors.

Gross Lesions and TB Infection

Lesions in Badgers

Among 357 badgers out of 13,620 (2.6%) necropsied showed TB-like lesions. Of these, 95 were found to be infected. Furthermore, only 21.5% of the 442 infected badgers showed TB-like lesions. Lesions were mostly found in the cephalic lymph nodes (retropharyngeal and submandibular) and the pulmonary tractus (lung, bronchial and mediastinal lymph nodes). In total, eight infected badgers had TB-like lesions on at least two internal organs and at least two lymph nodes. 16.2% of infected badgers (47/291) collected by targeted surveillance showed TB-like lesions, whereas in infected badgers collected by event-based surveillance, 31.0% (22/71) showed TB-like lesions ($p = 0.04$).

Lesions in Wild Boars

In all, 526 wild boars out of 7,838 (6.7%) collected by targeted surveillance showed TB-like lesions, and 77.8% of the infected

TABLE 6 | Apparent prevalence rates in wild boars in at-risk areas of France where infection has been found in wild boars in the 2012-2013-2014 period and the 2015-2016-2017 period [percentages are given with 95% confidence intervals (CI); in brackets number of infected/analyzed animals].

No. of the at-risk area (full name of the area)	P1 (2012–2013 and 2013–2014) *Culture*	P2 (2015–2016 and 2016–2017) *PCR*
	Apparent prevalence rates [95% CI] (No. of infected wild boar/no. analyzed)	
1 (Brotonne-Mauny forest)	1.5% [0.6–3.2%] (6/401)	1.3% [0.4–2.9%] (5/394)
2 (Côte-d'Or)	3.1% [1.7–5.1%] (15/483)	2.2% [1.0–4.2%] (9/404)
3 (Dordogne/Charente/ Charente-Maritime/Haute-Vienne/Corrèze/Gironde)	4.1% [2.4–6.4%] (17/419)	2.7% [1.7–4.1%] (21/770)
4 (Dordogne/Lot)	4.3% [1.9–8.2%] (8/188)	3.2% [1.6–5.7%] (11/341)
5 (Béarn)	2.1% [0.9–4.2%] (8/373)	4.4% [2.4–7.4%] (13/295)
9 (Lot-et-Garonne)	/	4.2% [1.6–8.9%] (6/143)
11 (Ariège/Haute-Garonne)	/	0.5% [0–2.9%] (1/189)

/: Targeted surveillance on badgers not required in the area.

wild boars showed TB-like lesions. Most of the TB-like lesions were found in the submandibular lymph nodes.

Lesions in Deer

Among the eight red deer found infected since 2011, six came from targeted surveillance and two from event-based surveillance (submitted by hunters because of visible TB-like lesions). Five red deer showed gross TB-like lesions: in the pulmonary system for three red deer, in retropharyngeal lymph nodes for three, in mesenteric lymph nodes for one and in the liver for one. Gross TB lesions were also observed in infected roe deer (19).

DISCUSSION

Organization of the Surveillance System

Surveillance of TB in wildlife on a national scale in France, coordinated by the Sylvatub system, has been implemented gradually since 2011 thanks to the strong contribution of stakeholders at the national or local levels. Thanks to the involvement of hunters, event-based surveillance through detailed game carcass examination has often enabled us to detect first cases of TB in wild ungulates before targeted surveillance is deployed. It has help to detect TB as early as possible.

However, the main challenge for Sylvatub lies in the involvement of volunteer actors (hunters, trappers, pest control officers) and local veterinary services in such a complex multi-partner network. The targeted surveillance recommended in the Level 2 and 3 departments required a particularly strong involvement of local volunteers to collect tissue samples of wild ungulates and to trap badgers, explaining why some targeted plans have only been partially implemented in some areas. And these volunteers are, for the large majority, not those who are directly impacted by TB in cattle (cattle breeders) but could be affected by negative consequences if infection is found in wildlife, as for example, the implementation of density control measures of wild ungulates. Furthermore, in some departments, surveillance has been renewed for many years, which leads to a weariness of local actors. It should also be noted that the cost of Sylvatub is important for the government since it amounts to about 1 million euros per year.

Sampling and Diagnostic Protocols

For each surveillance component, sampling was opportunistic and not performed randomly: for targeted surveillance it was based on trapper and hunter activity, and for event-based surveillance on different field actor interventions. Some areas or sectors were overrepresented whereas others were underrepresented depending on the number of volunteers, the intensity of their activity and the possibility to hunt. Moreover, samples collected were not strictly homogeneous from 1 year to the next, even within the same area.

For event-based surveillance, the collection of carcasses or the reporting of animals with TB-like lesions strongly depend on the awareness of actors in the field. We can reasonably expect that this awareness is generally greater for in the departments affected by TB (level 2 and 3 departments) which constitutes a selection bias.

In addition, wildlife surveillance must deal with unknown parameters such as densities, distribution, or the social behavior of animals. Surveillance must therefore adapt as well as possible to this variability and propose reasonable, realistic and attainable objectives but prevalence estimates are certainly biased. For example, it is difficult to set badger surveillance objectives without full knowledge of their densities and distribution. In practice, the samples planned in at-risk areas therefore had to be adjusted to the size of the area. We have set the design prevalence for sample size calculations at 3%. This threshold was chosen to be able to detect a relatively low prevalence while minimizing the sample size and therefore the cost. It could have affected the ability to detect TB in areas where TB is only present at prevalence below 3%, particularly in deer where prevalence seems lower than in the others species.

The amount of time dedicated to post-mortem examinations and their thoroughness influence the detection of visible lesions (5, 21). Here, wild ungulates were not always examined in a standardized way by hunters in the field. Even though training is provided, detection of lesions suggestive of TB by hunters in the field is less sensitive than the necropsy performed in the laboratory. Nevertheless, in some laboratories, necropsy of badgers or ungulates is sometimes performed without thoroughly inspecting all lymphatic nodes and organs. In addition, for wild ungulates, only organ blocks (head, lungs and mesenteric apparatus depending on the species and year) are transmitted to the local laboratories as part of targeted surveillance. For

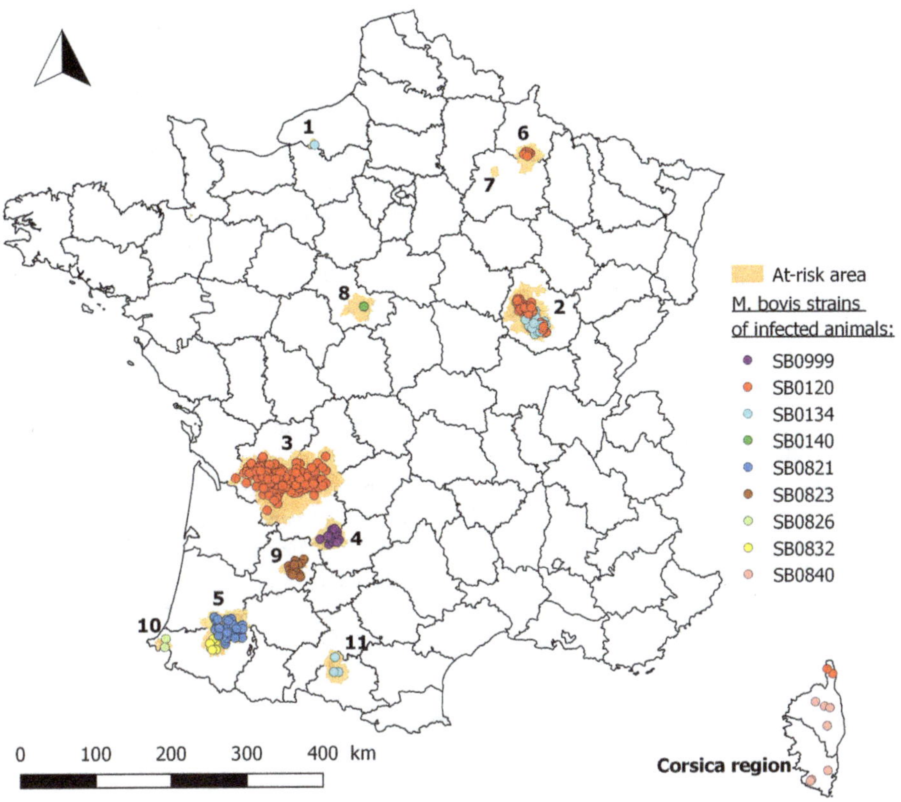

FIGURE 6 | Location of *M. bovis* strains in wildlife in France (*1*: Brotonne-Mauny forest; *2*: Côte-d'Or; *3*: Dordogne/Charente/Charente-Maritime/Haute-Vienne/Corrèze/Gironde; *4*: Dordogne/Lot; *5*: Béarn; *6*: Ardennes/Marne; *7*: Marne (Reims Mountain); *8*: Loir-et-Cher (Sologne); *9*: Lot-et-Garonne; *10*: Pays Basque; *11*: Ariège/Haute-Garonne).

all these reasons, the frequency of lesions has certainly been underestimated.

Since 2011, the protocol for sampling biological tissue and the composition of analyzed pools of tissues have changed. Before 2014, for badgers, salivary glands were sampled and mixed with lymphatic nodes. For wild boars, since 2014, only the cephalic lymph nodes have been sampled and analyzed whereas before the pulmonary lymph nodes were also analyzed. The purpose of these changes was to concentrate the tissue pools with the organs most likely to be contaminated by *M. bovis,* in order to increase diagnostic sensitivity. Unfortunately, the impact of these measures could not be assessed (22, 23).

Moreover, the type of analysis used for TB diagnosis changed from 2015: bacterial culture was used from 2011 to 2014 and then, from 2015, PCR was deployed. The year 2015 was a year of transition with the use of culture or PCR, depending on the local laboratory. Sensitivities were estimated in cattle populations by Courcoul et al. (14): on average 87.7% [82.5–92.3%] for PCR vs. 78.1% [72.9–82.8%] for culture. Culture sensitivity is probably lower when used for wild animals due to field conditions and the potential contamination and degradation of samples and because only a limited range of tissues are collected and analyzed from each wild animal. Furthermore, pooled samples are analyzed for wildlife, whereas cattle samples are analyzed separately. All together these factors lead to a decreased culture sensitivity estimated by about 30–40% and PCR sensitivity by about 10–20% (Boschiroli, personal communication) compared to those in cattle.

In order to calculate prevalence more accurately, we grouped the results into two periods: P1 (2012–2014—use of culture) and P2 (2016–2017—use of PCR), and we calculated apparent prevalence. These prevalence rates do not take into account the sensitivity of the two analytical methods. For comparison of results in badgers, the year 2012 was not taken into consideration because it was the first year of operation of the Sylvatub system with a protocol that was not always fully implemented. The year 2015 was also ruled out because of the use of both analytical methods, depending on the local laboratory.

M. bovis Infection in Wildlife

Distribution of Infected Wild Animals

All infected wild animals detected since 2012 have been found in the vicinity of cattle outbreaks (in at-risk areas up to 10 km from recent cattle outbreaks pastures), except for one wild boar found in Loir-et-Cher (Sologne), an area without known TB infection. The molecular profile of the *M. bovis* strain (SB0140; VNTR profile: 7 5 6 3 10 3 4 7) found in this wild boar was identical to that of a bovine animal slaughtered in Vendée (western France)

TABLE 7 | Genotype of *M. bovis* strains in wildlife in France.

No. of the at-risk area or region (full name of the area)	Spligotype	VNTR profile
1 (Brotonne-Mauny forest)	SB0134	7 4 5 3 10 4 5 10
2 (Côte-d'Or)	SB0120	5 5 4 1 11 4 5 6
		5 5 4 3 11 4 5 6
	SB0134	6 4 5 3 6 4 3 6
		6 5 5 3 6 4 3 6
3 (Dordogne/Charente/Charente-Maritime/Haute-Vienne/Corrèze/Gironde)	SB0120	5 3 5 3 9 4 5 6
4 (Dordogne/Lot)	SB0999	6 4 5 2 8 2 4 7
5 (Béarn)	SB0821	6 5 5 3 11 2 5s 8
	SB0832	6 5 5 3 11 2 4s 8
6 (Ardennes/Marne)	SB0120	5 3 5 6 11 4 6 8
8 (Loir-et-Cher)	SB0140	7 5 6 3 10 3 4 7
9 (Lot-et-Garonne)	SB0823	6 5 5 3 11 2 5s 6
10 (Pays Basque)	SB0826	6 6 3 3 10 2 5s 8
11 (Ariège/Haute-Garonne)	SB0134	6 5 5 3 6 4 5 6
Corsica region	SB0840	7 4 5 3 8 2 5s 4
	SB0120	4 5 5 3 11 4 5 7

in 1997. This profile is currently unknown outside of France, which appears to indicate that the infection originated within the country. However, cattle monitoring revealed no cases in herds located or grazing within 5 km of where the infected wild boar was found (844 cattle tested using the comparative intradermal tuberculin test, all negative) (24). Moreover, targeted surveillance in wild boar and red deer populations from open and closed areas (game parks) in a perimeter of 12 km around the index case has been implemented since the 2015–2016 hunting season without any infected animal having being discovered. There is no clear evidence about the origin of this case to date but it seems essential that the greatest vigilance be given to game parks and associated game movements. Infected wild boars were found in all at-risk areas except in the area of Ardennes-Marne (area 6) which is the only area where no infected wild boars were found despite 4 years of targeted surveillance.

Infected badgers were mainly found in infected areas. A few were found in buffer areas (2–7 km from recent cattle outbreaks pastures) and only five from TB-free areas surrounding buffer areas. These five infected badgers were collected by event-based surveillance very close to at-risk areas (<3.5 km), and four of these five badgers were collected in 2012 and 2013 when perimeters of at-risk areas were not well defined. The discovery of these badgers has led to strengthened surveillance in cattle and subsequent detection of bovine outbreaks. However, the absence of TB detection in TB-free areas should be interpreted with caution due to the limited sampling size. In the UK, infected badgers were also detected between 1972 and 1993 in TB-free areas. In Ireland, this prevalence was estimated to be 15% in places where TB had not been reported in cattle for 6 years (25).

All isolates obtained from infected wild animals exhibited the same genotypes that had already been found in isolates from cattle outbreaks in the same regions. In areas where two different genotypes are isolated in wildlife, we observe exactly the same two genotypes in cattle. Strains with the SB0120 or the SB0134 spoligotypes are present in cattle and wildlife in different regions in France albeit presenting different VNTR profiles (26, 27). These results highlight the epidemiological relationship between wildlife and cattle, and evidence that *M. bovis* infection spreads within a multi-species system in these areas as also observed in the UK, Ireland and Spain (28–31). The current risk is that complex reservoirs of *M. bovis* including one or more wild populations and the environment are locally constituted. Badger and wild boar are at the moment the two species most found infected (see sanitary results) and thus worrying in terms of maintenance community. But recent finding on red foxes in France (32) and in other regions of continental Europe (33) raises questions about the epidemiological role of foxes, and have motivated ongoing investigations in different endemic areas.

Location of Lesions

The location of lesions in badgers observed in France is consistent with previous studies carried out in the UK and in Ireland: the thoracic cavity (lungs and lymph nodes) and cephalic lymph nodes were the most common sites (3–5, 34, 35). As in these two countries, the presence of visible lesions only on lymph nodes was the most frequent finding.

With regard to wild boars, lesions are generally smaller and confined to the lymphatic nodes of the head (mainly submandibular lymph nodes) and are therefore less visible to hunters at the time of carcass examination. Systematic inspection of these lymph nodes in the laboratory or by a trained person is therefore essential.

The fact that the majority of infected deer have TB-like lesions and that these lesions are generally located in the pulmonary system makes it possible to suggest that surveillance by careful hunter examination and reporting observed lesions, remains a relevant and sensitive surveillance modality.

Prevalence of *M. bovis* Infection

Concerning deer, we have observed only a few *M. bovis*-positive cases since 2012 (eight red deer and five roe deer) in France, all of them from Côte-d'Or and Dordogne/Charente (areas 2 and 3) which are infected areas with large deer populations, the presence of numerous cattle-TB outbreaks, confirmed infection in badgers and wild boars. These observations suggest a more minor role of deer in the interspecific transmission of *M. bovis* in France compared to other species such as wild boars or badgers. These results are similar to those obtained in others European countries, especially in the Czech Republic, in Hungary where sporadic cases were observed in red deer or in Poland

and Italy in roe deer (36, 37). In Austria, red deer infected with *M. caprae* have been found since 1999 (38). In the UK, a large-scale study was conducted in 2007 and revealed a prevalence of 1.02% in red deer ($n = 196$) and 1.02% in roe deer ($n = 885$) (39).

The epidemiological situation of the Brotonne-Mauny forest (area 1) is special for France because of the very high prevalence level in red deer which were considered a TB maintenance host in the early 2000s (8, 9). This situation was also observed in southern Spain ($P = 27.4\%$, $n = 95$ in the Doñana National Park) (40) and in Portugal between 2009 and 2013 ($P = 38.3\%$, $n = 115$) (33).

The wild boar is considered a key maintenance host for tuberculosis in Spain with prevalence >50% in areas with high-density populations, such as in the Doñana National Park or in large hunting parks (22, 41). In Portugal, prevalence rates ranging from 6 to 46% have been observed (bacterial culture on a pool of lymph nodes) (42). Infected wild boars are commonly discovered in Germany, Italy and in several countries of Central Europe (43, 44).

In France, prevalence in wild boars is mostly lower [on average 3.04% in the 2011–2015 period (with culture) and 2.37% in the 2016–2017 period (with PCR)] than that observed in badgers in the same areas. This epidemiological situation is very different from that observed in south and central Spain where the wild boar is considered a key maintenance host for tuberculosis with prevalence >50% in areas with high-density populations, such as in the Doñana National Park or in large hunting parks (22, 41). In Portugal, prevalence rates ranging from 6 to 46% have been observed (bacterial culture on a pool of lymph nodes) (42). Infected wild boars are also commonly discovered in Germany, Italy and in several countries of Central Europe (43, 44).

Finally, outside the Sylvatub system, TB was also detected in 2012 in 7.3% of a wild boar population from a game park in the Marne, a cattle TB-free area (18). This detection raised questions on disease surveillance in captive wild animals, especially in game parks.

The prevalence observed in badgers in French infected areas was lower than that found in the bovine infection areas in the UK and Ireland. The prevalence rates estimated by culture in the UK during the randomized badgers culling trial, carried out between 1998 and 2006, varied widely (1.6–37.2%) depending on the *post-mortem* and culture methods used, with an average of 16.6% (3). In Ireland, 19.5 to 26.1% of the badgers analyzed by culture in the four study areas were found to be positive (45). A more recent study, in areas where there is high prevalence of bovine TB based on detailed *post-mortem* examination, histopathology, and culture in each specimen, reported a prevalence of 36.3% (4). Analysis of prevalence rates in ~5,000 badgers in Ireland revealed a decrease in the overall prevalence from 26 to 11% between 2007 and 2011 (46). In parallel, it should be noted that the herd prevalence in cattle in the UK and in Ireland is higher than in France (5–6 vs. 0.04%), and that all the analyzed badgers in these countries originated from areas with the highest prevalence in cattle (47).

In the north of Spain, in the provinces of Galicia and Asturias, where TB prevalence in cattle is between 0 and 4.3% depending on the district, badger prevalence rates between 6 and 7% are observed (28), which is similar to rates observed in some areas of France.

It is not possible to draw any conclusion on the relationship between the prevalence of TB in cattle herds and in surrounding badgers population due to important methodological differences. However, it would be also interesting to follow the relationship between the trends observed in some areas in cattle associated with disease control measures and the trend in the prevalence of these wild animal populations. Although the present dataset does not allow precise time comparison between P1 and P2 due to variations of sampling patterns and method for analyses, the ongoing surveillance may contribute to constitute consistent time series that may be analyzed for that concern. Nevertheless, in Côte-d'Or (area 2), if we considered that the apparent prevalence in P1 is underestimated because of the average sensitivity of the culture compared to that of the PCR, one can hypothesize that the prevalence has decreased in badgers from P1 to P2.

In Dordogne/Charente (area 3), where both event-based and targeted surveillance in badgers have been effective, we observe that badgers collected by event-based surveillance (mainly road-killed badgers) were more infected than those trapped. This could be explained by a lower vigilance of infected badgers and therefore increased collisions with vehicles. Moreover, movements of infected badgers are higher (48) and these infected badgers occupy larger home ranges (49, 50). These elements point to a greater probability of detecting infection by collecting road-killed individuals than by trapping.

Finally, we observed a higher prevalence in male than in female badgers, which corroborates several studies (51, 52). This has been interpreted as an influence of the aggressive behavior of males for the defense of the territories, and the attendance of several social groups during the rut period, resulting in a higher rate of infection in male badgers (52).

CONCLUSION

The implementation of a wide and important surveillance system as Sylvatub relies on the involvement, at the national or departmental level, of the main organizations involved in wildlife surveillance and field volunteers without whom this surveillance would not be possible. The detection of numerous cases of TB in free-ranging wildlife occurs in areas of cattle outbreaks with the same profile of *M. bovis* strains showing evidence that, in main endemic regions of France, TB circulates between cattle and wildlife. The current risk is that complex reservoirs of *M. bovis* including one or more wild populations and the environment are locally constituted. It is also worrisome to note the increase in the number of areas in which infected badgers or wild boars are found, partly due to a better surveillance over time. However, prevalence observed in France in badgers and wild boars are lower than those observed in the UK and in Ireland for badgers or in Spain for wild boars, and only sporadic cases have been detected in red deer and roe deer.

Wildlife surveillance contributes to the implementation of control strategies in wildlife and in cattle by allowing defining at-risk areas. It also allows adapting surveillance in cattle keeping in mind the multi-host aspect of the disease as well as targeting prevention actions and to follow their long-term efficiency. This information, complemented by scientific investigations and researches, are needed for conducting biosecurity measures in wildlife (control of artificial feeding, management of hunting waste, banning game release, wildlife populations reduction in highly infected TB areas), and in livestock (management of water points, protection of the food and barns for example). Convinced that wildlife can be an additional local factor of TB spread and maintenance, the French ministry in charge of agriculture has decided to make Sylvatub sustainable.

In parallel, evolvement of sampling strategies have been discussed in the aim to improve surveillance. In buffer areas, targeted surveillance will be replaced by *M bovis* detection in road-killed badgers. Another main development will concern wild boar in at-risk areas: serological testing for the detection of antibodies directed against *M. bovis* have been proposed as suitable tools for TB screening in wild boar populations (18, 53). ELISA method has been tested in comParison to PCR and culture in different areas in France with encouraging results (Richomme and Boschiroli, personal communication). It will be used as an alternative method to monitor the *M. bovis* exposure level in wild boars in the next years.

ETHICS STATEMENT

Samples were collected from animals trapped with appropriate permits, hunted legally during the hunting season with appropriate permits, shot legally because of severe debilitation, or found dead. All the samples included in this study were obtained from animals analyzed within an official context relating to TB surveillance in free-ranging wildlife. All sampling procedures complied with national and European regulations, and no specific ethics approval was therefore required.

AUTHOR CONTRIBUTIONS

JH, AF, ÉR, CR, M-LB, ÉF, LC, FC, IT, SP, and PH: Sylvatub conception and monitoring; ÉR: Data analysis; ÉR, M-LB, CR, and SD: Paper writing; CR, M-LB, SD, JH, ÉF, AF, LC, PJ, IT, SP, PH, and FC: Manuscript critical revision.

ACKNOWLEDGMENTS

The authors would like to thank the local state veterinary services, the local hunting federations, the local services of the National Game Hunting and Wildlife Agency, the local laboratories for analysis, the local Animal Health Defense Associations, and Julie Rivière, the first coordinator of the Sylvatub system from 2011 to 2012. We are grateful to all the trappers and their associations, Pest control officers and their associations and hunters of wild ungulates without whom the surveillance could not have taken place. Thank to Craig Stevens for his very useful comments on this article and his careful reading.

REFERENCES

1. World Organisation for Animal Health. *Terrestrial Animal Health Code.* 26 edn (2017).
2. Delahay RJ, Cheeseman CL, Clifton-Hadley RS. Wildlife disease reservoirs: the epidemiology of *Mycobacterium bovis* infection in the European badger (*Meles meles*) and other British mammals. *Tuberculosis* (2001) 81:43–9. doi: 10.1054/tube.2000.0266
3. Bourne FJ, Donnelly CA, Cox DR, Gettinby G, McInerney JP, Morrison WI, et al. *The Scientific Evidence, a Science Base for a Sustainable Policy to Control TB in Cattle, an Epidemiological Investigation into Bovine Tuberculosis.* Final Report of the Independent Scientific Group on Cattle TB. Department for Environment, Food and Rural Affairs, London (2007).
4. Murphy D, Gormley E, Costello E, O'Meara D, Corner LA. The prevalence and distribution of *Mycobacterium bovis* infection in European badgers (*Meles meles*) as determined by enhanced post mortem examination and bacteriological culture. *Res Vet Sci.* (2010) 88:1–5. doi: 10.1016/j.rvsc.2009.05.020
5. Corner LA, Murphy D, Gormley E. Mycobacterial infection in the Eurasian badger (*Meles meles*): the disease, pathogenesis, epidemiology and control. *J Comp Path.* (2011) 144:1–24. doi: 10.1016/j.jcpa.2010.10.003
6. Gortazar C, Ferroglio E, Höfle U, Frölich K, Vicente J. Diseases shared between wildlife and livestock: a European perspective. *Eur J Wildl Res.* (2007) 53:241–56. doi: 10.1007/s10344-007-0098-y
7. Cavalerie L, Courcoul A, Boschiroli ML, Réveillaud E, Gay P. Tuberculose bovine en France en 2014: une situation stable. *Bull Epidémiol Santé Anim.* (2014) 71:4–11.
8. Zanella G, Durand B, Hars J, Moutou F, Garin-Bastuji B, Duvauchelle A, et al. *Mycobacterium bovis* in wildlife in France. *J Wildl Dis.* (2008) 44:99–108. doi: 10.7589/0090-3558-44.1.99
9. Hars J, Richomme C, Rivière J, Payne A, Faure E, and Boschiroli ML. La tuberculose bovine dans la faune sauvage en France. Risques pour l'élevage bovin. *Bull Acad. Vet France* (2013) 166:216–221. doi: 10.4267/2042/51801
10. Payne A, Boschiroli ML, Gueneau E, Moyen JL, Rambaud T, Dufour B, et al. Bovine tuberculosis in ≪ Eurasian ≫ badgers (*Meles meles*) in France. *Eur J Wildl Res.* (2013) 59:331–9. doi: 10.1007/s10344-012-0678-3
11. Rivière J, Réveillaud E, Boschiroli ML, Hars J, Richomme C, Faure E, et al. Sylvatub: bilan d'une première année de surveillance dans la faune sauvage en France. *Bull Epidémiol Santé Anim.* (2013) 57:10–5.
12. Rivière J, Le Strat Y, Dufour B, Hendrikx P. Sensitivity of bovine tuberculosis surveillance in wildlife in France: a scenario tree approach. *PLoS ONE* (2015) 10:e0141884. doi: 10.1371/journal.pone.0141884

13. Lamarque F, Hatier C, Artois M, Berny P, Diedler C. Le réseau SAGIR, réseau national de suivi sanitaire de la faune sauvage française. *Epidemiol et Santé Anim* (2000) 37:21–30.
14. Courcoul A, Moyen JL, Brugère L, Faye S, Hénault S, Gares H, et al. Estimation of sensitivity and specificity of bacteriology, histopathology and PCR for the confirmatory diagnosis of bovine tuberculosis using latent class analysis. *PLoS ONE* (2014) 9:e90334. doi: 10.1371/journal.pone.0090334
15. Hénault S, Karoui C, Boschiroli ML. A PCR-based method for tuberculosis detection in wildlife. *Dev Biol.* (2006) 126:123–32.
16. Thierry D, Brisson-Noël A, Vincent-Lévy-Frébault V, Nguyen S, Guesdon JL, Gicquel B. Characterization of a *Mycobacterium tuberculosis* insertion sequence, IS6110, and its application in diagnosis. *J Clin Microbiol.* (1990) 28:2668–73.
17. Zhang J, Abadia E, Refregier G, Tafaj S, Boschiroli ML, Guillard B, et al. *Mycobacterium tuberculosis* complex CRISPR genotyping: improving efficiency, throughput and discriminative power of Bspoligotyping with new spacers and a microbead-based hybridization assay. *J Med Microbiol.* (2010) 59:285–94. doi: 10.1099/jmm.0.016949-0
18. Richomme C, Riviere J, Hars J, Boschiroli ML, Gueneau E, Fediaevsky A, et al. Tuberculose bovine: infection de sangliers dans un parc de chasse. *Bull Epidémiol Santé Anim.* (2013) 56:14–6.
19. Lambert S, Hars J, Réveillaud E, Moyen JL, Gares H, Rambaud T, et al. Host status of roe deer in bovine tuberculosis endemic areas. *Eur J Wildl Res.* (2017) 63:15. doi: 10.1007/s10344-016-1071-4
20. Hars J, Richomme C, Riviere J, Faure E, Boschiroli ML. Dix années de surveillance de la tuberculose bovine dans la faune sauvage française et perspectives. *Bull. Epidémiol. Santé Anim.* (2012) 52:2–6.
21. Crashaw TR, Griffiths IB, Clifton-Hadley MA. ComParison of a standard and detailed post mortem protocol for detecting Mycobacterium bovis in badgers. *Vet Rec.* (2008) 163:473–7. doi: 10.1136/vr163.16.473
22. Gortazar C, Vicente J, Gavier-Widen D. Pathology of bovine tuberculosis in the European wild boar (*Sus scrofa*). *Vet. Record* (2003) 152:779–80. doi: 10.1136/vr.152.25.779
23. Gavier-Widen D, Chambers MA, Palmer N, Newell DG, Hewinson RG. Pathology of natural *Mycobacterium bovis* infection in European badgers (*Meles meles*) and its relationship with bacterial excretion. *Vet Record.* (2001) 148:299–304.
24. Chevalier F, Hars J, Courcoul A, Hansen E, Boschiroli ML, Richomme C. Découverte d'un sanglier infecté par *M. bovis* en Sologne: investigations sur l'origine de l'infection et mesures de surveillance préconisées chez les ruminants domestiques et la faune sauvage. *Bull Epidémiol Santé Anim.* (2015) 72:12–6.
25. Anses. *Tuberculose Bovine et Faune Sauvage*. Rapport. Edition scientifique Anses (2011). Available online at: http://www.anses.fr/Documents/SANT2010sa0154Ra.pdf (Accessed 05 May, 2011).
26. Hauer A, Michelet L, De Cruz K, Cochard T, Branger M, Karoui C, et al. MIRU-VNTR allelic variability depends on Mycobacterium bovis clonal group identity. *Infect Genet Evol.* (2016) 45:165–9. doi: 10.1016/j.meegid.2016.08.038
27. Hauer A, De Cruz K, Cochard T, Godreuil S, Karoui C, Henault S, et al. Genetic evolution of *Mycobacterium bovis* causing tuberculosis in livestock and wildlife in France since 1978. *PLoS ONE* (2015) 10:e0117103. doi: 10.1371/journal.pone.0117103
28. Balseiro A, Rodriguez O, Gonzalez-Quiros P, Merediz I, Sevilla IA, Davé D, et al. Infection of Eurasian badgers (*Meles meles*) with *Mycobacterium bovis* and *Mycobacterium avium* complex in Spain. *Vet J.* (2011) 190:e21–5. doi: 10.1016/j.tvjl.2011.04.012
29. Jenkins HE, Woodroffe R, Donnely C, Cox DR, Johnston WT, Bourne FJ, et al. Effects of culling on spatial associations of *Mycobacterium bovis* infections in badgers and cattle. *J Appl Ecol.* (2007) 44:897–908. doi: 10.1111/j.1365-2664.2007.01372.x
30. Olea-Popelka FJ, Flynn O, Costello E, McGrath G, Collins JD, O'keeffe J, et al. Spatial relationship between *Mycobacterium bovis* strains in cattle and badgers in four areas in Ireland. *Prev Vet Med.* (2005) 71:57–70. doi: 10.1016/j.prevetmed.2005.05.008
31. Woodroffe R, Donnelly CA, Johnston WT, Bourne FJ, Cheeseman CL, Clifton-Hadley RS, et al. Spatial association of *Mycobacterium bovis* infection in cattle and badgers *Meles meles*. *J Appl Ecol.* (2005) 42:852–62. doi: 10.1111/j.1365-2664.2005.01081.x
32. Michelet L, De Cruz K, Hénault S, Tambosco J, Richomme C, Réveillaud É, et al. *Mycobacterium bovis* Infection of Red Fox, France. *Emerg Infect Dis.* (2018) 24:1150–3. doi: 10.3201/eid2406.180094
33. Matos AC, Figueira L, Martins MH, Pinto ML, Matos M, Coelho AC. New insights into *Mycobacterium bovis* prevalence in wild mammals in Portugal. *Transbound Emerg Dis.* (2016) 63:e313–22. doi: 10.1111/tbed.12306
34. Gallagher J, Clifton-Hadley RS. Tuberculosis in badgers; a review of the disease and its significance for others animals. *Res Vet Sci.* (2000) 69:203–17. doi: 10.1053/rvsc.2000.0422
35. Jenkins HE, Morrison WI, Cox DR, Donnelly CA, Johnston WT, Bourne FJ, et al. The prevalence, distribution and severity of detectable pathological lesions in badgers naturally infected with Mycobacterium bovis. *Epidemiol Inf.* (2008) 136:1350–61. doi: 10.1017/S0950268807009909
36. Pavlik I, Trcka I, Parmova I, Svobodova J, Melicharek I, Nagy G, et al. Detection of bovine and human tuberculosis in cattle and other animals in six Central European countries during the years 2000-2004. *Vet Med Praha* (2005) 50:291–9.
37. Chiari M, Zanoni M, Alborali LG, Zanardi G, Avisani D, Tagliabue S, et al. Isolation of *Mycobacterium caprae* (Lechtal Genotype) from Red Deer (*Cervus elaphus*) in Italy. *J. Wildlife Dis.* (2014) 50:330–3. doi: 10.7589/2013-06-135
38. Prodinger WM, Eigentler A, Allerberger F, Schönbauer M, Glawischnig W. Infection of Red Deer, Cattle, and Humans with *Mycobacterium bovis* subsp. *caprae* in Western Austria. *J Clin Microbiol.* (2002) 40:2270–2. doi: 10.1128/JCM.40.6.2270-2272.2002
39. Delahay RJ, Smith CG, Barlow AM, Walker N, Harris A, Clifton-Hadley RS, et al. Bovine tuberculosis in wild mammals in the South-West region of England: a survey of prevalence and semi quantitative assessment of the relative risk to cattle. *Vet J.* (2007) 173:287–301. doi: 10.1016/j.tvjl.2005.11.011
40. Gortazar C, Torres MJ, Vicente J, Acevedo P, Reglero M, de la Fuente J, et al. Bovine tuberculosis in Doñana Biosphere Reserve: the role of wild ungulates as disease reservoirs in the last Iberian lynx strongholds. *PLoS ONE* (2008) 3:e2776. doi: 10.1371/journal.pone.0002776
41. Vicente J, Barasona JA, Acevedo P, Ruiz-Fons JF, Boadella M, Diez-Delgado I, et al. Temporal trend of tuberculosis in wild ungulates from Mediterranean Spain. *Transbound Emerg Dis.* (2013) 60:92–103. doi: 10.1111/tbed.12167
42. Santos N, Correia-Neves M, Gebrehmichael S, Källenius G, Svenson SB, Almeida V. Epidemiology of *Mycobacterium bovis* infection in wild boar (*Sus scrofa*) from Portugal. *J Wildl Dis.* (2009) 45:1048–61. doi: 10.7589/0090-3558-45.4.1048
43. Mignone W, Ballardini M, Sanguinetti V, Bollo E, Dini V. La tuberculosi dei cinghiali (*Sus scrofa*) a vita libera in Liguria: Primi isolamenti di micobactteri e prtocollo di monitoraggio. *BIPAS* (1997) 16:79–84.
44. Machackova M, Matlova L, Lamka J, Smolik J, Melicharek I, Hanzlikova M, et al. Wild boar (*Sus scrofa*) as a possible vector of mycobacterial infections: review of literature and critical analysis of data from Central Europe between 1983 to 2001. *Vet Med.* (2003) 48:51–65.
45. Griffin JM, Williams DH, Kelly GE, Clegg TA, O'Boyle I, Collins JD. The impact of badger removal on the control of tuberculosis in cattle herds in Ireland. *Prev Vet Med.* (2005) 67:237–66. doi: 10.1016/j.prevetmed.2004.10.009
46. Byrne AW, Kenny K, Fogarty U, O'Keeffe JJ, More SJ, McGrath G, et al. Spatial and temporal analyses of metrics of tuberculosis infection in badgers (*Meles meles)* from the Republic of Ireland: trends in apparent prevalence. *Prev Vet Med.* (2015) 122:345–54. doi: 10.1016/j.prevetmed.2015.10.013
47. EFSA. *Modelling the Impact of a Change in MI Sensitivity on the Surveillance of bTB at the Country Level.* Supporting Publications, EN-450.40p (2013).
48. Vicente J, Delahay RJ, Walker NJ, Cheeseman CL. Social organization and movement influence the incidence of bovine tuberculosis in an undisturbed high-density badger Meles meles population. *J Anim Ecol.* (2007) 76:348–60. doi: 10.1111/j.1365-2656.2006.01199.x
49. Cheeseman C, Mallinson P. Behaviour of badgers (*Meles meles*) infected with bovine tuberculosis. *J Zool.* (1981) 194:284–9.
50. Garnett B, Delahay R, Roper T. Ranging behaviour of European badgers (*Meles meles*) in relation to bovine tuberculosis (*Mycobacterium bovis*) infection. *Appl Anim Behav Sci.* (2005) 94:331–40. doi: 10.1016/j.applanim.2005.02.013

51. Corner LA, Costello E, Lesellier S, O'Meara D, Gormley E. Experimental tuberculosis in the European badger (*Meles meles*) after endobronchial inoculation with *Mycobacterium bovis*: II. *Prog Infect Res Vet Sci.* (2008) 85:481–90. doi: 10.1016/j.rvsc.2008.03.003
52. Jenkins HE, Cox DR, Delahay RJ. Direction of association between bite wounds and *Mycobacterium bovis* Infection in Badgers: implications for transmission. *PLoS ONE* (2012) 7:e45584. doi: 10.1371/journal.pone.0045584
53. Boadella M, Lyashchenko K, Greenwald R, Esfandiari J, Jaroso R, Carta T, et al. Serologic tests for detecting antibodies against *Mycobacterium bovis* and *Mycobacterium avium subspecies paratuberculosis* in Eurasian wild boar (*Sus scrofa scrofa*). *J Vet Diagn Invest.* (2011) 23:77–83. doi: 10.1177/104063871102300111

10

A New Model to Calibrate a Reference Standard for Bovine Tuberculin Purified Protein Derivative in the Target Species

Klaas Frankena[1,2], Liesbeth Jacobs[3], Tonny van Dijk[3], Margaret Good[4], Anthony Duignan[5] and Mart C. M. de Jong[2]*

[1] Adaptation Physiology Group, Department of Animal Sciences, Wageningen University, Wageningen, Netherlands, [2] Quantitative Veterinary Epidemiology Group, Department of Animal Sciences, Wageningen University, Wageningen, Netherlands, [3] Thermofisher Scientific, Prionics Lelystad B.V., Lelystad, Netherlands, [4] Independent Researcher and Private Consultant, Dun Laoghaire, Ireland, [5] Department of Agriculture, Food and the Marine, Dublin, Ireland

***Correspondence:**
Klaas Frankena
klaas.frankena@wur.nl

Since 1986, use of a Bovine International Standard (BIS) for bovine tuberculin has been required to ensure national and international uniformity regarding the potency designation of bovine tuberculin Purified Protein Derivative (PPDb) preparations produced by multiple manufacturers. The BIS is the unique golden standard in the guinea pig potency assay, representing 100% potency, where potencies of production batches are calculated as relative potencies in comparison with the potency of the BIS which was set at 32,500 international Unit (IU) per mg. The stock supply and lifetime of the BIS is limited.The aim of this study was to develop a model to determine the potency of a newly produced in-house Reference Standard (RS) for PPDb with great accuracy in the target species (cattle) and to prove its precision and accuracy in the guinea pig potency test. First simulations were done to estimate the required number of cattle needed. Then, 30 naturally bTB infected cattle were subjected to a tuberculin skin test using multiple injections of both the RS and the BIS. Both were applied randomly in the same volume and concentration (1 dose). The potency of the RS against the BIS was directly derived from the least square means (LSMEANS) and was estimated as 1.067 (95% CI: 1.025–1.109), equal to a potency of 34,700 ± 1,400 IU/mg. In six guinea pig potency assays the RS was used to assign potencies to production batches of PPDb. Here, precision and accuracy of the RS was determined according to the parallel-line assay. Relative potencies were estimated by exponentiation of the common slope. The corresponding 95% confidence intervals were obtained according to Fieller's theorem. In sensitized guinea pigs, the relative potency of the RS against the BIS was 1.115 (95% CI: 0.871–1.432), corresponding to an absolute potency of 36,238 IU/mg (95% CI: 28,308–46,540).In conclusion: the method used to determine the potency of the RS against the BIS in naturally bTB infected cattle, resulted in a highly accurate potency estimate of the RS. The RS can be used in the guinea pig test to assign potencies to PPDb production batches with high precision and accuracy.

Keywords: ***mycobacterium bovis*, tuberculin, bovine international standard, new reference standard, potency estimation, guinea pigs, cattle**

INTRODUCTION

Bovine tuberculosis (bTB) is a zoonotic livestock infection most frequently caused by the bacterium *Mycobacterium bovis* which is often found to be endemic in cattle but which can infect several species of mammals and also marsupials. *Mycobacterium bovis*, belongs to a group of related Mycobacterium species, known as the *Mycobacterium tuberculosis* complex (MTBC), members of which cause tuberculosis in humans and multiple animal species including bovines (1, 2). TB in bovines is a chronic disease characterized by granulomatous lesions in multiple parts of the body and clinical signs such as coughing, reduced milk production etc. Infections can remain subclinical for many years, even if multiple organs are affected (3, 4).

Throughout the last century, extensive control programs resulted in eradication of bTB in many countries, including most EU Member States, Australia, Canada, Switzerland and many states in the USA. Important control measures in cattle include regular and systematic testing of cattle herds, compulsory slaughter of test-positive animals, movement restrictions out of infected herds and post-mortem slaughterhouse surveillance (5–7). However, bTB is still present in various countries, especially in those where a wildlife reservoir of *M. bovis* is present (8). To control and eradicate bTB, multiple tests have been developed to detect infected cattle. The widely used tuberculin skin tests are based on the development of a delayed type hypersensitivity reaction in cattle infected by a MTBC after an intradermal injection with bovine (*M. bovis*) tuberculin Purified Protein Derivative (PPDb) (9, 10). Details about the skin test are in Annex B Directive 64/432/EEC (10) and in OIE guidelines (9).

Since the development of the tuberculin skin tests in cattle, various companies worldwide commenced production of PPDb. To ensure national and international uniformity regarding the potency designation of the PPDb preparations it was essential to define a bovine tuberculin standard. In 1986, after multiple assays in both cattle and guinea pigs, the Bovine International Standard (BIS) was officially established by the World Health Organization (WHO) as the standard for PPDb. The BIS is freeze-dried and stored in glass ampoules, each ampoule containing 1.8 mg of PPDb. Based on the results of an international collaborative study, organized by the WHO, the activity of the contents of each ampoule was defined as 58,500 IU of PPDb (11, page 20), hence the ampoule contained 32,500 IU/mg PPDb Since 1987, the BIS is internationally distributed, on behalf of the WHO, by the International Laboratory for Biological Standards, Hertfordshire, England (11, 12).

Because the stock of the BIS is limited—and reported as seemingly being at the end of its lifetime due to formation of aggregates in some ampoules (13)—, the International Laboratory for Biological Standards encourages manufacturers of PPDb to produce their own Reference Standard (RS) to be used in the guinea pig and cattle potency test. The aim of this study was to determine the potency of a new RS for PPDb with great accuracy in the target species (cattle) and to prove its precision and accuracy in the guinea pig potency test, the prescribed release test for PPD. The new RS was comparable to the BIS in composition and potency in cattle and guinea pigs. A trial in natural bTB infected cattle was designed and performed to determine the potency of the RS in cattle with great precision and accuracy. In the guinea pig test the RS is used to assign potency to individual production batches of PPDb. The accuracy and precision of the RS in the assignment of the potency to production batches of PPDb in the guinea pig potency test was shown in 6 trials. Additionally, the potency of the new RS was compared with the BIS in sensitized guinea pigs.

METHODS

The study consisted of 2 parts: I. Calibration of the RS against the BIS in naturally bTB sensitized cattle. II. Prove of accuracy and precision of the RS in the guinea pig potency test. Here the RS is used to assign potency to individual production batches of PPDb.

Production of the Reference Standard

It was decided by Prionics Lelystad B.V. to produce the RS according to the same formula as was used for the BIS with respect to the *M. bovis* strain, volume of the vials, concentration of protein and buffer. Therefore, 15 L of homogenous bulk of PPDb, derived from *M. bovis AN5*, in glucose-phosphate buffer (R31 medium, Hyclone, UK) was formulated with a final concentration of 1 mg/mL (±0.05 mg). Formulation and sterile filtration was performed using Standard Operating Procedures with the exception of adding phenol to the formulated final product. The phenol concentration, due to the phenol present in the starting material of the concentrated tuberculin PPD, is estimated to be 0.03%. No extra phenol was added to the buffer used to formulate the final product. Phenol can evaporate during the freeze-dry process and is hazardous for the environment. The formulated final product was filled into 6 ml vials each vial containing 1.8 mL (±0.02). Freeze drying was done in a Klee Freeze Dryer using program TUB MSL/WSL (freezing of the samples for 3 h at −35°C; drying under vacuum at −33°C at 8.0E-2 mbar for 112 h; drying at 25°C at 1.0 E-2 mbar for 24 h). After freeze drying the vials were closed, capped, labeled and stored in sealed plastic bags at 2–8°C. Before use the content of a vial with the RS is reconstituted in 1.8 ml of Water For Injection (WFI) containing 0.42% phenol to give an end solution in R31 buffer of 0.45% phenol and 1 mg/mL of PPD.

Calibration of the RS Against the BIS in Naturally Infected Cattle

Cattle

The trial was carried out on the Longtown Veterinary Research Farm of the Central Veterinary Research Laboratory of the Department of Agriculture, Food and the Marine (DAFM) in Ireland. Thirty naturally infected steers, all between 14 and 24 months old, were selected from herds in which *M. bovis* infection was confirmed (see **Supplementary Material** for sample size calculation). Cattle which had given a positive skin response, in the single intradermal comparative tuberculin test (SICCT), i.e., showing an increase at the bovine site equal to 4 mm or more than any increase at the avian site, were selected. The time interval between the SICCT on the farms of origin and the study was at least 60 days. All animals also failed (tested positive in) the gamma interferon (y-IFN) Bovigam® test (Thermofisher Scientific, Lelystad) 2 weeks prior to the study, indicating they were responsive to tuberculin.

Trial Design and Testing Procedure in Cattle

For a RS to be considered as a valid standard, its potency must be estimated with high precision and accuracy. Therefore, the 95% confidence interval was set as the estimated potency ±10% of that potency.

In cattle, four injection sites at each side of the mid-neck are routinely used to perform a potency assay. Therefore, RS and BIS were applied twice on the left side and twice on the right side of the neck. Within the sides of the neck, the injections were randomly allocated to the four injection sites according to one of the 6 unique combinations. For each side, one of the 6 combinations was randomly selected using PROC SURVEYSELECT of SAS version 9.4 (14).

Four injection sites were marked and clipped, using a battery powered hair clippers, on both sides of the mid-neck of the 30 bovines, followed by measurement of the initial skinfold thickness with a caliper before injection. Subsequently cattle were injected (according to the randomization scheme) with a volume of 0.1 mL of BIS or RS at a concentration of 1.0 mg/ml. Skinfold thickness was measured again at 72 h post-injection and the increase in skinfold thickness developed between 0 and 72h was calculated. Injections and measurements were all performed by the same person (AD).

The cattle study was approved by the Health Products Regulatory Authority (HPRA), Dublin, Ireland (project authorization number: AE19113/P008).

Statistical Analysis

The differences in skinfold thickness were statistically analyzed at a significance level of 5% with a linear mixed model using the increase in diameter of skin at the injection sites (in mm) as outcome variable [PROC MIXED of SAS (14)]. Estimation method used was restricted maximum likelihood (REML) and variance component was specified as covariance structure. The initial model included tuberculin batch (RS, BIS), side (left, right) and site (1–4) of injection and animal was included as random effect. Relative potency can be derived directly from the least square means (LSMEANS) for both batches and its 95% CI from the 95% CI of the difference in LSMEANS. Next, the potency of the RS was calculated by multiplying the relative potency of the RS with the known potency of the BIS i.e. 32,500 IU/mg.

Proof of Accuracy and Precision of the RS in the Guinea Pig Potency Test

Guinea Pigs and Sensitization

Dunkin Hartley guinea pigs were obtained from ISO 9001 certified breeders of SPF guinea pigs. The guinea pigs were infected with 0.0008 mg of wet mass of living virulent *M. bovis* of strain AN5 by intramuscular injection of 0.5 ml into the left hind leg of each animal. Infection was 5 weeks prior to the skin test. At the moment of infection, the weight of the guinea pig was between 400 and 600 grams.

Trial Design and Assay Procedure

Tuberculin skin tests were performed in six trials (labeled T1 to T6) with each 9 guinea pigs. Per guinea pig four injection sites on both sides of the flanks were available. According to the incomplete balanced Latin square design three PPDb batches can be assayed per trial (production batches and/or standards). Batches (production batches and standards) are assayed in three dilutions which were randomly allocated to the injection sites according to the incomplete balanced Latin square design (15). This design can be analyzed as a parallel-line assay (16).

Five weeks after infection, flanks were shaved and treated with depilatory crème leaving enough space for 4 injection sites on each side. Subsequently each guinea pig received eight injections of 0.2 ml of bovine tuberculin PPD. Syringes were coded making persons involved in the GP trials blind for the precise content of any syringe. Diameters of delayed type hypersensitivity reactions, visible as reddish circles around the injection sites, were measured with calipers between 24 and 28 h later. For details of the procedure for skin testing in guinea pigs, see Annex B Directive 64/432/EEC (10), OIE guidelines (9) and the European Pharmacopeia Monograph 0536.

In the six trials, the potency of 4 production batches of PPDb was determined in the guinea pig potency assay using both the RS and the BIS as standard. The four production batches were respectively: A (batch 102402), B (batch 104008), C (batch 110404), and D (batch 112003). In each potency assay, BIS and RS were included and one of the tuberculin batches A–D. Batch A was used in three potency tests, batches B, C, and D each in one potency test. Furthermore, each PPDb was tested in three dilutions 1:200; 1:1,000 and 1:5,000 (concentrations for the RS and the BIS being 0.005, 0.001, and 0.0002 mg/ml. In general, these concentrations result in well measurable skin reactions and acceptable confidence limits (9). Also, these concentrations are 5-fold dilutions, being equidistant at the log scale.

Statistical Analysis

The goal of the analysis was to determine whether production batches get comparable potency estimates when assayed against either one of both standards (RS or BIS), additionally the relative potency of the RS to the BIS in guinea pigs was calculated. Guinea pig trials were statistically analyzed using generalized linear mixed models [PROC MIXED of SAS (14)] using diameter of skin reaction (in mm) as the outcome variable and guinea pig was included as random effect. Analysis was performed according to a parallel-line assay, as described by Finney (16), with pairs of tuberculins: Batches A, B, C, or D against either RS or BIS and RS against BIS. The independent variables were tuberculin batch (production batch or standard) (Batch), logarithm of the concentration (Logconc), square of Logconc (Logconc^2) and the interaction between Batch and Logconc (Batch*Logconc). Logconc^2 was included in the model to assess whether or not significant curvature was present. From the interaction Batch*Logconc it can be concluded whether or not both batches show parallel lines. Guinea pig (animal) was included as random effect. The assumption was that the diameter outcomes were directly proportional to the logarithm of the tuberculin concentration. For assaying the RS against the BIS a pooled analysis of all six trials was performed. Therefore, the variable Trial was added to the model as fixed effect, as well as the interaction between Batch and Trial. Insignificant variables ($p > 0.05$) were removed from the model using backward model building, except for Batch and Logconc, and Trial in case of the pooled analysis.

Relative potencies were estimated by exponentiation of the common slope. The corresponding 95% confidence intervals were obtained, according to Fieller's theorem (16) which is especially suited for interval estimation of ratios (17) using PROC IML of SAS (14). Finally, the relative potencies of the four additional tuberculin batches against RS were converted into actual potencies by multiplication with the potency estimate of RS from the cattle trial (which appeared to be 34,700 IU/mg). The relative potency of the RS against the BIS was converted to actual potency (expressed in IU) by multiplication with 32,500 IU which is the potency of BIS.

According to the regulations of the European Commission (10), the OIE (9) and the monograph 01/2008 /0536 of the European Pharmacopeia[1], potency testing of PPDbs in guinea pigs is only valid when the confidence limits are between 50 and 200% of the estimated potency. Furthermore, the estimated potency is not less than 66% and not more than 150% of the stated potency (9).

Guinea pig trials were approved by the Animal Ethic Committee (DEC) of the Animal Science Group of Wageningen University & Research (registration number 1625085300).

[1]European Pharmacopeia 9.0. *Monograph 01/2008/0536.*

RESULT

Cattle Trial

Descriptive Analysis

In total 240 observations were available, half of which were observations on RS injection sites and the other half on BIS injection sites. The average increase in skinfold thickness (between 0 and 72 h) was 6.88 mm (SD 2.81) and 6.48 mm (SD 2.61) for RS and BIS respectively.

Potencies

Statistical analysis showed that the variables Batch ($p = 0.01$) and Site ($p < 0.001$) were significantly related to the increase in skinfold thickness. LSMEANS for RS and BIS were 6.90 and 6.46 mm, respectively. The relative potency of RS against BIS (with stated potency of 32,500 IU/mg) was therefore estimated as 6.89540/6.4630 = 1.0669 (95% CI: 1.016–1.118) and the absolute potency of RS is then 1.067*32,500 = 34,674 IU/mg (95% CI: 33,020–36,335) or roughly 34,700 ± 1,650. This CI is smaller than the anticipated ±3,000 used in the simulation which is due to smaller variations between bovines (2.5 mm where 3.0 mm assumed) as well as within bovines (1.3 mm where 2.0 mm assumed). In the final model, the intra-class correlation due to the random bovine effect was 0.77.

Guinea Pig Trials

Descriptive Analysis

From all injections administered ($n = 432$), 34 resulted in a zero-response (diameter 0.00 mm). All originating from the lowest dose in the potency test (0.0002 mg/ml concentration). From historical data it is known that the lowest dose in the potency test can generate a zero-response. These were treated

TABLE 1 | Skin response (mm) of guinea pigs after injection with three concentrations of Bovine International Standard (BIS), Reference Standard (RS) and for production batches (A–D) using an incomplete balanced Latin square design; for RS and BIS data of six trials were pooled, for tuberculin A data of three trials were pooled.

Tuberculin batch	Concentration (mg/ml)	*N*	Mean	Std Dev	Minimum	Maximum
RS	0.0002	34	12.00	2.08	8.11	17.84
	0.001	48	15.70	1.92	10.31	18.97
	0.005	48	18.99	1.88	14.83	23.62
BIS	0.0002	36	12.04	1.81	7.25	16.16
	0.001	48	15.88	1.73	11.59	21.49
	0.005	48	18.67	2.00	14.90	24.75
A	0.0002	23	12.40	2.14	6.94	15.36
	0.001	24	16.07	1.40	13.58	18.69
	0.005	24	18.40	1.95	14.46	21.74
B	0.0002	4	12.75	3.68	9.20	17.90
	0.001	8	15.04	2.70	11.77	19.56
	0.005	8	20.23	1.65	17.64	22.47
C	0.0002	7	10.95	1.66	8.83	13.35
	0.001	8	15.78	2.37	12.69	20.05
	0.005	8	19.51	1.99	16.38	21.50
D	0.0002	6	12.02	1.63	9.85	14.12
	0.001	8	15.72	2.60	11.41	19.96
	0.005	8	19.69	0.97	18.10	20.85

as missing values and excluded from the analyses because there was no response to the lowest concentration of PPD. Besides that, inclusion of the zero-responses made the distribution of the outcome variable (diameter) non-Gaussian, preventing the valid use of generalized linear mixed models. Additionally, measurements of 36 skin reactions were labeled "weak" meaning they were measured with less accuracy due to an unclear distinction between the reddish hypersensitivity reaction and the normal skin. However, these measurements were not excluded from the analysis, as no clear decision rules exist when to exclude such observations. **Table 1** shows the average skin responses of all tuberculins as well as the corresponding minima, maxima and standard deviations. **Figure 1** shows the average responses of RS and BIS over the 6 trials.

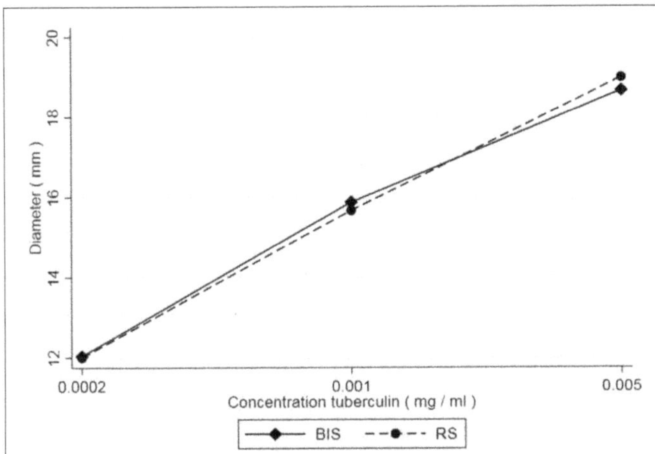

FIGURE 1 | Average skin responses (diameter) of guinea pigs ($n = 54$) after injection with 3 concentrations (equidistant on a log scale) of Bovine International Standard (BIS) and a Reference Standard (RS).

Parallel Line Assay

The initial model of the single trial analysis included the terms Batch, Logconc, Logconc^2, Site, and the interaction between Batch and Logconc. The effect of Site was not significant ($p > 0.05$) for any trial and was eliminated from the model. Logconc^2 was significant for the batch pair (A, BIS) in trial T2 and the interaction term Batch*Logconc was significant for (RS, BIS) and (A, RS) in T2 and for (RS, BIS) in T3. Therefore, these trials were deemed invalid and excluded from further analysis. The final models for T1 and T4-T6 included only Batch and Logconc as independent variables (**Table 2**).

Potencies

Table 2 displays the relative and absolute potencies and corresponding Fieller's 95% CI of RS compared to BIS, based on data of individual trials and of the four valid trials (T1, T4-T6) pooled. Potencies were not significantly different between RS and BIS because 1.0 is included in all confidence intervals of the relative potency of RS against BIS. The estimated potency of RS based on analysis of the pooled valid trials was 1.115*32,500 = 36,238 IU/mg (95% CI: 28,308–46,540).

Table 2 also shows the potency estimates of tuberculin batches A, B, C, and D against RS and BIS. These potency estimations were included to check whether the potency estimations of

TABLE 2 | Estimated relative and absolute potencies (IU/mg) of pairs of tuberculin batches with 95% CI's in six guinea pig trials.

Trial	Batch pair	N	Rel. pot. (95% CI)	Potency (95% CI)
T1	RS, BIS	48	1.230 (0.757–2.025)	39,975 (24,603–65,813)*
	A, BIS	48	1.233 (0.828–1.853)	40,073 (26,910–62,223)*
	A, RS	48	1.095 (0.739–1.627)	37,997 (25,643–56,457)**
T2	RS, BIS	48	Non-parallel	–
	A, BIS	48	Significant curvature	–
	A, RS	48	Non-parallel	–
T3	RS, BIS	45	Non-parallel	–
	A, BIS	45	0.782 (0.444–1.338)	25,415 (14,430–43,485)*
	A, RS	46	1.081 (0.760–1.542)	35,133 (24,700–50,115)**
T4	RS, BIS	41	1.132 (0.678–1.893)	39,280 (23,527–65,687)*
	C, BIS	43	1.103 (0.710–1.689)	35,848 (23,075–54,893)*
	C, RS	44	0.957 (0.639–1.417)	33,208 (22,173–49,170)**
T5	RS, BIS	39	0.954 (0.585–1.565)	31,005 (19,013–50,863)*
	D, BIS	42	1.181 (0.794–1.756)	38,383 (25,805–57,070)*
	D, RS	41	1.189 (0.766–1.827)	41,258 (26,580–63,397)**
T6	RS, BIS	41	1.131 (0.745–1.761)	36,785 (24,213–57,233)*
	B, BIS	42	0.975 (0.656–1.465)	31,688 (21,320–47,613)*
	B, RS	39	0.852 (0.559–1.285)	29,564 (19,397–44,590)**
T1, T4, T5, T6	RS, BIS	169	1.115 (0.871–1.432)	36,238 (28,308–46,540)*

*Relative potencies multiplied by 32,500 (potency assigned to BIS).

**Relative potencies multiplied by 34,700 (potency assigned to RS when calibrated against bis in cattle).*

these additional tuberculin batches against RS were more or less similar to the potency estimations against BIS, which will be the case if the potency estimate of RS as found in cattle is valid. Potencies estimated using RS differ between +2,900 (trial 5, batch B) to −2,700 (trial 4, batch D) compared to BIS. The overall effect of trial was not significant ($p = 0.16$) and also no significant differences were present between individual trials (all p-values > 0.16).

DISCUSSION

Dobbelaer et al. (18) stated that potency estimations in guinea pigs can differ significantly from the potencies in the natural host. Therefore, a cattle trial was designed, performed and analyzed to assign a potency to a reference standard (RS) PPDb. The suitability of the new RS as a *M. bovis* reference standard to assign potency to individual production batches of PPDb was assessed in the guinea pig potency test, the prescribed release test for PPD[1]. Data from tuberculin skin tests in naturally bTB infected cattle and *M. bovis* infected guinea pigs were used to determine the potency of RS compared to the potency of BIS.

To obtain an unbiased potency estimation of the RS, any interference with the potency estimation by the inclusion of other tuberculin batches or tuberculin concentrations, which are not used in practice, should be avoided. Therefore, the cattle trial solely included RS and BIS, in only one dose of 0.1 ml of 1 mg/ml (which is the standard dose of injection in the field) (18).

In the cattle trial, the potency of RS was slightly higher than the potency of BIS. When rounded to the nearest hundred, the potency estimate of RS was 34,700 IU/mg, indicating a difference of 6.8% compared to the potency of BIS.

In guinea pig trials, commonly two test tuberculins are assayed against a standard tuberculin and the common slope of these three tuberculins is then used to estimate the relative potencies of the test tuberculins against the standard tuberculin. However, the most unbiased estimation of the potency of a tuberculin should be solely based on observations of one tuberculin against the standard and by that preventing any influence of the third batch. Therefore, we applied pairwise estimations of potencies, i.e., RS against BIS and of production batches against either RS or BIS. The potency of RS was estimated at 36,238 IU/mg, indicating a difference of 10.3% compared to the potency of BIS. The relative potency estimate of batch A against BIS in trial T3 (TUB 13/009B_Ba) is remarkably lower compared to T1 (0.782 vs. 1.233, p-value of trial 0.06) while the relative potency of batch A against RS was very similar (1.081 vs. 1.095) (**Table 2**). This could be due to an aberrant quality of BIS in the particular ampoule used in trial T3. It is well known that the quality of BIS is decreasing after 30 years of storage. The relative potencies of the four production batches were somewhat lower against RS than against BIS in 3 out of the 4 valid trials.

The cattle model as described in this paper is shown to be an excellent model for precise estimation of the potency of a new RS. Therefore, it is highly recommended to determine the potencies of a new bovine RS in the natural host, i.e., in naturally bTB infected cattle.

However, according to the European Pharmacopeia the guinea pig potency test is the prescribed release test for production batches of bovine tuberculin PPD. Therefore, it was needed to show the suitability of the new RS needed in the guinea pig model as well. Our results are in accordance with the hypothesis of Dobbelaer et al. (18) that homologous tuberculins result in equal potencies in guinea pigs and in cattle. Indeed, the BIS, the RS and the four production batches used in this study are homologous tuberculins.

AUTHOR CONTRIBUTIONS

MdJ, KF, LJ, and TvD: conceptualization. KF, LJ, TvD, MG, and AD: data curation. KF and MdJ: formal analysis. MG, LJ, and MdJ: supervision. KF: Writing—original draft preparation..

REFERENCES

1. Maes M, Giménez JF, D'Alessandro A, Waard JH de. The stability of human, bovine and avian tuberculin purified protein derivative (PPD). *J Infect Dev Ctries* (2011) 5:781–5. doi: 10.3855/jidc.1689
2. Waters WR, Palmer MV, Buddle BM, Vordermeier HM. Bovine tuberculosis vaccine research: historical perspectives and recent advances. *Vaccine* (2012) 30:2611–22. doi: 10.1016/j.vaccine.2012.02.018
3. Neill SD, Bryson DG, Pollock JM. Pathogenesis of tuberculosis in cattle. *Tuberculosis* (2001) 81:79–86. doi: 10.1054/tube.2000.0279
4. de la Rua-Domenech R, Goodchild AT, Vordermeier HM, Hewinson RG, Christiansen KH, Clifton-Hadley RS. Ante mortem diagnosis of tuberculosis in cattle: a review of the tuberculin tests, gamma-interferon assay and other ancillary diagnostic techniques. *Res Vet Sci.* (2006) 81:190–210. doi: 10.1016/j.rvsc.2005.11.005
5. Caffrey JP. Status of bovine tuberculosis eradication programmes in Europe. *Vet Microbiol.* (1994) 40:1–4.
6. Clifton-Hadley R, Wilesmith J. An epidemiological outlook on bovine tuberculosis in the developed world. In: *Proceedings of the Second International Conference on Mycobacterium bovis.* Dunedin: University of Otago, (1995). p. 178–82.
7. Cousins DV. *Mycobacterium bovis* infection and control in domestic livestock. *Rev Sci Tech.* (2001) 20:71–85. doi: 10.20506/rst.20.1.1263
8. Hardstaff JL, Marion G, Hutchings MR, White PCL. Evaluating the tuberculosis hazard posed to cattle from wildlife across Europe. *Res Vet Sci.* (2014) 97:S86–93. doi: 10.1016/j.rvsc.2013.12.002.
9. OIE. *Manual of Diagnostic Tests and Vaccines for Terrestrial Animals 2017. OIE Biological Standards Commission. Chapter 2.4.6 Bovine Tuberculosis. (version adopted in May 2009).* (2017). Available online at: http://www.oie.int/fileadmin/Home/eng/Health_standards/tahm/2.04.06_BOVINE_TB.pdf (Last Accessed 25 May, 2018).
10. European Commission. *Council Directive of 26 June 1964 on Animal Health Problems Affecting Intra-Community Trade in Bovine Animals and Swine (64/432/EEC, With Later Amendments).* Office for Official Publications of the

European Communities, Consolidated legislation (CONSLEG): 1964L0432-18.12.2009. (2004). Available online at: http://eur-lex.europa.eu/LexUriServ/LexUriServ.do?uri=CONSLEG:1964L0432:20091218:EN:PDF (Accessed May 25, 2018).

11. World Health Organization Technical Report Series 760. *WHO Expert Committee on Biological Standardization.* (1987). Available online at: http://apps.who.int/iris/bitstream/handle/10665/39159/WHO_TRS_760_(part1).pdf;jsessionid=BEED81733CEF6F44EF158AC2B8DFBB42 (Accessed May 25, 2018).
12. O'Reilly LM, Haagsma J. Calibration of the Irish reference preparation for bovine PPD. In: *Proceedings of the Second International Conference on Animal Tuberculosis in Africa and the Middle-East.* Actes Editions, Rabat, (1997).
13. Bakker D. *Practicalities of the Immune-Based Diagnostic Assays for the Control of Bovine Tuberculosis. VI International M. bovis Conference.* Cardiff. (2014). Available online at: https://www.bcva.eu/system/files/resources/WEDNESDAY.pdf (Accessed May 25, 2018).
14. SAS Institute Inc. *Procedures Guide: Statistical Procedures.* Cary, NC: SAS Institute Inc. (2012).
15. Ai M, Li K, Liu S, Lin DKJ. Balanced incomplete Latin square designs. *J Stat Plan Infer.* (2013) 143:1575–82.
16. Finney DJ. *Statistical Method in Biological Assay, 3rd edn.* London: Griffin & Co (1978). p. 148–78.
17. Bebu I, Seillier-Moiseiwitsch F, Mathew T. Generalized confidence intervals for ratios of regression coefficients with applications to bioassays. *Biom. J.* (2009) 51:1047–58. doi: 10.1002/bimj.200900038
18. Dobbelaer R, O'Reilly LM, Génicot M, Haagsma J. The potency of bovine PPD tuberculin in guinea-pigs and in tuberculous cattle. *J Biol Stand.* (1983) 11:213–20.

11

A Retrospective Study on Bovine Tuberculosis in Cattle on Fiji: Study Findings and Stakeholder Responses

Elva Borja[1,2], *Leo F. Borja*[3], *Ronil Prasad*[3], *Tomasi Tunabuna*[3] *and Jenny-Ann L. M. L. Toribio*[1*]

[1] *The University of Sydney, Farm Animal Health, Sydney School of Veterinary Science, Sydney, NSW, Australia,* [2] *Vet Essentials, Suva, Fiji,* [3] *Ministry of Agriculture, Koronivia Research Station, Koronivia, Fiji*

***Correspondence:**
Jenny-Ann L. M. L. Toribio
jenny-ann.toribio@sydney.edu.au

Bovine tuberculosis (bTB) is globally significant due to its impacts on cattle production. A Brucellosis and Tuberculosis Eradication and Control (BTEC) program commenced in Fiji during the 1980's and has since been sustained by government funding and industry cooperation. A retrospective study of bTB data obtained during the Fiji BTEC program from 1999 to 2014 was undertaken at the University of Sydney with support from the Government of Fiji. It confirmed that bTB is well-established in dairy cattle farms in Naitasiri and Tailevu provinces of Central Division on the main island of Viti Levu, and suggested that the disease is present among cattle on farms in all or most provinces across three (Central, Northern, Western) of the four divisions in the country. It was evident that despite sustained efforts, disease reduction and containment was not being achieved. Reasons contributing to this situation included the appropriateness of the protocol for conduct of the single intradermal test (SID) in cattle, absence of regular quality assurance training of BTEC field staff, lack of standard procedures for bTB data collation and evaluation, unregulated cattle movements and the presence of stray cattle. The Fiji Ministry of Agriculture responded proactively to these findings by implementing revision to the use of the SID in cattle and refresher training for staff along with the Biosecurity Authority of Fiji who implemented cattle movement restriction. A subsequent apparent outbreak of bTB in some farms due to increased detection by the new test protocol raised concerns for the local dairy industry. To clarify the status and extent of bTB infection and the challenges faced by the industry, a stakeholder forum was held in May 2017, and a new BTEC strategy was formulated and endorsed by stakeholders. bTB remains a focus for cattle disease control by the government of Fiji. This case study highlights the challenges for bTB control in Fiji and underlines the importance of technical and social considerations to achieve success in disease control.

Keywords: bovine tuberculosis, disease control, surveillance, BTEC, Fiji

INTRODUCTION

Bovine tuberculosis (bTB) is a chronic bacterial disease of cattle caused mainly by *Mycobacterium bovis*, although other zoonotic members of the *M. tuberculosis* complex may be the cause, such as *M. caprae*, the common cause of bTB in central Europe (1). bTB results in serious economic losses for the livestock industry worldwide due to animal disposal, carcass confiscation, premature culling, low production and poor reproductive performance (2). Further infection in people results in disease that is predominantly extra-pulmonary but cannot be clinically distinguished from *M. tuberculosis* infection. Official estimates of human zoonotic TB cases due to *M. bovis* in 2016 stand at 147,000 new cases and over 12,500 deaths, mainly in Africa and South-East Asia (3).

In Fiji, bTB leads to decreased production and opportunity for local trade due to sick animals and early culling of potentially productive stock. The bTB situation in Fiji is becoming an increasing concern for industry stakeholders as the culling of stock further aggravates the low milk production in the country. Data in 2014 from cattle sent to slaughter after a positive skin test on farm showed that one in three reactors (animals with positive single intradermal test) had generalized TB, and 85% had some form of gross TB lesion at post-mortem examination. Successful eradication of bTB is recognized by the Government of Fiji to be of benefit to individual cattle owners and to the country in relation to trade and potentially to human health. Hardest hit is the dairy sector which has suffered the greatest loss of cattle numbers (4).

This paper provides a case study of bTB control in an endemically infected cattle population in the Pacific. It outlines the bTB control program in Fiji, presents the methods and results of a retrospective study of bTB from 1999 to 2014 in Fiji, discusses the actions of the Ministry of Agriculture and other government agencies in response to study findings, and considers the implications of this response for industry, and longer-term, for the eradication program. As bTB remains a high priority for cattle disease control by the Government of Fiji, this case study highlights the challenges for bTB control in Fiji and underlines the importance of technical and social considerations to achieve success in disease control.

bTB CONTROL IN Fiji

It is likely that bTB was introduced in Fiji through cattle brought in by European settlers during the 1830's (5). During the 1970's the deleterious effect of brucellosis and tuberculosis in local cattle farms was recognized and the need to establish a national control program voiced (6). Subsequently the Ministry of Agriculture (MOA) commenced the Fiji Bovine Brucellosis and Tuberculosis eradication and control (BTEC) program in the early 1980's with support from the Australian Government (6, 7) implementing dairy farm registration, cattle movement monitoring, and mandatory bTB testing and ear tagging of tested cattle, and carcass inspection at abattoir with compensation paid for condemnations at slaughter. These activities were based on property identification, animal tagging and surveillance programs of Australia (8) and the United Kingdom (9). However, the requirement for annual cattle farm registration is limited to dairy farms as the basis for legal sale of milk and milk products, with only some beef herds being voluntarily registered. Field testing was conducted annually although inconsistently between farms. Historical documentation on the BTEC program and bTB occurrence in Fiji is sparse with no information available prior to 1999. For example, the Animal Health Survey published in 1999 by the Secretariat of the Pacific Community (10) did not include a report for Fiji. Information about Fiji bTB from 1999 is limited to government reports and record books, and data reported to the World Organization for Animal Health (OIE) since Fiji became a member in 2007.

Cattle farms of all types (dairy and beef farms of individual farmers, school farms, village/settlement, government stations, middlemen) are included in the program and participation is mandatory although some farmers do not comply. There are no specific consequences for non-compliance other than ongoing transmission among cattle in non-compliant infected farms. All cattle aged 6 months and above are tested and have a metal tag with a unique number placed in the right ear to indicate the animal has been tested. The single intradermal test (SID) using purified protein derivative antigen from *M. bovis* (PPD-B) is administered at the caudal fold of the tail (CFT) with the result read 3 days after administration. Up to September 2014 a positive result was determined by the presence of a wheal not <4 mm in diameter. All log books and handwritten data collected from the field were filed by the Fiji Ministry of Agriculture in a government stock room. There was no written protocol for standard data management and analysis, and no systematic analysis of data to evaluate progress of bTB control over time. Quarterly and annual reports were prepared based on manual counts of records. Designated responsibility for the conduct of the bTB program was at the level of the division offices from 1999 to 2010 in an effort to increase surveillance coverage. This was centralized to the national office from 2011 to improve monitoring of the quality of testing.

Abattoir monitoring consists of carcass inspection for tubercle lesions by government meat inspectors at the two main abattoirs of the Fiji Meat Industry Board (FMIB) located in Nasinu, Central Division and Vuda, Western Division, respectively (11). Affected organs or whole carcasses are condemned based on the severity and location of tubercle lesions. Compensation to farmers is paid at slaughter of affected animal at a rate of FJD$1.60 per kg for the condemned part of the carcass and applies to animals detected through on-farm testing (reactors sent to slaughter) and to animals detected via carcass inspection at slaughter. Thus, this compensation is available to both farmers that comply with on-farm testing and those that do not. During 2015 the compensation rate was improved to equal the market price at the time of culling (12).

Farms with positive animals determined by on-farm testing or abattoir monitoring are classified as "Infected." BTEC requires an infected farm to be free from bTB for 3 consecutive SID tests held at a minimum of 3-months intervals to obtain "Restricted," "Provisionally clear," and "Clear" statuses, respectively. It requires a minimum of 9 months from the time of detection for a farm to complete three consecutive clear tests and obtain "Clear" (bTB-free) status.

The Fiji BTEC program, a long-term activity sustained by annual government funding and industry cooperation, demonstrates collective commitment to address bTB in the cattle population. To underpin a review of the BTEC program, a retrospective study of bTB surveillance data from 1999 to 2014 was conducted over 12 months during 2014–2015. The aim of the retrospective study was to document the progress of the BTEC program and to provide recommendations to strengthen it. The final results of the study were formally presented to Ministry of Agriculture in September 2016 and to the industry stakeholders during the BTEC Forum held in March 2017.

RETROSPECTIVE STUDY

Materials and Methods

Data Sources

This study was conducted using data collected by the BTEC program from 1999 to 2014. The Fiji Ministry of Agriculture granted approval for use of the Fiji BTEC data to conduct this study in March 2014. Hard copies of batch books, reactor books, field sheets, annual reports, memorandum and other documents related to bTB in Fiji were used to collate and cross-check data from 1999 to 2014. The dataset compiled by year included farm identification number, location, farm type, date of testing, total number of cattle tested, total number of cattle test positive and farm TB status. For 2011 to 2014, the dataset for each year listed tests conducted by individual animal tag number. The few bTB test results from species other than cattle (horse, pig) were excluded, as were farm record data on the number of cattle younger than 6 months. It was assumed that all TB test results were read 3 days after the date of tuberculin administration.

Records of carcass inspection at slaughter from 2011 to 2014 were obtained for FMIB abattoirs at Nasinu and Vuda. Individual cattle records for slaughtered bTB positive animals were identified, including reactors identified during on-farm testing and subsequently sent for slaughter, and other animals identified at slaughter via detection of lesions during carcass inspection. The dataset compiled included farm identification number, animal identification number, date of slaughter and type of lesion detected. Complete records were only available for the Nasinu abattoir.

Due to the absence of a formal national registration system for all cattle farms, no absolute total cattle number were available for use as a denominator to calculate the population coverage of testing or infection prevalence in this study. In place of this, cattle population estimates for 2011 to 2014 published in the World Animal Health Information Database (WAHIS Interface) (13) were used. However, no reliable cattle population numbers at the national and division level were available prior to 2011.

Data Transcription and Sorting

For each year from 1999 to 2014, data were transcribed from hard copy sources into a purpose-built spreadsheet in Microsoft Excel version 2003. *Farm ID spreadsheet* included farm registration number, farm name, farm location (division, province, district, village/settlement), farm type (dairy, beef, other), date of test, number of cattle on farm by age group, number of animals tested, number of animals tested positive, number of animals tested negative and TB status of farm. *Animal ID spreadsheet* included farm registration number, farm name, farm location (division, province, district, village/settlement), date of test, TB tag number, age-gender description (heifer, dry cow, lactating cow, bull, steer), and TB test result.

Data transcription was performed by BTEC personnel from May 2014 to May 2015. Data sorting and validation conducted by the first author produced a comprehensive inventory of cattle farms and farmers from 1999 to 2014. This was verified for dairy farms by matching farm registration number and farm name to the MOA dairy farm registration list, and for beef farms based on familiarity of BTEC staff with farmers and farm operations as there is no formal registration system for beef farms. The list identified 2,141 cattle holding facilities (dairy and beef farms of individual farmers, school farms, village/settlement, government stations, middlemen) including subsistence or irregular cattle farm operations. When needed, missing values for farm location were entered based on recall. This list was sent to MOA Economic Planning and Statistics Division (EP&S) to validate location details recorded for each farm. To ensure that all testing data were for bTB SID tests, a cross-check against records for bovine brucellosis testing was performed.

Data Analysis

Farm ID data from 1999 to 2014 and *Animal ID* data from 2011 to 2014 were available for analysis. Descriptive statistics for the number of positive farms and animals were calculated, and the number of positive animals detected through on-farm surveillance and abattoir monitoring were tabulated separately by division and by province per year.

Farm ID data were also analyzed to determine the number of tests conducted on infected farms each year and the status of each infected farm by year end. Within a calendar year, farms that had undergone one test with at least one reactor (SID test positive animal) were designated as "Infected." Farms that had undergone one test round with at least one positive result and undergone one follow up test within the same calendar year with no positive result were designated as "Restricted." Farms that had undergone two and three consecutive test rounds without any positive results were designated as "Provisionally clear" and "Cleared" farms, respectively.

For 2011 to 2014, the status of Infected farms from one calendar year to the next was investigated to identify farms that had positive cattle detected over consecutive years and did not attain cleared status within a period of two or more consecutive calendar years.

Results

From 1999 to 2014 ~2,141 cattle holding facilities were included in the BTEC program across the 4 divisions of Fiji (**Figure 1**). On average, 25,693 cattle (median: 27,562, range: 7,552–43,516) from 258 farms (median: 272, range: 96–438) were tested per year during these 16 years. The majority of animals tested were located in the Central Division with an average of 21,339 cattle (median: 25,102, range: 4,701–34,955) tested in this division every year from 1999. Less testing was undertaken elsewhere, with number of years testing conducted and total cattle numbers tested per division being for Western Division (16 years; median: 3,155, range: 139–9,064), Eastern Division (9 years; median: 28,

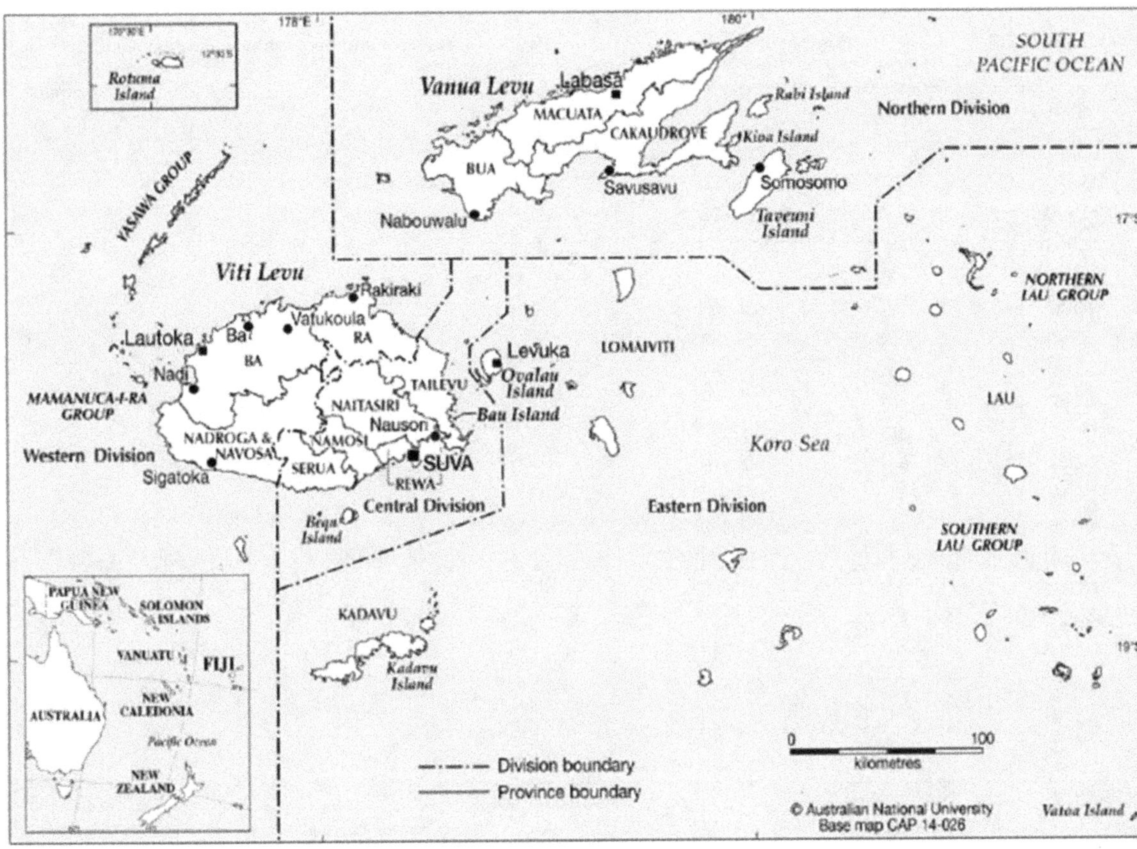

FIGURE 1 | Map of Fiji showing Division boundaries. Source: Maps Online, CartoGIS Services, ANU College of Asia and the Pacific, The Australian National University.

range: 0–397) and Northern Division (6 years; median: 0 range: 0–2,265).

Coverage of Fiji's BTEC Program

Cattle population numbers reported to the FAO and OIE required to estimate population coverage by the BTEC program were deemed unreliable prior to 2011 because the process used to estimate the reported numbers was not documented. For 2011 to 2014, the cattle population reported to the OIE based on data collated by a government veterinarian ranged between 40,008 and 44,388 cattle and the percentage of cattle tested ranged between 33.6 and 74.0%, with variation between years arising mainly from changes in the number of cattle tested. The total tested was markedly lower in 2004, 2006, 2007, 2010, 2011, and 2013, and for 2010 this aligned with a lower budget allocation compared to the previous year (**Table 1**).

bTB Positive Animals and Farms

A total of 2,823 TB positive cattle were identified from 1999 to 2014 with an average number of 176 (median 181.5) reactors per year (**Table 1**). The lowest number of positive cattle in a year was 17 from 7 positive farms in 2010, and the highest 721 reactors from 32 positive farms in 2014.

bTB positive cattle were identified in all four divisions of Fiji although the level of testing and the proportion of positive cattle varied between divisions (**Figure 2**).

For the Northern Division, testing was conducted in 1 of 4 provinces (Cakaudrove) in 6 years with positive cattle (termed reactors) detected in 1999 and 2004 (**Figure 2**). In 1999, 3 out of 9 (33%) farms tested in Cakaudrove province were positive (18 reactors). Testing was conducted only once on each positive farm and no further testing was scheduled in the Northern Division during the same year nor the following year to monitor the infected farms. In 2004, 1 out of 11 (9%) farms tested in the Northern Division was positive (4 reactors). This farm had been identified as infected in 1999 (15 of 18 reactors). No follow-up test was conducted to monitor this infected farm in 2004 or in 2005. No records were available to confirm if any of the reactors from the Northern Division were immediately culled.

In Eastern Division testing was conducted in 3 of 5 provinces (Kadavu, Lakeba Lau, Lomaiviti) in 9 years with three positive cattle from the two farms tested in Lomaiviti in 2005, and none in the other years (**Figure 2**). No further testing was conducted to monitor these two farms in 2005 or in 2006. No records were available to confirm if reactors were immediately culled from these farms.

In Western Division testing was conducted each year, and though usually undertaken in at least 2 of the 4 provinces

TABLE 1 | Budget for the Fiji BTEC program[a] and the number of farms and cattle tested for bovine tuberculosis by the program from 1999 to 2014.

Year	BTEC budget (USD)	Number of		Number and percentage with positive result			
		Farms tested	Animals tested	Farms		Animals	
				No.	%	No.	%
1999	36,450	373	38,870	56	15	220	1
2000	36,450	245	29,303	37	15	230	1
2001	72,900	299	26,277	50	17	293	1
2002	72,900	228	30,880	31	14	183	1
2003	72,900	170	27,506	26	15	121	0
2004	72,900	105	19,323	22	21	180	1
2005	72,900	438	41,591	34	8	192	0
2006	72,900	96	7,552	27	28	186	2
2007	114,079	98	9,569	23	23	61	1
2008	85,335	377	43,516	43	11	212	0
2009	718,065	417	32,160	11	3	39	0
2010	96,228	113	14,967	7	6	17	0
2011	437,400	136	14,916	14	10	60	0
2012	370,641	303	27,618	15	5	47	0
2013	364,500	324	17,439	11	3	61	0
2014	729,000	401	29,597	32	8	721	2
TOTAL	3,425,548	4,123	411,084	439		2,823	

[a] *Budget listed is the annual total for bovine brucellosis and bovine tuberculosis activities in the BTEC program.*

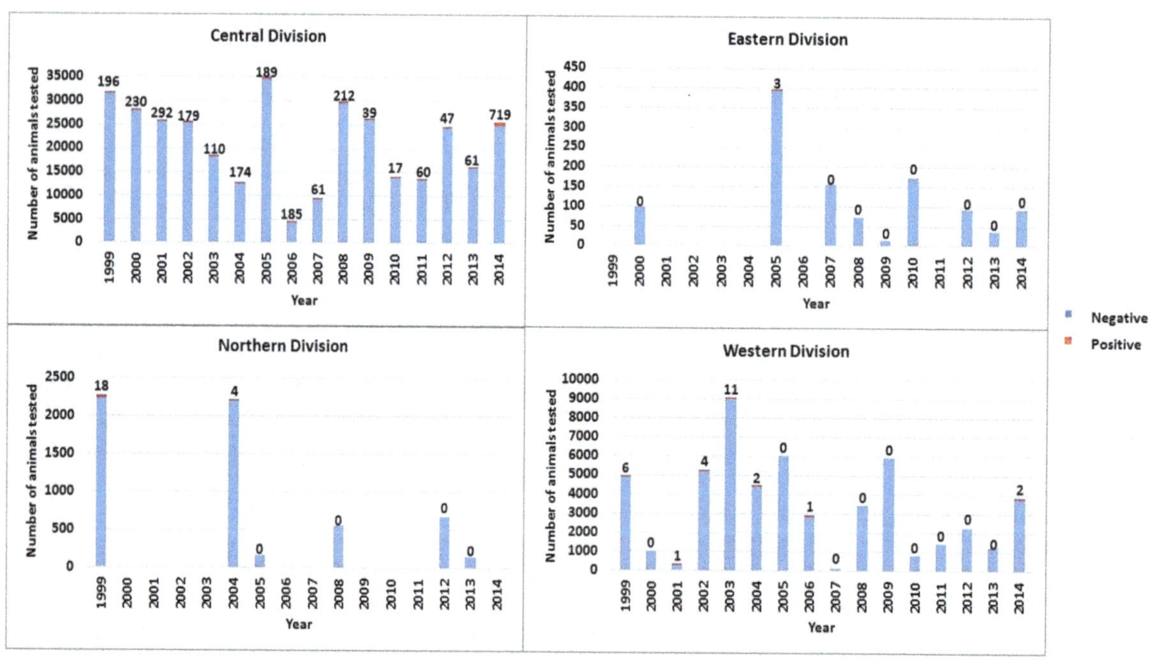

FIGURE 2 | Total number of cattle tested and number of bTB test positive cattle by division per year from 1999 to 2014 in Fiji.

annually for 16 years, most testing was conducted in Ba and Navosa/Nadroga provinces. Positive animals were detected in 7 of 16 years with the number and percentage of positive cattle ranging from 1 to 11 positive cattle or 0.04–2.27% (**Figure 2**). One farm was identified as positive in 2002 (all 4 out of total 4 reactors detected in this division in 2002 were located on this farm), 2003 (10 of total 11 reactors located on this farm), 2004 (2 of total 2 reactors located on this farm) and 2014 (2 of total 2 reactors located on this farm). No records were available from the abattoir at Vuda, in Western Division for this study to confirm if reactors were culled.

For Central Division, testing was conducted each year in the 5 provinces (Naitasiri, Namosi, Serua, Tailevu, Rewa) with positive cattle detected consistently (**Figure 2**), particularly in Tailevu province that had test positive cattle each of the 16 years with the highest number of positives recorded in 2014 (**Figure 3**). Seven hundred reactors were detected in Tailevu from 23 of the 147 farms tested (15.7%) in the province during 2014.

For the 16 years that testing was conducted in Naitaisiri province, reactors were detected each year except in 2010 and 2011 when lower numbers of cattle were tested (862 in 2010, 1,833 in 2011). For the other years, higher numbers were tested with 7,046 animals (3 reactors) tested in 2009, 5,044 animals (4 reactors) tested in 2012, 4,466 animals (2 reactors) in 2013, and 7,831 animals (6 reactors) tested in 2014.

Serua province had the second highest number of reactors (12 of 721 reactors) in 2014, compared to earlier years when Naitasiri commonly ranked next to Tailevu. Data showed that in 2014, reactors in Serua came from only 1 of 6 farms (17%) tested in the province.

Farm Types

An average of 168 dairy cattle (average: 168, median: 172.5, range: 16–717) were detected positive each year during the last 16 years compared to beef cattle (average: 3, median: 3, range: 0–18). Ninety-nine percent (2,685 of 2,690) of positive dairy animals detected from 1999 to 2014 were from Central Division.

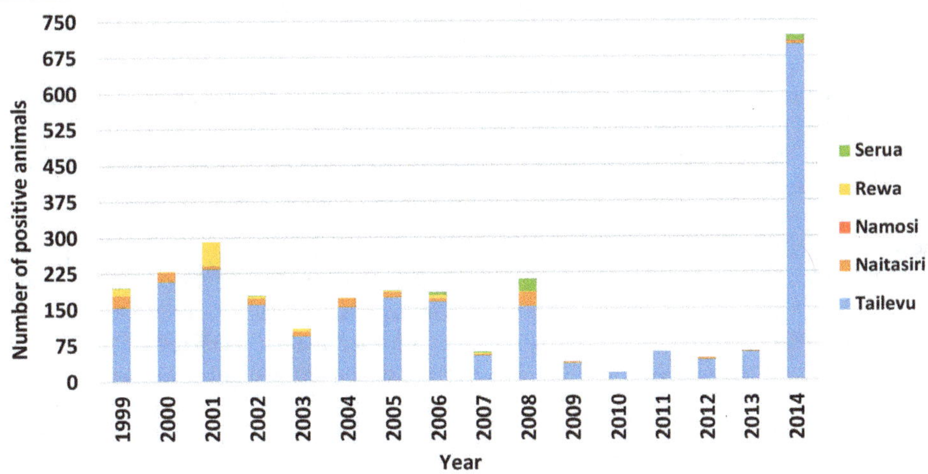

FIGURE 3 | Number of bTB test positive cattle per year in the five provinces of Central Division in Fiji from 1999 to 2014.

TABLE 2 | Number of cattle tested and of bTB test positive cattle by farm type from 1999 to 2014 in Central Division and Western Division Fiji.

Year	Central Division							Western Division						
	% Of positive animals			Number of animals tested				% Of positive animals			Number of animals tested			
	Beef	Dairy	Other[a]	Beef	Dairy	Other[a]	Total	Beef	Dairy	Other[a]	Beef	Dairy	Other[a]	Total
1999	0.2	0.7	0.3	919	23,598	7,195	31,712	0	0.5	0.1	982	396	3,515	4,893
2000	0	0.9	0.5	1,218	23,414	3,525	28,157	0	0	0	0	184	864	1048
2001	0.5	1.3	0.4	366	21,459	4,154	25,979	1.2	0	0	82	216	0	298
2002	0	0.8	0.3	662	23,064	1,935	25,661	0.1	0	0	4,900	0	319	5,219
2003	0	0.7	0.1	347	16,386	1,709	18,442	0.1	0.5	0	8,699	186	179	9,064
2004	0	1.4	0.9	387	12,110	214	12,711	0.2	0	0	1,029	17	3,363	4,409
2005	0.1	0.6	0	1,583	29,990	3,382	34,955	0	0	0	3517	132	2427	6076
2006	1.5	4.2	0	197	4,341	163	4,701	0	0.5	0	2,609	183	59	2,851
2007	0	0.7	0.4	304	7,662	1,308	9,274	0	0	0	0	0	73	73
2008	0.2	0.8	0	1,261	27,038	1,561	29,860	0	0	0	1,006	323	2,130	3,459
2009	0	0.2	0	904	24,559	716	26,179	0	0	0	1,695	4,134	97	5,926
2010	0	0.1	0.2	106	13,356	531	13,993	0	0	0	483	41	275	799
2011	0	0.5	0	453	12,776	263	13,492	0	0	0	1,102	0	322	1,424
2012	0.1	0.2	0.8	1,171	22,987	384	24,542	0	0	0	941	1,030	334	2,305
2013	0.5	0.4	0	560	15,173	286	16,019	0	0	0	122	1,037	68	1,227
2014	0.1	3.1	0.1	1,509	22,856	1,356	25,721	0.1	0	0	2,301	72	1,410	3,783

[a] *Farms with beef and/or dairy cattle that included school farms, villages/settlements, government stations and middlemen.*

For 1999 to 2014 in Central Division, a small proportion of dairy cattle tested positive every year (range 0.1–4.2%), from 0.1 to 1.5% of beef cattle tested positive in 8 of 16 years, and <1% of cattle from other farm types tested positive in 10 of 16 years (**Table 2**). In Western Division, lower proportions of positive cattle were detected in 4 of 14 years that beef cattle were tested, in 3 of the 13 years that dairy cattle were tested, and in 2 of the 15 years that cattle from other farms were tested (**Table 2**).

Among the dairy cattle that tested positive from 2011 to 2014 in Central Division, a high proportion were productive female cattle, for example, in 2011 when all test positive animals were dairy cattle, 61.7% were dairy cows and a further 16.7% were heifers selected to be milkers (**Table 3**).

Classification of bTB Infected Farms

Data show that from 1999 to 2014, no farms were cleared of bTB infection within a calendar year (**Table 4**).

Nine farms with positive cattle detected from 2011 to 2014 through on-farm testing and abattoir monitoring were all dairy farms situated in the localities of Waimaro and Namalata in Tailevu province (**Table 5**). Farms A and B had reactors consistently from 1999 to 2014. Except for Farms C and G, all other farms listed had their highest count of reactors in 2014. These farms are all located along an estimated 9.6 km stretch of the single major road in Tailevu.

Case Detection at Carcass Inspection

Each year from 2011 to 2014, cattle from Central, Western and Northern Divisions slaughtered at the FMIB Nasinu abattoir were found to have tubercle lesions during meat inspection (**Table 6**). The highest number of positive animals were from Tailevu province in Central Division with an average of 67 animals (268 total positives) detected in the abattoir per year. Although there was no reactor detected in Naitasiri during field testing in 2011 (**Figure 3**), three positive animals were detected at this abattoir. Further positive animals from the Northern Division were detected consistently from 2011 to 2014 with no on-farm detections despite testing conducted in 2012 and 2013 (**Figure 2**). Trace back of positive cattle from the Northern Division using the individual TB tag numbers showed that the 10 positive cattle had either read negative during on-farm testing or had never been tested on farm. This may imply that there are positive animals that are non-reactive to SID PPD-B affecting BTEC's proficiency in detection of infected animals in the field.

TABLE 3 | Number of bTB test positive cattle by age-gender group from 2011 to 2014 in Central Division Fiji.

Year	Heifer[a]	Dry cow[b]	Lactating cow[c]	Bull[d]	Steer[e]	No data	Total
2011	10	26	11	9	4	0	60
2012	14	8	17	4	4	0	47
2013	16	12	27	5	1	0	61
2014	134	212	260	76	33	4	719
Total	175	259	315	94	42	4	889

[a]*Heifer, female at least 6 months of age and not yet mated.*
[b]*Dry cow, adult female more than 12 months of age not being milked at time of test.*
[c]*Lactating cow, adult female more than 12 months of age being milked at time of test.*
[d]*Bull, adult uncastrated male.*
[e]*Steer, castrated male at least 6 months of age.*

Situation Analysis and Recommendations

The findings of the retrospective study confirmed that bTB had been endemic in Fiji for more than 16 years. Between 3 and 28% of farms tested per year in the BTEC program included cattle that tested positive to the SID test determined by the presence of a wheal size ≥4 mm until September 2014. This designation for a positive result at the highly specific interpretation of wheal ≥4 mm at the caudal fold was not adequate to identify sufficient positive animals for culling on infected farms to prevent ongoing bTB transmission.

There is clear evidence that bTB is well-established in the dairy cattle farms in Naitasiri and Tailevu provinces of Central Division on the main island of Viti Levu. While the strength of evidence for these provinces arises from a concentration of the BTEC program on-farm testing on the dairy farms in these two provinces, the abattoir monitoring results also support the conclusion of higher infection in these provinces at least for 2011–2014. Identification of SID test positive cattle in Central Division over multiple years also in beef farms (8 of 16 years) and other farm types (10 or 16 years) suggests that bTB infection is established throughout the cattle population.

Further the on-farm testing results and abattoir detections provide evidence that bTB is present among cattle farms in the other three divisions of the country, and in all 4 provinces of Western Division and in 3 of 4 provinces of Northern Division. Given the substantially lower numbers of dairy cattle in these other 3 divisions, this suggests that bTB is established at least among some beef cattle farms in Western Division and Northern Division.

From 1999 to 2014, the consistent positive status of a small number of farms and the fact that no farms were cleared of bTB infection within a calendar year (whilst acknowledging that a minimum of 9 months is required to progress from infected to clear status) is clear evidence that the test and cull plus quarantine procedures as applied for infected farms were inadequate to clear infection from a farm. The example of nine dairy farms located along one road in Tailevu province that were consistently positive for 2011–2014 exemplifies the situation with persisting infection.

The descriptive analysis of the BTEC data from 1999 to 2014 provided disturbing evidence that despite sustained efforts in on-farm testing and carcass inspection at abattoirs, BTB disease reduction and containment was not being achieved. This situation is well-illustrated although limitations of the 1999–2014 BTEC data, such as considerable variation in number of farms and animals tested between years and the positive SID designation based on wheal ≥4 mm, restricted the retrospective study to descriptive analyses.

Factors contributing to this situation and recommendations to strengthen the BTEC program are presented in **Table 7**. Further, given the need to identify bTB-free areas in Fiji that may be sources of replacement stock, surveillance sampling of farms in the provinces of Kadavu and Lakeba Lau in Eastern Division

TABLE 4 | Number of farms tested per division and total number of bTB positive farms from 1999 to 2014 with classification of these farms by the end of the calendar year.

Year	Farms tested	Central	Eastern	Northern	Western	Total Positive	Infected[a]	Restricted[b]	Provisionally clear[c]	Clear[d]
1999	373	49	0	3	4	56	47	9	0	0
2000	245	37	0	0	0	37	24	9	4	0
2001	299	49	0	0	1	50	40	8	2	0
2002	228	30	0	0	1	31	22	8	1	0
2003	170	24	0	0	2	26	24	2	0	0
2004	105	20	0	1	1	22	20	2	0	0
2005	438	32	2	0	0	34	20	9	5	0
2006	96	26	0	0	1	27	26	1	0	0
2007	98	23	0	0	0	23	23	0	0	0
2008	377	43	0	0	0	43	16	23	4	0
2009	417	11	0	0	0	11	8	2	1	0
2010	113	7	0	0	0	7	2	5	0	0
2011	136	14	0	0	0	14	12	2	0	0
2012	303	15	0	0	0	15	11	3	1	0
2013	324	11	0	0	0	11	10	1	0	0
2014	401	31	0	0	1	32	25	4	3	0
Total	4,123	460	2	4	11	439	330	88	21	0

[a] *Infected,farm with bTB positive cattle determined by on-farm testing or abattoir monitoring.*
[b] *Restricted,an infected farm after one negative round of testing.*
[c] *Provisionally free,an infected farm after two negative rounds of testing a minimum of 3 months apart.*
[d] *Clear,an infected farm declared bTB-free after three consecutive negative rounds of testing each a minimum of 3 months apart.*

TABLE 5 | Number of bTB positive cattle per year for the nine dairy farms in Tailevu province that were consistently positive for bovine tuberculosis from 2011 to 2014 detected through on-farm testing and carcass inspection at the abattoir.

Farm	Number of positive animals per year															
	1999	2000	2001	2002	2003	2004	2005	2006	2007	2008	2009	2010	2011	2012	2013	2014
A	10	43	34	31	27	48	18	21	7	19	10	5	21	6	36	76
B	2	53	11	27	8	4	29	16	2	28	5	2	7	14	20	199
C	9	9	10	15	5	10	1	12	1	1	0	0	8	3	23	11
D	0	2	4	4	0	5	4	6	2	3	6	0	6	6	5	43
E	11	9	20	5	2	41	31	20	4	39	0	2	17	23	17	53
F	0	6	11	1	0	0	10	7	2	10	0	1	18	4	16	66
G	6	6	10	6	0	8	3	13	0	0	0	0	7	6	1	4
H	23	18	77	6	26	8	7	22	6	15	9	0	31	11	12	76
I	0	0	0	0	0	1	4	0	0	4	0	0	4	3	1	24

should be conducted to confirm if these areas are bTB-free and permit declaration of a bTB-free zone in the country (14).

RESPONSES TO FINDINGS OF THE RETROSPECTIVE STUDY

The Fiji Ministry of Agriculture responded proactively to the findings of the retrospective study along with the Biosecurity Authority of Fiji (BAF) and the Fiji Cooperative Dairy Company Limited (FCDCL). The earliest responses commenced in late 2014 initiated following a preliminary analysis of the bTB records for 2011–2013. The response actions taken from 2014 to 2018 are described in detail below.

SOP for On-Farm Testing

The MOA updated the 2010 BTEC SOP in September 2014 and consequently implemented re-training of staff and calibration of BTEC field testing equipment. The revised protocol identified reactors as all animals that developed any size of wheal or redness in the SID injection site at the caudal fold 3 days after administration of PPD-B, following the OIE recommendation for detection of reactors in known infected farms (1). On the assumption that all cattle in Fiji are potentially bTB infected, this new protocol was applied to all farms, regardless of whether farms

TABLE 6 | Provinces with bTB positive cattle detected by meat inspectors at the FMIB Nasinu abattoir in Central Division, Fiji from 2011 to 2014.

Division	Province	Number of positive animals detected in the abattoir				
		2011	2012	2013	2014	Total
Central	Naitasiri	3	3	2	5	13
	Rewa	2	0	1	1	4
	Serua	1	0	0	0	1
	Tailevu	80	42	84	62	268
Northern	Bua	2	0	1	2	5
	Macuata	0	1	2	2	5
Western	Ba	1	0	1	0	2
	Navosa/Nadroga	0	6	6	2	14
	Ra	1	1	1	0	3
Grand Total		90	53	98	74	315

were previously identified as disease-free or infected (15, 16). This SOP change was implemented to improve the sensitivity of detection of infected animals in the field. A change that was needed for example due to identification at carcass inspection of some cattle with tubercle lesions that had previously tested negative using SID. A subsequent apparent outbreak of bTB in some farms was due to increased detection by the new test protocol, with a total of 721 reactors from 32 farms in 2014 compared to 61 reactors from 11 farms in 2013 (**Table 1**). This event raised concerns for the local dairy industry. The extent of infection in these farms was confirmed by post-mortem inspection of bTB reactors. For reactors at slaughter at FMIB Nasinu abattoir in Central Division, the percentages with generalized TB, gross TB lesions and no visible lesions were 33, 51, 16% in late 2014 ($n = 301$), and 26, 40, 34% in 2015 ($n = 1101$), respectively (17). The dairy sector experienced the greatest loss of cattle due to culling of reactors, and this had a serious economic impact for individual farmers and for the industry leading to a shortage of dairy cattle in the country, a reduction in the volume of milk produced, and an increase in the volume of imported processed milk (4). Dairy farmers with smaller, semi-commercial farms slowly converted to cash crops to supplement their dwindling income. In response to this serious situation, the MOA improved its compensation scheme in August 2015 to match current market prices per kg of condemned carcass. The purpose was to assist farmers recover quickly after losses from bTB (12).

Regulation of Cattle Movement

On 03 March 2016, as part of the disaster response of the Biosecurity Authority of Fiji post-Cyclone Winston a movement restriction on live animals was implemented to discourage movement of livestock without prior approval from the BAF or the Fiji National Disaster Management Office (18).

Subsequently on 13 January 2017 under section 77 of the Biosecurity Act 2008, the whole of Fiji was declared a biosecurity emergency area for Bovine Tuberculosis (*Mycobacterium bovis*) (19). During November 2017, the BAF and the MOA documented a movement control policy (20) to provide guidance on the implementation of cattle movement control. Movement of all calves and cattle within Fiji is strictly prohibited without prior authorization from BAF. Movement of cattle or calves without authorization is an offense attracting a maximum penalty of FJD 40,000 for individuals and FJD 200,000 for businesses or imprisonment. On 03 February 2018, the declaration was extended for continued implementation for a further 6 months.

National Stakeholder Forum

To clarify the status and extent of bTB infection and the challenges faced by the industry and to promote communication and collaboration in delivery of the BTEC program, a stakeholder forum was held in May 2017 with government MOA, Biosecurity Authority of Fiji (BAF) and Ministry of Health (MOH) representatives, Fiji industry stakeholders and relevant experts from Australia and New Zealand. Presentations highlighted the needs for a clear policy and strategy for bTB eradication and rehabilitation, action to address overlapping and unclear legislative and stakeholder responsibilities (particularly between MOA and BAF), immediate removal of infected cattle from farms, auditing and capacity building programmes, and a data recording system for monitoring, evaluation and learning (4). Stakeholders agreed that the BTEC Program requires further investment from the government to set up a stronger team structure with necessary equipment for disease surveillance and personnel with appropriate legal powers to effectively undertake its field operations. A draft BTEC strategy was developed during the forum and endorsed by stakeholders, and members for the BTEC planning committee designated to finalize the strategy document.

Documentation of Fiji Brucellosis and Tuberculosis Eradication Strategy

The Ministry of Agriculture further refined and finalized this strategy in early 2018. Input to this process included review and recommendations on meat hygiene, bTB control strategies and diagnostic test selection by a technical team under the Government of Chile funded project "Strengthening the institutions responsible for the inspection and certification

TABLE 7 | Factors contributing to this situation and recommendations to strengthen the BTEC program in Fiji.

Factor	Related to	Main recommendations
Insufficient consistency in the number and location of farms tested between years	Changes between years in government budget for the BTEC program eg reduction in 2006–2007 following political crisis in 2005/2006. Changes between years in budget allocation for bTB in the BTEC program eg reduction in 2009–2010 due to response to brucellosis detection after 13-years absence of detections (7). Insufficient number of BTEC field staff to conduct SID testing. No interrogation of BTEC records to inform plans for on-farm testing.	Ensure a consistent, adequate annual budget allocation for the BTEC program and the bTB component of it. Ensure adequate number of BTEC field staff. Implement a planning process for the BTEC program based on regular interrogation of bTB records with veterinary oversight. Establish a national database for data storage, manipulation and reporting.
Standard operating procedure for reading of SID test	Negative designation for any reaction at injection site <4 mm across all farms irrespective of status (unknown, infected, clear) will have led to a false negative result for some infected animals, such as cattle with chronic infection subsequently identified with tubercule lesions at abattoir carcass inspection and have impeded clearance of infection from infected farms.	Review of the SOP for reading of SID test particularly for known infected farms.
Inconsistent application of SOP for SID testing	Inadequate training and supervision of BTEC field staff.	Provide adequate training for BTEC field staff. Ensure adequate veterinarians in the BTEC program to supervise field staff.
Inconsistent application of SOP for test and cull and quarantine on infected farms	Inadequate training and supervision of BTEC field staff.	Provide adequate training for BTEC field staff. Ensure adequate veterinarians in the BTEC program to supervise field staff.
Unregulated cattle movements	Inadequate specification and implementation of cattle movement regulations.	Review of regulations on cattle movement administered by Biosecurity Authority of Fiji. Improve implementation of regulations by Biosecurity Authority of Fiji and consider involvement of harmonization with Ministry of Agriculture in implementation.
Stray cattle	Presence of stray cattle (untethered owned and unowned cattle grazing freely on public land and intruding on private land) acting to maintain infection in known infected areas.	Review of regulations on stray cattle administered by Biosecurity Authority of Fiji. Improve implementation of regulations by Biosecurity Authority of Fiji.

of agricultural products, and the coordination of the national system of food safety in Fiji" (21).

The goal of the Fiji BTEC Strategy is total eradication of bovine tuberculosis and brucellosis by 2037. The documented strategy lays out the direction for future implementation of the Fiji BTEC Program to attain the long term goal of official recognition by OIE of Fiji as free from both bovine brucellosis and bovine tuberculosis and maintaining this disease-free status (4). The strategy document includes specification on testing policy and strategy, zoning, reactor disposal and compensation, governance and operational management including staffing. It states a new role, full-time project manager, recognizing its importance for effective implementation of the BTEC program and an appointment effective June 2018 is being supported by the Fiji Dairy Industry Development Initiative [funded by New Zealand Ministry of Foreign Affairs and Trade (MFAT)].

Further Initiatives

Along with improvements to field testing and cattle movement control, opportunities for simultaneously improving the laboratory diagnostic capacity for bTB early detection and confirmatory diagnosis have been sought. The BTEC veterinarians and managers have established laboratory network links with Australia, India, New Zealand and Thailand to support diagnostic capacity building in Fiji. Under discussion with the World Organization for Animal Health (OIE) is funding for a Laboratory Twinning Program between FVPL and Animal and Plant Quarantine (QIA) Korea for proficiency testing and laboratory management training.

Concerned about the potential contribution of zoonotic TB to the human TB burden in Fiji, the MOA in collaboration with the Fiji Ministry of Health and Medical Services and the University of Sydney funded by the Marie Bashir Institute will undertake geospatial analysis of human tuberculosis cases and bTB-infected cattle farms, pilot TB surveillance of households in identified high risk areas for bTB exposure, and send samples from human extra-pulmonary cases and cattle cases for species determination. This investigation arises from concern about levels of extra-pulmonary tuberculosis (EPTB). During 2016 among the 312 notified human TB cases, 29% were classified as extra-pulmonary tuberculosis, nearly double the 15% of extra-pulmonary tuberculosis cases among the global total of human TB notifications in 2016 (3, 22). The contribution of bTB to these EPTB cases in Fiji is unknown because the routine diagnostics used do not distinguish pathogen species. There is suspicion of involvement due to the practice of raw milk consumption in some households that own cattle.

DISCUSSION

When the preliminary analysis of 2011–2013 bTB records indicated wide spread endemic infection, the Fijian government acted swiftly in September 2014 to revise SOP for SID testing. This was followed up by actions from 2014 to 2018 that have enhanced identification of infected cattle farms and removal of infected cattle, strengthened implementation of restrictions on cattle movements, and led to the endorsement of a new Fiji Brucellosis and Tuberculosis Eradication Strategy. These are critical steps on the journey to reduce bTB in the national cattle herd, and then subsequently to progress to bTB eradication. This staged process of bTB reduction and containment followed by eradication can be guided by the lessons learnt by other countries on the road to bTB control and eradication, such as Australia, Ireland and New Zealand. The generic components, first of bTB control and containment while ensuring continuity of the industry, and second of bTB eradication and proof of freedom must be contextualized to the bTB situation in Fiji. A policy based on contemporary scientific evidence and international best practice in bTB control needs to be accompanied by specific research in Fiji, given its particular geoclimatic and cultural features. It is crucial for the Fijian government and the dairy and beef industries to be aware that the current policy will need to be modified over time and the commitment to implementation maintained when the BTEC program transitions to the final eradication stage. Industry concern about an increasing proportion of SID test positive cattle with no visible lesions at slaughter is expected with continuation of current SOPs. This provides an example of a situation where technical expertise is required to inform future decisions on test protocol, and where specific research would be beneficial to determine if false positive cases are present and to understand the basis and the extent of these. The international community also needs to consider its role in supporting the Fijian government and industry to attain bTB freedom for the benefit of animal and human health in the Pacific. As Fiji serves as a regional hub, providing live animal stocks and animal products to the neighboring island countries, addressing bTB in Fiji supports the long-term goals of sustainable livelihood and food security in the Pacific island region.

The case study of bTB control in Fiji offers lessons within a Pacific context about the importance of the following technical and social aspects to achieve success in animal disease control.

1. Objective, ongoing assessment of bTB distribution using agreed performance measures (such as bTB farm incidence, reactors per thousand tests, number and proportion of reactors removed) is internationally accepted as essential for critical assessment of progress toward control and eradication (8). This requires a national database for data storage, manipulation and reporting plus data sharing with other national systems for cattle movement and farm registration. It is timely that the NZ MFAT funded project Fiji Dairy Industry Development Initiative has extended its project coverage to include development of web-based database which will link the BTEC geospatial and farm registration information with the agriculture census information of the Economic Planning and Statistics Division of the Ministry of Agriculture. Funding to progress has been approved and the database is now at the planning stage.
2. Robust and accurate diagnostics able to minimize false farm or animal designation given bTB prevalence level at the relevant stage of the control and eradication process must be applied. Selection of the most appropriate diagnostic test/s given the stage of control program and the field conditions for animal testing requires expertise in test protocols. Understanding is needed of the costs of false designation to bTB maintenance and spread (in relation to false negative animals/farms) and to unnecessary loss of productive animals and prohibition to trade (in relation to false positive animals/farms). The Fiji MOA recognizes that early identification of infected farms and infected animals is critical. To date the SID PPD-B in the caudal fold is the single diagnostic applied in the Fiji BTEC program due principally to its low cost and practical suitability to on-farm conditions. While the combination of SID test in the caudal fold (assuming use of potent tuberculin) and carcass inspection at slaughter is reasonable for detection of infected farms, a more sensitive testing regime is needed to support eradication from known infected farms. Thus, the MOA is considering application of other diagnostics, such as the interferon-γ test as a confirmatory test for SID positive animals in known infected farms, and increased use of culture to confirm status of lesions identified at abattoir carcass inspection. A cost-benefit analysis on the use of single intradermal comparative tuberculin test (SICTT) and interferon-γ [with sensitivity when applied in parallel approaching 93% (23)] in place of SID for cattle on known infected farms to aid control and eradication whilst maintaining a milking herd to permit business continuity is recommended.
3. Quality control (QC), the managerial process to compare actual and desired performance of a service or product, will act to ensure an animal disease control program is meeting its objective at the best possible return for the funds invested (24, 25). When disease detection is based on diagnostic procedures with aspects that have subjective interpretation, such as the SID PPD-B and post-mortem inspection (26), quality control will contribute to improve accuracy and consistency in detection. The Irish bTB eradication program with QC applied inputs (personnel, training, SOP, equipment, tuberculin, reagents, computerized recording system), performance (post-mortem surveillance, field surveillance) and outputs (test results, program delivery), provides a model for consideration. For example, the National Handbook of the Irish program that states the national policy and SOP for veterinary management of herds under restriction due to bTB is revised every 3 years to ensure continued improvement and refinement of program activities (27). Given the reliance on SID in the caudal fold and carcass inspection at slaughter for infected farm detection in Fiji, QC

should particularly focus on checking tuberculin potency and standardized training and competency testing of government meat inspectors.

4. Farmer cooperation with control and surveillance activities is vital for the success of animal disease programs. Active participation requires farmer knowledge of bTB risk and impact on cattle production and health, and farmer confidence that BTEC requirements are feasible and effective. Strengthening incentives, such as compensation for culling of positive animals will encourage more farmer cooperation. Effective communication about bTB via farmer targeted and general community campaigns is required to generate farmer action and community support. Clear messaging is proving challenging for bTB due to confusion about tuberculin skin test performance, the involvement of wildlife reservoirs in some countries, and local cultures and beliefs, particularly in countries where despite sustained control programs bTB remains endemic, such as Spain and the United Kingdom. Recent qualitative research involving farmers and veterinarians in Spain articulated the link between farmer non-participation in on-farm testing and distrust of official veterinary services and with farmer perception of little benefit to be gained from bTB freedom (28).

CONCLUSION

The Government of Fiji has demonstrated sustained commitment to reduce bTB in the cattle population. The determination to succeed in a resource limited setting with challenging field conditions is to be commended. The history of bTB control elsewhere shows that the use of tuberculin tests (SID PPD-B and/or SICTT) needs to be relevant to the context (29) and the purpose of their application communicated clearly to avoid confusion and farmer disengagement (28). Guidance from the international animal health community is essential to inform refinement to the Fiji BTEC Strategy on the journey to a bTB-free Fiji.

AUTHOR CONTRIBUTIONS

EB collated and analyzed the data for the retrospective study. RP assisted EB with collation and entry of the bTB data 1999–2014. LB, RP, and TT assisted with interpretation of the findings of the retrospective study. All authors contributed to the content and the preparation of this manuscript.

ACKNOWLEDGMENTS

The authors gratefully acknowledge the Fiji Ministry of Agriculture for granting permission to conduct the retrospective study of the 1999–2014 Fiji BTEC data and the BTEC personnel that performed the data transcription. The first author completed the retrospective study in partial fulfillment for the requirements of the Master of Veterinary Public Health Management degree at The University of Sydney.

REFERENCES

1. OIE. Bovine tuberculosis. In: OIE, editor. *Manual of Diagnostic Tests and Vaccines for Terrestrial Animals*, 7th ed., Chapter 2.4.6, Paris: World Organisation for Animal Health (2012). p. 1–16.
2. Alarcon GJ. Efficacy of a vaccine formula against tuberculosis in cattle. *PLoS ONE* (2013) 8:e76418. doi: 10.1371/journal.pone.0076418
3. WHO. *Global Tuberculosis Report 2017.* Geneva: World Health Organisation (2017).
4. AH&P. *BTEC Strategic Plan. Brucellosis & Tuberculosis Eradication & Control Strategy.* Suva: Ministry of Agriculture (2018).
5. McMillan R. *Cyclopedia of Fiji (1987 ed.).* Ann Arbor, MI: University of Michigan: R. McMillan (1907).
6. FVPL. *2014-2016 Public Sector Investment Program.* Suva: Fiji Veterinary Pathology Laboratory AH&P Ministry of Agriculture (2013).
7. Tukana A, Warner J, Hedlefs R, Gummow B. The history of brucellosis in the Pacific Island countries and territories and its re-emergence. *Prev Vet Med.* (2015) 122:14–20. doi: 10.1016/j.prevetmed.2015.10.005
8. More SJ, Good M. Understanding and managing bTB risk: perspectives from Ireland. *Vet Microbiol.* (2015) 176:209–18. doi: 10.1016/j.vetmic.2015.01.026
9. EU. *Eradication Programme for Bovine Tuberculosis-United Kingdom. 2009/470/3C.* SANCO/10361/2014. Brussels: European Commission (2014).
10. Martin T, Epstein V. *The Animal Health Status Survey.* Secretariat of the Pacific Community, Animal health and Production. Noumea: Secretariat of the Pacific Community (1999).
11. FVPL. *General Operations–BTEC.* BTEC SOP. Suva: Fiji Veterinary Pathology Laboratory AH&P Ministry of Agriculture (2010).
12. AH&P. Memorandum: rate of compensation–TB positive cattle. In: Borja LF, editor. *Memorandum.* Suva: Animal Health & Production Division Ministry of Agriculture (2015).
13. OIE (Ed.). *World Organisation for Animal Health.* Retrieved from WAHIS Interface (2015).
14. Borja E. *Retrospective Study on Bovine Tuberculosis in the Cattle Population of Fiji.* University of Sydney, Faculty of Veterinary Science. Sydney: University of Sydney (2015).
15. FVPL. *2014 Annual Report, Fiji Veterinary Pathology Laboratory–Animal Health & Production.* Suva: Ministry of Agriculture (2014).
16. FVPL. *BTEC Standard Operating Procedure.* BTEC SOP. Suva: Fiji Veterinary Pathology Laboratory (2014).
17. Tunabuna T. *Bovine Tuberculosis in Fiji–Current Situation. BTEC Stakeholder Forum, 03–04 May 2017, Suva* (2017).
18. BAF. *BAF Restricts Movement of Live Animals/Carcass and Bee Hives & Equipment within Fiji During Emergency Period.* Biosecurity Notice on Movement of Animals in Emergency Period. Suva: Biosecurity Authority of Fiji (2016).
19. Sayed-Khayum A. *Extension of Declaration of Biosecurity Emergency Area for Bovine Tuberculosis.* Gazette Supplement of the Government of Fiji. Suva: Government of Fiji (2017).
20. MOA. *Movement Control Regulation.* Movement Control Policy. Suva: Ministry of Agriculture (2017).
21. MOA. *Report: Chile Training Needs Analysis.* Suva: Ministry of Agriculture (2017).
22. WHO. *Tuberculosis Country Profile 2016.* Suva: World Health Organisation (2016).
23. Gormley E, Doyle MB, Fitzsimons T, McGill K, Collins JD. Diagnosis of Mycobacterium bovis infection in cattle by use of the gamma-interferon (Bovigam1) assay. *Vet Microbiol.* (2006) 112:171–9. doi: 10.1016/j.vetmic.2005.11.029
24. Duignan A, Good M, More SJ. Quality control in the national bovine tuberculosis eradication programme in Ireland. *Sci Tech Rev OIE* (2012) 31:845–60. doi: 10.20506/rst.31.3.2166
25. Sheridan M. Progress in tuberculosis eradication in Ireland. *Vet Microbiol.* (2011) 151:160–9. doi: 10.1016/j.vetmic.2011.02.040

26. Clegg TA, Duignan A, More SJ. The relative effectiveness of testers during field surveillance for bovine tuberculosis in unrestricted low-risk herds in Ireland. *Prev Vet Med.* (2015) 119:85–9. doi: 10.1016/j.prevetmed.2015.02.005
27. Good M, Duignan A. *Veterinary Handbook for Herd Management in the Bovine TB Eradication Programme.* Dublin: Department of Agriculture, Food and the Marine (2016).
28. Ciaravino G, Ibarra P, Casal E, Lopez S, Espluga J, Casal J, et al. Farmer and veterinarian attitudes towards the bovine tuberculosis eradication programme in Spain: what is going on in the field? *Front Vet Sci.* (2017) 4:202. doi: 10.3389/fvets.2017.00202
29. Good M, Bakker D, Duignan A, Collins DM. The history of *in vivo* tuberculin testing in bovines: tuberculosis, a "One Health" issue. *Front Vet Sci.* (2018) 5:59. doi: 10.3389/fvets.2018.00059

12

Baiting and Feeding Revisited: Modeling Factors Influencing Transmission of Tuberculosis among Deer and to Cattle

Melinda K. Cosgrove [1*], *Daniel J. O'Brien* [1] *and David S. L. Ramsey* [2]

[1] *Wildlife Disease Laboratory, Michigan Department of Natural Resources, Lansing, MI, United States,* [2] *Department of Environment, Land, Water and Planning, Arthur Rylah Institute for Environmental Research, Heidelberg, VIC, Australia*

Correspondence:
Melinda K. Cosgrove
cosgrovem1@michigan.gov

Although tuberculosis caused by *Mycobacterium bovis* (bTB) is endemic in white-tailed deer (*Odocoileus virginianus*) in northeastern Michigan, USA, baiting and feeding of deer continue despite a regulatory ban. Previous modeling suggests aggregation at bait sites slows the rates at which harvest and/or vaccination decrease bTB prevalence, prolongs time to eradication, and increases the likelihood that once eradicated, bTB will re-establish following an incursion. However, the extent to which specific factors such as food density, attractiveness to deer, and persistence on the landscape influence bTB transmission is unknown. We used an individual-based, spatially-explicit stochastic simulation model of bTB in deer and cattle to investigate effects of feed density, attractiveness, and spatial and temporal persistence on bTB prevalence in deer and the probability of breakdowns in adjacent cattle herds. Because hunter harvest remains key to controlling bTB in deer, and harvest rates are in long term decline, we modeled these feeding-associated factors at harvest rates prevailing both when the model was developed (2003–2007) and in 2018. Food placement at randomized locations vs. fixed sites had little effect on bTB prevalence in deer, whereas increasing the probability that deer move to food piles (attractiveness) had the greatest effect of factors studied on both prevalence and herd breakdowns. Reducing food pile density reduced prevalence, but decreased herd breakdowns only modestly. Consistent availability of food over longer periods of time, as would occur with supplemental winter feeding or persistent recreational feeding, increased both prevalence in deer and cattle herd breakdowns dramatically. Though perhaps implausible to the public, altering how bait and feed for deer are used can reduce cattle herd breakdowns. Baiting and feeding bans have contributed to declining bTB prevalence, but non-compliance and continued legal sales of feed impede eradication. Requiring hunters to move food piles is unlikely to mitigate effects on transmission and is not a useful management tool. Compared to baiting, winter supplemental feeding or extended recreational feeding is likely to magnify bTB transmission by prolonging temporal availability. Because attractiveness of feed is influenced both by type of feed and deer behavior, research to quantify factors influencing deer movement to food should be a priority.

Keywords: baiting, cattle, feeding, management, *Odocoileus virginianus*, simulation model, tuberculosis, white-tailed deer

INTRODUCTION

Infectious disease management in a wildlife reservoir is a contentious issue, especially when changes in human behavior are necessary. While there may be general agreement that control measures are warranted, the specific actions adopted are often controversial. The elimination of human-provided supplemental food for wildlife is of notable debate. Although the use of supplemental food for wildlife is recognized as a mechanism for both inter- and intra-species disease transmission (1–7), disagreements regarding the potential benefits vs. consequences related to this practice are still prevalent. Nonetheless, zoonotic diseases can have serious ecological and economic impacts (5, 8) and the disease management strategies chosen influence the magnitude of the impacts. Advocates for the use of supplement food as bait (an attractant during legal hunting seasons) argue that baiting is necessary to increase and maintain harvest for disease control, yet evidence for this is lacking (9, 10). However, the use of bait increases deer concentrations around these sites, increasing contact rates and so the potential for disease transmission. Supplemental food used in winter to (theoretically) aid survival can have similar consequences (5–7).

In Michigan, baiting and feeding of white-tailed deer (*Odocoileus virginianus*) is recognized as one of the biggest risks for transmission of tuberculosis caused by *Mycobacterium bovis* (bTB) (4, 8, 11, 12). In the wake of extensive logging and the decimation of deer populations by market hunting that occurred in the 1800s, large tracts of land were bought into private ownership and "hunt clubs" were established, both to conserve what deer remained and to provide populations for sport hunting and sustainable harvest. In the 1920's deer numbers in the northern Lower Peninsula of Michigan rose dramatically, in part due to lower harvest pressure on privately owned lands effectively maintained as refuges, and winter starvation became common (13, 14). In an attempt to reduce starvation, supplemental feeding became prevalent, yet starvation continued as the biological carrying capacity of the marginal habitat had been exceeded (13). During this same time, bTB reactor rates in cattle across the state were relatively high, reaching 20–30% in some counties (15, 16). Although Michigan was later successful in lowering bTB reactor rates in cattle and was eventually declared bTB free in 1979, contact between infected cattle and concentrated numbers of deer had been occurring for decades. Large scale supplemental feeding increased in the 1980's as competition increased between private land owners to attract deer to their property. It is hypothesized that spillover of bTB from cattle to deer occurred sometime during the 1950s to 1960s (17, 18), although deer were not recognized as a maintenance host until the 1990's (11). By that time bTB had become self-sustaining in the free-ranging deer herd and persists to the present day (11, 19).

Although bTB is endemic in deer in northeast Lower Michigan, winter feeding and baiting of deer continue despite a regulatory ban, albeit at lower levels than historically practiced. The sale of bait and feed remains legal and widespread, even where its use is banned (8). The current economic value of these sales is thought to be substantial. In 1995, it was estimated that baiting and supplemental feeding generated $15 million for Michigan farmers (20), and predictably, bans are typically opposed by farmers gaining from the sale of crops otherwise unmarketable for human consumption. This presents a persistent struggle to eradicate a contagious disease in the face of exacerbating practices. Previous modeling, using estimated levels of current baiting practices, suggests aggregation at bait sites slows the rates at which harvest and/or vaccination decrease bTB prevalence, prolongs time to eradication, and increases the likelihood that once eradicated, bTB will re-establish following an incursion (21). However, not well known are the extent to which specific factors such as feed site density, attractiveness to deer, and persistence on the landscape influence bTB transmission among deer and between deer and cattle.

Both direct and indirect interactions between livestock and wildlife have been well documented as a source of disease transmission (22–26). Increased bTB reactor rates in livestock resulting from alterations in supplemental food use for deer could be associated as well. We used an existing spatially-explicit model of bTB in deer and cattle (27) to evaluate how altering supplemental food density, attractiveness, and temporal and spatial persistence impact bTB prevalence in deer and the rate of cattle herd breakdowns.

MATERIALS AND METHODS

Study Area

We conducted simulations over a 48 x 51 km land area in the northeastern Lower Peninsula of Michigan consisting mainly of Deer Management Unit (DMU) 452 [12, 27, **Figure 1**]. Deer Management Unit 452 includes parts of Alcona, Alpena, Montmorency, and Oscoda counties, is ~148,018 ha (1,480 km^2), and comprised of 93% privately-owned land and 7% public land (28, 29). Topography, habitat, and deer management practices are described elsewhere (12, 30, 31). Historically, this area has defined the core outbreak area for bTB in Michigan (8).

The Model

We used an individual-based spatially-explicit stochastic simulation model of bTB in white-tailed deer and cattle for all simulations. The structure, parameters, testing, validation, and assumptions of the model are described at length elsewhere (12, 27, 31). We used two Geographic Information System (GIS) layers to distribute deer and cattle across the landscape and account for movements and spatial concomitance that facilitate bTB transmission among deer and from deer to cattle. We used a deer layer that quantifies winter habitat potential for deer (as a surrogate for biological carrying capacity) to spatially distribute deer throughout the landscape (12, 31–33). We added a second layer that incorporated cattle producer locations, pasture areas, and cattle densities for all farms within and directly adjacent to DMU 452 to approximate cattle distribution (27). The model was originally calibrated to closely approximate steady-state age and sex specific bTB prevalence matched to long-term bTB surveillance data for deer from 2003–2007 (12, 31) and cattle herd breakdown rates 2003–2012 (27). A cattle herd breakdown is defined as a herd having at least one bTB reactor in the herd during whole herd testing.

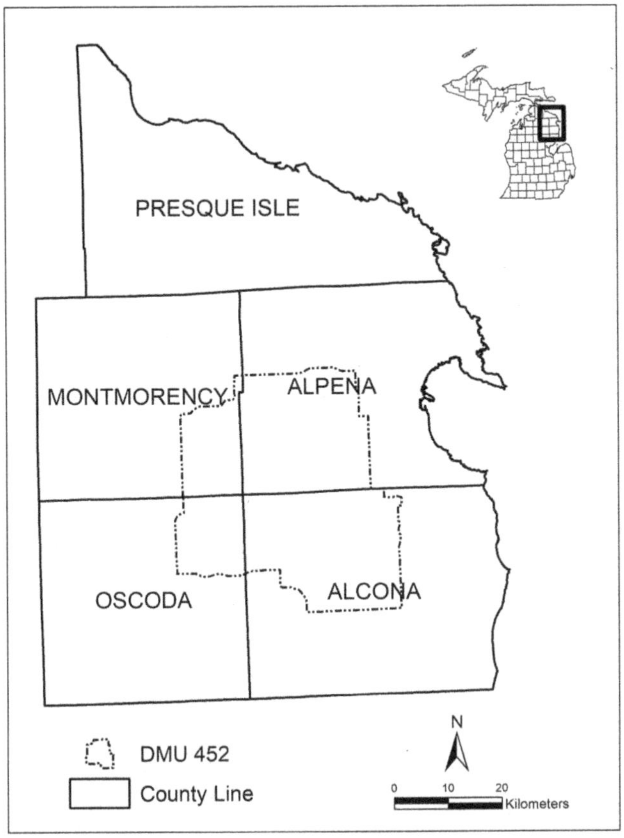

FIGURE 1 | Simulation model study area, Deer Management Unit (DMU) 452, in northeastern Lower Peninsula of Michigan, USA.

Because rates of hunter harvest have declined over the last two decades, primarily due to demographic factors (34), the model was recalibrated in 2018 to adjust bTB transmission rates to accommodate current harvest rates. Briefly, sex- and age-specific harvest rates for DMU 452 were estimated from MDNR deer hunter harvest survey data via the sex-age kill method (35). Using those harvest rates, simulations were run to calibrate the sex-specific transmission rate parameters (betas) so that the predicted sex-specific bTB prevalence closely approximated field prevalence rates recorded from 2012–2016.

The baseline model simulates aggregation of deer around supplemental food sources by estimating the movement of a deer to the food source based on the location of the food source within its home range (12, 31). During each time step (2 months), each deer conducts a search of habitat cells within its home range. If a food pile is encountered, there is assumed to be a 0.2 probability of a change in the deer's current location to the food pile if it occurs at the center of its home range. That probability declines as a half normal function of the distance of the food pile from the home range center and was zero for food piles outside the home range. Food piles were randomly distributed across the landscape. Supplemental food was available from September to December, coinciding with deer hunting seasons in Michigan when bait is used.

In this study, we define supplemental food in two ways: (1) Baiting—the autumnal use of food to attract deer in an attempt to aid harvest; and (2) Feeding—the use of food for deer outside of legal hunting seasons (e.g., to facilitate wildlife viewing, or in an effort to aid winter survival). Our previous modeling suggests that aggregation of deer at food sites has a substantial effect on bTB transmission (12). However, that work only investigated the effects of the presence or absence of bait. The spatial nature of the model affords the ability to assess a variety of parameters associated with baiting and feeding. We altered four different supplemental food parameters to evaluate the effect on bTB prevalence in deer and cattle herd breakdowns over a 30-year period. Other model parameters were kept at default values as described previously (12, 27, 31). We ran each scenario under the original and current harvest rates for 5,000 replicates, discarding simulations for the first 50 and 150 years, respectively, (burn-in period). Due to the stochastic nature of the model, the burn-in period was required to ensure bTB and cattle breakdown rates had stabilized prior to changing the parameters under investigation. For comparison to our treatments, we conducted baseline simulations for both the original and current age- and sex-specific bTB transmission and harvest rates.

Simulated Scenarios

Food Pile Density

Baiting and feeding is illegal in DMU 452 and has been since 1999 with limited use allowed in 2001 (8). However, a non-compliance rate of ~25% was estimated for hunters in the area (36). By dividing the number of potential baiters (determined from deer hunting license sales; see (12)) by the area of DMU 452, the bait pile density was set at 0.02/ha. We evaluated the effect of reducing the non-compliance rate by 50% (e.g., via more stringent enforcement) which in turn reduced the bait pile density to 0.01/ha.

Food Pile Attractiveness

We define bait attractiveness as the probability that a deer will visit a bait pile if the bait pile is located within the center of the deer's home range. Attractiveness is influenced by both feed type and deer behavior and is thus difficult to quantify with certainty. Consequently, we evaluated three arbitrary variations of this probability: 0.05, 0.1, and 0.5, which were considered to be plausible bounds on the likely attractiveness of bait to deer, assuming the odds of deer being attracted to accessible bait are 50:50 or lower.

Spatial Persistence

Most hunters have preferred hunting locations and often establish permanent tree stands or deer blinds at these locations from which they hunt each year. In turn, if the hunter uses bait, the food piles are located in approximately the same location every year. We simulated the effect of requiring hunters to move food piles to new locations each year by randomizing pile locations, thus potentially affecting contact rates between habituated deer.

Temporal Persistence

Supplemental feeding commonly takes place during winter months when the public attempts to supplement reduced natural food sources for wild deer. This type of feeding can potentially aid winter survival, thus increasing deer densities to a level that exceeds the biological carrying capacity of the habitat. Both supplemental and prolonged recreational feeding (typically for the purposes of viewing) can unnaturally congregate deer for extended periods and in turn increase the probability of disease transmission. We evaluated the effects of prolonged food provision by humans on bTB prevalence and cattle herd breakdowns by expanding the temporal duration of food piles for two different time frames: September–February and September–April. The former simulates feeding through the most severe months of winter in Michigan, and the latter supplementing food through the entire winter.

Analysis

We used R (version 3.0.2, R Foundation for Statistical Computing, Vienna, Austria) for analyzing model output. Summary plots were generated for deer (bTB prevalence) over the simulated 30-year time frame. We compared output from the baseline simulation (no change to current deer management) to output from the simulations evaluating changes in baiting and feeding practices, to detect the direction and magnitude of influence on prevalence and herd breakdowns. Changes in bTB prevalence are expressed as absolute differences in year 30 vs. year zero of each simulation.

RESULTS

The baseline simulation for the original harvest rates resulted in a 0.001 decrease in deer prevalence after 30 years, and no change in prevalence over 30 years under the current harvest rates (**Figures 2, 3**). Cattle herd break downs were 2.8 per year on average under the original harvest rates and 3.4 per year under the current rates for the baseline simulations after 30 years (**Table 1**).

Food Pile Density

Reducing the baiting non-compliance rate (and thus food pile density) by 50% reduced bTB prevalence in deer by ~0.005 under both harvest rates, and reduced cattle herd breakdowns by an average of ~1.5 per year under both harvest rates (**Table 1**).

Food Pile Attractiveness

Under the original harvest rates, reducing the probability that a deer visited a bait pile within its home range to 0.05 and 0.1, reduced prevalence by ~0.007 and 0.008 respectively, and by ~0.012 and 0.011 under the current harvest rates (**Figure 2**). Increasing the probability of visitation to a bait pile to 0.5 increased prevalence by 0.06 and 0.069 for the original and current harvest rates respectively. Cattle herd breakdowns were reduced to ~1 breakdown every 2 years under the original harvest rates and ~1 breakdown every 5 years under the current harvest rates for the visitation probability of 0.05. For the visitation probability of 0.1, breakdowns were reduced to ~1 breakdown every 2 years under both harvest rates (**Table 1**). However, increasing the probability of visitation to 0.5, increased herd breakdowns dramatically, ~22 per year under original harvest and ~19 per year under current harvest rates.

Spatial Persistence

Changes in harvest rates notwithstanding, randomizing the location of bait piles each year had a negligible effect on bTB prevalence (0.002 decrease) in deer and on cattle herd breakdowns (**Table 1**).

Temporal Persistence

Extending the time supplemental food was available by 2 months (i.e., through February) increased bTB prevalence by ~0.019 and 0.028 for the original and current harvest rates, respectively (**Figure 3**). When food was available through April, prevalence increased by ~0.051 and 0.061, respectively. Cattle herd breakdowns were approximately triple for both harvest rates after a 2-month increase in supplemental food (**Table 1**). Breakdowns were 5–7 times higher after a 4-month extension of supplemental food.

DISCUSSION

Over the 10 years since our model was first developed, there has been a decreasing trend in deer harvest, requiring the recalibration of our model. We simulated our scenarios under both old and new harvest rates, to illustrate the effect of this harvest reduction, and to enable comparisons to our previously reported findings. Many of the scenarios simulated under the current harvest rates showed increased bTB impacts as compared to the original harvest rates, emphasizing that hunter harvest remains an important factor controlling bTB in deer. Yet, hunter retention and recruitment are recognized as being in critical decline, and this may have detrimental effects for wildlife disease management (37–40). For density dependent diseases, such as bTB in deer, population control of wildlife reservoirs is crucial. However, after more than 20 years of providing increased harvest opportunity in DMU 452, harvest has likely been saturated and further extending harvest opportunity is unlikely to increase harvest (12). A survey of hunters and livestock producers in northeast Lower Michigan more than a decade ago indicated that only 23% of resident hunters supported a further reduction in deer numbers, whereas and somewhat surprisingly, only 57% of livestock producers in the area were in support of further reductions (41). Future bTB management in Michigan must take into consideration what can realistically be accomplished given the likelihood that reductions in harvest experienced over the past two decades are permanent. Thus far, policymakers have been reluctant to entertain other potential options for bTB control such as culling or vaccination, likely because prevalence in the deer population could be kept low via hunter harvest alone. However, as demographic changes continue to reduce the number of deer hunters (34), harvest may no longer be as efficacious as in the past.

In addition to deer density reduction, prohibiting the use of bait and feed for deer is generally one of the first control strategies

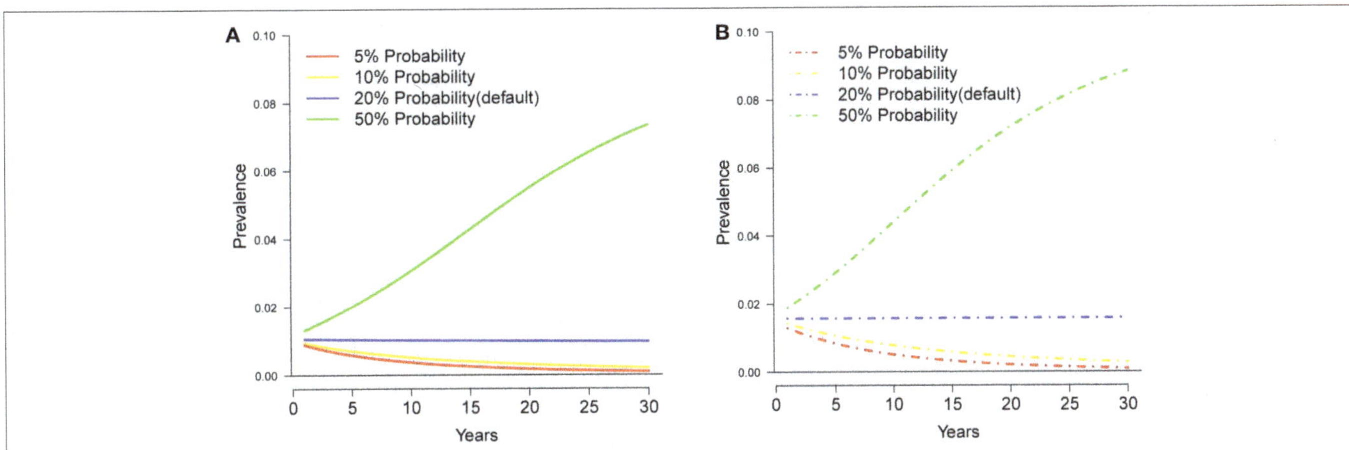

FIGURE 2 | Tuberculosis prevalence in white-tailed deer over 30 years under different probabilities of deer movement to a supplemental food pile, assuming original **(A)** and current **(B)** harvest rates.

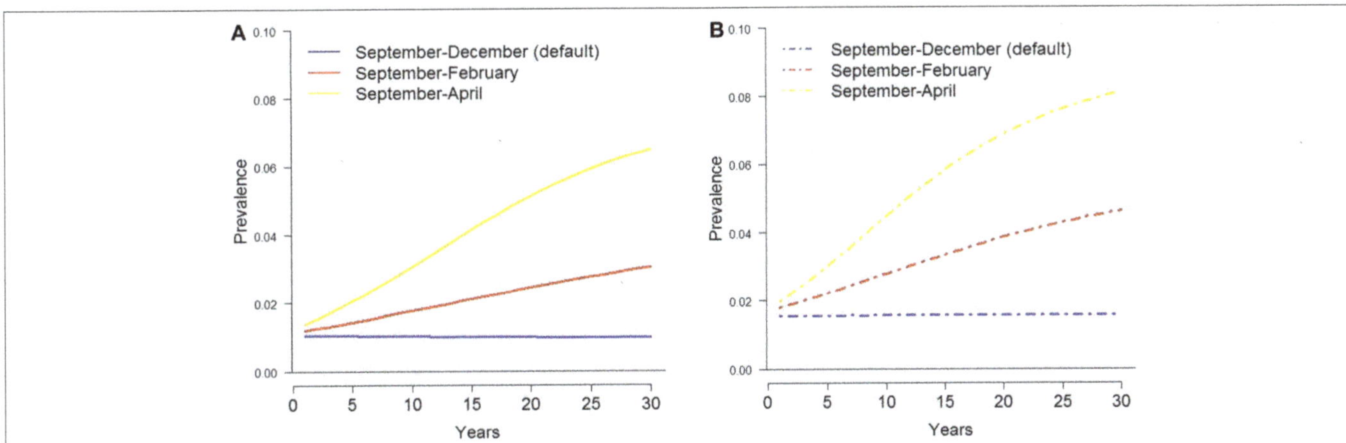

FIGURE 3 | Tuberculosis prevalence in white-tailed deer over 30 years under extended temporal availability of supplemental food piles, assuming original **(A)** and current **(B)** harvest rates.

implemented to limit disease transmission (5). However, a complete ban, in practice, is usually unattainable. Baiting and feeding bans have contributed to declining bTB prevalence in Michigan, but non-compliance, problematic prosecution of violators, and continued legal sales of feed impede eradication. Consequently, attempting to keep the non-compliance rate as low as possible becomes the goal. Even if a 50% reduction of the estimated non-compliance rate in DMU 452 could be achieved, our results show that only modest decreases in bTB prevalence and herd breakdowns would result. While we did not examine the effect of an increased non-compliance rate and an increase in food density, a resurgence in baiting may be occurring in DMU 452. Observations by MDNR field staff have noted an increase in supplemental feed sales (pers. comm. B. Mastenbrook). Moreover, it is not clear that a decreasing number of hunters will necessarily result in fewer bait sites on the landscape. If younger hunters are more likely to employ bait than the older hunters who are gradually leaving the hunting population, it is conceivable that the amount of bait on the landscape may not mirror the decline in hunter numbers.

If a complete prohibition of bait could be achieved, the benefits realized could be diminished by reduced hunter participation (42). In Michigan, there is a cultural significance to deer hunting, and traditions of deer hunting in some regions of the state have long included the use of bait (8, 42). Because reducing deer density is currently the primary strategy for bTB control, the willingness of hunters to harvest deer in endemic areas is crucial for success. If hunters are reluctant to hunt without bait due to the perceived increase in hunter effort, or if hunters choose to hunt elsewhere, baiting bans could potentially decrease harvest further. Following the 2001 hunting season in Michigan, a segment of hunters indicated through surveys that they eliminated or decreased their hunting activities due to the baiting ban (10, 42–44). However, participation and antlerless harvest were similar between DMU 452 and the remainder of the state where baiting remained legal (42). Notably, evidence

TABLE 1 | Average number of cattle herd breakdowns per year under the original and current deer harvest rates after 30 simulated years.

Scenario*	Harvest rates	
	Original	**Current**
Baseline	2.8	3.4
Density 0.1	1.5	1.9
Prob 0.05	0.6	0.2
Prob 0.1	0.6	0.6
Prob 0.5	22.4	18.9
Random	2.5	3.0
Sept-Feb	9.3	9.8
Sept-Apr	20.2	17.9

Scenarios: Density 0.1 = Food Pile Density (0.01 food piles/ha); Prob 0.05, 0.1, 0.5 = Food Attractiveness (probabilities of deer moving to a food pile); Random = Spatial Persistence (randomizing food pile locations annually); Sept-Feb, Sept-Apr = Temporal Persistence (extension of time food piles are available).

suggests that in general, baiting does not increase harvest (9, 10, 20, 45).

Even if minimal baiting was allowed in an attempt to maintain hunter satisfaction, a method to mitigate the increased disease transmission resulting from supplemental food has not yet been found (6, 7). We simulated requiring hunters to move bait piles to new locations each year, but the practice had a negligible effect on bTB prevalence and herd breakdowns and is thus unlikely to be a useful management tool. Previous research has shown deer in northeast Lower Michigan to have a high fidelity to baited areas, but not to specific bait locations (46). Effectiveness notwithstanding, requiring hunters to move their bait sites is likely to be impractical. In DMU 452, thousands of hunters are spread over a 1,480 km^2 area, >90% of which is privately-owned land. The effort necessary to enforce such an approach is not feasible and would arguably be more constructively applied to enforcing a strict baiting ban.

The more attractive a bait pile, the more likely a deer is to move to it. In our simulations attractiveness had a considerable impact on bTB prevalence and cattle herd breakdowns. Reducing the likelihood of a deer moving to a bait pile had a desirable impact on prevalence. However, increasing the probability of visitation to a bait pile resulted in 3.5-fold increase in prevalence and an average of 19 cattle herd breakdowns per year after 30 years. Hunters deliberately use bait piles to attract deer. Thus, expecting hunters to use less "attractive" bait defeats the purpose of using bait in the first place. However, attractiveness is also driven by deer behavior. Although supplemental food influences deer behavior (6, 46), quantifying that influence is difficult. Our modeling results are sensitive to variation in this parameter [see (12), Appendix A) and research to better quantify the combined effect of food attractiveness and deer behavior would be valuable.

Compared to baiting, winter supplemental feeding or extended recreational feeding is likely to magnify bTB transmission by prolonging temporal availability. In our simulations, each 2-month extension of food availability increased bTB prevalence 2–3% and herd breakdowns increased dramatically (**Table 1**). The longer food sites are maintained, the greater the cumulative transmission of disease over time (6, 7, 47). These simulations suggest that even 5 years of feeding throughout the winter increased prevalence by more than 50%. Although historic large-scale winter feeding (11) has decreased significantly, a resurgence of this practice could wipe out gains made in bTB control to date after only a few years. Should managers ever allow winter feeding to become widespread again, knowing the likely consequences, the temporal window during which it is allowed must be a critical consideration.

Our temporal persistence scenarios extended the time bait was available on the landscape to simulate winter feeding, a reasonable but imperfect approximation. Bait is used theoretically to aid harvest in autumn. Winter feed sites occur without harvest and generally contain a greater quantity of food than bait sites, potentially attracting more deer to the site. Yet there are usually fewer feed sites in winter than bait sites during the hunting seasons. Historic winter feed site locations were documented previously via aerial surveys when winter feeding was extensive. Future research could incorporate these sites into our model as a new GIS layer to more precisely estimate site densities for comparison against these results.

Our model does not explicitly account for indirect transmission of bTB resulting from environmental contamination; if it did, we hypothesize that both prevalence of bTB in deer and the number of cattle herd breakdowns would likely increase, although the magnitude of those increases is uncertain. Deer infected with *M. bovis* shed infectious bacteria in oronasal secretions (48), and food items contaminated by infected deer are infectious for susceptible deer (49). In a field setting, bait and supplemental feed sites facilitate both the contamination of feedstuffs and surrounding soil with saliva and nasal secretions of deer feeding there (**Figure 4**), and so act as an efficient source of bTB transmission even after both the infected deer, and perhaps the feed itself, are gone. Experimental studies conducted both under laboratory (50) and Michigan outdoor (51, 52) conditions have shown that *M. bovis* can remain viable on feedstuffs for days to several months, depending on the substrate and ambient conditions such as temperature, humidity, and shade. That said, efforts to isolate the bacteria from documented deer feeding sites in Michigan have thus far proven unsuccessful (53). Although yet to be explicitly shown in Michigan field settings, research from other bTB-infected ecosystems has elegantly demonstrated the efficacy of environmental substrates such as watering holes as sources of bTB exposure (54). To parameterize indirect environmental transmission in our model, further research to determine the visitation rates of deer to sites where food was once, but is no longer, present would be necessary, along with rates of soil ingestion. Persistence times for *M. bovis* could be drawn from existing distributions of bacterial survival on foodstuffs (50). Alternatively, a value for indirect transmission could be estimated arbitrarily, and subjected to sensitivity analysis as in previous work (12). In any case, our model has demonstrated the importance of bait piles for bTB transmission in WTD, notwithstanding the additional risk due to environmental contamination.

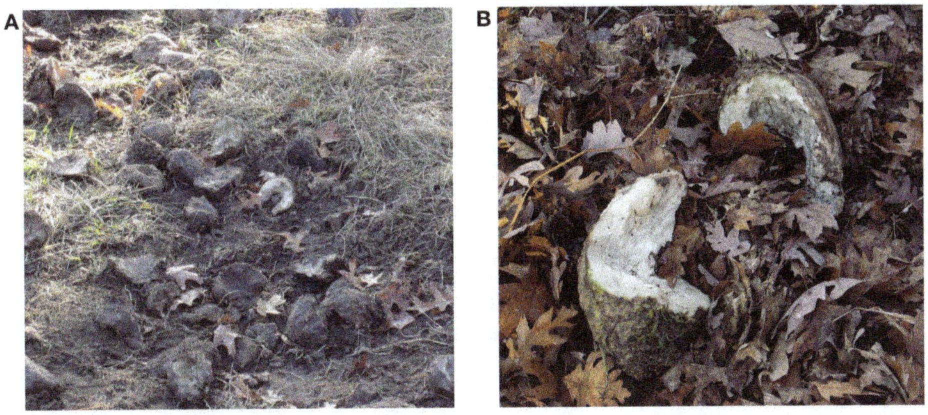

FIGURE 4 | Sugar beets (*Beta vulgaris* subsp. *vulgaris* convar. *vulgaris* var. *altissima*) in an illegal deer baiting site, Alcona County, Michigan. **(A)** Hoof traffic exposes soil which may act as a source of indirect exposure to *M. bovis* when contaminated by infected deer. **(B)** Teeth marks on sugar beets partially eaten by deer. *M. bovis* likely survives for extended periods on these foodstuffs under the cold, wet conditions typical of autumn and winter in northeastern Michigan.

No matter how feed sites are used, their presence, and potentially their past presence, increases bTB prevalence (12). Aggregation, crowding, increased competition, exposure to unrelated individuals, and increased predator-prey interactions are a few of the consequences of feed sites (5–7, 46, 55). These effects in turn increase stress and lower immune response, increasing susceptibility to disease (7, 56). Supplemental feed is often of lower quality than naturally available food and does not provide complete nutrition (57), leading to deficiencies and lowered immune response. Feeding deer to aid winter survival can be successful if begun early, but resulting increased survival and fecundity can increase densities, increasing bTB transmission. Feeding later in winter after nutritional deficits are realized often does not aid survival because body condition is often too poor to be reversed, putting these deer at even greater disease risk (57).

Our results indicate that altering how bait and feed for deer are used can reduce, or increase, cattle herd breakdowns, which is frequently implausible to the public. Discussions regarding the use of bait and feed are often considered of relevance only to bTB transmission among deer. While not effective as the sole management tool (27), how food provided by humans for deer impacts broader issues of bTB eradication from cattle must be considered by both regulators and agricultural producers. While deer bait and feed provide a market for crops that have limited marketability as human food, agricultural stakeholder groups should carefully consider the trade-offs between income generated for crop farmers vs. the economic costs of herd breakdowns to the cattle industry and the larger agricultural economy. Such introspection has largely been lacking in Michigan thus far.

Managing disease in deer must not preclude the use of other means of disease management for livestock. Increased biosecurity on farms in areas where bTB is endemic should remain a priority. Brook et al. (25) argue that a "bottom-up" approach for reducing transmission risk at the wildlife-livestock interface would be more practical and effective. This approach tailors risk mitigation to the individual farm level, taking into consideration spatial overlap and resources, winter feeding areas, animal behavior, fencing, and farm management, in contrast to relying primarily on wildlife culling or harvest, disease testing, baiting and feeding regulations, and cattle depopulation. Clearly, changing farm management can reduce disease transmission between wildlife and livestock substantially (23, 25, 26, 58–60). Our model includes a parameter to account for the proportional reduction in deer-to-cattle contact likely to be afforded by increased biosecurity [see Equation 1 in (27)]. For this study, we chose to hold that parameter at its default value of 1 (unmitigated deer to cattle contact). While heightened biosecurity could help reduce the effects of increased deer baiting and feeding, previous work suggests quite a high level of biosecurity would be necessary in order to have a high probability of reducing herd breakdowns [Figure 10 in (27)]. Although increased biosecurity alone is unlikely to eliminate herd breakdowns in the absence of broader measures to control bTB in deer (27), improving farm management in conjunction with altering supplemental food use for wildlife may facilitate reductions in interspecies bTB transmission.

CONCLUSION

The use of supplemental food for deer continues to be one of the biggest regulatory challenges to bTB eradication in Michigan. As long as widespread baiting and feeding continue, successful eradication of bTB is likely unattainable. As wildlife managers learn to compensate for the decline in hunter numbers and adjust to changes in hunter demographics, the challenges for disease management become more complex. Even if a low level of bTB in deer is acceptable to the public, the ever present and serious risks to livestock remain problematic. Our modeling results demonstrate that a link between supplemental feeding of deer and occurrence of bTB in livestock exists and that feeding has implications not only for deer. Wildlife management necessarily involves managing people and their behaviors as well as wildlife populations. Disease management programs need to include educating people on how perceived short-term benefits from the use of bait and feed can lead to adverse long-term consequences. Convincing people not only to change their own behavior, but to also encourage others to do so, requires a culture change. Invoking this change is one of the most difficult challenges wildlife disease managers face.

AUTHOR CONTRIBUTIONS

DR developed and recalibrated the model. DO provided the project concept and design. MC conducted the simulations, analyzed output, and drafted the manuscript. All authors contributed to intellectual material, manuscript review, and editing, and have approved the submitted manuscript.

ACKNOWLEDGMENTS

The authors are grateful to A. Locher for allowing use of habitat potential data from which the habitat layers of the deer model are constructed.

REFERENCES

1. Becker DJ, Hall RJ. Too much of a good thing: resource provisioning alters infectious disease dynamics in wildlife. *Biol Lett.* (2014) 10:20140309. doi: 10.1098/rsbl.2014.0309
2. Becker DJ, Streicker DG, Altizer S. Linking anthropogenic resources to wildlife-pathogen dynamics: a review and meta-analysis. *Ecol Lett.* (2015) 18:483–95. doi: 10.1111/ele.12428
3. Brown RD, Cooper SM. The nutritional, ecological, and ethical arguments against baiting and feeding white-tailed deer. *Wildlife Soc Bull.* (2006) 34:519–24. doi: 10.2193/0091-7648(2006)34[519:TNEAEA]2.0.CO;2
4. Miller R, Kaneene JB, Fitzgerald SD, Schmitt SM. Evaluation of the influence of supplemental feeding of white-tailed deer (*Odocoileus virginianus*) on the prevalence of bovine tuberculosis in the Michigan wild deer population. *J Wildlife Dis.* (2003) 39:84–95. doi: 10.7589/0090-3558-39.1.84
5. Sorensen A, van Beest FM, Brook RK. Impacts of wildlife baiting and supplemental feeding on infectious disease transmission risk: a synthesis of knowledge. *Prev Vet Med.* (2014) 113:356–63. doi: 10.1016/j.prevetmed.2013.11.010
6. Thompson AK, Samuel MD, Van Deelen TR. Alternative feeding strategies and potential disease transmission in Wisconsin white-tailed deer. *J Wildlife Manage.* (2008) 72:416–21. doi: 10.2193/2006-543
7. Murray MH, Becker DJ, Hall RJ, Hernandez SM. Wildlife health and supplemental feeding: a review and management recommendations. *Biol Conserv.* (2016) 204:163–74. doi: 10.1016/j.biocon.2016.10.034
8. O'Brien DJ, Schmitt SM, Fitzgerald SD, Berry DE, Hickling GJ. Managing the wildlife reservoir of *Mycobacterium bovis*: the Michigan, USA, experience. *Vet Microbiol.* (2006) 112:313–23. doi: 10.1016/j.vetmic.2005.11.014
9. Van Deelen TR, Dhuey B, McCaffery KR, Rolley RE. Relative effects of baiting and supplemental antlerless seasons on Wisconsin's 2003 deer harvest. *Wildlife Soc Bull.* (2006) 34:322–8. doi: 10.2193/0091-7648(2006)34[322:REOBAS]2.0.CO;2
10. Frawley BJ. *Deer Baiting in the Northeast Lower Peninsula of Michigan.* Wildlife Division Report No. 3372. Lansing, MI: Michigan Department of Natural Resources (2002). p. 14.
11. Schmitt SM, Fitzgerald SD, Cooley TM, Bruning-Fann CS, Sullivan L, Berry D, et al. Bovine tuberculosis in free-ranging white-tailed deer from Michigan. *J Wildlife Dis.* (1997) 33:749–58. doi: 10.7589/0090-3558-33.4.749
12. Ramsey DSL, O'Brien DJ, Cosgrove MK, Rudolph BA, Locher AB, Schmitt SM. Forecasting eradication of bovine tuberculosis in Michigan white-tailed deer. *J Wildl Manage.* (2014) 78:240–54. doi: 10.1002/jwmg.656
13. Bartlett IH. *Whitetails: Presenting Michigan's Deer Problem.* Lansing, MI: Michigan Department of Conservation, Game Division, and Franklin DeKleine Company (1938).
14. Jenkins DH, Bartlett IH. *Michigan Whitetails.* Lansing, MI: Michigan Department of Conservation, Game Division (1959).
15. State Departement of Agriculture, Livestock Disease Control, Bovine Tuberculosis Eradication. *First Annual Report For the Fiscal Year ending June 30, 1922.* Lansing, MI: Michigan State Department of Agriculture (1922). pp. 71–82.
16. State Department of Agriculture, Livestock Disease Control, Bovine Tuberculosis Eradication. *Second Biennial Report For the Fiscal Years ending June 30, 1925 and 1926.* Lansing, MI: Michigan State Department of Agriculture (1926). pp. 42–60.
17. McCarty CW, Miller MW. A versatile model of disease transmission applied to forecasting bovine tuberculosis dynamics in white-tailed deer populations. *J Wildlife Dis.* (1998) 34:722–30. doi: 10.7589/0090-3558-34.4.722
18. Salvador LCM, O'Brien DJ, Cosgrove MK, Stuber TP, Schooley A, Crispell J, et al. Implications for disease management at the wildlife-livestock interface: using whole-genome sequencing to study the role of elk in bovine tuberculosis transmission in Michigan. *USA Mol Ecol.* (2018).
19. O'Brien DJ, Schmitt SM, Fitzgerald SD, Berry DE. Management of bovine tuberculosis in Michigan wildlife: current status and near term prospects. *Vet Microbiol.* (2011) 151:179–87. doi: 10.1016/j.vetmic.2011.02.042
20. Winterstein SR. *Michigan Hunter Opinion Surveys. Report to Michigan Department of Natural Resources*, Wildlife Division. East Lansing, MI: Michigan State Unviersity, Department of Fisheries and Wildlife, (1992).
21. Ramsey DSL, O'Brien DJ, Smith RW, Cosgrove MK, Schmitt SM, Rudolph BA. Management of on-farm risk to livestock from bovine TB in white-tailed deer in Michigan, USA. In: *VI International M. bovis Conference, Animal Health and Veterinary Laboratories Agency & British Cattle Veterinary Association*, Poster abstracts-wildlife reservoirs. Cardiff (2014).
22. Berentsen AR, Miller RS, Misiewicz R, Malmberg JL, Dunbar MR. Characteristics of white-tailed deer visits to cattle farms: implications for disease transmission at the wildlife-livestock interface. *Eur J Wildlife Res.* (2014) 60:161–70. doi: 10.1007/s10344-013-0760-5
23. Ribeiro-Lima J, Carstensen M, Cornicelli L, Forester JD, Wells SJ. Patterns of cattle farm visitation by white-tailed deer in relation to risk of disease transmission in a previously infected area with bovine tuberculosis in minnesota, USA. *Transboun Emerg Dis.* (2017) 64:1519–29. doi: 10.1111/tbed.12544
24. Brook RK. *Historical Review of Elk-agriculture Conflicts in and Around Riding Mountain National Park.* Canada: Human-Wildlife Conflicts (2009) 3:72–87.
25. Brook RK, Vander Wal E, van Beest FM, McLachlan SM. Evaluating use of cattle winter feeding areas by elk and white-tailed deer: implications for managing bovine tuberculosis transmission risk from the ground up. *Prev Vet Med.* (2013) 108:137–47. doi: 10.1016/j.prevetmed.2012.07.017
26. Lavelle MJ, Kay SL, Pepin KM, Grear DA, Campa H, VerCauteren KC. Evaluating wildlife-cattle contact rates to improve the understanding of dynamics of bovine tuberculosis transmission in Michigan, USA. *Prev Vet Med.* (2016) 135:28–36. doi: 10.1016/j.prevetmed.2016.10.009
27. Ramsey DSL, O'Brien DJ, Smith RW, Cosgrove MK, Schmitt SM, Rudolph BA. Management of on-farm risk to livestock from bovine tuberculosis in Michigan, USA, white-tailed deer: Predictions from a spatially-explicit stochastic model. *Prev Vet Med.* (2016) 134:26–38. doi: 10.1016/j.prevetmed.2016.09.022

28. Hickling GJ. *Dynamics of Bovine Tuberculosis in Wild White-tailed Deer in Michigan, Wildlife Division Report No. 3363.* Michigan Department of Natural Resources, Wildlife Division, Lansing, MI. (2002). pp. 34.
29. Michigan Center for Geogrpahic Information, *Michigan (Lower Peninsula) GAP Land Stewardship Coverage* (2001).
30. Cosgrove MK, Campa III H, Schmitt SM, Marks DR, Wilson AS, O'Brien DJ. Live-trapping and bovine tuberculosis testing of free-ranging white-tailed deer for targeted removal. *Wildlife Res.* (2012) 39:104–11. doi: 10.1071/WR11147
31. Cosgrove MK, Campa III H, Ramsey DSL, Schmitt SM, O'Brien DJ. Modeling vaccination and targeted removal of white-tailed deer in Michigan for bovine tuberculosis control. *Wildlife Soc Bull.* (2012) 36:676–84. doi: 10.1002/wsb.217
32. Felix AB, Campa H, Millenbah KF, Winterstein SR, Moritz WE. Development of landscape-scale habitat-potential models for forest wildlife planning and management. *Wildlife Soc Bull.* (2004) 32:795–806. doi: 10.2193/0091-7648(2004)032[0795:DOLHMF]2.0.CO;2
33. Felix AB, Walsh DP, Hughey BD, Campa H, Winterstein SR. Applying landscape-scale habitat-potential models to understand deer spatial structure and movement patterns. *J Wildlife Manage.* (2007)71:804–10. doi: 10.2193/2006-366
34. Winkler R, Warnke K. The future of hunting: an age-period-cohort analysis of deer hunter decline. *Popul Env.* (2013) 34:460–80. doi: 10.1007/s11111-012-0172-6
35. Mattson KM, Moritz WE. Evaluating differences in harvest data used in the sex-age-kill deer population model. *J Wildlife Manage.* (2008) 72:1019–25. doi: 10.2193/2006-219
36. Rudolph BA. *Enforcement, Personal Gains, and Normative Factors Associated With Hunter Compliance and Cooperation With Michigan white-tailed Deer and Bovine Tuberculosis Management Interventions.* Dissertation. Department of Fisheries and Wildlife, Michigan State University, East Lansing, MI. (2012)
37. Brown TL, Decker DJ, Riley SJ, Enck JW, Lauber TB, Curtis PD, et al. The future of hunting as a mechanism to control white-tailed deer populations. *Wildlife Soc Bull.* (2000) 28:797–807. Available online at: https://www-jstor-org.proxy2.cl.msu.edu/stable/3783834
38. Enck JW, Decker DJ, Brown TL. Status of hunter recruitment and retention in the United States. *Wildlife Soc Bull.* (2000) 28:817–24. Available online at: https://www-jstor-org.proxy2.cl.msu.edu/stable/3783836
39. Everett MW, Gore ML. Measuring flow in Michigan youth firearm deer hunters: implications for measurement and practice. *Loisir Soc.-Soc Leis.* (2015) 38:100–9. doi: 10.1080/07053436.2015.1007579
40. Ryan EL, Shaw B. Improving hunter recruitment and retention. *Human Dimens Wildlife* (2011) 16:311–7. doi: 10.1080/10871209.2011.559530
41. Dorn ML, Mertig AG. Bovine tuberculosis in Michigan: stakeholder attitudes and implications for eradication efforts. *Wildlife Soc Bull.* (2005) 33:539–52. doi: 10.2193/0091-7648(2005)33[539:BTIMSA]2.0.CO;2
42. Rudolph BA, Riley SJ, Hickling GJ, Frawley BJ, Garner MS, Winterstein SR. Regulating hunter baiting for white-tailed deer in michigan: biological and social considerations. *Wildlife Soc Bull.* (2006) 34:314–21. doi: 10.2193/0091-7648(2006)34[314:RHBFWD]2.0.CO;2
43. Frawley BJ. *Factors Affecting the Sale of Antlerless Deer Hunting Licenses in the Northeast Lower Peninsula, Wildlife Division Report No. 3373.* Michigan Department of Natural Resources, Lansing, MI. (2002). pp. 18.
44. Frawley BJ. *Michigan Deer Harvest Survey Report - 2001 Seasons, Wildlife Division Report No. 3371.* Michigan Department of Natural Resources, Lansing, MI. (2002). pp. 37.
45. Langeanu E, Flegler EJ, Hill HR. Deer Hunters' Opinion Survey. Wildlife Division Report No. 3012. Lansing, MI: Michigan Department of Natural Resources (1984). pp. 18.
46. Garner MS. *Movement Patterns and Behavior at Winter Feeding and Fall Baiting Stations in a Population of White-tailed Deer Infected With Bovine Tuberculosis in the Northeatstern Lower Peninsula of Michigan.* Dissertation. Department of Fisheries and Wildlife, Michigan State University, East Lansing, Michigan (2001).
47. Mejia-Salazar MF, Waldner CL, Ten Hwang Y, Bollinger TK. Use of environmental sites by mule deer: a proxy for relative risk of chronic wasting disease exposure and transmission. *Ecosphere* (2018) 9:18. doi: 10.1002/ecs2.2055
48. Palmer MV, Whipple DL, Olsen SC. Development of a model of natural infection with *Mycobacterium bovis* in white-tailed deer. *J Wildlife Dis.* (1999) 35:450–7. doi: 10.7589/0090-3558-35.3.450
49. Palmer MV, Waters WR, Whipple DL. Shared feed as a means of deer-to-deer transmission of *Mycobacterium bovis*. *J Wildlife Dis.* (2004) 40:87–91. doi: 10.7589/0090-3558-40.1.87
50. Palmer MV, Whipple DL. Survival of *Mycobacterium bovis* on feedstuffs commonly used as supplemental feed for white-tailed deer (*Odocoileus virginianus*). *J Wildlife Dis.* (2006) 42:853–8. doi: 10.7589/0090-3558-42.4.853
51. Fine AE, Bolin CA, Gardiner JC, Kaneene JB. A study of the persistence of *Mycobacterium bovis* in the environment under natural weather conditions in Michigan, USA. *Vet Med Int.* (2011) 2011:765430. doi: 10.4061/2011/765430
52. Kaneene JB, Hatttey JA, Bolin CA, Averill J, Miller R. Survivability of *Mycobacterium bovis* on salt and salt-mineral blocks fed to cattle. *Am J Vet Res.* (2017) 78:57–62. doi: 10.2460/ajvr.78.1.57
53. Fine AE, O'Brien DJ, Winterstein SR, Kaneene JB. An effort to isolate *Mycobacterium bovis* from environmental substrates during investigations of bovine tuberculosis transmission sites (cattle farms and wildlife areas) in Michigan, USA. *ISRN Vet Sci.* (2011) 2011:787181. doi: 10.5402/2011/787181
54. Barasona JA, Vicente J, Diez-Delgado I, Aznar J, Gortázar C, Torres MJ. Environmental presence of *Mycobacterium tuberculosis* complex in aggregation points at the wildlife/livestock interface. *Transbound Emerg Dis.* (2017) 64:1148–58. doi: 10.1111/tbed.12480
55. Blanchong JA, Scribner KT, Epperson BK, Winterstein SR. Changes in artificial feeding regulations impact white-tailed deer fine-scale spatial genetic structure. *J Wildlife Manage.* (2006) 70:1037–43. doi: 10.2193/0022-541X(2006)70[1037:CIAFRI]2.0.CO;2
56. Forristal VE, Creel S, Taper ML, Scurlock BM, Cross PC. Effects of supplemental feeding and aggregation on fecal glucocorticoid metabolite concentrations in elk. *J Wildlife Manage.* (2012) 76:694–702. doi: 10.1002/jwmg.312
57. Putman RJ, Staines BW. Supplementary winter feeding of wild red deer Cervus elaphus in Europe and North America: justifications, feeding practice and effectiveness. *Mammal Rev.* (2004) 34:285–306. doi: 10.1111/j.1365-2907.2004.00044.x
58. Barasona JA, VerCauteren KC, Saklou N, Gortazar C, Vicente J. Effectiveness of cattle operated bump gates and exclusion fences in preventing ungulate multi-host sanitary interaction. *Prev Vet Med.* (2013) 111:42–50. doi: 10.1016/j.prevetmed.2013.03.009
59. Gortazar C, Diez-Delgado I, Barasona JA, Vicente J, Fuente JDL, Boadella M. The wild side of disease control at the wildlife-livestock-human interface: a review. *Front Vet Sci.* (2015) 1:27. doi: 10.3389/fvets.2014.00027
60. Martinez-Lopez B, Barasona JA, Gortazar C, Rodriguez-Prieto V, Sanchez-Vizcaino JM, Vicente J. Farm-level risk factors for the occurrence, new infection or persistence of tuberculosis in cattle herds from South-Central Spain. *Prev Vet Med.* (2014) 116:268–78. doi: 10.1016/j.prevetmed.2013.11.002

13

Association of *Fasciola gigantica* Co-Infection with Bovine Tuberculosis Infection and Diagnosis in a Naturally Infected Cattle Population

Robert F. Kelly[1,2], Rebecca Callaby[1], Nkongho F. Egbe[3], Diana J. L. Williams[4], Ngu Ngwa Victor[5], Vincent N. Tanya[6], Melissa Sander[7], Lucy Ndip[8], Richard Ngandolo[9], Kenton L. Morgan[10], Ian G. Handel[1,2], Stella Mazeri[1], Adrian Muwonge[1] and Barend M. de C Bronsvoort[1†]*

[1] The Roslin Institute, Royal (Dick) School of Veterinary Studies, University of Edinburgh, Midlothian, United Kingdom, [2] Royal (Dick) School of Veterinary Studies, University of Edinburgh, Midlothian, United Kingdom, [3] Microbiology and Parasitology Unit, Faculty of Allied Medical Science, University of Calabar, Calabar, Nigeria, [4] Veterinary Parasitology, Institute of Infection and Global Health and School of Veterinary Science, Liverpool, United Kingdom, [5] School of Veterinary Medicine and Sciences, University of Ngaoundere, Ngaoundere, Cameroon, [6] Cameroon Academy of Sciences, Yaoundé, Cameroon, [7] Tuberculosis Reference Laboratory Bamenda, Hospital Roundabout, Bamenda, Cameroon, [8] Laboratory of Emerging Infectious Diseases, University of Buea, Buea, Cameroon, [9] Laboratoire de Recherches Vétérinaires et Zootechniques de Farcha, N'Djamena, Chad, [10] Institute of Ageing and Chronic Disease and School of Veterinary Science, University of Liverpool, Neston, United Kingdom

***Correspondence:**
Barend M. de C Bronsvoort
mark.bronsvoort@roslin.ed.ac.uk

† These authors have contributed equally to this work

Bovine tuberculosis (bTB), caused by *Mycobacterium bovis*, remains a major livestock and public health problem in both high and low-income countries. With the current absence of an effective vaccine, control in cattle populations is reliant on regular testing and removal of positive animals. However, surveillance and control are hampered by imperfect diagnostic tests that have poorly described properties in naturally infected populations. Recent research in cattle co-infected with the temperate liver fluke, *Fasciola hepatica*, has raised concerns about the performance of the intradermal skin test in high fluke incidence areas. Further, recent studies of parasitic co-infections have demonstrated their impact on Th1 and Th2 responses, concurrent disease pathology and susceptibility to mycobacterial infections. Here we report for the first time the association of co-infection with the tropical liver fluke, *Fasciola gigantica*, with the presence of bTB-like lesions and the IFN-γ response in naturally infected African cattle. After adjusting for age and sex we observed a complex interaction between fluke status and breed. Fulani cattle had a higher risk of having bTB-like lesions than the mixed breed group. The risk of bTB-like lesions increased in the mixed breed group if they had concurrent evidence of fluke pathology but was less clear in the coinfected Fulani breed. Further, we observed a slight decline in the IFN-γ levels in fluke infected animals. Finally we explored factors associated with IFN-γ false negative results compared to the presence of bTB-like lesions. Fulani cattle had a higher risk of having a false negative result compared to the mixed breed group. Further, the mixed breed cattle had an increased risk of being false negative if also co-infected with fluke. Interesting, as with the risk of bTB-like lesions, this association was less clear in the Fulani cattle with weak evidence of a slight decrease in risk of having a false negative test result when fluke pathology positive. This interesting interaction where different breeds appear to have different responses to co-infections is intriguing but further work is needed to confirm and understand more clearly the possible confounding effects of different other co-infections not measured here, breed, management or exposure risks.

Keywords: bovine tuberculosis, *M. bovis*, co-infection, *F. gigantica*, fasciolosis, Cameroon, diagnostic tests, interferon-γ

INTRODUCTION

In natural populations, individuals are usually infected with multiple pathogens, also known as "co-infections," rather than single infections (1). In the presence of multiple co-infections, the immune response observed to an individual pathogen, across a population, is variable. This has been shown to depend on the combination of infections and their differing interactions with the host immune system and other infections (2). Like many infectious diseases, *Mycobacterium bovis* infection has been studied in isolation until relatively recently. Co-infections with *Fasiola hepatica* have been implicated as a potential reason for poor bTB diagnostic test performance and disagreement between tests (3). More specifically, co-infections with *F. hepatica* have been shown to down-regulate the Th1 responses (with a resultant dampening of the IFN-γ response), with subsequent predominance of Th2 responses, in order for the parasite to survive and reproduce (4–8).

Bovine tuberculosis (bTB), caused by the bacterium *M. bovis*, is both a major veterinary and public health disease of cattle and other livestock. It is an important zoonosis (9, 10) causing pulmonary and extra-pulmonary disease in people and is responsible for an estimated 3% of human tuberculosis globally (11) amounting to an estimated 147,000 zoonotic cases per year, of which 70,000 are in sub-Saharan Africa (www.who.int/tb/areas-of-work/zoonotic-tb/en/). In many high-income countries, such as the United Kingdom and New Zealand, compulsory bTB "test and slaughter" programs coupled with compensation have been successful in reducing transmission of *M. bovis* in livestock populations (12–14). Diagnostic testing involves detection of immune responses in the early stages of infection, such as dominant Th1 responses (15), to remove bTB positive animals as soon possible. Ante-mortem diagnostic tests, such as the single intradermal comparative cervical test (SICCT) or the interferon-γ (IFN-γ) assay, are based on detecting the Th1 immune response to *M. bovis* (16). However, the variable sensitivity of the SICCT (55.1-93.5%) and the IFN-γ assay (73-100%), which rely on detecting this Th1 response, particularly in late stage disease when a Th2 immune response dominates, can lead to false negative cattle persisting within the population (17) resulting in continuing transmission and larger outbreaks.

Although the co-infection relationship has yet to be fully elucidated, various studies have demonstrated that *F. hepatica* co-infection is associated with a reduced Th1 immune response (3) and a reduced mycobacterial burden (18), which potentially leads to the underestimation of bTB prevalence (19). This is particularly important when using the IFN-γ assay to detect bTB positive cattle. IFN-γ is a cytokine which is produced as part of the Th1 immune response to *M. bovis* infection (20). It has been demonstrated that *F. hepatica* infections down-regulate IFN-γ pro-inflammatory cytokine responses in favor of Th2 cytokine induction and an IgG1 response (21). When using the IFN-γ assay to detect bTB infected animals, the presence of *F. hepatica* co-infection can lead to a reduction in IFN-γ response below the diagnostic test cut-off leading to false negative results (22). However, the extent of bTB misdiagnosis using the IFN-γ assay in bTB endemic cattle populations co-infected with other *Fasciola* species, remains unquantified. In addition, although similar immune evasion and modulation strategies to *F. hepatica* have been identified in bovine *F. gigantica* infections, the effect of co-infection with *F. gigantica* on bTB immune responses has been minimally investigated (23).

This paper reports the first study of co-infection with *F. gigantica* (23) in bTB infected cattle under natural conditions in a tropical African population. Bovine tuberculosis (24–26) and *F. gigantica* (27–29) infections are endemic in cattle populations in Cameroon and are currently poorly controlled, providing an opportunity to study their interaction within a natural transmission setting. The data used for this analysis were a subset of data that were generated from a larger study of *M. bovis* epidemiology in Cameroonian cattle (26, 29, 30). We describe the association of *F. gigantica* co-infection with the presence of observable bTB-like lesions and diagnostic test results using the IFN-γ assay.

METHODS

Abattoir Cross-Sectional Study

Data were collected at the Ngaoundere municipal abattoir in the Adamawa Region, a major cattle-producing area of Cameroon (**Figure 1**). The details of study design and sample collection are reported elsewhere (26) and were based on collection of bTB-like lesion material for culture. In brief, based on previous estimates of bTB-like lesions from the North West Region of Cameroon (31) we assumed a prevalence of lesions of ~5% and calculated a target sample size of ~1000 cattle to ensure recovery of at least 25 isolates assuming a 50% recovery from culture. This would allow the within abattoir prevalence of 5% to be estimated with a precision of ±1.3% at 95% confidence. During sampling, cattle were cast for slaughter by the butchers, after which the

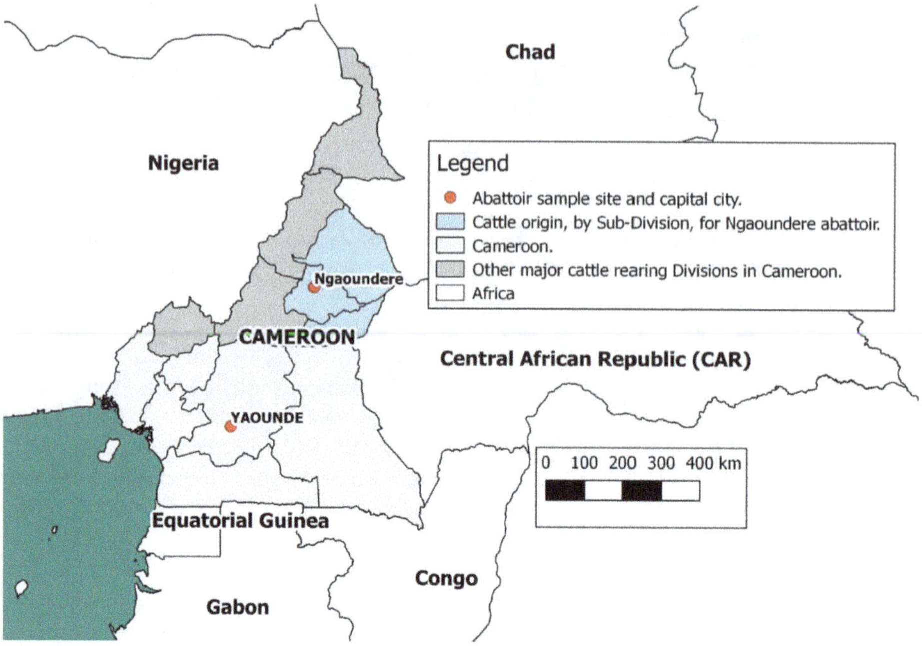

FIGURE 1 | Map of Cameroon showing the location of the Ngaoundere abattoir and the catchment areas of cattle feeding into it. This figure was generated using QGIS 2.2 and shp files obtained from the GADM database of Global Administrative Areas.

research team tagged the animal, collected a heparinized blood sample and recorded animal-level data on owner/butcher, sex, breed as reported by the butcher, dentition score (DS) as an estimation of age (32) and market of origin as reported by the butcher. Post mortem meat inspection was carried out by local Ministry of Livestock, Fisheries and Industrial Agriculture (MINEPIA) inspectors who examined the carcass and offal for presence of granulomatous bTB-like lesions and evidence of liver damage/cirrhosis. Once identified by the veterinary inspectors, the research team collected up to 3 macroscopic bTB-like lesions from different anatomical sites per animal into sterile 25ml universal tubes using forceps and scalpel blades. Lesion grades were also recorded following identification and tissue samples taken (33, 34). Matching numbered tags issued by the research team were used to link animal data, blood samples, meat inspection of the carcass, offal (including the liver) and head. In addition to the tissue samples for culture from animals with lesions, a number of animals classed as non-lesioned by the meat inspectors were randomly sampled (using random number generator www.Random.org) and a single retropharyngeal lymph node per animal collected for culture as controls.

Tissue samples (lesioned lymph nodes) were stored in the vapor phase in liquid nitrogen dry shippers (Taylor-Wharton) and shipped to the Tuberculosis Reference Laboratory (TBRL) Bamenda. Upon arrival at the TBRL the samples were stored at -80°C until processed. Heparinised blood samples were stored in a coolbox at the abattoir (ranging between 10°C to 26°C) and then taken to the lab and kept at room temperature prior to being stimulated in the IFN-γ assay (Bovigam®) described below. Animal data recorded on paper in the abattoir, was transferred to a relational Microsoft Access database where the results could be linked back to individual animals.

Diagnostic Tests

Fasciola Pathology at Meat Inspection

All carcases were inspected for evidence of *F. gigantica* infection by MINEPIA meat inspectors. The meat inspectors examined the liver systematically to identify gross pathology associated with *Fasciola* infection by slicing down the common bile duct with an additional 1–2 slices through the liver parenchyma. Once an animal was identified to have gross fasciolosis related pathology, the liver was graded by a member of the research team and scored 0–3 (35). A score of 0 = no visible pathology; 1 = low grade pathology with minimal damage to the parenchyma of the liver through migratory fibrotic/ cirrhotic tracts from the parasite, thickening of bile ducts with a few *F. gigantica* parasites noted in bile ducts; 2 = moderate grade pathology with *F. gigantica* species parasites found in the bile ducts and up to approximately half the liver having evidence of fibrosis/ cirrhosis; 3 = severe grade pathology with the majority of the liver is noted to have extensive fibrosis/ cirrhosis without having to cut the surface of the liver. For this analysis the score was converted into a presence (positive) or absence (negative) of *F. gigantica* pathology for subsequent analysis.

Mycobacterial Culture and Typing

The tissue samples were prepared and cultured as previously described (26) following the World Organization of Animal Health (OIE) guidelines with minor modifications. Briefly, samples were processed, inoculated into a Mycobacterial Growth

Indicator Tubes (MGIT) and incubated for 8 weeks on the BACTEC MGIT 960 automated culture system (Becton, Dickinson and Company, 1 Becton Drive, Franklin Lakes, NJ, USA) following the manufacturer's instructions. A further 2 cultures were prepared by inoculating 0.1 ml (2 drops) of prepared sample onto each of two Lowenstein Jensen (LJ) slopes (one supplemented with pyruvate and the other with glycerol). These were observed weekly for up to 12 weeks. A smear was made with 3% formal saline from any observed growth on the LJ media and any MGIT indicated positive tube. The smears were heat-fixed, stained by the Ziehl-Neelsen (ZN) method (36) and microscopically observed for the presence of acid fast bacilli (AFB). All acid fast bacilli were typed using the Hain GenoType® MTBC assay and GenoType® Mycobacterium CM/AS kit (Hain Lifescience®,GmbH, Nehren, Germany) (26). Animals were classed as confirmed bTB cases (as opposed to having a bTB-like lesion) if one or more lesions were positive by one or more culture methods confirmed by the Hain Genotype® test.

Interferon-Gamma Assay

The IFN-γ ELISA (Bovigam®) was conducted as per published protocol (37, 38). Briefly within 6–12 h of collection three aliquots of heparinised blood, per animal, were incubated with either avian PPD, bovine PPD (Prionics® Lelystad Tuberculin PPD) or PBS for 24 h at 37°C in a portable polystyrene egg incubator (http://www.theincubatorshop.co.uk) run in the field. Following incubation samples were centrifuged at 300g for 10 minutes, the plasma was aliquotted and stored at −20°C in a portable travel freezer (Waeco CF50 12V/240 fridge freezer)). Plasma samples were transported at −20°C to the LEID and the IFN-γ ELISA was conducted as per the published protocol. The acceptable averaged negative bovine OD value was <0.130 and positive bovine control was >0.700. Animals with a bovine stimulated sample optical density of ≥0.1 above that of the avian PPD sample were classified as test positive and interpreted as the animal being infected with *M. bovis*.

Statistical Analysis

The proportions of cattle with bTB-like lesions, a positive IFN-γ result and liver fluke pathology were calculated and various co-infection definitions were explored using *Fasciola* pathology and one of the bTB outcomes (positive IFN-γ, bTB-like lesion or *M. bovis* culture positive).

Multivariable logistic regression (MLR) models were developed to explore the association between fluke infection and bTB status using a number of different definitions including IFN-γ, bTB-like lesion and *M. bovis* culture results. Animal-level explanatory variables (breed, dentition score and sex) were always included in the models as fixed effects to control for confounding. Model selection was based on the AIC and the best model was selected using the lowest AIC and ΔAIC (39). MLR models were constructed using the *brglm* function in the *brglm* package (40) with AIC and ΔAIC calculated using the *modavg* function from the *AICcmodavg* package (41). Predicted probabilities and their standard errors were calculated from each model for specific covariate patterns using the *predict* function and used to produce 95% confidence intervals for plotting.

Some variables were simplified due to small numbers of observations in some categories. The dentition score (DS) was simplified from number of permanent teeth to a binary age category based on the approximate relationship between age and eruption of permanent incisors in cattle. DS <2 was categorized as "<3 years old" and DS of ≥2 was categorized as "≥3 years old." The breed variable was simplified to "mixed" (collapsing mixed breed, where the butchers were unsure of the breed cross and Gudali to a single category) or "Fulani" (collapsing Red and White Fulani to a single category).

RESULTS

Summary Statistics

During a 4 week period in August 2013, 935 cattle were examined at the Ngaoundere abattoir. The details of bacterial culture results have been presented elsewhere (26). A total of 173 records were dropped due to missing data (at random) due to the hectic nature of the sampling in the abattoir environment which resulted in occasional failure to collect a blood sample or link samples to a carcass. A further 30 animals from one day were dropped from this analysis due to missing IFN-γ results giving a final dataset of 732 animals.

During the sampling period 10.7% (78/732) of animals had visible bTB-like lesions observed. The proportion of animals with evidence of liver fluke infection was 49.6% (363/732) and the proportion of animals positive by the IFN-γ assay was 6.6% (48/732). The distribution of the prevalances of bTB-like lesion, liver fluke pathology and IFN-γ based on animal dentition (as a measurable proxy for age) are given in **Figure 2**. Exploratory bivariate relationships between the variables of interest (age, breed, sex, lesion status, fluke status and IFN-γ status) were checked prior to inclusion in the multivariable models (**Figure 3A**). Breed and fluke status were strongly associated with presence of visible bTB-like lesions and breed was strongly associated with IFN-γ status. There was an association between breed and the ordinal distribution of fluke pathology scores (χ^2 test p-value <0.001) but the odds ratios did not change across pathology scores above zero so the effect is captured by collapsing the fluke score into a binary variable (**Figure 3B**).

Association of *F. gigantica* Co-infection With Bovine Tuberculosis-Like Lesions

A multivariable logistic regression (MLR) model of the association between visible lesion and fluke status was developed (**Table 1**). This suggests a complex interaction between breed and *F. gigantica* pathology status with the probability of observing visible TB-like lesions in cattle in this setting. Fulani cattle had a higher risk of having observable bTB-like lesions than the mixed breed group. However, the risk in the mixed breed group increased if they also had fluke pathology. This association ith fluke pathology was less clear in Fulani cattle. For example, an adult, female, mixed breed animal, that had no fluke pathology had a ∼ 5.2% (95% CI: 2.5–7.8) probability of having a TB-like lesion compared to ∼ 27.7% (95% CI: 16.8–38.4) for a Fulani animal (**Figure 5A**). The presence of fluke increased this risk in mixed breed animals to ∼ 12.0% (95% CI: 7.7–16.3) while the

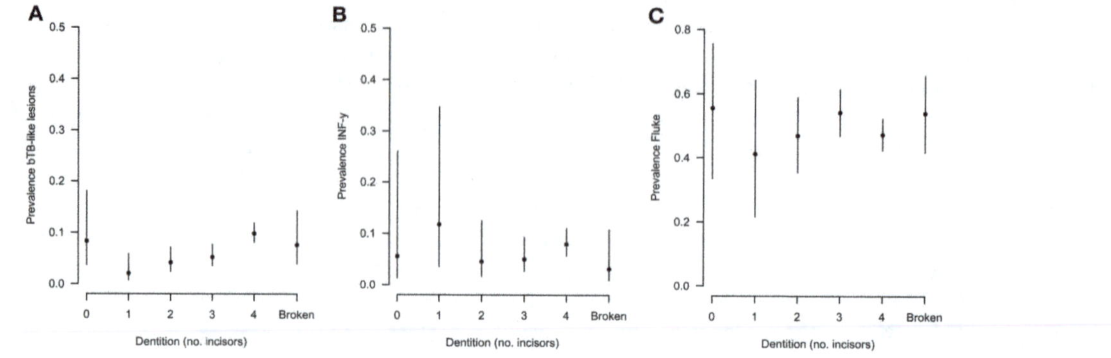

FIGURE 2 | Distribution of **(A)** lesion, **(B)** fluke, and **(C)** IFN-γ prevalences based on animal dentition for Ngaoundere abattoir ($n = 732$).

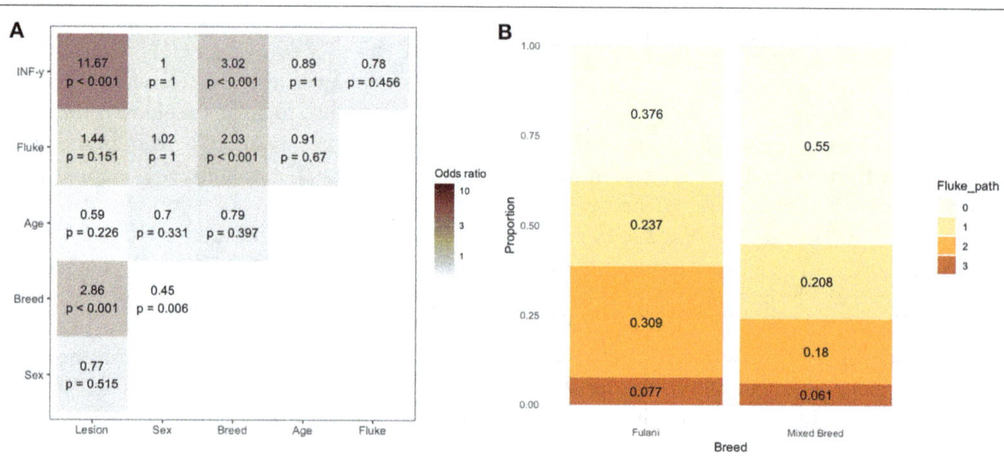

FIGURE 3 | (A) Bivariable odds ratios and *p*-values for pairwise associations of variables of interest for inclusion in multivariable models. **(B)** Proportion of Fulani ($n = 194$) and mixed breed ($n = 538$) classified cattle sampled in Ngaoundere abattoir by *F. gigantica* pathology score. Legend: Lesion, lesion status (positive/negative); sex, male/female; Breed, Fulani/mixed; Age, <3 years/≥3 years; Fluke, fluke pathology status (positive/negative); IFN-γ, IFN-γ test positive/negative.

risk declined (although the evidence is weaker) in Fulani cattle to ~ 15.6% (95% CI: 8.8–22.2). The age and sex terms were included to control for confounding but do not appear to be important for this model.

Impact of *F. gigantica* co-infection on IFN-Gamma Responses

The association between IFN-γ result and *F. gigantica* pathology status was investigated. The raw PPD-B minus PPD-A difference in ELISA OD readings were explored in the subset of animals which were confirmed *M. bovis* culture positive (n = 53). The raw difference is plotted, stratified by *F. gigantica* pathology status in **Figure 4** where there is some evidence of a dampening of the IFN-γ response with a smaller variance in the fluke pathology positive group. When the outlying high value for the fluke pathology positive group is removed the variances are statistically significantly different (Mann-Whitney test $p < 0.001$, $n = 52$).

A multivariable linear regression model of the raw PPD-B minus PPD-A difference was developed (with the outlying value dropped) and after accounting for age, sex and breed there was a small mean decrease in the difference of −0.02 (−0.04 to 0.00) in OD value in the fluke pathology positive animals (**Table 2**). A multivariable logistic regression model for IFN-γ binary test

TABLE 1 | Multivariable logistic regression model for the presence of TB lesions at slaughter ($n = 732$).

Variable	Levels	Odds ratio	95% CI
Sex	Female	1	
	Male	1.17	0.50–2.47
Age	≥3 years	1.00	
	<3 years	0.60	0.25–1.26
Breed	Mixed	1	
	Fulani	7.00	3.36–14.95
Fluke	Negative	1	
	Positive	2.51	1.32–4.98
Breed*Fluke		0.19	0.07–0.51

*Key: Lesion, TB lesion result (Positive or negative); Sex, Sex of cattle (Male or Female); Age, Age of cattle by dentition score (<3 years or ≥3 years); Fluke, F. gigantica pathology score; Breed, Breed of cattle (Mixed breed or Fulani breed); *Interaction between variables.*

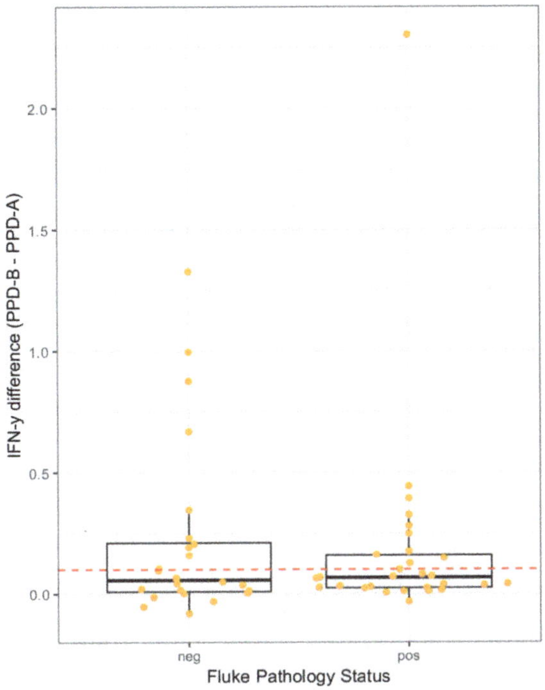

FIGURE 4 | IFN-γ response (PPD-B minus PPD-A) stratified by *F. gigantica* pathology status (neg, no pathology; pos, evidence of fluke pathology) in the subset of *M. bovis* culture positive cattle ($n = 53$). Individual cattle; Orange circles. Dashed red line IFN-γ recommended test cut-off of 0.1.

TABLE 2 | Multivariable regression model for the raw IFN-γ PPD-B minus PPD-A difference ($n = 731$).

Variable	Levels	Coef	95% CI
Sex	Female	1	
	Male	–0.01	–0.46 to 0.02
Age	≥3 years	1	
	<3 years	–0.01	–0.31 to 0.02
Breed	Mixed	1.00	
	Fulani	0.02	0.13 to 1.46
Fluke	Negative	1	
	Positive	–0.02	–1.92 to 0.01

Key: IFN-γ, IFN-γ assay result (PPD-B - PPD-A); Sex, Sex of cattle (Male or Female); Age, Age of cattle by dentition score (<3 years or ≥3 years); Fluke, F. gigantica pathology score; Breed, Breed of cattle (Mixed breed or Fulani breed).

TABLE 3 | Multivariable logistic regression model for the raw IFN-γ PPD-B minus PPD-A difference (n=731).

Variable	Levels	Odds ratio	95% CI
Sex	Female	1	
	Male	0.91	0.28–2.29
Age	≥3 years	1	
	<3 years	0.99	0.38–2.22
Breed	Mixed	1.00	
	Fulani	3.18	1.73–5.85
Fluke	Negative	1	
	Positive	0.62	0.33–1.13

Key: IFN-γ, IFN-γ assay result (Positive or negative); Sex, Sex of cattle (Male or Female); Age, Age of cattle by dentition score (<3 years or ≥3 years); Fluke, F. gigantica pathology score; Breed, Breed of cattle (Mixed breed or Fulani breed).

status and fluke pathology status was also developed including age, breed and sex as potential confounders (**Table 3**). Both these regression models give some weak support for an association between the IFN-γ result and *F. gigantica* pathology status, with fluke pathology positive cattle more likely to have a lower OD value difference and to be IFN-γ negative. The association using the binary test results suggest an adult, female, mixed breed cow had a ∼ 5.6% (95%: 3.1–8.1) probability of testing positive which dropped to ∼ 3.5% (95%: 1.7-5.6) if infected with liver fluke compared to a Fulani, adult, female animal which had a ∼ 16.3% (95%: 8.7–24.0) of testing positive which dropped to ∼ 11.1% (95%: 5.9–16.2) if fluke pathology positive (**Figure 5B**).

Factors Associated With a False Negative IFN-γ Test Result When Compared to TB-Like Lesion

Using the subset of results where the IFN-γ test result was negative ($n = 684$) a new variable was generated where a IFN-γ test result was classified as a false negative if there was an observed bTB-like lesion ($n = 54$) and true negative if there was no lesion observed ($n = 630$). A multivariable logistic regression analysis to explore the association with fluke pathology was conducted including sex, age and breed as confounders. In addition, for this model the presence or absence of non-tubercular mycobacteria (NTM), based on the Haines typing from cultured samples from lesions, was also included as a known potential confounder for being lesion positive but test negative. The final model is given in **Table 4**. Again the best fitting model includes an interaction between fluke pathology status and breed. The baseline probability of being a false negative IFN-γ test result in adult, female, non-tubercular mycobacterium negative (NTM), fluke pathology negative mixed breed cows was ∼ 4.3% (95%: 1.9–6.7) which increased to ∼ 10.4% (95%: 6.3–14.5) if they had fluke pathology. In comparison IFN-γ test negative Fulani cattle had a ∼ 16.0% (95%: 6.3–25.6) probability of being a false negative which declined to ∼ 8.5% (95%: 3.1–14.0) if fluke pathology positive (**Figure 5C**). An NTM infection also was also associated with a large increased risk of giving a false negative IFN-γ result.

DISCUSSION

It is well recognized, though still poorly studied, that co-infecting pathogens can have a range of synergistic or antagonist effects. For example, (42) showed African buffalo co-infected with strongyle nematodes had a dampened Th1 response which facilitated bTB invasion and establishment of infection. Interactions between bovine tuberculosis and the temperate liver fluke *F. hepatica* have been shown in the United Kingdom (3, 19)

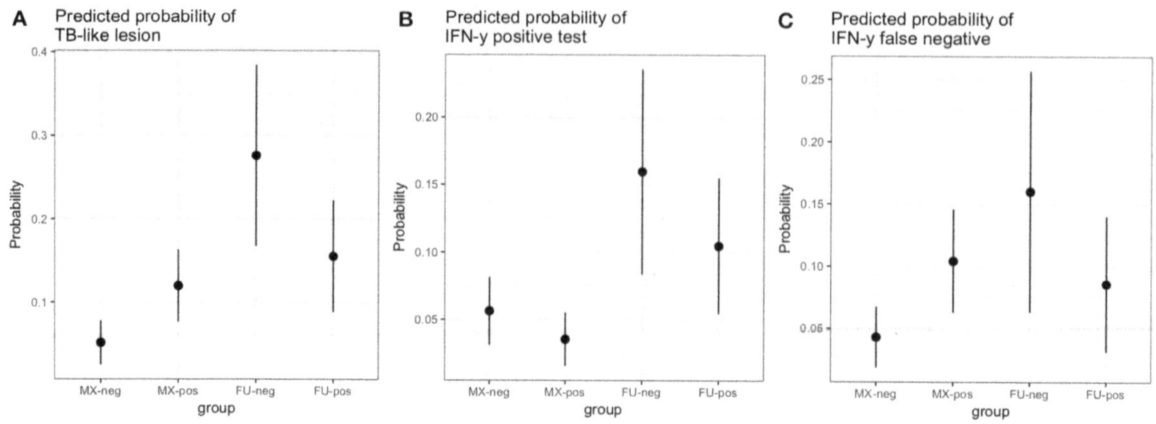

FIGURE 5 | Predicted probabilities for an adult female animal by breed (MX, mixed breed; FU, Fulani) and fluke status (neg, no fluke pathology; pos, evidence of fluke pathology) based on the logistic regression models described in the results section.

TABLE 4 | Multivariable logistic regression model ($n = 684$) for being IFN-γ false negative result conditioned on having a negative IFN-γ test result and using observable TB-like lesions as the true state (gold standard).

Variable	Level	Odds ratio	95% CI
Sex	Female	1	
	Male	0.97	0.31–2.46
Age	≥3 years	1	
	<3 years	0.68	0.24–1.57
NTM	Negative	1	
	Positive	15.29	3.32–75.7
Breed	Mixed	1	
	Fulani	4.23	1.68–10.44
Fluke	Negative	1	
	Positive	2.59	1.28–5.49
Breed*Fluke		0.19	0.06–0.64

*Key: Lesion, TB lesion result (Positive or negative); Sex, Sex of cattle (Male or Female); Age, Age of cattle by dentition score (<3 years or ≥3 years); Fluke, F. gigantica pathology score; Breed, Breed of cattle (Mixed breed or Fulani breed); NTM, non-tubercular mycobacterium; *Interaction between variables.*

but less is known about the interactions of bovine tuberculosis and the tropical fluke *F. gigantica*. Despite the ecological, genetic and antigen differences between these two species, both species appear to evade and modulate the host immune response to infection (43). Here we have examined the association between both bTB-like lesion occurrence and the Bovigam (*M. bovis specific*) IFN-γ response in a naturally *F. gigantica* infected cattle population in Africa.

The levels of fluke infection were very high in this abattoir population with nearly 50% of animals showing liver pathology consistent with fluke infections and/or adult fluke identified in the bile ducts. Previous studies have identified an association with visible bTB-like lesions and being fluke positive in slaughter cattle populations such as in Zambia (44). Further, in experimental infections in mice it has been shown that mice infected with *M. tuberculosis* have higher bacterial loads and TB lesion pathology when co-infected with the trematode *S. mansoni* (45). It is proposed that the fluke infection suppresses the Th1 response resulting in a reduced level of IFN-γ. In cattle, previous studies have reported that co-infection results in a lower bacterial load but no qualitative or quantitative differences in tuberculous lesions of *M. bovis* (18).

In the present study, we observed a complex interaction between cattle breed and liver fluke pathology status and the presence of visible bTB-like lesions. There is strong support for an increased risk of having bTB-like lesions in Fulani cattle compared to the mixed breed group. In Cameroon, Fulani cattle have been reported to have a higher prevalence of bTB than other breeds (31) but this study was from the Northwest Region. One explanation may be to do with differing responses in different cattle/host genotypes. It has been reported in the UK that Holstein cattle with the INRA111 genotype appeared to be less likely to develop bTB (46). Similarly, in Ethiopia comparing Holstein cattle and indigenous zebu *B. indicus* cattle, researchers found that Holstein cattle were more susceptible (33).

The presence of fluke pathology in the mixed breed group was associated with an increased risk of visible lesions. In Fulani cattle, which are more likely to have bTB-like lesions, co-infection with fluke was not associated with an increased risk but potentially a reduced probability of having visible bTB-like lesions, although the evidence was weak for this association in Fulani cattle. Our study relied on the butchers classification of breed recorded in the hectic environment of the slaughterhouse. There is the possibility that their classification was incorrect in some cases, however, this is more likely to reduce the chances of observing an association. To improve on this we are currently genotyping the subset of cattle from which we collected lymph nodes for culture (both lesioned and the random sample of non-lesioned lymph nodes). Alternatively, the breed association may be due to confounding by other unobserved variables such as differing management between breeds or differences in exposures interacting with different genotypes of *M. bovis*. However, these are more difficult to untangle.

The IFN-γ assay is particularly useful to detect early (1-4 weeks post infection) *M. bovis* infections as part of control programs often in combination with the SICCT (20, 47). Previous studies have demonstrated that *F. hepatica* co-infection can down-regulate IFN-γ responses to *M. bovis* infection (21, 22). In this African cattle population there was weak evidence of a reduced IFN-γ response (reduced variance in the raw PPD-B - PPD-A value) in fluke infected animals conditional on having been bTB culture positive. This reduction in IFN-γ was also weakly observed in the linear regression analysis (on the continuous test result) and in the logistic regression analysis (on the binary result). However, we did observed a moderate association between increased IFN-γ levels and breed, with Fulani cattle having a higher probability of testing positive. Given the higher rates of infection observed in the lesion data, this is not surprising. This represents relatively weak evidence for a decline in test sensitivity in fluke infected animals and increased risk of leaving potential bTB positive animals in a herd. However, the prevalence of bTB was relatively low in this relatively small study, meaning the power to detect these effects is less than ideal and further larger studies are needed to confirm these findings.

In order to further explore this potential decline in test sensitivity, we looked at the subset of IFN-γ test negative animals (based on the binary cut-off of 0.1 as recommended by the manufacturers). Using visible bTB-like lesions as the comparison test, which we know from culture results from these cattle is reasonably specific (sp=69.7%) and sensitive (95.8%), (with a positive predictive value of 65.1% and negative predictive value of 96.6% calculated from (30) for this sample), we looked at factors associated with false negative results in the IFN-γ negative subset of animals. The risk of false negative results was strongly associated with NTM infections. This is to be expected as we know that lesions are an imperfect predictor of *M. bovis* and that a number of these animals with lesions had NTMs based on culture results (30). Interestingly, having accounted for a major source of the disagreement, there again remained a complex interaction between breed and fluke status. In the mixed breed animals the risk of being a false negative increased from $\sim$ 4% to $\sim$ 10% consistent with suppression of the Th1 response by fluke infections. Also Fulani cattle had higher rates of false positives compared to the mixed breed group but Fulani cattle with fluke pathology had a drop in risk from $\sim$ 16% to $\sim$ 8.5%, although the statistical support for this decline is weak. Again, this may be due to different host genetics, management or exposures and needs further investigation.

More work is needed to understand these interactions between co-infecting pathogens. Variation in immune interaction of the host, with *M. bovis* and *Fasciola gigantica*, at different stages in the pathogenesis of one pathogen may affect the pathogenesis of the other (48, 49). One possible explanation for this complexity may be that we have not accounted for other confounding co-infections. Conducting studies to look at all possible co-infections can become extremely complex, expensive and logistically challenging (50). There have been a number of co-infection studies including nematode infections in buffalo (42) and fluke in cattle (19) with evidence of associations with bTB-like lesions or interference with IFN-γ test results, however, a recent paper failed to find a statistical association with fluke or bovine viral infections (51) in European cattle, although they did find an association with paratuberculosis co-infections, which were associated with an increased probability of observing visible bTB-like lesions.

It is clear that co-infections can have complex impacts on test diagnostics and pathogen invasion and this may have important implications for control programmes. As one bacillus is sufficient to establish *M. bovis* infection within a host (52), leaving any infected animals behind in a control programme has the potential to maintain transmission and there was evidence here that in the mixed breed group at least, fluke infections were associated with an increased risk of a false negative IFN-γ result. Certainly, test and slaughter programs are likely to continue to play their part in bTB control in high income settings and certain wildlife control settings. Mitigating against *Fasciola spp.* co-infections (or other co-infections such as paratuberculosis) or being able to incorporate the likely impact on test performance may improve ante-mortem diagnostic test sensitivity within cattle or wildlife populations.

In conclusion, this study explored the association between co-infection with the tropical liver fluke *F. gigantica* on the pathology and detection of *M. bovis* infections in a natural ecological setting in African cattle. We have shown a complex association between the presence of visible bTB-like lesions in carcasses and the presence of concurrent *Fasciola* infections which appears to be also affected by breed. Furthermore, we have shown that the IFN-γ response may be slightly dampened down in *F. gigantica* infected cattle although further data are needed to confirm this. However, it does appear to be sufficient to increase the false negative risk in the mixed breed group at lest in this population. The reduction in sensitivity of the IFN-γ assay by *Fasciola spp.* co-infection could have profound effects on bTB control and eradication programs as *Fasciola spp.* are present worldwide (53). Given the complexity of determining whether animals are truly *M. bovis* infected, there is a need to develop more subtle and sophisticated algorithms for interpretation of individual animal bTB diagnostic test results that use the raw test readings as well as other animal and related herd variables.

ETHICS STATEMENT

This study did not involve the experimental use of any live vertebrate but reports the results of a pre-slaughter blood sampling and post mortem examinations of cattle for bovine tuberculosis carried out by the local veterinary inspectors in a commercial abattoir in Cameroon. Samples for culture were collected from carcases in accordance with best practice guidelines to minimize contamination. Local approval was given by the Head of Epidemiology at the Ministry of Livestock, Fisheries and Animal Industries responsible for supervision of activities at commercial slaughterhouses in each administrative Division. This project and the protocols had ethical approval from the University of Edinburgh Ethical Review Committee (Animal (Scientific Procedures) Act, 1986) (ERC No: OS02-13).

AUTHOR CONTRIBUTIONS

BB, RK, LN, VT, KM, RN, MS, and NE: conceived and designed the study; RK, SM, NV, NE, and AM: performed the field work; RK, BB, IH, SM, and RC: analyzed the data; RK, BB, IH, SM, MS, and DW: contributed reagents, expertise, materials, analysis tools; RK and BB: wrote the first draft paper; All authors read and contributed to the final draft of the paper.

ACKNOWLEDGEMENTS

The authors thank the Wellcome Trust (WT094945) for funding this research project. BB also thanks the BBSRC for their support through the Institute Strategic Programme (BB/J004235/1).The funders had no role in study design, data collection and analysis, decision to publish, or preparation of the manuscript. Importantly we would like to thank all the cattle keepers, the butchers and their staff in the abattoirs, the MINEPIA veterinary center staff and delegates without whom this study would not have been possible.

REFERENCES

1. Cox FEG. Concomitant infections, parasites and immune responses. *Parasitology* (2011) 122:S23–S38.
2. Vaumourin E, Vourc'h G, Gasqui P, Vayssier-Taussat M. The importance of multiparasitism: examining the consequences of co-infections for human and animal health. *Parasit Vectors* 8:545. doi: 10.1186/s13071-015-1167-9
3. Flynn RJ, Mulcahy G, Elsheikha HM. Coordinating innate and adaptive immunity in *Fasciola hepatica* infection: implications for control. *Vet Parasitol.* (2010) 169:235–40. doi: 10.1016/j.vetpar.2010.02.015
4. Brady MT, Neill SMO, Dalton JP, Mills KHG. *Fasciola hepatica* suppresses a Protective Th1 Response against *Bordetella pertussis Fasciola hepatica* suppresses a protective Th1 Response against *Bordetella pertussis. Infect Immun.* (1999)67:5372–8.
5. O'Neill SM, Mills KHG, Dalton JP. *Fasciola hepatica* cathepsin L cysteine proteinase suppresses Bordetella pertussis-specific interferon-gamma production *in vivo*. *Paras Immunol.* (2001) 23:541–7. doi: 10.1046/j.1365-3024.2001.00411.x
6. Donnelly S, O'Neill SM, Sekiya M, Mulcahy G, Dalton JP. Thioredoxin peroxidase secreted by *Fasciola hepatica* induces the alternative activation of macrophages. *Infect Immun.* (2005) 73:166–73. doi: 10.1128/IAI.73.1.166-173.2005
7. Flynn RJ, Irwin JA, Olivier M, Sekiya M, Dalton JP, Mulcahy G. Alternative activation of ruminant macrophages by *Fasciola hepatica*. *Veter Immunol Immunopathol.* (2007) 120:31–40. doi: 10.1016/j.vetimm.2007.07.003
8. Flynn RJ, Mulcahy G. The roles of IL-10 and TGF-β in controlling IL-4 and IFN-γ production during experimental *Fasciola hepatica* infection. *Int J Parasitol.* (2008)38:1673–80. doi: 10.1016/j.ijpara.2008.05.008
9. O'Reilly LM, Daborn CJ. The epidemiology of *Mycobacterium bovis* infections in animals and man: a review. *Tubercle Lung Dis.* (1995) 76(Suppl. 1):1–46. doi: 10.1016/0962-8479(95)90591-X
10. Thoen C, Lobue P, de Kantor I. The importance of *Mycobacterium bovis* as a zoonosis. *Veter Microbiol.* (2006) 112:339–45. doi: 10.1016/j.vetmic.2005.11.047
11. Cosivi O, Grange JM, Daborn CJ, Raviglione MC, Fujikura T, Cousins D, et al. Zoonotic tuberculosis due to *Mycobacterium bovis* in developing countries. *Emerging Infect Dis.* (1999)4:59–70. doi: 10.3201/eid0401.980108
12. Palmer MV, Waters WR. Advances in bovine tuberculosis diagnosis and pathogenesis: what policy makers need to know. *Veter Microbiol.* (2006) 112:181–90. doi: 10.1016/j.vetmic.2005.11.028
13. Torgerson PR, Torgerson DJ. Public health and bovine tuberculosis : what's all the fuss about? (2009):67–72. doi: 10.1016/j.tim.2009.11.002
14. Bezos J, Casal C, Romero B, Schroeder B, Hardegger R, Raeber AJ, et al. Current ante-mortem techniques for diagnosis of bovine tuberculosis. *Res Veter Sci.* (2014) 97(Suppl.):S44–52. doi: 10.1016/j.rvsc.2014.04.002
15. McNair J, Welsh MD, Pollock JM. The immunology of bovine tuberculosis and progression toward improved disease control strategies. *Vaccine* (2007)25:5504–11. doi: 10.1016/j.vaccine.2007.02.037
16. de la Rua-Domenech R, Goodchild aT, Vordermeier HM, Hewinson RG, Christiansen KH, Clifton-Hadley RS. Ante mortem diagnosis of tuberculosis in cattle: a review of the tuberculin tests, gamma-interferon assay and other ancillary diagnostic techniques. *Res Veter Sci.* (2006) 81:190–210. doi: 10.1016/j.rvsc.2005.11.005
17. Schiller I, Oesch B, Vordermeier HM, Palmer MV, Harris BN, Orloski Ka, et al. *Bovine tuberculosis*: a review of current and emerging diagnostic techniques in view of their relevance for disease control and eradication. *Transbound Emerg Dis.* (2010) 57:205–20. doi: 10.1111/j.1865-1682.2010.01148.x
18. Garza-Cuartero L, O'Sullivan J, Blanco A, McNair J, Welsh M, Flynn RJ, et al. *Fasciola hepatica* infection reduces *Mycobacterium bovis* burden and mycobacterial uptake and suppresses the pro-inflammatory response. *Paras Immunol.* (2016) 38:387–402. doi: 10.1111/pim.12326
19. Claridge J, Diggle P, Mccann CM, Mulcahy G, Flynn R, Mcnair J, et al. *Fasciola hepatica* is associated with the failure to detect bovine tuberculosis in dairy cattle. *Nat Commun.* (2012) 853:1–8. doi: 10.1038/ncomms1840
20. Pollock JM, Welsh MD, McNair J. Immune responses in bovine tuberculosis: towards new strategies for the diagnosis and control of disease. *Veter Immunol Immunopathol.* (2005) 108:37–43. doi: 10.1016/j.vetimm.2005.08.012
21. Flynn RJ, Mulcahy G, Welsh M, Cassidy JP, Corbett D, Milligan C, et al. Co-infection of cattle with *Fasciola hepatica* and *Mycobacterium bovis*-immunological consequences. *Transbound Emerg Dis.* (2009) 56:269–74. doi: 10.1111/j.1865-1682.2009.01075.x
22. Flynn RJ, Mannion C, Golden O, Hacariz O, Mulcahy G. Experimental *Fasciola hepatica* infection alters responses to tests used for diagnosis of bovine tuberculosis. *Infect Immun.* (2007) 75:1373–81. doi: 10.1128/IAI.01445-06
23. Dalton JP, Robinson MW, Mulcahy G, O'Neill SM, Donnelly S. Immunomodulatory molecules of *Fasciola hepatica*: candidates for both vaccine and immunotherapeutic development. *Veter Parasitol.* (2013) 195:272–85. doi: 10.1016/j.vetpar.2013.04.008
24. Awah-Ndukum J, Tchoumboue J, Niba AT. Prevalence of bovine tuberculosis at the SODEPA Douala abattoir, Cameroon (1995–2003). *Cameroon J Exp Biol.* (2006) 1:116–120. doi: 10.4314/cajeb.v1i2.37938
25. Awah Ndukum J, Kudi AC, Bradley G, Ane-Anyangwe IN, Fon-Tebug S, Tchoumboue J. Prevalence of bovine tuberculosis in abattoirs of the littoral and Western highland regions of cameroon: a cause for public health concern. *Veter Med Int.* (2010) 2010:495015. doi: 10.4061/2010/495015
26. Egbe NF, Muwonge A, Ndip L, Kelly RF, Sander M, Tanya V, et al. Abattoir-based estimates of mycobacterial infections in Cameroon. *Sci Reports* (2016)6:24320. doi: 10.1038/srep24320
27. Ntonifor HN, Ndaleh WN. Prevalence of liver fluke infections and other gastrointestinal tract parasites in slaughtered cattle in Douala, Cameroon. *Bull Animal Health Prod Afr.* (2012) 60:438–444.
28. Ngole IU, Ndamukong KJN, Mbuh JV. Short communication internal parasites and haematological values in cattle slaughtered in buea subdivision of Cameroon. *Health (San Francisco)* (2003) 35:409–13.
29. Kelly RF, Hamman SM, Morgan KL, Nkongho EF, Ngwa VN, Tanya V, et al. Knowledge of bovine tuberculosis, cattle husbandry and dairy practices amongst pastoralists and small-scale dairy farmers in Cameroon. *PLOS ONE* (2016) 11:e0146538. doi: 10.1371/journal.pone.0146538
30. Egbe NF, Muwonge A, Ndip L, Kelly RF, Sander M, Tanya V, et al. Molecular epidemiology of *Mycobacterium bovis* in Cameroon. *Sci Reports* (2017) 7:4652. doi: 10.1038/s41598-017-04230-6
31. Awah-Ndukum J, Kudi AC, Bradley G, Ane-Anyangwe I, Titanji VPK, Fon-Tebug S, et al. Prevalence of bovine tuberculosis in cattle in the

highlands of Cameroon based on the detection of lesions in slaughtered cattle and tuberculin skin tests of live cattle. *Veterin Med Int.* (2012) 57:59–76. doi: 10.17221/5252-VETMED

32. Cahn, C M , Line SE. Dental development. In: Kahn CM, editor. *Merck Veterinary Manual, 9th Edn.* Philadelphia, PA: National Publishing Inc. (2005). p. 137–140.
33. Ameni G, Aseffa A, Engers H, Young D, Gordon S, Hewinson G, et al. High prevalence and increased severity of pathology of bovine tuberculosis in Holsteins compared to zebu breeds under field cattle husbandry in central Ethiopia. *Clin Vaccine Immunol.* (2007) 14:1356–61. doi: 10.1128/CVI.00205-07
34. Ameni G, Aseffa A, Engers H, Young D, Hewinson G, Vordermeier M. Cattle husbandry in Ethiopia is a predominant factor affecting the pathology of bovine tuberculosis and gamma interferon responses to mycobacterial antigens. *Clin Vaccine Immunol.* (2006) 13:1030–6. doi: 10.1128/CVI.00134-06
35. Charlier J, De Meulemeester L, Claerebout E, Williams D, Vercruysse J. Qualitative and quantitative evaluation of coprological and serological techniques for the diagnosis of fasciolosis in cattle. *Veter Parasitol.* (2008) 153:44–51. doi: 10.1016/j.vetpar.2008.01.035
36. Lumb R, Van Deun A, Bastian I, Fitz-Gerald M. *Laboratory Diagnosis of Tuberculosis by Sputum Microscopy: The Handbook* (2013). Available online at: http://www.stoptb.org/wg/gli/assets/documents/TB%20MICROSCOPY%20HANDBOOK_FINAL.pdf
37. Schiller I, Vordermeier HM, Waters WR, Whelan AO, Coad M, Gormley E, et al. Bovine tuberculosis: effect of the tuberculin skin test on *in vitro* interferon gamma responses. *Veter Immunol Immunopathol.* (2010) 136:1–11. doi: 10.1016/j.vetimm.2010.02.007
38. Prionics. *Mycobacterium bovis Gamma Interferon Test Kit for Cattle BOVIGAM*. Lelystad (2012).
39. Dahoo I, Martin W, Stryhn H. Logistic regression. In: McPike SM, editor. *Veterinary Epidemiologic Research, 2nd Edn.* Charlottetown, PE: VER Inc. (2009). p. 395–426.
40. Kosmidis I. brglm: *Bias Reduction in Binary-Response Generalized Linear Models.* R package version 0.6.1 (2017). Available online at: http://www.ikosmidis.com/software.html
41. Mazerolle MJ. *AICcmodavg: Model Selection and Multimodel Inference Based on (Q)AIC(c).* Package Version 2 0-3 R (2015). Available online at: http://cran.r-project.org/package=AICcmodavg
42. Ezenwa VO, Etienne RS, Luikart G, Beja-Pereira A, Jolles AE. Hidden consequences of living in a wormy world: nematodeinduced immune suppression facilitates tuberculosis invasion in African buffalo. *Am Natl.* (2010) 176:613–24. doi: 10.1086/656496
43. Piedrafita D, Raadsma HW, Prowse R, Spithill TW. Immunology of the host-parasite relationship in fasciolosis (*Fasciola hepatica* and *Fasciola gigantica*). *Can J Zool.* (2004) 82:233–50. doi: 10.1139/z03-216
44. Munyeme M, Mweemba HM, Nambota A, Muma JB, Phiri, A M, Nalubamba KS. The Nexus between Bovine Tuberculosis and Fasciolosis Infections in Cattle of the Kafue Basin Ecosystem in Zambia: implications on Abattoir Surveillance. *Veter Med Int.* (2012) 2012:1–6. doi: 10.1155/2012/921869
45. Frantz FG, Rosada RS, Peres-Buzalaf C, Perusso FRT, Rodrigues V, Ramos SG, et al. Helminth coinfection does not affect therapeutic effect of a DNA vaccine in mice harboring tuberculosis. *PLOS Neglect Trop Dis.* (2010) 4:e700. doi: 10.1371/journal.pntd.0000700
46. Driscoll EE, Hoffman JI, Green LE, Medley GF, Amos W. A preliminary study of genetic factors that influence susceptibility to bovine tuberculosis in the British cattle herd. *PLoS ONE* (2011) 6:e18806. doi: 10.1371/journal.pone.0018806
47. Collins JD. Tuberculosis in cattle: strategic planning for the future. *Veter Microbiol.* (2006) 112:369–81. doi: 10.1016/j.vetmic.2005.11.041
48. Eswarappa SM, Estrela S, Brown SP. Within-Host dynamics of multi-species infections : facilitation, competition and virulence. *PLoS ONE* (2012) 7:e38730. doi: 10.1371/journal.pone.0038730
49. Pathak AK, Pelensky C, Boag B, Cattadori IM. Immuno-epidemiology of chronic bacterial and helminth co-infections: observations from the field and evidence from the laboratory. *Int J Parasitol.* (2012) 42:647–55. doi: 10.1016/j.ijpara.2012.04.011
50. Thumbi SM, Bronsvoort BMDC, Poole EJ, Kiara H, Toye PG, Mbole-Kariuki MN, et al. Parasite Co-Infections and Their Impact on Survival of Indigenous Cattle. *PLoS ONE* (2014) 9:e76324. doi: 10.1371/journal.pone.0076324
51. Byrne AW, Graham J, Brown C, Donaghy A, Guelbenzu-Gonzalo M, McNair J, et al. Modelling the variation in skin-test tuberculin reactions, post-mortem lesion counts and case pathology in tuberculosis-exposed cattle: effects of animal characteristics, histories and co-infection. *Transbound Emerg Dis.* (2018) 65:844–58. doi: 10.1111/tbed.12814
52. Neill SD, O'Brien JJ, Hanna J. A mathematical model for Mycobacterium bovis excretion from tuberculous cattle. *Veter Microbiol.* (1991) 28:103–9. doi: 10.1016/0378-1135(91)90102-L
53. Charlier J, Vercruysse J, Morgan E, van Dijk J, Williams DJL. Recent advances in the diagnosis, impact on production and prediction of *Fasciola hepatica* in cattle. *Parasitology* (2014) 141:326–35. doi: 10.1017/S0031182013001662

14

Whole Genome Sequencing of *Mycobacterium bovis* Isolated from Livestock in the United States, 1989–2018

Kathy Orloski[1]*, *Suelee Robbe-Austerman*[2]*, *Tod Stuber*[2], *Bill Hench*[3] and *Mark Schoenbaum*[3]

[1] U.S. Department of Agriculture, Animal and Plant Health Inspection Service, Veterinary Services, Centers for Epidemiology and Animal Health, Fort Collins, CO, United States, [2] National Veterinary Services Laboratories, U.S. Department of Agriculture, Animal and Plant Health Inspection Service, Veterinary Services, Ames, IA, United States, [3] U.S. Department of Agriculture, Animal and Plant Health Inspection Service, Veterinary Services, Fort Collins, CO, United States

***Correspondence:**
Kathy Orloski
kathy.a.orloski@aphis.usda.gov
Suelee Robbe-Austerman
suelee.robbe-austerman@aphis.usda.gov

The United States official bovine tuberculosis (bTB) eradication program has utilized genotyping for *Mycobacterium bovis* isolates since 2000 and whole genome sequencing was implemented in 2013. The program has been highly successful, yet as bTB prevalence has reached historic lows, a small number of new bTB-affected cattle herds occur annually. Therefore, understanding the epidemiology of bTB transmission is critically important, in order to target limited resources for surveillance and achieve eradication. This evaluation described the diversity and epidemiology of *M. bovis* isolates identified in the USA livestock. Isolates from animals within the bTB endemic area of Michigan were excluded. Broad diversity was found among 1,248 isolates, collected from affected cattle and farmed cervids herds and fed cattle during 1989–2018. Nearly 70% of isolates from 109 herds/cases during 1999–2018 were European clonal complex 1 and 30% were European clonal complex 2. The sources of infection based on the herd investigation were known for 41% of herds/cases and 59% were not epidemiologically linked to another USA origin herd. Whole genome sequencing results were consistent with the investigation findings and previously unrecognized links between herds and cases were disclosed. For herds/cases with an unknown source of infection, WGS results suggested several possible sources, including undocumented cattle movement, imported cattle and humans. The use of WGS in new cases has reduced the time and costs associated with epidemiological investigations. Within herd SNP diversity was evaluated by examining 18 herds with 10 or more isolates sequenced. Forty percent of isolates had not diverged or accumulated any SNPs, and 86% of the isolates had accumulated 3 or fewer SNPs. The results of WGS does not support a bTB reservoir in USA cattle. The bTB eradication program appears to be highly effective as the majority of herds/cases in the USA are unique strains with limited herd to herd transmission.

Keywords: ***Mycobacterium bovis*, bovine tuberculosis, genotyping, whole genome sequencing, bovine, cervid**

INTRODUCTION

Mycobacterium bovis (bTB) has a broad host range, causing economic loss to beef and dairy production and infecting humans and wildlife. Therefore, most developed countries and many developing countries have national bovine tuberculosis eradication programs in livestock. The United States (USA) began a national eradication program for *M. bovis* infection in cattle in 1917. At the program's inception, the apparent prevalence of bTB was 5% of cattle, as estimated by positive responses to the caudal fold tuberculin skin test (CFT) (1). The program's history has been documented elsewhere, including the reduction of prevalence in cattle to <0.005% of cattle herds today (2, 3).

During 2001 to 2011, 92 U.S. cattle herds were infected with *M. bovis*, in an estimated cattle population of 87 million head on 913,000 operations (3). During 1991–2004, there were 41 bTB-affected farmed cervid herds (4, 5). State and Federal veterinarians conduct extensive investigations when bTB is detected; routinely investigating animals that arrived and left the herd within the last 5 years. The program's cornerstone activities are national surveillance for cattle, bison and farmed cervids and quarantine of bTB-affected herds until the infection is no longer detected in individual animals. Despite these efforts, each year there are 2–15 affected cattle herds (3). Affected farmed cervid herds occur sporadically, with the most recent occurrence in 2009. As the USA bTB prevalence has reached historic lows, understanding the epidemiology of bTB transmission is critically important, in order to target limited resources for surveillance and achieve eradication. Challenges to the final eradication of bTB in the USA include a wildlife reservoir in white-tailed deer in northeastern Michigan, sporadic occurrences in dairies and beef herds, bTB in imported feeder cattle, and limitations in the ability to trace animals (3, 6).

Genotyping of *M. bovis* isolates has been in use since 2000 in the official USA bTB eradication program, beginning with IS*6110* based restriction fragment length polymorphism analysis, then adding spoligotyping in 2004 and multiple loci variable number tandem repeat analysis in 2008. These results showed that strains in the USA were highly diverse in both genotypes and geographical locations, with overlap in strains between USA origin and Mexican origin cattle. However, the low resolution of these genotyping methods failed to identify transmission paths (7). Whole genome sequencing is useful at elucidating sources of infection, resolving indistinguishable genotypes identified by other methods and potentially estimating when a new strain was introduced (8, 9). Whole genome sequencing (WGS) was implemented at NVSL on an experimental basis in 2012 and for official program use in January 2013, when WGS replaced traditional spoligotyping and VNTR. The laboratory was able to provide WGS results within the same time frame as traditional genotyping (typically within 4–6 weeks from tissue submission), which was then used to inform the field investigation. Several training programs and webinars were done to prepare the staff for interpreting results (10).

The objectives of this paper are to characterize *M. bovis* isolates identified in the USA from livestock and captive/farmed wildlife, and describe the molecular epidemiology of *M. bovis* in bTB-affected cattle herds in the USA. This information will assist animal health officials and the cattle industry in understanding the transmission of *M. bovis* and use this information for disease prevention.

METHODS

Isolate Selection

Because all official bTB eradication program laboratory diagnostics were performed at the United States Department of Agriculture (USDA), National Veterinary Services Laboratories (NVSL), all isolates archived and maintained at that facility up to May 2018 were sequenced. Prior to 2000, there were no procedures in place to permanently archive isolates, consequently a limited number of isolates prior to 2000 were available. After 2000, nearly all *M. bovis* isolates that were obtained through official bTB program activities from livestock and other animals residing on premises with bTB-infected cattle or farmed cervids were available. In addition, *M. bovis* and *M. caprae* isolates originating from clinical specimens that were submitted to the NVSL were included. Clinical specimens are defined as those originating from diagnostic submissions from animals that are not legally covered by official bTB eradication program regulations. For example, animals in zoological collections or laboratory animals. These isolates originated from other domestic and captive animals residing in the USA that were not under bTB eradication program regulatory authority. Official USDA records detailing the epidemiological investigations that occurred during federal fiscal years 1999 through June 2018 were correlated with the corresponding sequenced isolates. Because a complete list of confirmed bTB-affected herds was not available prior to 1999, results for isolates identified before 1999 were analyzed separately within this paper. Also included in the paper were five reference isolates, AF2122/97 (Biosample: ERS1462286), Ravenel (Biosample: SAMN04448492), BCG (Biosample: SAMN06847294), AN5 (Biosample: SAMN04448491), and 94-1MIDNRdeerAlp (Biosample: SAMN04386752) (the index Michigan deer isolate). See **Supplemental File 1** for isolate metadata. All samples were collected and tested under the authority of the Code of Federal Regulations (CFR) enacted to guide the State-Federal Cooperative bovine tuberculosis eradication program as outlined in 9 CFR part 49, 50.

Official Program Standards

Official program activities include ongoing slaughter surveillance, live animal testing, and investigations of bTB-affected herds. These activities are described in the USDA, Bovine Tuberculosis Eradication, Uniform Methods and Rules (11), and are summarized elsewhere (8, 9, 12, 13). Briefly, antemortem testing is performed on cattle, bison and farmed cervids for a number of reasons, such as entry to a show or sale, state entry requirements, and as part of bTB-affected herd investigations. The CFT is the primary test for cattle and bison, and the single cervical tuberculin skin test (SCT) and the Dual Path Platform (DPP®) are the primary tests in farmed cervids. Secondary tests are administered to responders. Slaughter surveillance in cattle and bison consists of standardized carcass inspection conducted at federally inspected slaughter establishments (14).

When bTB is suspected, an official investigation is conducted by state and federal animal health regulatory officials (11). This investigation collects information about the premises where the animal resided (city, county, state) and its movements prior to confirming infection. The investigation includes adjacent, contact and possible source herds for the affected herd. Bovine tuberculosis affected herds are classified as epidemiologically linked based on investigative evidence. Investigative evidence includes but is not limited to slaughter establishment records, records of animal movement, such as a bill of sale or certificate of veterinary inspection or other official documents. These records are used to determine where an infected animal resided over time, identify potentially exposed animals and herds and look for the source of infection. Herds exposed through animal movements from a bTB-affected herd are tested, and exposed animals are removed, necropsied and sampled.

Case Definitions

Adult cattle were defined as sexually intact animals >2 years of age, whereas fed cattle are defined as castrated or spayed animals without regard to age that are raised for the purpose of beef production. Another type of cattle are those animals used for roping and other performance events. Castration status has precedence over age, for example, a 4-year-old castrated steer is classified as a fed animal. Slaughter surveillance targets culled adult cattle because these are more likely to exhibit lesions suspicious of bTB (15). bTB-affected herds were classified by production type, including beef, dairy, mixed (beef and dairy), event cattle (roping, rodeo animals), farmed cervids, and unknown.

The case definition used for classifying an animal as confirmed infected with *M. bovis* was either a histologic diagnosis of compatible for mycobacteriosis with a positive polymerase chain reaction (PCR) test performed on formalin fixed tissue using primers for IS*6110* to identify *M. tuberculosis* complex, or bacteriological isolation of *M. bovis*. Affected herds are confirmed when an animal from within the herd is confirmed with bTB. When this criterion cannot be met, the singleton animal (generally found as a result of slaughter surveillance) was defined as a case. The source of infection for affected herds was based on the results of epidemiological investigations as being either unknown, or another USA herd. The latter classification was applied when there was documented animal movement or the potential for fence line or other direct contact. Outbreaks were defined as two or more bTB-affected herds or cases with a documented exposure, such as animal movement between premises.

To identify the likely source, (likely external to the USA or internal transmission within USA) we conservatively estimated that a USA origin strain would not be tlikely to be exported and established in another country after the USA's national bTB prevalence was below 0.5%, which occurred around 1960. Consequently herds that could have shared a common ancestor within the last 60 years would more likely be internal transmission rather than importation. Using the average reported SNP mutation rate of 0.3 SNP/year (16), suggests a reasonable cutoff point of 20 SNPs. Consequently, we considered isolates that were within 20 SNPs of sharing a common ancestor with USA origin cattle to originate from USA and isolates that were within 20 SNPs of sharing a common ancestor with Mexican origin cattle isolates to have originated from Mexico. If more than 20 SNPs had accumulated since sharing a common ancestor with an isolate in the database, we considered the source unknown. Isolates from Michigan cattle within the known endemic area and all Michigan wildlife were excluded.

Laboratory Methods

During slaughter inspection or when bTB test positive animals are euthanized and necropsied, granulomatous-appearing lesions are collected and submitted to the laboratory for histologic examination, PCR testing and mycobacterial culture (17). For some bTB test positive animals, if no visible lesions are observed during necropsy, representative head, abdominal, and thoracic lymph nodes are collected and tested (9, 11, 13). For herds with many bTB infected animals, generally at least 10 isolates were collected and sequenced and in some herds many more were sequenced when sufficient resources existed.

To obtain the WGS, isolates were sequenced on a MiSeq instrument (Illumina, San Diego, CA, United States) using 2 × 250 paired-end chemistry and the Nextera XT library preparation kit (Illumina, San Diego, CA, United States). FASTQ files were put through the NVSL in-house pipeline (https://github.com/USDA-VS). Reads were aligned to the reference genome AF2122/97, NCBI accession number NC_002945 (18), using BWA (19) and post-processing of the alignment was done using Samtools (20). BAM files were processed based on Genome Analysis Toolkit (GATK)'s "best practice" workflow (21, 22). SNPs were called using GATK's HaplotypeCaller with ploidy set to 2, outputting SNPs to variant call format (VCF) files. PPE-PGRS and repeat regions were filtered as well as SNPs that uniformly had QUAL scores < 150 across isolates. To identify SNP calls that were heterozygous, a SNP with an allele call of AC = 1 was relabeled using the International Union of Pure and Applied Chemistry guidelines for ambiguous calls. In order to manage and more accurately analyze this large and diverse dataset, a small number of isolates representing the diversity of the entire dataset were ran through the pipeline. High quality SNPs were identified that clustered the isolates into smaller more manageable groups. Groups were created based on the number of isolates as well as the evolutionary distance. Because these groupings were based on convenience for analysis purposes, they were not necessarily similar in evolutionary distance. For example, group 23 and 24 are very closely related, but because there were so many isolates in that clustered closely together, 2 groups were made. Individual SNPs tables and phylogenetic trees were then created for each group after removing all uninformative SNPs that were homogeneous between the grouped isolates. Because of this process, the reference AF2122, worked as the outgroup isolate for all individual groups. SNPs were then further verified manually using Integrative Genomics Viewer (23) and additional filtering of problematic SNPs was performed on a group by group basis using the SNP tables. Phylogenetic trees were created using RAxML (24) and the GTRCATI model with default settings and accuracy of the phylogenetic tree was confirmed using the manually validated SNP table.

Data Analysis

We examined WGS results for *M. bovis* isolates from cattle and farmed cervid breeding herds and individual animal cases detected through surveillance in the USA, and described the diversity of the isolates within herds and between herds. We identified the most recent common ancestor (MRCA) in the herd. Then, the most closely related isolate was selected from the NVSL WGS database, based on having the fewest number of single nucleotide polymorphisms (SNP) differences, when compared to the herd or case isolate. A pairwise comparison of SNPs to the MRCA was recorded. For herds with *M. bovis* isolates from multiple bTB confirmed infected animals, the tip with the shortest branch length to the tree root was used for the comparison. The most closely related isolates were grouped based on information about the animal or human from which the isolate was obtained. For example, whether the isolate was from imported cattle or a confirmed bTB-affected herd in the USA.

RESULTS

Sequencing was performed on 1,248 isolates, this included 154 that were published previously (8, 9). Of these, 185 isolates were collected during 1989–1998, and 1,063 were collected during 1999–2018. The *M. bovis* isolates separated into 24 major phylogenetic groups (**Figure 1**). Twelve *M. bovis* isolates were obtained from clinical specimens submitted to NVSL (four non-human primates, one jaguar, one elephant, one domestic cat, one brocket deer, 4 unknown species from zoological collections). There were four *M. caprae* isolates from three non-human primates and one rhinoceros residing in zoological collections.

bTB-Affected Herds and Slaughter Cases in Culled Adult Cattle

There were 83 bTB-affected herds, and 26 cases in infected adult domestic cattle during 1999–2018 (**Supplemental Table 1**). An isolate was not available for two additional cattle herds that are not included in this analysis. The production types included 54 beef herds/cases (49.5%), 37 dairies (33.9%), 3 event/rodeo (2.8%), 3 mixed purpose (2.8%), 11 farmed cervids (10.1%), and one herd of an unknown production type. The herds/cases were located in 21 States (Arizona, California, Colorado, Indiana, Iowa, Kansas, Kentucky, Michigan, Minnesota, Mississippi, North Dakota, Nebraska, New Mexico, New York, Ohio, Oklahoma, Oregon, South Dakota, Texas, Washington, Wisconsin).

There were 563 bTB isolates from these 109 herds/cases (**Supplemental Table 1**). No herds were identified with more than one strain. Seventy-six (69.7%) of the herds/cases were European clonal complex 1 (EU1) strains, 32 (29.4%) were European clonal complex 2 (EU2) strains, and one herd was infected with a strain not identified within a clonal complex (group 8) (**Supplemental Table 1**, **Table 1**). Groups 8 and 14 contain isolates associated with outbreaks in USA and Canada farmed cervid herds (4, 5, 25, 26). The number of isolates per herd ranged from one to 48, (median 2, mean 5), and 52/83 herds (62.7%) had more than one isolate (**Supplemental Table 1**).

Within herd SNP diversity was evaluated by examining the 18 herds with 10 or more isolates sequenced, identifying the common ancestor, or index sequence, and then counting the number of SNPs accumulated from the index sequence (**Table 2**). Forty percent of isolates had not diverged or accumulated any SNPs, 86% of the isolates had accumulated 3 or fewer SNPs and no cattle herds contained isolates that had accumulated more than 6 SNPs (**Table 2**). These accumulated SNPs may be unique to a single isolate or found in a cluster of isolates within a herd. The highest diversity occurred in two herds, a 2009 farmed cervid herd with 28 isolates and 35 SNPs, and a 2017 cattle herd with 25 SNPs among 13 isolates. Based on the epidemiologic investigation, both herds were likely infected for several years.

Despite all of the retrospective data and epidemiological investigations that have been conducted in the USA, we were able to attribute multiple transmission events to a single cow only one time. In this instance, a cow with disseminated TB lesions was sold into a feedlot and exposed a group of cows for <30 days. Within 90 days of exposure, all exposed cows were slaughtered and 6 were identified with lesions. The isolate sequence recovered from a pooled sample of the lesions from the index cow along with the 6 isolate sequences recovered from exposed cows are shown in **Table 3**. In this event, four different SNP profiles were transmitted to these 6 cows.

The sources of infection based on the investigation results were known for 45/109 (41.3%) of herds/cases (epidemiologically linked via animal movement or adjacent premises contact) and 64 were not epidemiologically linked to another USA origin herd. There was only one documented case of transmission from Mexico, in a roping steer newly imported from Mexico that was found to be infected during a herd test for interstate movement. These 45 herds with a known infection source were associated with 14 outbreaks. Eight outbreaks involved two herds each, two outbreaks involved three herds, one outbreak involved five herds (13), one involved six herds (five herds occurred before 1999) and one outbreak in Minnesota involved 12 herds (8).

The source of infection could not be determined epidemiologically for 64 herds/cases.The most recent common ancestor was within 20 SNPs of a Mexican origin animal for 22 (34.9%) of USA herds/cases suggesting Mexico may be the source (**Supplemental Table 1**). Twelve cases/herds were within 20 SNPs of unknown origin fed cattle and 20 were within 20 SNPs other USA herds/cases. Isolates from the remaining nine herds/cases, were >20 SNPs from the most recent common ancestor, therefore, no conclusive linkage was found by genetic sequencing or epidemiology. Interestingly, only one of these 64 herds/cases were within 5 SNPs of Mexican origin fed cattle slaughtered in the USA. One additional isolate from a dairy cow was indistinguishable from a worker in the same dairy that was initially diagnosed with bTB, and the dairy was subsequently tested (27).

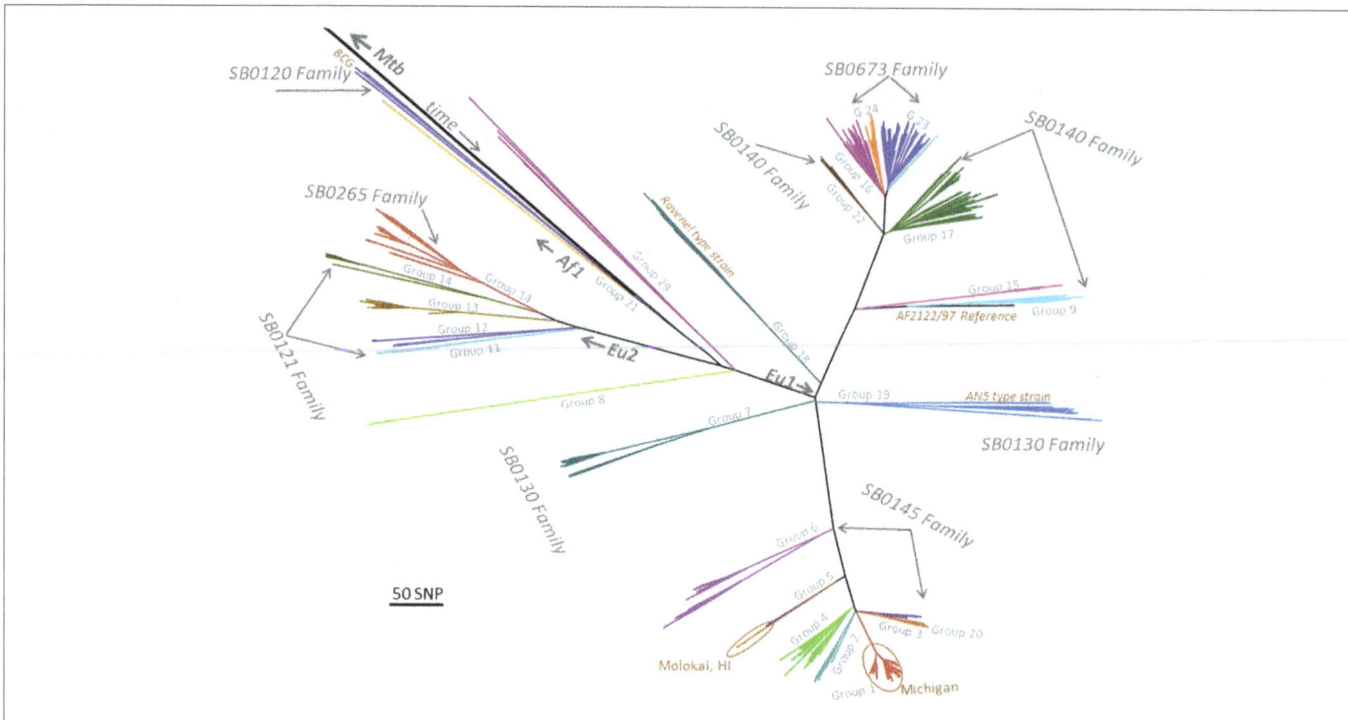

FIGURE 1 | Low resolution phylogenetic tree representing 1,248 *Mycobacterium bovis* isolates and major spoligotyping families. MTBC, M. tuberculosis complex; EU1, European clonal complex 1; EU2, European clonal complex 2; Af1, African complex 1; SNP, single nucleotide polymorphism; BCG, bacille Calmette-Guerin; HI, Hawaii; AN5, *M. bovis* AN5 strain.

There was one extensive outbreak involving two closely related clusters within phylogenetic group 14. Group 14 consists of USA farmed cervids and cattle and Canada farmed cervids (4, 5, 25, 26). The first cluster involved 1 farmed cervid herd (Nebraska), three cattle herds [Nebraska, South Dakota (2)], and 1 cattle case in Nebraska during 2009–2013. The cattle herds and case were epidemiologically linked by animal movement or fence line contact and the source herd was a bTB-affected cervid herd [(26), USDA Veterinary Services, unpublished information]. The second cluster, when limited to known animal movement or fence line contact consisted of three cervid (Indiana) and two cattle herds during 2009-2017 (Indiana, Michigan). One of the three Indiana cervid herds (2009) was the source herd. However, three additional cattle herds (Indiana (2), Kentucky) and 3 cases (Indiana (2), Arizona) occurred during 2009-2017, but did not have documented links to the second cluster. Isolates from these six herds/cases are either indistinguishable or have 1-2 SNPs from the 2009 index farmed cervid herd and other group 14 isolates, indicating undocumented animal movements or contacts occurred.

During 1989–1998, there were 50 bTB isolates obtained from 24 affected herds, representing 12 cattle and 12 farmed cervid herds (**Supplemental Table 1**). These isolates were from 11 States, including Hawaii, Missouri, Montana, New Mexico, New York, Oklahoma, Puerto Rico, Texas, Virginia, Vermont, and Wisconsin. One hundred bTB-affected herds occurred during this time; therefore, isolates were not available for 76 herds. Existing isolates from 1989–1998 separated into 10 major phylogenetic groups (groups 5, 6, 8, 9, 13, 14, 16, 19, 21, 24). Seven of these groups contained isolates recovered from Mexico origin cattle (groups 6, 9, 13, 14, 16, 19, 24), while three did not (groups 5, 8, 21). Four groups were not represented after 1998 (groups 5, 9, 21, 24). The Hawaii isolate was obtained from a beef herd in 1997. The most closely related isolate to the beef herd were from feral swine, obtained during wildlife surveillance efforts there during 2007–2009.

Group 7, subgroup B, provides examples of WGS results (**Supplemental File 2**). Substantial diversity exists among the 108 isolates, which is typical of the phylogenetic groups. There are two outbreaks, one involving three South Dakota beef herds, and the second involving five Colorado beef and dairy herds [an isolate was not available for one herd, (13)]. For the Colorado outbreak, 12 isolates were sequenced with two unique SNPs; however, the majority of nearly 90 isolates from the index dairy herd were not sequenced due to resource limitations. For the South Dakota outbreak, 30 isolates from the index herd (designated 17-A in the isolate name) were sequenced, with 20 unique SNPs. Isolates from three additional animals sold to other herds (herds 17-B and 17-C) from the index herd had the same SNP pattern as isolates from animals in the index herd. In addition to the two outbreaks, Group 7 includes a single beef herd infection and several single animal cases. The single beef herd occurred in Oklahoma in 2007, for which one fed steer from this herd was found in a Kansas feedlot. There is one case in an adult beef cow found through slaughter surveillance that traced to New Mexico in 2004. This case could not be linked to a bTB-affected herd. The isolate from this animal is only one SNP different

TABLE 1 | Whole genome sequencing group for 83 bTB-affected herds and 26 cases during 1999-2018.

Whole genome sequencing group	Number of herds and cases	Percent of total
EUROPEAN CLONAL COMPLEX 1		
2	2	1.8
3	1	0.9
4	1	0.9
6	12	11.0
7	11	10.1
16	8	7.3
17	21	19.3
19	1	0.9
20	3	2.8
22	2	1.8
23	13	11.9
No associated clonal complex		
8	1	0.9
EUROPEAN CLONAL COMPLEX 2		
11	1	0.9
12	2	1.8
13	6	5.5
14	24	22.0
Total	109	100.0

from the 2007 Oklahoma herd. It is hypothesized the 2004 case originated from the Oklahoma herd; however, investigative information is no longer available. A second, unrelated case found through slaughter surveillance occurred during 2005 in a Nebraska beef cow, in which bTB could not be confirmed in the herd of origin. The most closely related isolates to this beef cow are from unknown (1992) and Mexican (2012) origin fed cattle slaughtered in the US (10 and 12 SNPs, respectively). Other group 7 isolates include 36 cases in fed cattle from 1991–2012; many of these were imported from Mexico and slaughtered in Texas. Finally, there are 18 results for isolates from cattle in Mexico.

Slaughter Cases in fed Cattle

There were a total of 521 confirmed bTB cases in fed cattle found through slaughter inspection during 1990–2018 (**Figure 2**). These isolates separated into 19 phylogenetic groups (**Table 4**). One isolate had a mixed infection. When considered by country of origin, 276 (53.0%) were from Mexico, the country of origin could not be determined for 223 (42.8%) and 22 (4.2%) occurred in USA origin cattle. An additional two cases in fed cattle from Canada slaughtered in Washington State were classified in group 23 (data not shown). Twenty of the USA origin cases separated into six phylogenetic groups and originated from six known bTB-affected herds. One case was untraceable and one case was under investigation at the time of this report. The country of origin could not be determined for 223 isolates from fed cattle. The most common reason that country of origin cannot be determined is because official animal identification was not available and the infected animal had been comingled with both USA and Mexican origin cattle in pastures or feedlots prior to slaughter (VS unpublished). Twenty-four isolates (4.6%) were from cases that occurred during 1989–1993, representing a small fraction of 1,504 bTB feedlot investigations that were reported during 1989–1993 (28).

Four groups (9, 15, 18, 24) were represented in fed cattle cases but not bTB-affected herds and cases, and one group was found in a farmed cervid herd but not in fed cattle (group 8). The five largest groups are 7, 13, 16, 17, and 23, and contain 72.3% of isolates from fed cattle. In comparison, the five largest groups are 6, 7, 14, 17, and 23, containing 65.4% of affected herds and cases during 1989–2018.

Spoligotyping

A comparison of spoligotyping and whole genome sequencing results are shown in **Figure 1**. There are six spoligotyping families that occur in the USA and each WGS group falls within one spoligotype family. Spoligotyping family SB0673 contains WGS Groups 16, 23, and 24; SB0120 contains Group 21; SB0121 contains Groups 11-14; SB0140 contains Groups 9, 17, 17 and 22; SB0130 contains Groups 7 and 19; and, SB0145 contains Groups 1-6 (**Figure 1**).

DISCUSSION

Consistent with previous reports, broad diversity exists among USA bTB isolates detected in cattle and farmed cervids (7). Not unexpectedly, many of the fed cattle isolates were from imported cattle, and contain even more diversity. WGS results do not support a bTB reservoir in USA cattle. The bTB eradication program appears to be highly effective as the majority of herds/cases in the USA are unique strains with limited herd to herd transmission. Two major exceptions occurred outside the endemic area of Michigan: the first in farmed cervid herds that subsequently spilled into cattle herds (15 herds/cases from 2009 to 2018) and the second in Minnesota where bTB spilled over into the local white-tailed deer and 12 cattle herds were affected (8). Farmed cervids are subject to official bTB program requirements including surveillance, and no bTB-affected cervid herds have occurred since 2009.

In all cases, WGS results corroborated investigative evidence of herd-to-herd transmission events. Not unexpectedly, there was less SNP diversity between epidemiologically linked herds, almost half these herds had no unique SNPs and the maximum number of unique SNPs was four (**Supplemental Table 1**). Nearly half of the herd to herd transmission events had a SNP genotype that had been found in the source herd.

WGS results also discovered previously unrecognized links between herds and cases. Isolates from 12 herds/cases with an unknown source of infection were within three SNPs of other USA herds/cases during 2009–2018, including six herds/cases clustering within the group 14 outbreak. In another example, the isolate from a 2010 bTB-infected Holstein cow from an Ohio

TABLE 2 | The number of single nucleotide polymorphisms (SNPs) from the common ancestor genotypes among bTB-affected herds with >10 isolates, United States, 1999–2018.

	Number of SNPs								
Herd name	0	1	2	3	4	5	6	7	8
2001 TX beef (%)	100	0	0	0	0	0	0	0	0
2002 TX dairy (%)	45	27	0	27	0	0	0	0	0
2003 CA dairy (%)	54	23	8	15	0	0	0	0	0
2007 NM dairy (%)	64	29	7	0	0	0	0	0	0
2009 IN cervid A (%)	0	17	0	0	33	33	17	0	0
2009 NE cervid (%)	0	37	11	4	11	15	19	0	4
2010 CO dairy A (%)	83	17	0	0	0	0	0	0	0
2012 CA dairy B (%)	75	25	0	0	0	0	0	0	0
2013 CA dairy (%)	47	27	20	7	0	0	0	0	0
2013 MI Dairy (%)	23	6	64	6	0	0	0	0	0
2014 TX dairy (%)	4	78	6	10	2	0	0	0	0
2015 TX organic dairy (%)	36	28	23	4	6	2	0	0	0
2016 IN beef (%)	13	0	4	29	38	13	4	0	0
2016 IN Longhorn (%)	23	8	31	8	23	0	8	0	0
2016 NM dairy A (%)	19	29	38	10	5	0	0	0	0
2017 NM Dairy A (%)	82	18	0	0	0	0	0	0	0
2017 SD beef A (%)	39	21	6	21	9	3	0	0	0
2017 SD beef D (%)	14	52	29	5	0	0	0	0	0
(%)	**40**	**24**	**14**	**8**	**7**	**4**	**3**	**0**	**0**

Green, the number of unique SNPs did not occur; Light to dark red, the proportion of isolates that had 0–8 unique SNPs (lower to higher proportion).

TABLE 3 | Example of accumulated single nucleotide polymorphisms (SNPs) resulting from multiple transmission events from one animal, 2018.

Genome position based on the reference NC_002945.4	1999500	1021045	241655	1147922
Reference call	**C**	**C**	**C**	**C**
18-0522_SD_IA_Fed-Cow-Index	S*	C	C	C
18-1919_SD_IA_Fed-Cow	**G**	C	C	C
18-1930_SD_IA_Fed-Cow	**G**	C	C	C
18-1932_SD_IA_Fed-Cow	**G**	**T**	C	C
18-1927_SD_IA_Fed-Cow	**G**	**T**	C	C
18-1922_SD_IA_Fed-Cow	C	C	**T**	C
18-1904_SD_IA_Fed-Cow	C	C	C	**T**

**S Designates a heterogenous SNP call containing both cytosine and guanine. The colors indicate a unique SNP from the reference call.*

dairy had one additional SNP from a single isolate obtained from a 2008 New Mexico dairy cow (**Supplemental Table 1**). Investigative evidence indicated the 2010 Ohio dairy cow originated from New Mexico though no direct links could be found to the 2008 herd. These findings raise the possibility of undocumented animal movements or exposure. A pathways analysis of 12 bTB-affected California dairy herds based predominantly on herd investigations, concluded that with one exception, *M. bovis* occurred because of independent introductions from sources outside the system (12).

Most of the isolates recovered from imported fed cattle are not closely related to isolates from USA herds, with only one of the 109 herds/cases within 5 SNPs of an imported fed steer, despite having nearly complete representation of fed cattle and affected herds during 1999–2018. This suggests there may be other vectors transmitting bTB to the USA national herd such as humans or even imported dairy products (29, 30). It may also be possible to have undetected residual strains from historical cases. In one example, 11 years elapsed between bTB detection in epidemiologically linked California dairy herds (12). Alternatively, a limitation of this analysis are missing isolates from bTB-infected animals not detected through surveillance activities. Slaughter surveillance in the USA has an estimated sensitivity of detecting a bTB affected herd in 1 year of 3.2% in small beef herds (1-49 head), to 50.6% in large dairies (>500 head) (31). A Bayesian molecular clock phylogenetic analysis of the Minnesota outbreak reported the median time to the most recent common ancestor was 1999 (range 1991, 2005) for isolates from the Minnesota outbreak (3 SNPs) and its mostly closely related isolate, a 2012 Texas beef herd (8 SNPs) (8). We were unable to determine if there were two introductions into the USA of a closely related genotype from Mexico, or if common ancestors were present in the USA, possibly as early as 1991, but were not present in the NVSL database.

The most closely related isolates to some affected herds are from fed cattle that occurred earlier in time than the affected herds, many prior to 1999. We hypothesized that if imported cattle were the source of infection for affected herds, we would find closely related isolates among imported fed cattle and

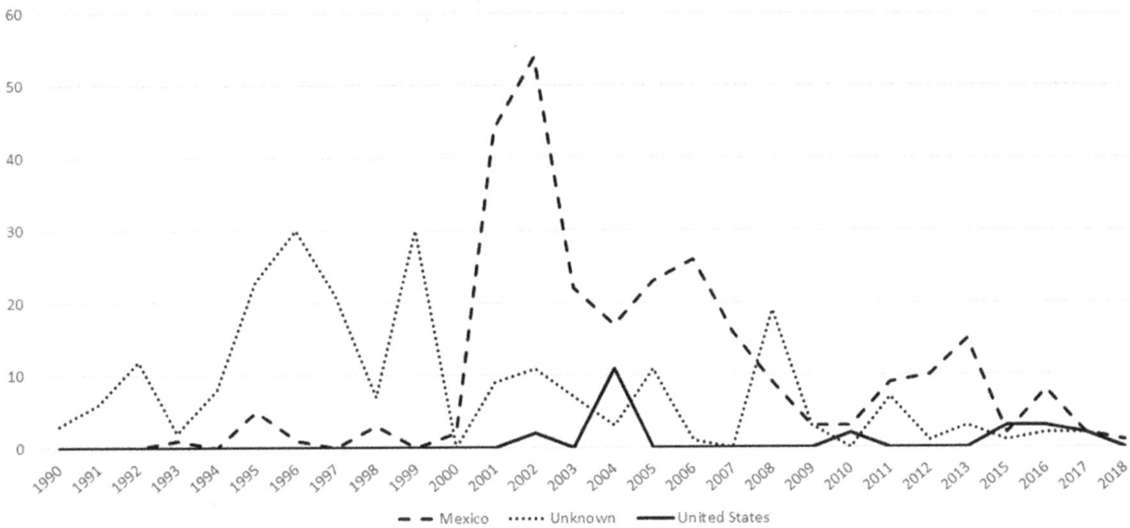

FIGURE 2 | Number of bTB cases that have whole genome sequencing results, by year and country of animal's origin for fed cattle slaughtered in the U.S, federal fiscal years 1990-2018 ($n = 521$).

TABLE 4 | Number of isolates by whole genome sequencing group and country of animal's origin for fed cattle slaughtered in the U.S, 1990–2018.

Group	Mexico	Unknown	USA	Total
Mixed	0	1	0	1
2	6	3	0	9
3	1	0	0	1
4	7	7	0	14
6	15	10	1	26
7	24	21	0	45
9	7	1	0	8
11	1	0	0	1
12	3	2	0	5
13	17	23	1	41
14	8	3	6	17
15	5	9	0	14
16	17	12	4	33
17	49	69	0	118
18	2	0	0	2
19	4	1	0	5
20	1	2	0	3
22	9	7	0	16
23	83	46	10	139
24	17	6	0	23
Total	276	223	22	521

affected herds/cases during 1999–2018. That pre-1999 fed cattle cases are the closest match to some post-1999 affected herds/cases is noteworthy, because the pre-1999 isolates from fed cattle represent only a small fraction of the cases that occurred (28). There was a substantially higher risk of bTB introduction from Mexican origin cattle during 1983–1993, compared to today (28).

Limited diversity occurred within most herds, with the majority of isolates having three or fewer SNPs. This may be useful in guiding epidemiologic investigations. For example, additional unique SNPs may indicate that an intermediary herd exists. The estimated SNP occurrence per genome per year ranges from 0.147 (32) to 0.53 (2.5% lower 0.22, 97.5% upper 0.94, (16). Applying these to the time frames and SNPs reported here may indicate a common exposure for the isolates with five or fewer SNPs, while separate introduction events may be more likely for isolates with >5 SNPs. The unique SNPs observed among animals within a herd may represent strain variation caused by animal to animal transmission, or an actual mutation. In the one example we observed, four different SNP profiles were transmitted to six cows exposed for 30 days to a single bTB-infected beef cow. Thacker et al. (33) reported that a single SNP genotype was recovered in 80% of affected tissues from experimentally infected white tailed deer. The inoculum and isolates from the remaining animals contained different WGS genotypes, some with the same SNP, and it was hypothesized that the SNP was not a mutation but was present though undetected in the original inoculation.

The use of WGS in new cases has focused epidemiological investigations and significantly reduced time and costs associated with these investigations and reduced the burden on livestock producers. Whole genome sequencing results for a 2013 case in a California Holstein heifer without animal identification enabled resources to focus on testing an epidemiologically linked herd (**Supplemental Table 1**). If these results had not been available, as many as 60 herds that had contributed cattle to the slaughter lot of the bTB infected case would have been administered a whole herd test. However, care must also be taken that the scope of the investigation not be prematurely limited by WGS results, at the risk of missing cases. WGS results provided critical information that enabled the successful detection of bTB spread to cattle from the 2009 NE infected farmed cervid herd (26). In another case, whole genome sequencing evidence linked three bTB-affected cattle operations to the index herd in the absence of cattle movements between the premises (9).

bTB prevalence in dairies is approximately twice that of beef herds (3). The risk factors for disease transmission among beef and dairy herds in the USA are unknown. The WGS results reported here may be useful in guiding future work to identify risk factors for bTB transmission. General trends in the beef and dairy industries during the study period include a decrease in the number of beef and dairy cattle and cattle operations during 1993–2008, while the average herd size has increased (34–36). The magnitude of this change was greater in dairy operations, where the number of operations declined 58.4% during 1991–2006, while the average dairy herd size doubled from 54 to 122 cows (36). Larger dairies continue to increase in herd size, and almost 30% of dairy operations introduced new cattle. Similarly, almost 35% of cow-calf beef operations introduced new cattle, most commonly weaned beef bulls and weaned steers (34).

Transmission from human workers to cattle has been hypothesized, especially for dairy cattle operations because of intensive management practices (12). In 2013, a USA dairy worker was diagnosed with bTB. The dairy herd was tested and bTB was confirmed in three animals (27). One animal was infected with the identical strain as the worker. While the direction of transmission could not be determined, this case suggests the possibility of human to animal transmission, as no other sources of exposure for the cattle could be identified. An evaluation of human and cattle *M. bovis* isolates from Baja California, Mexico found that 155 isolates from cattle and 17 from humans clustered into seven major groups (37). The human isolates were interspersed among the cattle isolates, and cheese is the suspected source of exposure of *M. bovis* for humans. In these examples from the USA and Mexico, direct or indirect contact between the human and animal subjects occurred; however, as noted previously, closely related isolates should not be used to imply transmission events, in the absence of epidemiologic linkages.

All isolates were sequenced for some herds, particularly those with a small number of bTB infected animals, but because of resource limitations, a smaller proportion of available isolates were sequenced for larger herds with dozens or hundreds of bTB infected animals. This limitation may bias these results by potentially under reporting the number of SNPs in herds with large numbers of infected animals, or conversely, fail to document if limited SNPs are present despite extensive within herd transmission.

CONCLUSION

Whole genome sequencing has become a cost effective, essential tool for the USA official bTB eradication program, providing information that increases the success and efficiency of the extensive investigations that occur when bTB is confirmed in cattle and farmed cervids. The isolates that occur among USA livestock are diverse, and the lack of diversity within herds support that a reservoir does not exist in the USA cattle population, although transmission of one strain has continued to occur from farmed cervids to cattle herds. The source of infection is unknown for approximately half of bTB-affected herds, and WGS results suggest several possible sources, including undocumented cattle movement, imported cattle, as well as humans or unpasteurized dairy products.

AUTHOR CONTRIBUTIONS

SR-A and TS performed WGS and provided summarized results. KO and SR-A compiled and analyzed the summarized WGS results. KO and SR-A wrote the paper. BH and MS provided epidemiological information. BH and MS reviewed/edited the paper.

ACKNOWLEDGMENTS

We thank Drs. Pauline Nol and Michael Carter for reviewing the manuscript.

REFERENCES

1. Olmstead AL, Rhode PW. The Tuberculous cattle trust: disease contagion in an era of regulatory uncertainty. *J Econ History* (2004) 64:929–63. doi: 10.1017/S0022050704043049
2. Palmer MV, Waters WR. Bovine tuberculosis and the establishment of an eradication program in the united states: role of veterinarians. *Vet Med Internat.* (2011) 2011:816345. doi: 10.4061/2011/816345
3. Portacci K, Lombard J, Schoenbaum M, Orloski K, Camacho M. The occurrence of *M. bovis* cases in U.S. cattle, 2001–2011. In: Thoen CO, Steele JH. editors. *Zoonotic Tuberculosis: Mycobacterium bovis and Other Pathogenic Mycobacteria.* Ames, IA; West Sussex, UK; Oxford, UK: John Wiley and Sons (2014). Pp. 253–61.
4. Gilsdorf M, Judge L, Ebel ED. Current challenges to and impacts on the U.S. national bovine tuberculosis eradication program: *Mycobacterium bovis* outbreaks in alternative species and surveillance performance. In: Thoen CO, Steele JH, Gilsdorf MJ. editors. *Mycobacterium bovis Infection in Animals and Humans.* Blackwell Publishing (2006) pp. 211–25.
5. Essey MA, Vantiem JS. Mycobacterium bovis infection in farmed Cervidae: an eradication program. In: Thoen CO and Steele JH. editors. *Mycobacterium bovis Infection in Animals and Humans,* Ames: Iowa State University Press (1995). pp. 145–57.
6. United States Department of Agriculture (March 2006). *Veterinary Services Progressive Bovine Tuberculosis Eradication Strategic Plan.* Animal and Plant Health Inspection Service, Veterinary Services.
7. Tsao K, Robbe-Austerman S, Miller RS, Portacci K, Grear DA, Webb C. Sources of bovine tuberculosis in the United States. *Infect Genetics Evol.* (2014) 28:137–43 doi: 10.1016/j.meegid.2014.09.025
8. Glaser L, Carstensen M, Shaw S, Robbe-Austerman S, Wunschmann A, Grear D, et al. Descriptive epidemiology and whole genome sequencing

analysis for an outbreak of bovine tuberculosis in beef cattle and white-tailed deer in northwestern minnesota. *PLoS ONE* (2016) 11:e0145735. doi: 10.1371/journal.pone.0145735
9. Bruning-Fann CS, Robbe-Austerman S, Kaneene JB, Thomsen BV, Tilden JD Jr, Ray JS, et al. Use of whole-genome sequencing and evaluation of the apparent sensitivity and specificity of antemortem tuberculosis tests in the investigation of an unusual outbreak of *Mycobacterium bovis* infection in a Michigan dairy herd. *J Am Vet Med Assoc.* (2017) 241:206–16. doi: 10.2460/javma.251.2.206
10. Robbe-Austerman S. Interpreting whole genome sequencing results. (2014) USDA, APHIS, VS. Available online at: http://www.screencast.com/users/NVSL
11. USDA (2004). *Bovine Tuberculosis Eradication. Uniform Methods and Rules.* Animal and Plant Health Inspection Service, Veterinary Services.
12. McCluskey B, Lombard J, Strunk S, Nelson D, Robbe-Austerman S, Naugle A, et al. Mycobacterium bovis in California dairies: a case series of 2002-2013 outbreaks. *Prevent Vet Med.* (2014) doi: 10.1016/j.prevetmed.2014.04.010
13. Francisco TI, Orloski KA, Roberts NJ. Investigation of a *Mycobacterium bovis* outbreak in cattle at a Colorado dairy in 2010. *J Am Vet Med Assoc.* (2014) 244:805–12. doi: 10.2460/javma.244.7.805
14. USDA (2015). *Inspection, sampling and disposition of cattle for tuberculosis (TB).* Food Safety Inspection Service Directive 6240.1.
15. Brooks-Pollock E, Conlan AJK, Mitchell AP, Blackwell, McKinley TJ, Wood JLN. Age-dependent patterns of bovine tuberculosis in cattle. *Vet Res.* (2013) 44:97. doi: 10.1186/1297-9716-44-97
16. Crispell J, Zadoks RN, Harris SR, Paterson B, Collins DM, de-Lisle GW, et al. Using whole genome sequencing to investigate transmission in a multi-host system: bovine tuberculosis in New Zealand. *BMC Genomics* (2017) 18:180. doi: 10.1186/s12864-017-3569-x
17. Robbe-Austerman S, Bravo DM, Harris B. Comparison of the MGIT 960, BACTEC 460 TB and solid media for isolation of Mycobacterium bovis in United States veterinary specimens. *BMC Vet Res.* (2013) 9:74. doi: 10.1186/1746-6148-9-74
18. Malone KM, Farrell D, Stuber TP, Schubert OT, Aebersold R, Robbe-Austerman S, et al. Updated reference genome sequence and annotation of Mycobacterium bovis AF2122/97. *Genome Announc.* (2017) 5:e00157–17. doi: 10.1128/genomeA.00157-17
19. Li H, Durbin R. Fast and accurate short read alignment with Burrows-Wheeler transform. *Bioinformatics* (2009) 25: 1754–60. doi: 10.1093/bioinformatics/btp324PMID:19451168
20. Li H, Handsaker B, Wysoker A, Fennell T, Ruan J, Homer N, et al. The sequence alignment/map format and SAMtools. *Bioinformatics* (2009b) 25:2078–79. doi: 10.1093/bioinformatics/btp352PMID:19505943
21. McKenna A, Hanna M, Banks E, Sivachenko A, Cibulskis K, Kernytsky A, et al. The Genome Analysis Toolkit: a MapReduce framework for analyzing next-generation DNA sequencing data. *Genome Res.* (2010) 20:1297–303. doi: 10.1101/gr.107524.110
22. Van der Auwera GA, Carneiro MO, Hartl C, Poplin R, Del Angel G, Levy-Moonshine A, et al. From FastQ data to high-confidence variant calls: the genome analysis toolkit best practices pipeline. *Curr Protoc Bioinformat.* (2013) 43:11.0. 1–33. doi: 10.1002/0471250953.bi1110s43
23. Robinson JT, Thorvaldsdottir H, Winckler W, Guttman M, Lander ES, Getz G, et al. Integrative genomics viewer. *Nat Biotechnol.* (2011) 29:24–6. doi: 10.1038/nbt.1754
24. Stamatakis A. RAxML version 8: a tool for phylogenetic analysis and post-analysis of large phylogenies. *Bioinformatics* (2014) 30:1312–3. doi: 10.1093/bioinformatics/btu033
25. Andrievskaia O, Duceppe M-O, Lloyd D. Genome sequences of five Mycobacterium bovis strains isolated from farmed animals and wildlife in Canada. *Genome Announc.* (2018) 6:e00258–18. doi: 10.1128/genomeA.00258-18.
26. Waters WR, Stevens GE, Schoenbaum MA, Orloski KA, Robbe-Austerman S, Harris NB, et al. Bovine tuberculosis in a nebraska herd of farmed elk and fallow deer: a failure of the tuberculin skin test and opportunities for serodiagnosis. *Vet Med Int.* (2011) 2011:953985. doi: 10.4061/2011/953985
27. Pritschet D, Cochran D. We Herd You Had TB. *North Dakota Public Health Nursing Conference.* (2015) Available onlne at: http://www.ndhealth.gov/ch/conference/nd_public_health_nursing_conference_%207-16-15.pdf (Accessed on April 1, 2018).
28. National Research Council. *Livestock Disease Eradication, Evaluation of the Cooperative State-Federal Bovine Tuberculosis Eradication Program.* National Academy Press Committee on Bovine Tuberculosis. Washington DC: National Research Council (1994). Available online at: https://www.nap.edu/catalog/9144/livestock-disease-eradication-evaluation-of-the-cooperative-state-federal-bovine
29. Harris NB, Payeur J, Bravo D, Osorio R, Stuber T, Farrell D, et al. Recovery of *Mycobacterium bovis* from soft fresh cheese originating from Mexico. *Appl Environ Microbiol.* (2006) 73:1025–28. doi: 10.1128/AEM.01956-06
30. Rodwell TC, Kapasi AJ, Moore M, Milian-Suazo F, Harris B, Guerrero LP, et al. Tracing the origins of *Mycobacterium bovis* tuberculosis in humans in the USA to cattle in Mexico using spoligotyping. (2010) 14(Suppl. 3):e129–35. doi: 10.1016/j.ijid.2009.11.037
31. USDA (2009). *Analysis of Bovine Tuberculosis Surveillance in Accredited Free States.* Animal and Plant Health Inspection Service, Veterinary Services.
32. Biek R, O'Hare A, Wright D, Mallon T, McCormick C, Orton RJ, et al. Whole genome sequencing reveals local transmission patterns of *Mycobacterium bovis* in sympatric cattle and badger populations. *PLoS Pathog.* (2012) 8:e1003008. doi: 10.1371/journal.ppat.1003008
33. Thacker TC, Palmer MV, Robbe-Austerman S, Stuber TP, Waters WR. Anatomical distribution of *Mycobacterium bovis* genotypes in experimentally infected white-tailed deer. *Vet Micro.* (2015) 180:75–81. doi: 10.1016/j.vetmic.2015.07.006
34. USDA (2009). Beef 2007-08, Part II: Reference of Beef Cow-calf Management Practices in the United States, 2007–08 USDA:APHIS:VS, CEAH. Fort Collins, Colorado. #N512.0209
35. USDA (2008). *Beef 2007–08, Part III: Changes in the U.S. Beef Cow-Calf Industry, 1993–2008.* USDA:APHIS:VS, CEAH. Fort Collins, Colorado #518.0509
36. USDA (2008). Dairy 2007, Part II: Changes in the U.S. Dairy Cattle Industry, 1991–2007 USDA-APHIS-VS, CEAH. Fort Collins, Colorado. #N481.0308
37. Sandoval-Azuara SE, Muniz-Salazar R, Perea-Jacobo R, Robbe-Austerman S, Perera-Ortiz A, Lopez-Valencia G, et al. Whole genome sequencing of *Mycobacterium bovis* to obtain molecular fingerprints in human and cattle isolates from Baja California, Mexico. *Int J Infect Dis.* (2017) 48–56, doi: 10.1016/j.ijid.2017.07.012

15

Genetic Diversity and Potential Paths of Transmission of *Mycobacterium bovis* in the Amazon: The Discovery of *M. bovis* Lineage Lb1

*Paulo Alex Carneiro [1,2], Cristina Kraemer Zimpel [3,4], Taynara Nunes Pasquatti [5], Taiana T. Silva-Pereira [3], Haruo Takatani [6], Christian B. D. G. Silva [6], Robert B. Abramovitch [4], Ana Marcia Sa Guimaraes [3], Alberto M. R. Davila [7], Flabio R. Araujo [8] and John B. Kaneene [1]**

[1] Center for Comparative Epidemiology, College of Veterinary Medicine, Michigan State University, East Lansing, MI, United States, [2] Amazonas State Federal Institute, Manaus, Brazil, [3] Laboratory of Applied Research in Mycobacteria, Department of Microbiology, Institute of Biomedical Sciences, University of São Paulo, São Paulo, Brazil, [4] Department of Microbiology and Molecular Genetics, Michigan State University, East Lansing, MI, United States, [5] Dom Bosco Catholic University, Campo Grande, Brazil, [6] Agência de Defesa Agropecuaria Do Amazonas, Manaus, Brazil, [7] Computational and Systems Biology Laboratory, Oswaldo Cruz Institute and Graduate Program in Biodiversity and Health, FIOCRUZ, Rio de Janeiro, Brazil, [8] Embrapa Gado de Corte, Campo Grande, Brazil

***Correspondence:**
John B. Kaneene
kaneenej@msu.edu

Bovine tuberculosis (bTB) has yet to be eradicated in Brazil. Herds of cattle and buffalo are important sources of revenue to people living in the banks of the Amazon River basin. A better understanding of *Mycobacterium bovis (M. bovis)* populational structure and transmission dynamics affecting these animals can significantly contribute in efforts to improve their sanitary status. Herein, we sequenced the whole genome of 22 *M. bovis* isolates (15 from buffalo and 7 from cattle) from 10 municipalities in the region of the Lower Amazon River Basin in Brazil and performed phylogenomic analysis and Single Nucleotide Polymorphism (SNP)-based transmission inference to evaluate population structure and transmission networks. Additionally, we compared these genomes to others obtained in unrelated studies in the Marajó Island (n = 15) and worldwide (n = 128) to understand strain diversity in the Amazon and to infer *M. bovis* lineages. Our results show a higher genomic diversity of *M. bovis* genomes obtained in the Lower Amazon River region when compared to the Marajó Island, while no significant difference was observed between *M. bovis* genomes obtained from cattle and buffalo ($p \geq 0.05$). This high genetic diversity is reflected by the weak phylogenetic clustering of *M. bovis* from the Lower Amazon River region based on geographic proximity and in the detection of only two putative transmission clusters in the region. One of these clusters is the first description of inter-species transmission between cattle and buffalo in the Amazon, bringing implications to the bTB control program. Surprisingly, two *M. bovis* lineages were detected in our dataset, namely Lb1 and Lb3, constituting the first description of Lb1 in South America.

Most of the strains of this study (13/22) and all 15 strains of the Marajó Island carried no clonal complex marker, suggesting that the recent lineage classification better describe the diversity of *M. bovis* in the Amazon.

Keywords: tuberculosis, bovine TB transmission, clonal complex, whole genome sequencing, spoligotype, *Mycobacterium bovis*, bovine tuberculosis

INTRODUCTION

Mycobacterium bovis (M. bovis) is a member of the *Mycobacterium tuberculosis* complex (MTBC) and is the leading causative agent of bovine tuberculosis (bTB), an OIE (World Organization for Animal Health) notifiable disease that affects mainly cattle, buffalo, and other domesticated and wild animals, but can also be transmitted to humans (zoonotic TB) (1, 2). bTB is distributed worldwide but has very low prevalence in most industrialized countries and has even been eradicated in few nations. However, the disease remains a major problem in developed countries with wildlife reservoirs that end up transmitting the pathogen to domestic livestock and vice-versa, and in developing countries where inefficient bTB control programs result in high disease endemicity and spread (1, 2). In the Brazilian Amazon, few studies aiming to better understand bTB's epidemiology were performed (3–6). The prevalence within animals in the area ranged from 0.1% (4) to 5.4% (6) and the major risk factors associated with bTB were the introduction of new animals into the herds (4), the buffalo species, herds with more than 100 animals, and the presence of cattle and buffalo in the same farm (6).

MTBC members evolved from a most recent common ancestor with *M. canettii*, and are characterized as clonal species demonstrating high genomic similarity (7). Currently, the use of whole-genome sequencing (WGS) to understand tuberculous mycobacteria populational structure is widespread and provided the basis for outbreak tracing and phylogenetic analysis resulting in the classification of human-adapted MTBC into 8 lineages, with *M. tuberculosis* accounting for L1 to L4 and L7-L8, and *Mycobacterium africanum* comprising of L5 and L6 (8, 9). On the other hand, *M. bovis* has been historically classified by Clonal Complexes (CCs), which are identified by genomic deletions, few Single Nucleotide Polymorphism's (SNPs), and/or spoligotypes patterns (10). Accordingly, four different *M. bovis* CCs have been described presenting distinct geographical distribution patterns: African 1 and 2 restricted to Africa, European 2 commonly found in the Iberian Peninsula, and European 1 distributed globally (11–14). With the advent of WGS, recent studies at a global scale provided insights into the population structure and evolution of *M. bovis* lineages (9), showing that CCs do not represent the whole genomic diversity of the isolates (9, 15, 16) and suggesting the existence of at least four *M. bovis* lineages, named Lb1 through Lb4, and three "unknown groups" (9). With the populational structure of *M. bovis* based on WGS starting to be unveiled, additional studies covering different geographic locations are needed to better comprehend worldwide disease spread and to provide new insights regarding the use of genomes to understand disease transmission at the herd and farm levels.

Molecular epidemiological investigation has proved to be a useful tool for TB control and surveillance, which allows us to better understand the dynamics of disease transmission and precisely identify the infectious agent (17). In addition, the knowledge regarding strain diversity within host species has special contribution in areas under risk of zoonotic TB occurrence, thereby providing new insights in strain distribution that may help establishing strategic measures for TB control and prevention (18, 19). In Brazil, few and dispersed molecular epidemiologic studies of *M. bovis* have been reported (20–24), and the WGS characterization of the pathogen is just starting to be unraveled (24–26). While few studies focused on areas of high dairy herd productivity (25, 26), a recent study evaluating *M. bovis* genomes obtained from buffalo and cattle of the Marajó Island, Northern Brazil, was performed and showed the existence of a monophyletic group without CC classification (24). Therefore, the aim of this study was to apply whole-genome and SNP-based phylogenomic analyses to obtain novel information regarding the genetic diversity of *M. bovis* strains circulating in buffalo and cattle from the region of the Lower Amazon River Basin. We believe that such information will guide policy development and strategies to contain the disease in livestock, and thus reduce the risk associated with transmission to humans.

MATERIALS AND METHODS

M. bovis Isolate Selection

A total of 24 *M. bovis* isolates were selected, representing one herd of each municipality involved in two previous studies (6, 20) that obtained a total of 63 *M. bovis* isolates from Amazonas State (12 from cattle and 45 from buffalo) and from Pará State (5 from cattle and 1 from buffalo). The selection of *M. bovis* isolates maintained the proportionality according to species (cattle and buffalo) and the local prevalence from the previous studies (6, 20). Accordingly, these isolates were from tissue samples of 8 cattle and 16 buffalos collected at the slaughterhouse from herds with or without known tuberculin skin test (TST) status originating from 12 different municipalities: Alenquer (n = 1), Apui (n = 1), Autazes (n = 1), Careiro da Varzea (n = 1), Itacoatiara (n = 2), Manacapuru (n = 1), Novo Ceu (n = 8), Parintins (n = 3), Prainha (n = 2), Presidente Figueiredo (n = 1), and Urucara (n = 3). Samples were collected from June 2016 to October 2017.

DNA Extraction

M. bovis isolates were reactivated in Stonebrink media and incubated until positive growth at 37°C. DNA extractions from colonies suggestive of *M. bovis* for genomic sequencing were performed according to the protocol of van Embden et al. (27), with modifications. Initially, for inactivation, 2-3 colonies were resuspended in 400 μl TE buffer (10 mM Tris-HCI and 1 mM ethylenediaminetetraacetic acid—EDTA, pH 8.0) and heated at 80°C for 30 min. Subsequently, 50 μl of lysozyme (10 mg/ml) were added and incubated at 37°C for 1 h. Then, 75 μl of 10% SDS (sodium dodecyl sulfate) and 10 μl of proteinase K (10 mg/ml) were added and incubated at 65°C for 10 min. Next, 100 μl of 5M NaCl (sodium chloride) and 100 μl of CTAB (cetyltrimethylammonium bromide) were added, followed by stirring and incubation at 65°C for 10 min. After that, 750 μl chloroform/isoamyl alcohol (24:1) were added, stirred and centrifuged at 12,000 g for 5 min. The aqueous phase (surface) was transferred to another tube, 450 μl of isopropanol were added and incubated at −20°C for 30 min and then centrifuged again at 12,000 g for 15 min at room temperature. The supernatant was discarded, and the pellet washed once with 1 ml of ice-cold ethanol (70%) with centrifugation at 12,000 g for 5 min. After drying the tube by evaporation at room temperature, the DNA was resuspended in 20 μl of TE buffer and stored in a freezer at −20°C. The quality and concentration of the extracted DNAs were evaluated using Nanodrop (Thermo Fisher Scientific). Procedures were performed in a Biosafety Level 3 Laboratory located at the Embrapa Gado de Corte, Campo Grande, Brazil.

Genome Sequencing

WGS was performed at the NGS multi-user platform of Oswaldo Cruz Foundation (FIOCRUZ), Rio de Janeiro, Brazil. Briefly, DNA quantification was performed using the Qubit™ dsDNA HS Assay Kit (Thermo Fisher Scientific, Waltham, USA) and the Agilent High Sensitivity DNA Kit (Agilent, California, USA). WGS of *M. bovis* isolates was carried out on a HiSeq instrument (Illumina, San Diego, CA) using HiSeq Rapid SBS Kit v2 (200 cycles) chemistry and the Nextera DNA Flex Library preparation kit (Illumina, San Diego, CA) according to the manufacturer's instructions. Sequencing reads were deposited in Sequence Read Archive (BioProject number PRJNA675550), NCBI and accession numbers are described in **Supplementary Data Sheet 1**.

Genome Quality Assessment and Regions of Difference Identification

Obtained reads were trimmed using a Trimmomatic version 0.38 (28) for adapters and low-quality base removal (sliding window 5:20). Trimmed reads were then evaluated for reads size, per

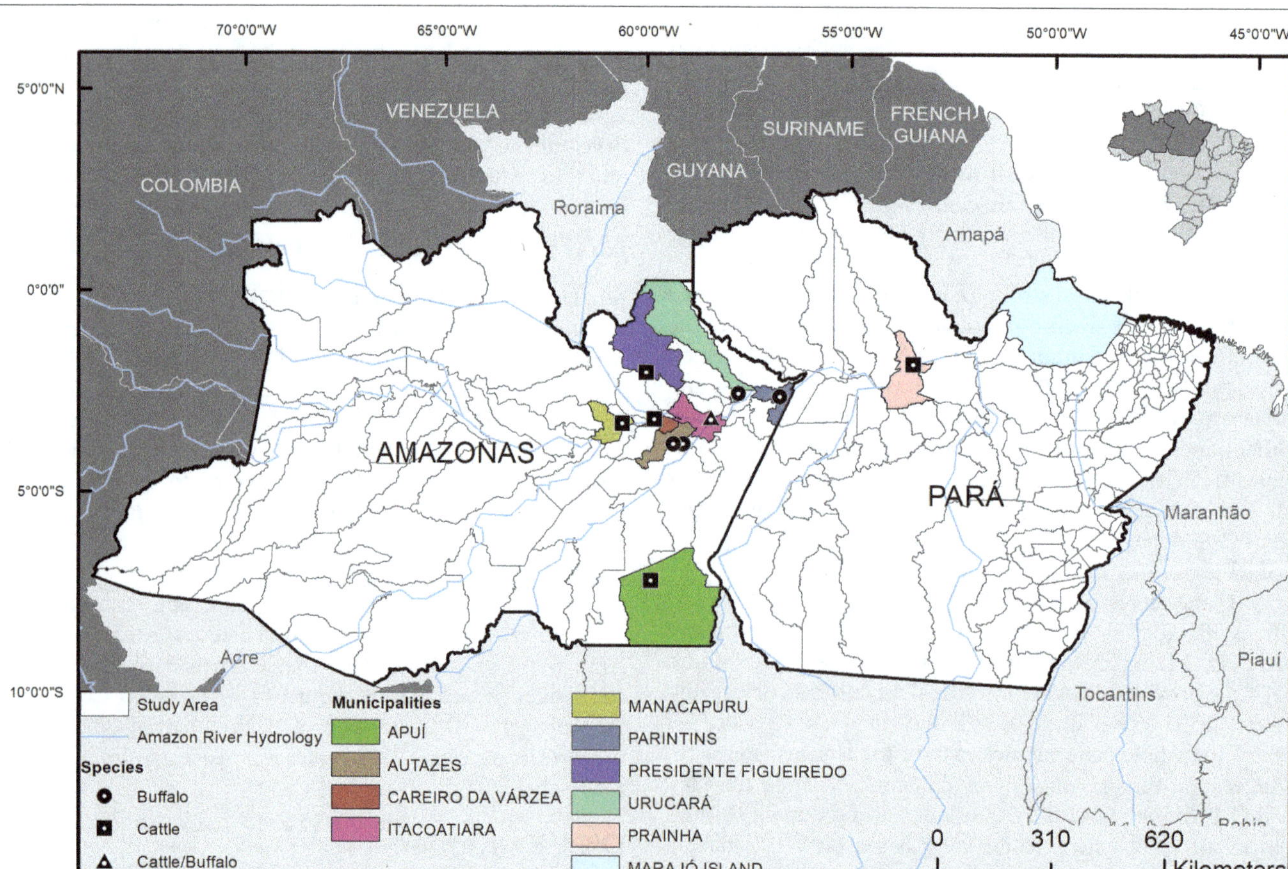

FIGURE 1 | Geographic origin and host species of the *Mycobacterium bovis* isolates from municipalities of Lower Amazon River Basin, Brazil. Isolates were selected from 63 *M. bovis* strains previously isolated from cattle and buffalo (6, 20).

base and read sequence quality, presence of adapters, and GC content using FastQC (29). The GC content had to be around 65% (which is common to mycobacterial genomes) and without multiple peaks (i.e., possible contamination with sequences of different GC content) per quality criteria.

As to confirm that genomes were from *M. bovis*, reads were mapped against *M. tuberculosis* H37Rv using Burrows-Wheeler Aligner (bwa-mem) (30) and the positions according to reference genome of RD1 (4,354,000–4,358,331 nt), RD4 (1,696,017–1,708,748 nt), and RD9 (2,330,880–2,332,100 nt) were evaluated for coverage as previously described (31). The genome was considered as *M. bovis* species when RD1 was absent (i.e. region was intact) and RD4 and RD9 were present (i.e. regions were deleted) (32). Obtained coverage against *M. tuberculosis* H37Rv was also used as quality criteria, considering 95% as a minimum mapping percentage for a genome to be included in the analysis.

Spoligotyping and Clonal Complexes

Spoligotypes were also investigated *in silico* using SpoTyping (31). Identified genetic spacers were processed in the *M. bovis* Spoligotype Database (www.mbovis.org) to retrieve a spoligotype pattern and SB number. The CCs African 1 (Af1) and 2 (Af2) and European 1 (Eu1) and 2 (Eu2) were evaluated as previously described (9). Briefly, the SNP in the *guaA* gene was investigated in the bam files generated from read mapping against *M. tuberculosis* H37Rv, by checking the position 3,813,236. For the RDs, the same bam files were used to investigate read depth using samtools depth (33) and GNU parallel 2018 (34) for the following regions: RDEu1 (1,768,074–1,768,878 nt), RDAf1 (665,042–668,394 nt), and RDAf2 (680,337–694,429 nt) also as described previously (9).

Variant Calling

Trimmed *M. bovis* reads were mapped against *M. bovis* AF2122/97 (NC_002945.4) using bwa-mem (30). Duplicated reads were removed using Picard v2.18.23 (https://github.com/broadinstitute/picard). SNPs were called using Samtools v1.9 mpileup (33) and VarScan v2.4.3 mpileup2cns (35), selecting read depth of 7, mapping quality and minimum base quality of 20, and strand bias filter on, followed by annotation using snpEFF (36). INDELs (insertions and deletions), as well as SNPs from repetitive regions (PE/PPE, transposases, integrases, maturase, phage and repetitive family 13E12 genes) were removed from the analysis using a previously described awk command (9). Genomes were also evaluated based on the number of heterogenous SNPs, considering 15% as a maximum amount for a genome to be included in the analysis.

Phylogenetic Reconstruction

As to evaluate genetic diversity of *M. bovis* in the geographic region, 15 quality-approved *M. bovis* genomes previously sequenced and obtained from cattle and buffalo of the Marajó Island (24) (ENA accession number ERP116404) were used to evaluate the phylogenetic relatedness with the *M. bovis* genomes sequenced in this study. The Marajó Island is geographically close to the targeted region analyzed herein (**Figure 1**), together with the Lower Amazon River Basin are the regions of major concentration of bufallo in the country, and these *M. bovis* genomes (24) were the only strains of the North of Brazil sequenced up until this study. These genomes were quality-assessed and SNPs were obtained as described above. A matrix of concatenated SNPs of the *M. bovis* genomes was constructed as described (9) and used to estimate a maximum likelihood (ML) phylogeny. RAxML version 8.2.12 (37) was used to construct this phylogenetic tree, selecting the GTRCAT model and autoMRE for best-scoring ML tree and a maximum of 1,000 bootstrap inferences. Genomes of *Mycobacterium caprae* (*M. caprae*) (ERR1462591, ERR1462625, ERR1462617, ERR1462581) were also included in the SNP matrix to serve as outgroup.

TABLE 1 | Distribution of *Mycobacterium bovis* in Amazon by municipality, host, and spoligotype.

Municipality	Species	Spoligotype
Apui	Cattle	SB0822
Autazes	Buffalo	Unknown*
Careiro da Varzea	Cattle	SB0295
Itacoatiara	Buffalo	SB0295
	Cattle	SB0295
Manacapuru	Cattle	SB0822
Novo Ceu	Buffalo	SB0822 (3)
	Buffalo	SB1190 (2)
	Buffalo	SB0295 (2)
	Buffalo	SB0121
Parintins	Buffalo	SB0822 (2)
	Buffalo	SB1800
Prainha	Cattle	SB0822
	Cattle	SB0295
Presidente Figueiredo	Cattle	SB0822
Urucara	Buffalo	SB1800
	Buffalo	SB0822
TOTAL		22

**Unknown spoligotype pattern: we have submitted the pattern to M.bovis.org database, but up until this publication, a new SB number has not been provided.*

Minimum Spanning Tree

A pairwise SNP-distance matrix and a minimum spanning tree were constructed using PHYLOViZ (38) with default parameters and using a concatenated SNP matrix of the *M. bovis* genomes as input.

Phylogenomic Analysis With Lineage Representatives of *M. bovis* Genomes

Mycobacterium bovis genomes obtained from this study and those from Marajó Island (24) were compared against a collection of 106 genomes representing the four *M. bovis* lineages (Lb1–Lb4) and unknown groups 1, 2, and 3 from a recent study that evaluated worldwide distribution and evolution of *M. bovis* genomes (9) (**Supplementary Data Sheet 1**). In addition, 21 quality-approved *M. bovis* genomes from France (39), which include representatives of the recently suggested CC called European 3 (40), were also included in the analysis

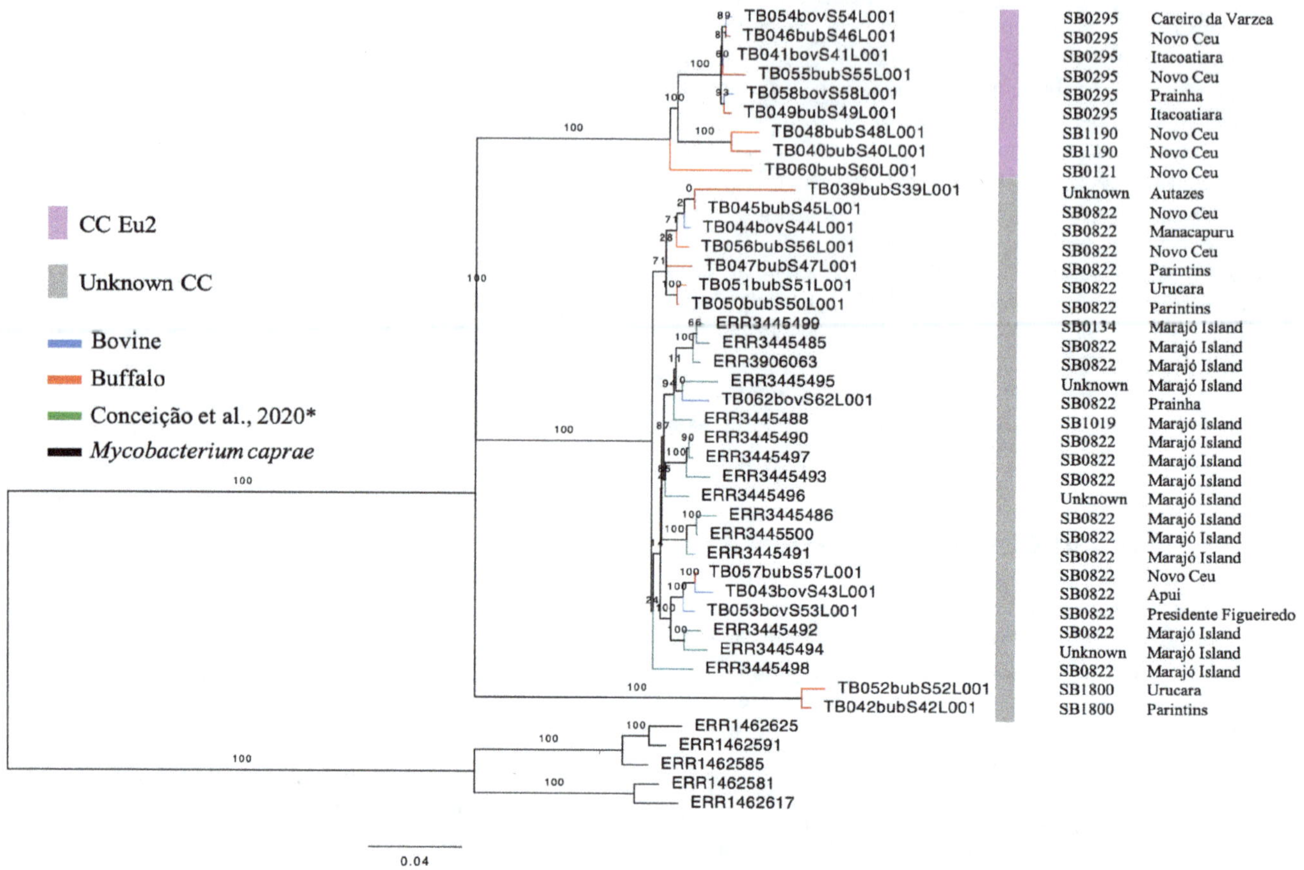

FIGURE 2 | Phylogenetic analysis of *Mycobacterium bovis* genomes from North of Brazil. Maximum likelihood (ML) phylogenetic tree from concatenated SNPs (single nucleotide polymorphisms) of *Mycobacterium bovis* genomes sequenced in this study and by Conceição et al. (24) from Marajó Island. Blue tips: *M. bovis* genomes obtained from cattle and sequenced in this study; red tips: *M. bovis* genomes obtained from buffalo and sequenced in this study; green tips: *M. bovis* genomes from unknown hosts sequenced by Conceição et al. (24) and obtained from cattle or buffalo from Marajó Island, Pará; black tips: *Mycobacterium caprae* genomes (outgroup). Purple bar, *M. bovis* genomes carrying markers of European 2 clonal complex; gray bar, *M. bovis* genomes carrying no markers of known clonal complexes. SB, spoligotype patterns. The phylogenetic tree was generated using RAxML and annotated using FigTree v1.4.3 (43). Horizontal bar shows substitutions per nucleotide. *unknown spoligotype pattern: we have submitted the pattern to M.bovis.org database, but up until this publication, a new SB number has not been provided.

(**Supplementary Data Sheet 1**). Genomes of *M. caprae* and *M. tuberculosis* H37Rv (outgroup) (**Supplementary Data Sheet 1**) were included to construct the phylogenetic tree using the ML approach as described above.

Pairwise SNP-Comparisons

From the SNP-distance matrix, pairwise distances distributions between *M. bovis* genomes obtained from cattle vs. buffalo (Amazon dataset) and between *M. bovis* genomes originating from the Lower Amazon River Basin and Marajó Island were compared using the non-parametric Mann Whitney-test in R software. A result was considered statistically significant when p-value ≤ 0.05.

RESULTS

Out of the 24 *M. bovis* isolates sequenced, two were excluded because of low coverage against the reference genome of *M. tuberculosis* H37Rv or >15% heterogeneous SNPs. These occurred because one isolate resulted in only 38 Kb of sequencing (i.e., failed to be properly sequenced) and the other showed the presence of mixed-strain infection, respectively. The 22 remaining quality-approved *M. bovis* genomes originated from 10 municipalities: Apui ($n = 1$), Autazes ($n = 1$), Careiro da Varzea ($n = 1$), Itacoatiara ($n = 2$), Manacapuru ($n = 1$), Novo Ceu ($n = 8$), Parintins ($n = 3$), Prainha ($n = 2$), Presidente Figueiredo ($n = 1$), and Urucara ($n = 2$) (**Figure 1**).

The genotypic characterization by spoligotyping revealed 5 distinct profiles (**Table 1**). The predominant spoligotype was SB0822, detected in 10 isolates, followed by SB0295, representing 6 isolates; the patterns SB1190 and SB1800 were identified in 2 isolates each; the pattern SB0121 had one representative; and one isolate without described spoligotype pattern. Surprisingly, out of 19 *M. bovis* isolates previously typed using an experimental technique (20),

Number of SNPs

0	250	500	750

	ERR3445485	ERR3445486	ERR3445488	ERR3445490	ERR3445491	ERR3445492	ERR3445493	ERR3445494	ERR3445496	ERR3445497	ERR3445498	ERR3445499	ERR3445500	ERR3906063	TB039bubS39L001	TB040bubS40L001	TB041bovS41L001	TB042bubS42L001	TB043bovS43L001	TB044bovS44L001	TB045bubS45L001	TB046bubS46L001	TB047bubS47L001	TB048bubS48L001	TB049bubS49L001	TB050bubS50L001	TB051bubS51L001	TB052bubS52L001	TB053bovS53L001	TB054bovS54L001	TB055bubS55L001	TB056bubS56L001	TB057bubS57L001	TB058bovS58L001	TB060bubS60L001	TB062bovS62L001	NC_002945.4
ERR3445485	0	94	60	76	91	91	89	94	81	78	82	25	86	29	169	572	529	621	96	92	100	532	100	565	536	90	87	617	97	536	533	100	94	525	544	71	565
ERR3445486	94	0	92	96	43	97	79	92	95	100	88	93	26	93	151	592	547	635	92	86	82	550	76	575	556	86	81	607	107	554	527	98	106	539	552	95	559
ERR3445488	60	92	0	68	69	79	87	86	61	70	86	51	76	53	183	566	525	613	100	90	96	528	94	569	530	76	87	627	79	530	543	92	82	529	548	65	579
ERR3445490	76	96	68	0	75	77	35	84	59	8	84	67	76	75	171	556	515	607	98	88	92	518	88	561	520	72	85	619	77	520	535	88	76	521	542	81	573
ERR3445491	91	43	69	75	0	82	98	91	70	77	91	84	23	80	176	569	526	614	107	83	87	529	81	572	533	67	78	628	84	533	546	81	83	532	549	90	582
ERR3445492	91	97	79	77	82	0	94	49	82	79	85	80	89	90	172	565	524	614	77	103	101	527	95	568	529	89	100	614	66	529	532	105	67	528	547	100	570
ERR3445493	89	79	87	35	98	94	0	87	84	37	95	90	97	90	164	587	546	634	91	97	91	549	87	578	551	93	96	610	100	551	530	109	103	542	555	94	560
ERR3445494	94	92	86	84	91	49	87	0	83	86	82	85	92	97	167	566	525	617	72	108	92	528	86	571	530	90	103	609	75	530	525	108	70	537	550	105	563
ERR3445496	81	95	61	59	70	82	84	83	0	61	83	72	75	74	178	557	518	608	95	85	89	521	87	562	523	59	72	624	76	523	538	85	75	524	541	80	578
ERR3445497	78	100	70	8	77	79	37	86	61	0	88	71	80	77	173	556	515	607	98	88	92	518	94	561	520	76	85	619	79	520	535	88	82	521	540	87	573
ERR3445498	82	88	86	84	91	85	95	82	83	88	0	87	90	93	157	564	521	611	88	90	92	524	88	555	530	84	85	603	97	528	521	96	84	525	536	85	555
ERR3445499	25	93	51	67	84	80	90	85	72	71	87	0	85	22	174	565	522	612	103	97	99	525	95	568	529	83	94	620	86	527	538	97	87	528	549	72	572
ERR3445500	86	26	76	76	23	89	97	92	75	80	90	85	0	81	171	576	533	621	104	82	88	536	82	575	540	70	77	629	87	540	547	84	86	535	552	89	581
ERR3906063	29	93	53	75	80	90	90	97	74	77	93	22	81	0	178	575	532	620	99	89	97	535	93	570	539	81	86	624	86	537	542	95	85	532	547	62	576
TB039bubS39L001	169	151	183	171	176	172	164	167	178	173	157	174	171	178	0	597	552	640	145	125	121	555	139	580	561	143	132	608	182	559	532	139	165	550	557	158	458
TB040bubS40L001	572	592	566	556	569	565	587	566	557	556	564	565	576	575	597	0	153	697	568	564	570	156	574	69	150	552	559	711	561	158	173	560	554	165	208	565	675
TB041bovS41L001	529	547	525	515	526	524	546	525	518	515	521	522	533	532	552	153	0	652	525	521	527	13	529	154	17	511	514	666	522	15	30	515	509	20	165	520	630
TB042bubS42L001	621	635	613	607	614	614	634	617	608	607	611	612	621	620	640	697	652	0	611	609	613	655	615	698	661	601	604	40	610	661	672	607	597	664	681	612	703
TB043bovS43L001	96	92	100	98	107	77	91	72	95	98	88	103	104	99	145	568	525	611	0	80	74	528	82	557	532	82	73	593	51	530	509	94	24	523	534	81	553
TB044bovS44L001	92	86	90	88	83	103	97	108	85	88	90	97	82	89	125	564	521	609	80	0	22	524	62	549	528	44	35	605	91	526	523	32	80	519	528	71	563
TB045bubS45L001	100	82	96	92	87	101	91	92	89	92	92	99	88	97	121	570	527	613	74	22	0	530	44	569	534	46	51	605	97	532	521	38	82	539	546	87	563
TB046bubS46L001	532	550	528	518	529	527	549	528	521	518	524	525	536	535	555	156	13	655	528	524	530	0	532	161	20	514	517	669	523	12	31	522	512	27	172	527	633
TB047bubS47L001	100	76	94	88	81	95	87	86	87	94	88	95	82	93	139	574	529	615	82	62	44	532	0	571	538	48	57	605	95	536	523	60	80	541	548	85	563
TB048bubS48L001	565	575	569	561	572	568	578	571	562	561	555	568	575	570	580	69	154	698	557	549	569	161	571	0	163	553	542	694	568	163	162	557	555	152	191	548	658
TB049bubS49L001	536	556	530	520	533	529	551	530	523	520	530	529	540	539	561	150	17	661	532	528	534	20	538	163	0	516	523	675	525	24	39	524	518	21	174	529	639
TB050bubS50L001	90	86	76	72	67	89	93	90	59	76	84	83	70	81	143	552	511	601	82	44	46	514	48	553	516	0	13	613	75	516	527	44	62	523	532	67	571
TB051bubS51L001	87	81	87	85	78	100	96	103	72	85	85	94	77	86	132	559	514	604	73	35	51	517	57	542	523	13	0	602	88	521	516	47	71	512	521	60	560
TB052bubS52L001	617	607	627	619	628	614	610	609	624	619	603	620	629	624	608	711	666	40	593	605	605	669	605	694	675	613	602	0	626	675	648	619	613	664	673	608	671
TB053bovS53L001	97	107	79	77	84	66	100	75	76	79	97	86	87	86	182	561	522	610	51	91	97	523	95	568	525	75	88	626	0	527	540	91	31	528	547	90	586
TB054bovS54L001	536	554	530	520	533	529	551	530	523	520	528	527	540	537	559	158	15	661	530	526	532	12	536	163	24	516	521	675	527	0	37	522	516	29	174	527	637
TB055bubS55L001	533	527	543	535	546	532	530	525	538	535	521	538	547	542	532	173	30	672	509	523	521	31	523	162	39	527	516	648	540	37	0	535	529	32	171	526	610
TB056bubS56L001	100	98	92	88	81	105	109	108	85	88	96	97	84	95	139	560	515	607	94	32	38	522	60	557	524	44	47	619	91	522	535	0	78	527	536	79	577
TB057bubS57L001	94	106	82	76	83	67	103	70	75	82	84	87	86	85	165	554	509	597	24	80	82	512	80	555	518	62	71	613	31	516	529	78	0	521	534	71	573
TB058bovS58L001	525	539	529	521	532	528	542	537	524	521	525	528	535	532	550	165	20	664	523	519	539	27	541	152	21	523	512	664	528	29	32	527	521	0	163	518	628
TB060bubS60L001	544	552	548	542	549	547	555	550	541	540	536	549	552	547	557	208	165	681	534	528	546	172	548	191	174	532	521	673	547	174	171	536	534	163	0	525	635
TB062bovS62L001	71	95	65	81	90	100	94	105	80	87	85	72	89	62	158	565	520	612	81	71	87	527	85	548	529	67	60	608	90	527	526	79	71	518	525	0	566
NC_002945.4	565	559	579	573	582	570	560	563	578	573	555	572	581	576	458	675	630	703	553	563	563	633	563	658	639	571	560	671	586	637	610	577	573	628	635	566	0

FIGURE 3 | Pairwise single nucleotide polymorphism (SNP)-distance between *Mycobacterium bovis* genomes of Northern Brazil. Genomes of *M. bovis* from the Lower Amazon River Basin (sequenced in this study) and from Marajó Island [sequenced by Conceição et al. (24)] are included. Genomes starting with ERR are from Marajó Island, while genomes starting with TB are from the Lower Amazon River Basin. NC_002945.4: reference genome *Mycobacterium bovis* AF2122/97. Pairwise comparisons were generated from concatenated SNP matrix using PHYLOViZ (38).

12 were discordant. Disagreement between *in silico* and experimental spoligotyping has been previously described (41, 42). Finally, comparing hosts, our results show a higher number of spoligotypes patterns in buffalo when compared to cattle (**Table 1**). Given the low sample size, further studies should be conducted to confirm if buffalo have consistently higher diversity of spoligotype patterns when compared to cattle in this region.

Among the CCs, only the CC Eu2 was found among 41% (9/22) of the isolates. The remaining 13 samples (59%) were not identified as belonging to any known CC (i.e., Eu1, Eu2, Af1, or Af2). Within buffalo, 40% (6/15) of the samples were Eu2, 60% (9/15) had no CC marker. Within cattle, 42.8% (3/7) of the samples demonstrated the marker of CC Eu2, and the remaining of the isolates (4/7) were not classified within any described CC. In the generated phylogenetic tree, with *M. bovis* strains from the Lower Amazon River Basin and Marajó Island, the host classes (buffalo and cattle) are found dispersed among different clades (**Figure 2**), while *M. bovis* genomes from Marajó Island clustered together, appearing more closely related, and genomes from different Amazonas municipalities did not follow a clear clustering pattern according to geographic region.

Pairwise-SNP comparisons (**Figures 3**, **4**) and minimum spanning tree (**Figure 5**) of the *M. bovis* genomes obtained herein and from the Marajó Island (24) showed a highly diverse genomic dataset, with pairwise SNP-distances varying from 8 to 711 (from 8 to 100 among *M. bovis* genomes from Marajó Island and from 12 to 711 among *M. bovis* genomes of the Amazon) (**Figure 3**). Although the overall distribution was not significantly different (**Figure 4A**), *M. bovis* genomes from the Lower Amazon River region tend to show higher pairwise SNP-distances than *M. bovis* genomes from the Marajó Island (**Figure 3**). There was also no significant difference of *M. bovis* genetic diversity distribution using the dataset from the Lower Amazon River region as a function of host (**Figure 4B**; host information from Marajó Island was not available in ENA).

Reflecting this high diversity, based on current *M. tuberculosis*-based SNP threshold to infer recent transmission

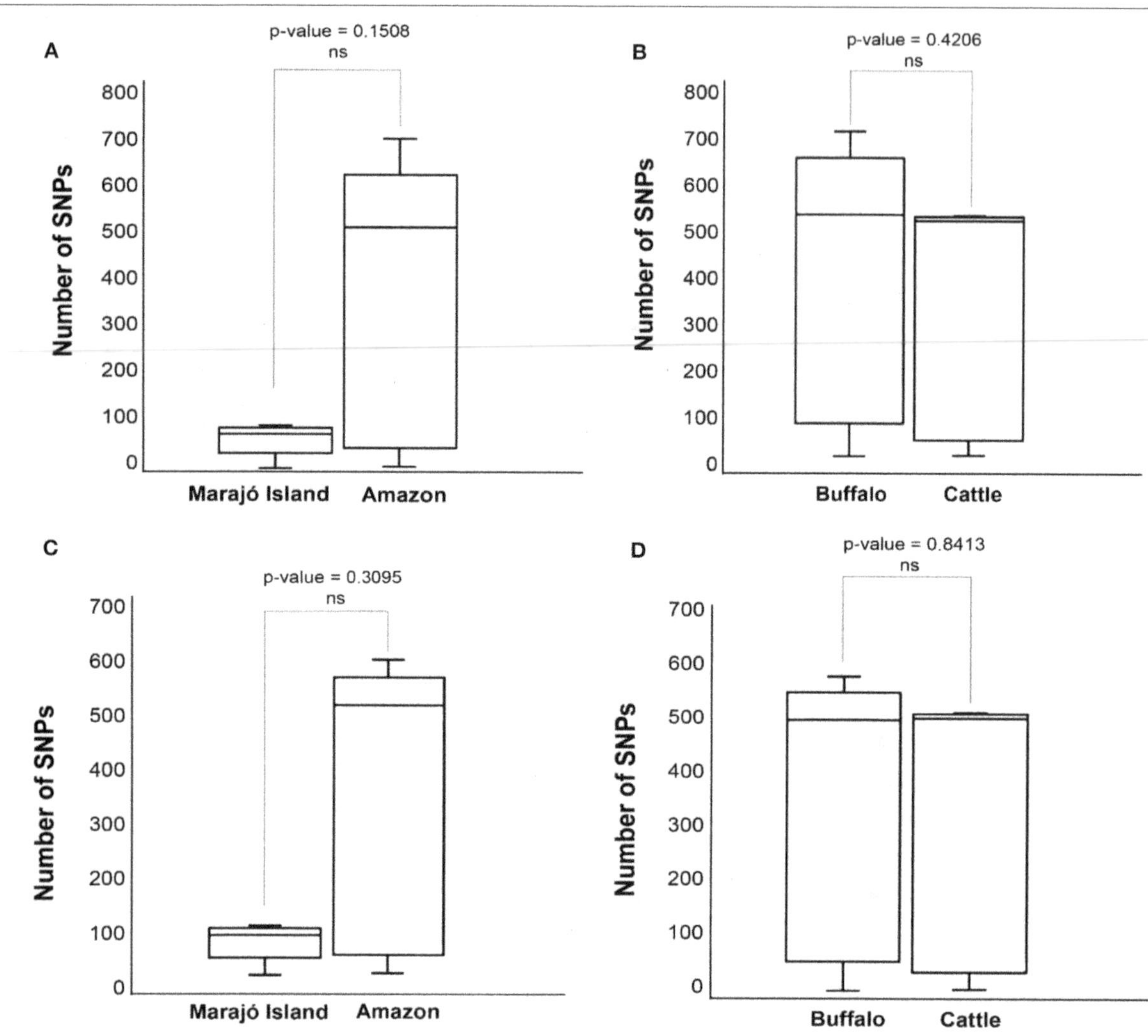

FIGURE 4 | Distributions of pairwise single nucleotide polymorphism (SNP)-distance distance of *Mycobacterium bovis* genomes Northern Brazil. **(A)** Comparison of *M. bovis* pairwise SNP-distance between genomes originating from the Lower Amazon River Basin (sequenced in this study) and from Marajó Island [sequenced by Conceição et al. (24)]. **(B)** Comparison of *M. bovis* pairwise SNP-distance between genomes obtained from buffalo and cattle in the Lower Amazon River Basin. **(C)** Comparison of *M. bovis* lineage 3 (Lb3) pairwise SNP-distance between genomes originating from the Lower Amazon River Basin (sequenced in this study) and from Marajó Island [sequenced by Conceição et al. (24)]. **(D)** Comparison of *M. bovis* Lb3 pairwise SNP-distance between genomes obtained from buffalo and cattle in the Lower Amazon River Basin.

links (~12 SNPs) (44–46), only three possible active transmission clusters can be observed, one in Marajó Island (host unknown), one connecting the municipalities of Urucará and Parintins (between two buffalo, TB051 and TB050), and one connecting the municipalities of Careiro da Várzea, Novo Céu and Itacoatiara (involving cattle and buffalo, TB54, TB46, and TB41), demonstrating recent transmission between different herds and hosts (**Figure 5**). Isolates comprising each transmission clusters also had the same spoligotype pattern (SB0822, SB0822, and SB0295, respectively).

Based on the proposed four major global lineages of *M. bovis* (Lb1, Lb2, Lb3, and Lb4) (7) our setting would be composed by two lineages, Lb1 with two buffalo isolates (TB052 and TB042) and Lb3 with six buffalo and three cattle isolates with the CC marker Eu2 and seven buffalo and four cattle isolates without CC markers (**Figure 6** and **Table 2**). All isolates from Marajó Island were also identified as being from Lb3 without a CC marker. The presence of Lb1, infecting two buffalo, is the first description of this *M. bovis* lineage in Brazil and requires further investigation into the actual origin of these isolates.

In order to evaluate if the high genetic diversity observed in *M. bovis* from the Lower Amazon River region was only due to the presence of the two highly divergent Lb1 genomes, we compared the distributions of pairwise-SNP distances between the Lower Amazon River region and Marajó Island for the Lb3 only (**Figure 4C**). No significant difference in *M. bovis* genetic diversity was observed (**Figure 4C**). However, the maximum SNP-distance between two genomes observed in the Marajó Island was 100, while in the *M. bovis* genomes of the Amazon (Lb3 only) continued to be high. There was also no

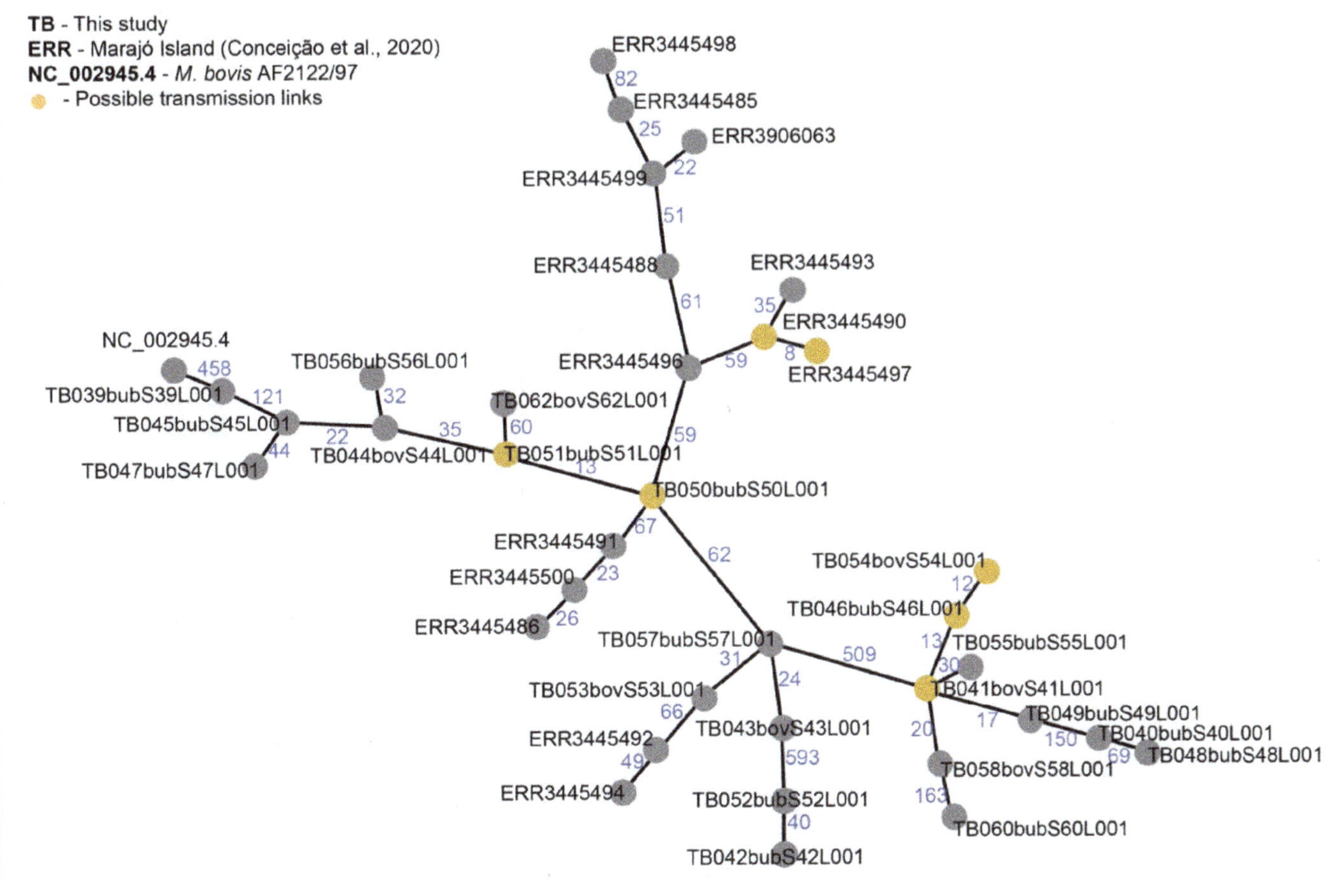

FIGURE 5 | Minimum spanning tree (MST) of *Mycobacterium bovis* genomes from Northern Brazil. Genomes of *M. bovis* from Amazonas state (sequenced in this study, starting with TB) and from Marajó Island [sequenced by Conceição et al. (24), starting with ERR] are included. NC_002945.4: reference genome *Mycobacterium bovis* AF2122/97. Nodes represent *M. bovis* genomes and edges the number of SNPs separating two genomes. Orange nodes represent possible transmission links using an approximate cut-off of 12 single nucleotide polymorphisms (SNP) distance between two *M. bovis* genomes. MST was generated from a concatenated SNP matrix using PHILOViZ (38). Possible transmission links: TB054, TB046 and TB041 are from the municipalities of C. da Varzea, Novo Ceu and Itacoatiara; TB051 and TB050 are from Urucará and Parintins; ERR3445490 and ERR3445497 are from Marajó Island.

significant difference in the genetic diversity of *M. bovis* Lb3 when comparing genomes obtained from cattle and buffalo (**Figure 4D**).

DISCUSSION

To investigate the clonality and population structure of *M. bovis* in the study area at first, we relied on the use of spoligotyping in the characterization of 22 *M. bovis* isolates from 15 buffalo and 7 cattle from June 2016 to October 2017. The spoligotype SB0822 in Brazil was first described in our previous study (20) and we agree with the recent study in Marajó Island in Pará state (24) which seems to demonstrate that SB0822 is the predominant spoligotype in the Amazon region, opposite to a national study with 143 samples from 10 states that found only one occurrence of SB0822 (21). Moreover, SB0822 has been previously described in France (47), cattle in Spain (48) and Portugal (49), and buffalo in Colombia (50), and overall agree with the history of the livestock in the region where the first animals introduced came from Cape Verde (a former Portugal's colony) initially to Marajó Island and from there expanded to the floodplains of the Lower Amazon, on the banks of the Amazon River (51).

Our results also show a higher number of spoligotype patterns of *M. bovis* in the Lower Amazon River Basin compared to the Marajó Island, which can be explained due to the frequent movement of animals in our area of study and the isolation of the herds in the Marajó Island. It is important to highlight that the diversity of *M. bovis* found within buffalo in our sampling is unlikely a result of recent introduction of animals from other Brazilian states since there has been no buffalo imported from other states to the Amazon region and this is probably maintained by constant reinfection from reservoir animals. Accordingly, SB0121 (the most prevalent spoligotyping in Brazil) was found in only one sample, which may reflect the low transit of animals from other states to the area of this study.

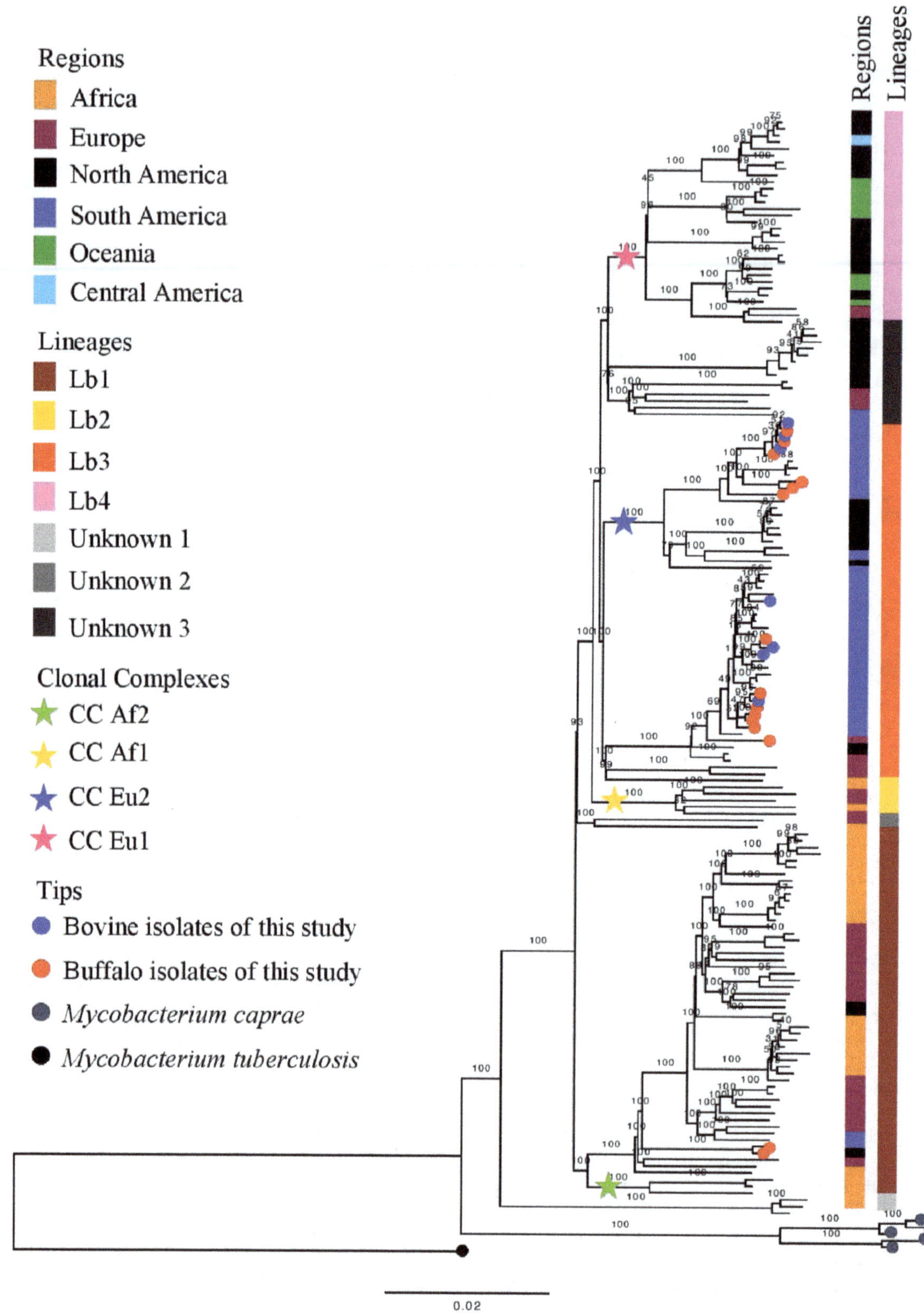

FIGURE 6 | Phylogenetic analysis of *Mycobacterium bovis* lineages. Maximum likelihood (ML) phylogenetic tree from concatenated SNPs (single nucleotide polymorphisms) of *Mycobacterium bovis* genomes from North of Brazil [Amazon, this study, and Marajó Island from Conceição et al. (24)] and worldwide isolates. *Mycobacterium caprae* genomes were included in the analysis, and *Mycobacterium tuberculosis* H37Rv was used as outgroup. The phylogenetic tree was generated using RAxML and annotated using FigTree v1.4.3 (43). Horizontal bar shows substitutions per nucleotide. Lineages are classified according to Zimpel et al. (9).

TABLE 2 | Distribution of *Mycobacterium. bovis* in Amazon by municipality, year, host, clonal complexes, and lineages.

Municipality	Year	Host species	Lb1	Lb3	
				Eu2	No CC marker
Apui	2017	Cattle	-	-	1
Autazes	2017	Buffalo	-	-	1
Careiro da Várzea	2017	Cattle	-	1	-
Itacoatiara	2017	Buffalo	-	1	-
	2017	Cattle	-	1	-
Manacapuru	2017	Cattle	-	-	1
Novo Ceu	2016	Buffalo	-	5	3
Parintins	2017	Buffalo	1		2
Prainha	2017	Cattle	-	1	1
Presidente Figueiredo	2017	Cattle	-	-	1
Urucara	2017	Buffalo	1	-	1
TOTAL			2	9	11

Eu2, Clonal Complex European 2; CC, Clonal Complex; Lb1 and Lb3, lineages of Mycobacterium bovis 1 and 3.

Our results show overall higher genetic diversity of *M. bovis* genomes obtained from different municipalities of Lower Amazon River region when compared to the Marajó Island. This is most likely due to the geographic isolation of the island with lower chances of animal importation over time. We also show possible transmission links between buffalo and cattle from different herds but from close geographic proximity. As wildlife reservoirs have not been identified in Brazil thus far, this transmission may have occurred due to infected animal transit and/or introduction into different herds, showing the presence of a two-host system allowing inter-species transmission in the region.

The detection of an inter-species transmission link, the intertwined phylogenetic dispersal of *M. bovis* obtained from cattle and buffalo, and the absence of significant difference in *M. bovis* genetic diversity in cattle *vs.* buffalo suggest that contact rate between different hosts and consequent geographic proximity likely played a more important role in determining the host range of *M. bovis* in this region than host species, agreeing with recent studies (10, 24). Currently the most accepted hypothesis is that *M. bovis* is not a specialized pathogen, i.e., can affect several host species irrespective of its genetic makeup. However, we cannot neglect the possibility of differential host susceptibility to different strains or lineages of *M. bovis*, which may allow one particular strain or lineage to thrive in a specific host. Herein and in the study in Marajó Island (24), for instance, there is only 40% power to determine a possible significant difference in distribution of *M. bovis* strains between buffalo and cattle. Therefore, studies with a higher sample size comparing the dynamics of *M. bovis* infection within buffalo and cattle are needed to definitively clarify this research question.

The results from our study support the fact that current CCs cannot represent the whole diversity of *M. bovis* strains. Interestingly, this is the first time that is described in Brazil isolates of *M. bovis* originating from the *M. bovis* lineage Lb1 (9). In a recent global phylogenomic study of *M. bovis*, strains of Lb1 were shown to emerge from older nodes than Lb3 in the phylogenetic tree and were detected in Eritrea, Ethiopia, Tanzania, Uganda, Tunisia, France, Spain, Italy, Switzerland, and the United States (9). However, some strains identified in this lineage carry the CC Af2 marker (9) which is found at high frequency in bTB cases from East Africa (12), demonstrating the important ties of this lineage to the African continent. One hypothesis to be looked at is that due to the proximity of these countries with Portugal and its colonies; these strains might have been first introduced in the Amazon region during Brazil colonization.

Results from this study, along with others (9, 16, 39, 40), can be used to refine the understanding of *M. bovis* lineage Lb1. With current genomic data, this lineage is composed of two main clusters: one made of *M. bovis* genomes carrying the CC Af2 marker, and the other without known CC markers (9, 16). Herein, the Lb1 cluster without CC Af2 marker includes 19 out of the 21 French *M. bovis* genomes of SB0120 sequenced by Hauer et al. (39) and included in this study. Recently, Branger et al. (52) suggested that this phylogenetic cluster be called CC European 3, also based on their previous work (39). In this study and in others (9, 16), this cluster is composed of *M. bovis* genomes of many spoligotype patterns (e.g., SB0120, SB0134, SB0828, SB0948, SB1517; **Supplementary Data Sheet 1**) and of BCG vaccine strains (16, 39). Although 19 specific SNPs have been provisionally suggested to be specific of Lb1 (9) and 5 SNPs of its non-Af2 cluster [i.e., CC Eu3; cluster I in Hauer et al. (39)], further studies using comprehensive global datasets should be conducted to confirm or identify definitive genetic markers. The remaining two French *M. bovis* genomes, SRR7851366 and SRR7851376, grouped with genomes of Lb3 and "unknown 3" group, respectively; their disparate position on the phylogenetic tree corroborates the finding of Hauer et al. (39).

The finding of isolates from Marajó Island belonging to Lb3 without CC marker reinforces the previously described (24) existence of a unique *M. bovis* clade in the island that was likely introduced in a single event. In contrast, our results suggest that *M. bovis* was introduced into the Lower Amazon River region as three different events, for which the temporal order remains to be evaluated. One introduction is related to the neighbor cities of Parintins and Urucara, with strains Lb1. Another introduction occurred with Lb3 strains without the CC Eu2 marker, probably with the same origin from the Marajó Island. And finally, an additional introduction is observed with Lb3 strains carrying the CC Eu2 marker, likely from cattle imported from other states and spreading to buffalo. In 2019, a study with 90 samples of cattle lesions suggestive of bTB from the states of Goias, Mato Grosso, Mato Grosso do Sul, Minas Gerais, São Paulo, Tocantins, and Pará found that 14.4% (13/90) belonged to the CC Eu1 and 81.1% (73/90) to the CC Eu2, while 4.65% (4/90) were not identified as any of the four known complexes (53). As the isolates without CC markers were not classified into lineages, the data collected seems insufficient to reveal the true epidemiological picture of the bTB in Brazil. Knowing the genetic profile and understanding the transmission routes of *M. bovis* in the Amazon and elsewhere is essential in order to focus on public health and veterinary resources to contain bTB.

A limitation of this study is the sample size. The small number of *M. bovis* isolates may not be representative of the whole bacterial and animal populations of the Lower Amazon River Basin. Results must be interpreted in light of this fact, and efforts should continue to isolate and study additional *M. bovis* strains from the region.

From our study, we can make the following conclusions: (1) The *M. bovis* CCs classification cannot cover the whole diversity of *M. bovis* strains present in the Amazon region; (2) The presence of *M. bovis* strains Lb1 infecting buffalo requires further investigation into the actual origin of these isolates, showing that the true global diversity of *M. bovis* strains remains to be discovered, likely influenced by cattle trade over history; and (3) The *M. bovis* classification in lineages by SNP-based phylogenetic analyses seems to better cover the diversity of *M. bovis* strains present in the Amazon region compared to CC classification.

ETHICS STATEMENT

Ethical review and approval was not required for the animal study because no animal was used in this study.

AUTHOR CONTRIBUTIONS

PC and JBK designed experiments, coordinated the research team, interpreted the data, wrote and revised the manuscript. HT and CS coordinated field sampling. CS coordination of field sampling. RA reviewed the manuscript. CZ designed experiments, assessed reads quality, performed phylogenomic analysis, interpreted the data, wrote and revised the manuscript. TTP performed pairwise SNP comparisons, constructed the minimum spanning tree, and interpreted the data. AG designed experiments, supervised CZ and TTP, interpreted the data, wrote and revised the manuscript. FA and TNP cultured *M. bovis*, and performed PCR and DNA extraction. AD performed whole genome sequencing. All authors contributed to the article and approved the submitted version.

FUNDING

This work was supported by the Center for Comparative Epidemiology, the College of Veterinary Medicine (Edward and Roberta Sterner Fund), and the Center for Latin American and Caribbean Studies at Michigan State University; CAPES foundation (Procedures: 00199999.000963/2014-03 and 88887.508739/2020-00), Embrapa (Process: 02.13.10.008.00.00), Brazilian National Council for Scientific and Technological Development (CNPq: Process 443235/2014-7), Mato Grosso do Sul Research Foundation (FUNDECT: Procedures 59/300,121/2015, TO: 085/2015 and 59/300.104/2017 SIAFEM 027282), and São Paulo Research Foundation (FAPESP 2016/26108-0, 2019/10896-8, 2017/04617-3).

ACKNOWLEDGMENTS

The authors would like to acknowledge Cheyenne Lei for the map design, Gisele Olivas de Campos Leguizamon for technical support, and the CEFAP (Research Facility) of the Institute of Biomedical Sciences, University of São Paulo, Brazil for computer core services.

REFERENCES

1. Thoen CO, Steele JH, Gilsdorf MJ. *Mycobacterium bovis Infection in Animals and Humans.* 2nd ed Ames, IA: Blackwell Publishing (2008).
2. Chambers MA, Gordon SV, Olea-Popelka F, Barrow PA. *Bovine Tuberculosis.* Wallingford, Oxfordshire: CABI (2018).
3. Barbosa JD, da Silva JB, Rangel CP, da Fonseca AH, Silva NS, Bomjardim HA, et al. Tuberculosis prevalence and risk factors for water buffalo in Pará, Brazil. *Trop Anim Health Prod.* (2014) 46:513–7. doi: 10.1007/s11250-013-0521-1
4. Vendrame FB, Amaku M, Ferreira F, Telles EO, Filho JHHG, Gonçalves VSP, et al. Epidemiologic characterization of bovine tuberculosis in the State of Rondônia, Brazil. *Semin Agrar.* (2016) 37:3639–46. doi: 10.5433/1679-0359.2016v37n5Supl2p3639
5. Silva T, Brasil T, Moraes R, Melo L. First record of bovine tuberculosis in the state of Acre, Brazil. *Ciência Anim.* (2019) 29:152–7. Available online at: https://www.cabdirect.org/cabdirect/abstract/20203160502
6. Carneiro PAM, Takatani H, Pasquatti TN, Silva CBDG, Norby B, Wilkins MJ, et al. Epidemiological study of *Mycobacterium bovis* infection in buffalo and cattle in Amazonas, Brazil. *Front Vet Sci.* (2019) 6:434. doi: 10.3389/fvets.2019.00434
7. Supply P, Marceau M, Mangenot S, Roche D, Rouanet C, Khanna V, et al. Genomic analysis of smooth tubercle bacilli provides insights into ancestry and pathoadaptation of *Mycobacterium tuberculosis. Nat Genet.* (2013) 45:172–9. doi: 10.1038/ng.2517
8. Malone KM, Gordon SV. *Mycobacterium tuberculosis* complex members adapted to wild and domestic animals. In: Gagneux S, editor. *Strain Variation in the Mycobacterium tuberculosis Complex: Its Role in Biology, Epidemiology and Control.* Cham: Springer (2017). p. 135–54.
9. Zimpel CK, Patané JSL, Guedes ACP, de Souza RF, Silva-Pereira TT, Camargo NCS, et al. Global distribution and evolution of *Mycobacterium bovis* lineages. *Front Microbiol.* (2020) 11:843. doi: 10.3389/fmicb.2020.00843
10. Guimaraes AMS, Zimpel CK. *Mycobacterium bovis*: from genotyping to genome sequencing. *Microorganisms.* (2020) 8:667. doi: 10.3390/microorganisms8050667
11. Müller B, Hilty M, Berg S, Carmen Garcia-Pelayo M, Dale J, Boschiroli ML, et al. African 1, an epidemiologically important clonal complex of *Mycobacterium bovis* dominant in Mali, Nigeria, Cameroon, and Chad. *J Bacteriol.* (2009) 191:1951. doi: 10.1128/JB.01590-08
12. Berg S, Garcia-Pelayo MC, Müller B, Hailu E, Asiimwe B, Kremer K, et al. African 2, a clonal complex of *Mycobacterium bovis* epidemiologically important in East Africa. *J Bacteriol.* (2011) 193:670–8. doi: 10.1128/JB.00750-10

13. Smith NH, Berg S, Dale J, Allen A, Rodriguez S, Romero B, et al. European 1: a globally important clonal complex of *Mycobacterium bovis*. *Infect Genet Evol.* (2011) 11:1340–51. doi: 10.1016/j.meegid.2011.04.027
14. Rodriguez-Campos S, Schürch AC, Dale J, Lohan AJ, Cunha MV, Botelho A, et al. European 2—A clonal complex of *Mycobacterium bovis* dominant in the Iberian Peninsula. *Infect Genet Evol.* (2012) 12:866–72. doi: 10.1016/j.meegid.2011.09.004
15. Orloski K, Robbe-austerman S, Stuber T, Hench B, Schoenbaum M. Whole genome sequencing of *Mycobacterium bovis* isolated from livestock in the United States, 1989-2018. *Front Vet Sci.* (2018) 5:253. doi: 10.3389/fvets.2018.00253
16. Loiseau C, Menardo F, Aseffa A, Hailu E, Gumi B, et al. An African origin for *Mycobacterium bovis*. *Evol Med Public Heal.* (2020) 2020:49–59. doi: 10.1093/emph/eoaa005
17. Pérez-Lago L, Navarro Y, García-de-Viedma D. Current knowledge and pending challenges in zoonosis caused by *Mycobacterium bovis*: a review. *Res Vet Sci.* (2014) 97:S94–100. doi: 10.1016/j.rvsc.2013.11.008
18. Smith NH, Dale J, Inwald J, Palmer S, Gordon SV, Hewinson RG, et al. The population structure of *Mycobacterium bovis* in Great Britain: clonal expansion. *Proc Natl Acad Sci USA.* (2003) 100:15271–5. doi: 10.1073/pnas.2036554100
19. Drewe JA, Smith NH. Molecular epidemiology of Mycobacterium bovis. In: Thoen CO, Steele JH, Kaneene JB, editors. *Zoonotic Tuberculosis: Mycobacterium bovis and Other Pathogenic Mycobacteria*, third edition. Ames, IW: Wiley Blackwell (2014). p. 79–88.
20. Carneiro PAM, Pasquatti TN, Takatani H, Zumárraga MJ, Marfil MJ, Barnard C, et al. Molecular characterization of *Mycobacterium bovis* infection in cattle and buffalo in Amazon Region, Brazil. *Vet Med Sci.* (2020) 6:133–41. doi: 10.1002/vms3.203
21. Figueiredo Rocha VC, de Souza-Filho AF, Ikuta CY, Hildebrand e Grisi Filho JH, de Azevedo Issa M, Coelho Mota PMP, et al. High discrimination of *Mycobacterium bovis* isolates in Brazilian herds by spoligotyping. *Prev Vet Med.* (2020) 179:104976. doi: 10.1016/j.prevetmed.2020.104976
22. Zimpel CK, Brandão PE, de Souza Filho AF, de Souza RF, Ikuta CY, Ferreira Neto JS, et al. Complete genome sequencing of *Mycobacterium bovis* SP38 and comparative genomics of *Mycobacterium bovis* and *M. tuberculosis* strains. *Front Microbiol.* (2017) 8:2389. doi: 10.3389/fmicb.2017.02389
23. Carvalho RCT, Vasconcellos SEG, Issa MDA, Filho PMS, Mota PMPC, De Araújo FR, et al. Molecular typing of *Mycobacterium bovis* from cattle reared in midwest Brazil. *PLoS ONE.* (2016) 11:1–16. doi: 10.1371/journal.pone.0162459
24. Conceição ML, Conceição EC, Furlaneto IP, Silva SP, Guimarães AES, Gomes P, et al. Phylogenomic perspective on a unique *Mycobacterium bovis* clade dominating bovine tuberculosis infections among cattle and buffalos in Northern Brazil. *Sci Rep.* (2020) 10:1747. doi: 10.1038/s41598-020-58398-5
25. Anzai EK. *Sequenciamento do genoma completo do Mycobacterium bovis como instrumento de sistema de vigilância no Estado de Santa Catarina.* São Paulo: University of São Paulo (2019).
26. Patané JSL, Martins J, Castelão AB, Nishibe C, Montera L, Bigi F, et al. Patterns and processes of *Mycobacterium bovis* evolution revealed by phylogenomic analyses. *Genome Biol Evol.* (2017) 9:521–35. doi: 10.1093/gbe/evx022
27. van Embden JD, Cave MD, Crawford JT, Dale JW, Eisenach KD, Gicquel B, et al. Strain identification of *Mycobacterium tuberculosis* by DNA fingerprinting: recommendations for a standardized methodology. *J Clin Microbiol.* (1993) 31:406–9. doi: 10.1128/JCM.31.2.406-409.1993
28. Bolger AM, Lohse M, Usadel B. Trimmomatic: a flexible trimmer for illumina sequence data. *Bioinformatics.* (2014) 30:2114–20. doi: 10.1093/bioinformatics/btu170
29. Andrews S. FastQC: *A Quality Control Tool for High Throughput Sequence Data* [Online] (2010). Available online at: http://www.bioinformatics.babraham.ac.uk/projects/fastqc/ (accessed January 23, 2021).
30. Li H, Durbin R. Fast and accurate long-read alignment with Burrows-Wheeler transform. *Bioinformatics.* (2010) 26:589–95. doi: 10.1093/bioinformatics/btp698
31. Faksri K, Xia E, Tan JH, Teo YY, Ong RTH. *In silico* region of difference (RD) analysis of *Mycobacterium tuberculosis* complex from sequence reads using RD-analyzer. *BMC Genomics.* (2016) 17:1–10. doi: 10.1186/s12864-016-3213-1
32. Warren RM, Pittius NCG, Barnard M, Hesseling A, Engelke E, Kock M, et al. Differentiation of *Mycobacterium tuberculosis* complex by PCR amplification of genomic regions of difference. *Int J Tuberc Lung Dis.* (2006) 10:818–22.
33. Li H. A statistical framework for SNP calling, mutation discovery, association mapping and population genetical parameter estimation from sequencing data. *Bioinformatics.* (2011) 27:2987–93. doi: 10.1093/bioinformatics/btr509
34. Tange O. *GNU Parallel.* (2018). Available online at: https://www.gnu.org/software/parallel (accessed January 23, 2021).
35. Koboldt DC, Zhang Q, Larson DE, Shen D, McLellan MD, Lin L, et al. VarScan 2: somatic mutation and copy number alteration discovery in cancer by exome sequencing. *Genome Res.* (2012) 22:568–76. doi: 10.1101/gr.129684.111
36. Cingolani P, Platts A, Wang LL, Coon M, Nguyen T, Wang L, et al. A program for annotating and predicting the effects of single nucleotide polymorphisms, SnpEff. *Fly (Austin).* (2012) 6:80–92. doi: 10.4161/fly.19695
37. Stamatakis A. RAxML version 8: a tool for phylogenetic analysis and post-analysis of large phylogenies. *Bioinformatics.* (2014) 30:1312–3. doi: 10.1093/bioinformatics/btu033
38. Francisco AP, Vaz C, Monteiro PT, Melo-Cristino J, Ramirez M, Carriço JA. PHYLOViZ: phylogenetic inference and data visualization for sequence based typing methods. *BMC Bioinformatics.* (2012) 13:87. doi: 10.1186/1471-2105-13-87
39. Hauer A, Michelet L, Cochard T, Branger M, Nunez J, Boschiroli M-L, et al. Accurate phylogenetic relationships among *Mycobacterium bovis* strains circulating in France based on whole genome sequencing and single nucleotide polymorphism analysis. *Front Microbiol.* (2019) 10:955. doi: 10.3389/fmicb.2019.00955
40. Branger M, Loux V, Cochard T, Boschiroli ML, Biet F, Michelet L. The complete genome sequence of *Mycobacterium bovis* Mb3601, a SB0120 spoligotype strain representative of a new clonal group. *Infect Genet Evol.* (2020) 82:104309. doi: 10.1016/j.meegid.2020.104309
41. Xia E, Teo Y-Y, Ong RT-H. SpoTyping: fast and accurate *in silico* Mycobacterium spoligotyping from sequence reads. *Genome Med.* (2016) 8:19. doi: 10.1186/s13073-016-0270-7
42. Coll F, Mallard K, Preston MD, Bentley S, Parkhill J, McNerney R, et al. SpolPred: rapid and accurate prediction of Mycobacterium tuberculosis spoligotypes from short genomic sequences. *Bioinformatics.* (2012) 28:2991–3. doi: 10.1093/bioinformatics/bts544
43. Rambaut A. *FigTree v1.4.3* (2012). Available online at: http://tree.bio.ed.ac.uk/software (accessed January 4, 2021).
44. Walker TM, Ip CLC, Harrell RH, Evans JT, Kapatai G, Dedicoat MJ, et al. Whole-genome sequencing to delineate *Mycobacterium tuberculosis* outbreaks: a retrospective observational study. *Lancet Infect Dis.* (2013) 13:137–46. doi: 10.1016/S1473-3099(12)70277-3
45. Hatherell HA, Colijn C, Stagg HR, Jackson C, Winter JR, Abubakar I. Interpreting whole genome sequencing for investigating tuberculosis transmission: a systematic review. *BMC Med.* (2016) 14:1–13. doi: 10.1186/s12916-016-0566-x
46. Merker M, Kohl TA, Niemann S, Supply P. The evolution of strain typing in the *Mycobacterium tuberculosis* complex. *Adv Exp Med Biol.* (2017) 1019:79–93. doi: 10.1007/978-3-319-64371-7_3
47. *The Mycobacterium bovis Spoligotype Database.* Available online at: http://www.Mbovis.org (accessed January 4, 2021).
48. Romero B, Aranaz A, Sandoval Á, Álvarez J, de Juan L, Bezos J, et al. Persistence and molecular evolution of *Mycobacterium bovis* population from cattle and wildlife in Doñana National Park revealed by genotype variation. *Vet Microbiol.* (2008) 132:87–95. doi: 10.1016/j.vetmic.2008.04.032
49. Matos F, Cunha MV, Canto A, Albuquerque T, Amado A, Botelho A. Snapshot of *Mycobacterium bovis* and *Mycobacterium caprae* infections in livestock in an area with a low incidence of bovine tuberculosis. *J Clin Microbiol.* (2010) 48:4337–9. doi: 10.1128/JCM.01762-10

50. Jojoa-Jojoa J, Maira Wintaco M, Francisco Osorio R, Puerto-Castro G, Guerrero-Guerrero M. First approach to molecular epidemiology of bovine tuberculosis in Colombia. Rev. *MVZ Cordoba.* (2016) 21:5222–36. doi: 10.21897/rmvz.32
51. Lourenço Júnior JB, Garcia AR. Produção Animal No Bioma Amazônico : Atualidades E Perspectivas. In: *An. Simpósios da 43a Reun. Anu. da SBZ* Joao Pessoa, PB (2006). p. 42–60.
52. Branger M, Hauer A, Michelet L, Karoui C, Cochard T, De Cruz K, et al. Draft genome sequence of *Mycobacterium bovis* strain D-10-02315 isolated from wild boar. *Genome Announc.* (2016) 4:e01268–16. doi: 10.1128/genomeA.01268-16
53. Sales ÉB, de Alencar AP, Hodon MA, Soares Filho PM, de Souza-Filho AF, et al. Identification of clonal complexes of *Mycobacterium bovis* in Brazil. *Arch Microbiol.* (2019) 201:1047–51. doi: 10.1007/s00203-019-01674-4

16

A Meta-Analysis of the Effect of Bacillus Calmette-Guérin Vaccination against Bovine Tuberculosis: Is Perfect the Enemy of Good?

Sreenidhi Srinivasan[1,2], *Andrew J. K. Conlan*[3], *Laurel A. Easterling*[4], *Christian Herrera*[1,2], *Premanshu Dandapat*[5], *Maroudam Veerasami*[6], *Gobena Ameni*[7], *Naresh Jindal*[8], *Gopal Dhinakar Raj*[9], *James Wood*[3], *Nick Juleff*[10], *Douwe Bakker*[11], *Martin Vordermeier*[12,13] and *Vivek Kapur*[1,2]*

[1] Department of Animal Science, The Pennsylvania State University, University Park, PA, United States, [2] The Huck Institutes of the Life Sciences, The Pennsylvania State University, University Park, PA, United States, [3] Disease Dynamics Unit, Department of Veterinary Medicine, University of Cambridge, Cambridge, United Kingdom, [4] School of Veterinary Medicine, University of Pennsylvania, Philadelphia, PA, United States, [5] Indian Veterinary Research Institute, Eastern Regional Station, Kolkata, India, [6] Cisgen Biotech Discoveries Pvt Ltd, Chennai, India, [7] Aklilu Lemma Institute of Pathobiology, Addis Ababa University, Addis Ababa, Ethiopia, [8] Department of Veterinary Public Health and Epidemiology, Lala Lajpat Rai University of Veterinary and Animal Sciences, Hisar, India, [9] Translational Research Platform for Veterinary Biological, Tamil Nadu University of Veterinary and Animal Sciences, Chennai, India, [10] The Bill & Melinda Gates Foundation, Seattle, WA, United States, [11] Technical Consultant and Independent Researcher, Lelystad, Netherlands, [12] Animal and Plant Health Agency, Addlestone, United Kingdom, [13] Centre for Bovine Tuberculosis, Institute for Biological, Environmental and Rural Sciences, University of Aberystwyth, Aberystwyth, United Kingdom

Correspondence:
Vivek Kapur
vkapur@psu.edu

More than 50 million cattle are likely exposed to bovine tuberculosis (bTB) worldwide, highlighting an urgent need for bTB control strategies in low- and middle-income countries (LMICs) and other regions where the disease remains endemic and test-and-slaughter approaches are unfeasible. While Bacillus Calmette-Guérin (BCG) was first developed as a vaccine for use in cattle even before its widespread use in humans, its efficacy against bTB remains poorly understood. To address this important knowledge gap, we conducted a systematic review and meta-analysis to determine the direct efficacy of BCG against bTB challenge in cattle, and performed scenario analyses with transmission dynamic models incorporating direct and indirect vaccinal effects ("herd-immunity") to assess potential impact on herd level disease control. The analysis shows a relative risk of infection of 0.75 (95% CI: 0.68, 0.82) in 1,902 vaccinates as compared with 1,667 controls, corresponding to a direct vaccine efficacy of 25% (95% CI: 18, 32). Importantly, scenario analyses considering both direct and indirect effects suggest that disease prevalence could be driven down close to Officially TB-Free (OTF) status (<0.1%), if BCG were introduced in the next 10-year time period in low to moderate (<15%) prevalence settings, and that 50–95% of cumulative cases may be averted over the next 50 years even in high (20–40%) disease burden settings with immediate implementation of BCG vaccination. Taken together, the analyses suggest that BCG vaccination may help accelerate control of bTB in endemic settings, particularly with early implementation in the face of dairy intensification in regions that currently lack effective bTB control programs.

Keywords: BCG vaccine, bovine tuberculosis, efficacy, cattle, control program

INTRODUCTION

Bovine tuberculosis (bTB) is a chronic infectious disease of cattle that is predominantly caused by *Mycobacterium bovis*, a zoonotic agent (1). The disease remains endemic in most low- and middle-income countries (LMICs) where it negatively impacts livestock productivity and represents a significant threat to public health. A live attenuated strain of *M. bovis*, the "Bacille de Calmette et Guérin" (BCG), has been used for experimental vaccination of cattle against bTB since 1913, well before its first trials in humans (2). Following Calmette and Guérin's promising early reports demonstrating safety of BCG and BCG-induced protection of cattle against experimental challenge with *M. bovis*, several trials were carried out in different countries in the early 20th century to better define its efficacy (3). Despite the repeated demonstration of BCG vaccine-induced protection in cattle, field use was not pursued because of the incomplete protection reported and, more importantly, because as a live attenuated vaccine, BCG sensitizes animals to the current World Organisation for Animal Health (OIE)-recommended purified protein derivatives (PPD)-based skin tests. This compromises the specificity of the standard tuberculin skin test and results in an inability to differentiate infected from vaccinated animals (DIVA) (4). Therefore, bTB control programs that use the OIE-prescribed tuberculin skin test also prohibit the use of BCG vaccination (5).

In the last decade, research in the field has focused on identifying antigens that are present in *M. bovis* and absent or not immunogenic in BCG. In particular, the antigens ESAT-6, CFP10 and Rv3615c have shown promise for differential diagnosis of bTB (4, 6, 7). The DIVA capability of these antigens has been demonstrated in both experimental and naturally infected animals, hence enabling the use of BCG vaccination as part of future bTB control programs (8, 9).

In order to assess the potential utility of BCG vaccination as a component of future bTB control programs, accurate estimates of its efficacy are first required. We sought to address this major knowledge gap through a systematic review and meta-analysis of the existing literature on efficacy of BCG vaccination against bTB in cattle. Vaccines can protect populations through two main modes of action—reducing the susceptibility of vaccinates to infection or by reducing the potential for transmission by vaccinates after infection. The latter effect is particularly relevant for BCG vaccination where reduction in pathology has been reported more frequently (10, 11) than sterilizing immunity. However, also estimating reduction in infectiousness requires either large scale field trials or carefully designed natural transmission studies (11). The vast majority of published efficacy studies of BCG in cattle have used experimental challenge models with a relatively high infectious dose that can only measure a reduction in susceptibility rather than assess the impact on transmission.

For our quantitative meta-analysis, we therefore focus on the effect of the vaccine to reduce susceptibility to infection (vaccine efficacy, ε_S) defined by the presence or absence of visible lesions and/or confirmed by culture. We also review the evidence that supports what the possible range of efficacy BCG may offer in terms of a reduction in infectiousness (ε_I) and explore the implications for disease control using a conceptual dynamic transmission model.

RESULTS

Characteristics of Included Studies

A total of 1,392 articles were screened, and 24 articles were included in the analyses (**Figure 1**) (12–35). In the instance that an article evaluated different doses and strains of BCG, different routes of vaccine administration, breeds of cattle, etc., each was considered as separate strata level data and included as a unique study. For instance, the study by Wedlock et al. (20) was extracted into three strata level data, representing the three different strains or variants of BCG tested (BCG Danish 1331, BCG Danish 1331 freeze-dried and BCG Pasteur 1173P2) (20). In total, 49 strata level data were extracted from the 24 publications included in the systematic review. The included publications spanned the time period from 1972 to 2018, and represented a total of 1,902 vaccinates compared against 1,667 control animals. All included studies are summarized in **Table 1**.

Meta-Analysis

A funnel plot of the log risk ratio against standard error was constructed to assess potential publication bias (**Figure 2**). This revealed a large degree of asymmetry suggesting the presence of publication bias. There was no obvious difference in symmetry between random-effects (RE) and fixed-effects (FE) funnel plots. Similarly, visual inspection of the predicted vs. empirical observations (Normal Q-Q plot) also did not show any major differences in data fit for RE and FE models (**Supplementary Figure 1**).

Given the suggestion of publication bias in the data, we focus on the RE model, which adjusts for variability between individual studies, as the more appropriate model to assess the relative risk

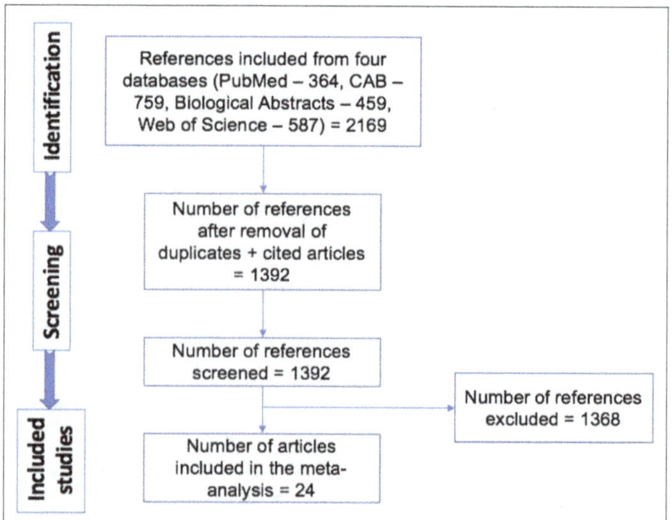

FIGURE 1 | Schematic representation of literature selection procedure for the systematic review of BCG efficacy against bTB.

TABLE 1 | List of strata-level data ($n = 49$) extracted from a total of 24 publications for inclusion in our meta-analysis.

Database #	Authors	Source	Location	Tpos	Tneg	Cpos	Cneg	BCG dose	Route	Method	Infection measurement method	Sample allocation method
101	Wedlock et al. (20)_1	BCG Pasteur 1173P2	New Zealand	9	1	10	0	1–4 × 10^6 CFU	Subcutaneous	Experimental	Culture	Stratified Random Sample
101	Wedlock et al. (20)_2	BCG Danish 1331	New Zealand	8	2	10	0	1–4 × 10^6 CFU	Subcutaneous	Experimental	Culture	Stratified Random Sample
101	Wedlock et al. (20)_3	BCG Danish freeze-dried	New Zealand	9	1	10	0	1–4 × 10^6 CFU	Subcutaneous	Experimental	Culture	Stratified Random Sample
120	Buddle et al. (17)	BCG Pasteur 1173P2	New Zealand	16	2	7	2	1 × 10^5 CFU	Subcutaneous	Experimental	Culture	Stratified Random Sample
579	Ameni et al. (35)	BCG Danish 1331	Ethiopia	14	9	22	4	1–4 × 10^6 CFU	Subcutaneous	Natural	Culture	Random Sample
802	Buddle et al. (16)	BCG Pasteur 1173P2	New Zealand	5	4	5	4	5 × 10^5 CFU	Subcutaneous	Experimental	Culture	Random Sample
826	Buddle et al. (14)_1	BCG Pasteur 1173P2	New Zealand	5	11	10	5	6 × 10^4 CFU	Subcutaneous	Experimental	Culture	Not specified
826	Buddle et al. (14)_2	BCG Pasteur 1173P2	New Zealand	4	12	10	5	6 × 10^6 CFU	Subcutaneous	Experimental	Culture	Not specified
828	Buddle et al. (15)_1	BCG Pasteur 1173P2	New Zealand	4	5	6	3	2 × 10^5 CFU	Subcutaneous	Experimental	Culture	Random Sample
828	Buddle et al. (15)_2	BCG Pasteur 1173P2	New Zealand	4	5	6	3	2 × 10^3 CFU	Subcutaneous	Experimental	Culture	Random Sample
828	Buddle et al. (15)_3	BCG Pasteur 1173P2	New Zealand	3	6	6	3	2 × 10^5 CFU	Intratracheal	Experimental	Culture	Random Sample
956	Berggren (13)	BCG Glaxo	Malawi	75	129	82	128	8–26 × 10^6 CFU	Subcutaneous	Natural	Culture	Alternate calves vaccinated
1065	Wedlock et al. (22)	BCG Pasteur 1173P2	New Zealand	5	5	7	3	1 × 10^6 CFU	Subcutaneous	Experimental	PM	Stratified Random Sample
1080	Buddle et al. (21)_1	BCG Pasteur 1173P2	New Zealand	3	7	7	3	1 × 10^6 CFU	Subcutaneous	Experimental	PM	Stratified Random Sample
1080	Buddle et al. (21)_2	BCG Pasteur 1173P2	New Zealand	2	8	7	3	1 × 10^9 CFU	Oral	Experimental	PM	Stratified Random Sample
1080	Buddle et al. (21)_3	BCG Pasteur 1173P2	New Zealand	3	7	7	3	*	Subcutaneous and oral	Experimental	PM	Stratified Random Sample
1213	Buddle et al. (18)_1	BCG Pasteur 1173P2	New Zealand	6	4	10	0	1 × 10^6 CFU	Subcutaneous	Experimental	Culture	Random Sample
1213	Buddle et al. (18)_2	BCG Pasteur 1173P2	New Zealand	9	1	10	0	1 × 10^6 CFU	Subcutaneous	Experimental	Culture	Random Sample
1213	Buddle et al. (18)_3	BCG Pasteur 1173P2	New Zealand	8	2	10	0	1 × 10^6 CFU	Subcutaneous	Experimental	Culture	Random Sample
1263	De Klerk et al. (24)	BCG Pasteur 1173P2	South Africa	8	6	9	4	3.2 × 10^7 CFU	Intramuscular	Combined	Culture	Random Sample
1266	Ameni et al. (23)	BCG Danish 1331	Ethiopia	4	9	11	3	1 × 10^6 CFU	Subcutaneous	Natural	Culture	Random Sample
1296	Thom et al. (28)_1	BCG Danish 1331	UK	6	3	8	1	1–4 × 10^6 CFU	Subcutaneous	Experimental	Culture	Stratified Random Sample
1296	Thom et al. (28)_2	BCG Danish 1331	UK	9	0	9	0	1–4 × 10^6 CFU	Subcutaneous	Experimental	Culture	Stratified Random Sample
1303	Parlane et al. (31)_1	BCG Danish 1331	New Zealand	14	2	16	1	2–8 × 10^6 CFU	Subcutaneous	Experimental	PM	Stratified Random Sample
1303	Parlane et al. (31)_2	BCG Danish 1331	New Zealand	11	4	16	1	2–8 × 10^6 CFU	Subcutaneous	Experimental	PM	Stratified Random Sample
1304	Buddle et al. (29)_1	BCG Danish 1331	New Zealand	2	7	10	0	1–4 × 10^5 CFU	Subcutaneous	Experimental	PM	Stratified Random Sample
1304	Buddle et al. (29)_2	BCG Danish 1331	New Zealand	3	6	10	0	1–4 × 10^6 CFU	Subcutaneous	Experimental	PM	Stratified Random Sample
1337	Buddle et al. (33)	BCG Danish 1331	New Zealand	6	6	7	5	1.5 × 10^6 CFU	Subcutaneous	Experimental	PM	Stratified Random Sample
1358	Nugent et al. (34)_1	BCG Danish 1331	New Zealand	0	30	8	122	1 × 10^8 CFU	Oral	Natural	PM	Random Sample
1358	Nugent et al. (34)_2	BCG Danish 1331	New Zealand	1	33	8	122	3 × 10^5 CFU	Subcutaneous	Natural	PM	Random Sample
1358	Nugent et al. (34)_3	BCG Danish 1331	New Zealand	3	169	9	108	1 × 10^8 CFU	Oral	Natural	PM	Random Sample
1358	Nugent et al. (34)_4	BCG Danish 1331	New Zealand	11	166	12	74	1 × 10^8 CFU	Oral	Natural	PM	Random Sample
1358	Nugent et al. (34)_5	BCG Danish 1331	New Zealand	12	156	26	83	1 × 10^8 CFU	Oral	Natural	PM	Random Sample

(Continued)

TABLE 1 | Continued

Database #	Authors	Source	Location	Tpos	Tneg	Cpos	Cneg	BCG dose	Route	Method	Infection measurement method	Sample allocation method
1358	Nugent et al. (34)_6	BCG Danish 1331	New Zealand	4	93	8	81	1×10^8 CFU	Oral	Natural	PM	Random Sample
1366	Buddle et al. (19)_1	BCG Pasteur 1173P2	New Zealand	6	4	9	1	1×10^8 CFU	Oral	Experimental	PM	Stratified Random Sample
1366	Buddle et al. (19)_2	BCG Pasteur 1173P2	New Zealand	7	3	9	1	1×10^9 CFU	Oral	Experimental	PM	Stratified Random Sample
1366	Buddle et al. (19)_3	BCG Pasteur 1173P2	New Zealand	5	5	9	1	1×10^6 CFU	Subcutaneous	Experimental	PM	Stratified Random Sample
1371	Hope et al. (27)_1	BCG Danish 1331	UK	7	0	7	0	2×10^6 CFU	Subcutaneous	Experimental	PM and Culture	Not specified
1371	Hope et al. (27)_2	BCG Pasteur 1173P2	UK	3	4	7	0	2×10^6 CFU	Subcutaneous	Experimental	PM and Culture	Not specified
1373	Lopez-Valencia et al. (25)	BCG Tokyo	Mexico	6	59	15	51	1×10^6 CFU	Subcutaneous	Natural	Skin test and IFNg assay	Alternate calves vaccinated
1379	Buddle et al. (26)_1	BCG Danish 1331	New Zealand	2	7	6	4	1×10^6 CFU	Subcutaneous	Experimental	PM	Stratified Random Sample
1379	Buddle et al. (26)_2	BCG Danish 1331	New Zealand	5	4	6	4	1×10^8 CFU	Oral	Experimental	PM	Stratified Random Sample
1379	Buddle et al. (26)_3	BCG Danish 1331	New Zealand	5	4	6	4	1×10^7 CFU	Oral	Experimental	PM	Stratified Random Sample
1379	Buddle et al. (26)_4	BCG Danish 1331	New Zealand	6	3	6	4	1×10^6 CFU	Oral	Experimental	PM	Stratified Random Sample
1383	Dean et al. (30)	BCG Danish 1331	UK	4	6	9	1	1×10^6 CFU	Subcutaneous	Experimental	Culture	Not specified
1385	Dean et al. (32)_1	BCG Danish 1331	UK	8	2	8	1	1×10^6 CFU	Subcutaneous	Experimental	Culture	Random Sample
1385	Dean et al. (32)_2	BCG Danish 1331	UK	5	5	8	1	5×10^5 CFU	Subcutaneous and endobronchial	Experimental	Culture	Random Sample
1385	Dean et al. (32)_3	BCG Danish 1331	UK	5	5	8	1	1×10^6 CFU	Endobronchial	Experimental	Culture	Random Sample
1410	Nugent et al. (36)	BCG Danish 1331	New Zealand	2	518	8	289	3×10^5 CFU	Subcutaneous	Natural	PM and Culture	Block Randomization

**Buddle et al. (21)_3 used a combination of Oral and Subcutaneous BCG; Study no. 1263 (24) was performed in buffaloes. Tpos and Cpos are animals classified as positive for bTB in vaccinates and controls, respectively. Tneg and Cneg are animals that remained negative for bTB in vaccinates and controls, respectively.*

Multiple strata level data extracted from a single study are represented with numbers at the end in the Author column. For example, Database #101, Wedlock et al had 3 strata level data represented as Wedlock et al._1, Wedlock et al._2 and Wedlock et al._3. Buddle_a is Reference (14) and Buddle_b is Reference (15). a1, a2, and b1, b2 are strata level data of those respective studies.

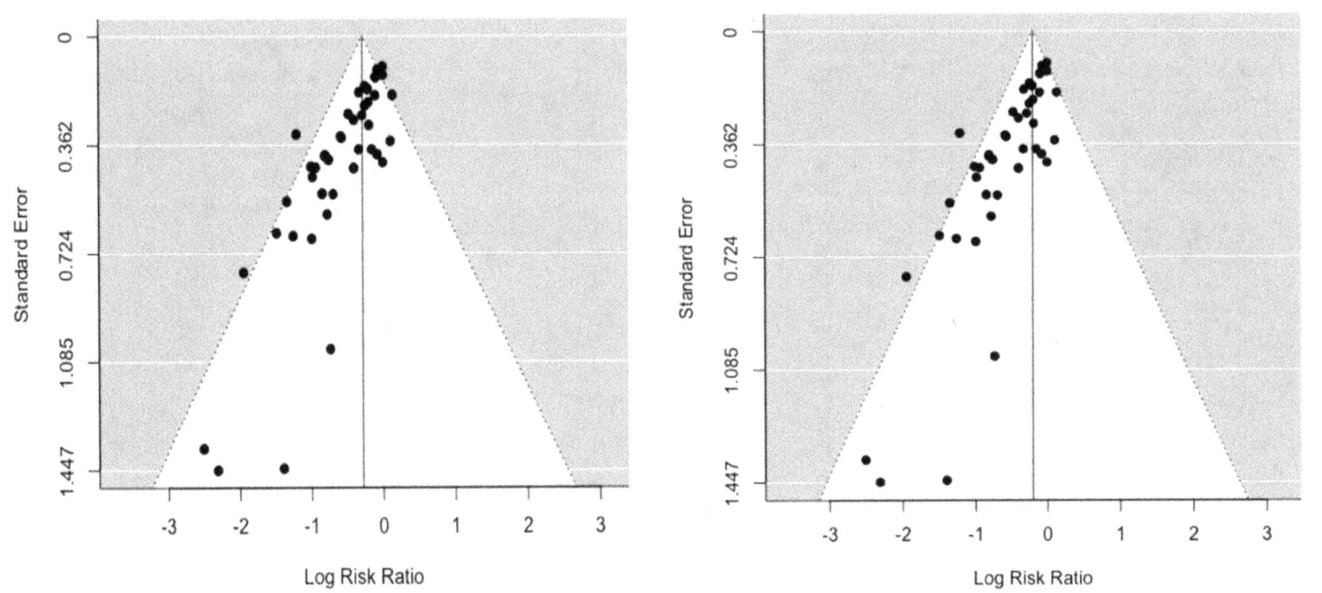

FIGURE 2 | Funnel plots (left: RE; right: FE) of the log risk ratio against standard error demonstrate potential publication bias.

ratio (RR). The relative risk ratio is defined as the probability of an outcome in an exposed group to that in an unexposed group (37). The RE model estimated RR to be 0.75 (95% CI: 0.68, 0.82), suggesting a 25% reduction in risk of infection (vaccine efficacy, ε_S) as measured by PM and/or culture in BCG vaccinates compared to control animals. Cochran's (Q) value ($Q = 76.1$, $df = 50$, and $p = 0.01$) and Higgins statistic ($I^2 = 32.1\%$) were computed to test for heterogeneity ($I^2 < 50\%$ represents low heterogeneity). While both the Q value and I^2 statistic are classical measures of heterogeneity, neither is comprehensive since Cochran's (Q) suffers low power and I^2 is imprecise in the case of meta-analyses of relatively small numbers of included studies. We used a forest plot to graphically summarize the variation in RR between studies (**Figure 3**).

To explore the potential impact of publication bias on the estimated RR, we carried out a sensitivity analysis using the trim and fill method (38). This is an algorithmic method to adjust for publication bias in a meta-analysis by imputing the values of missing studies (39). Here, the estimated number of missing studies on the right side of the funnel plot was found to be 21 (**Figure 4**). The Paul-Mantel method was used due to convergence issues with the maximum likelihood based methods (Maximum-Likelihood (ML), Restricted Maximum-Likelihood (40) and Empirical Bayes (EB) estimators). The adjusted RR estimate per this sensitivity analysis was found to be 0.84 (95% CI: 0.73, 0.98).

Meta-Regression

Several important biological factors varied between published studies, which *a priori* could have an impact on the estimated vaccine efficacy. Such confounding factors could also potentially lead to systematic patterns of bias as shown by the funnel plot analysis. We therefore constructed a multivariable meta-regression model using these factors to explore whether they could improve model fit and to assess the relative effect of these biological variables on estimates of vaccine efficacy. The factors included BCG source, dose, route, whether or not revaccination was performed, and challenge method (**Table 2**).

An omnibus test of all the moderator variables (QM = 23.7, df = 13, $p = 0.03$) indicates that the explained variance by the model is greater than the unexplained variance. However, this amounts to only 49.1% of the total heterogeneity and only one moderator (BCG Glaxo source) has a RR significantly different than 1 (at the 95% level). Given the relatively small sample sizes, reflective of the logistical constraints of experimental studies, this lack of statistical significance is unsurprising and does not rule out the potential biological importance of these variables and highlights the critical need for additional well-powered investigations to better assess the impact of these confounders on overall vaccine efficacy.

Implications for bTB Control

To explore the implications of the estimated efficacy of vaccination of $\varepsilon_S \sim 25\%$ for disease control, we carried out scenario analyses using a conceptual herd level transmission dynamic model. Given the potential density dependence of transmission rates of bTB within herds, intensification of production in emerging dairy industries is a particular concern for LMICs (41). Thus, we consider a scenario with an initial herd size of 30 but growing in size at a rate of 15% per year to 134 animals after 50 years. Motivated by estimates from India we consider an initial bTB prevalence (5, 10, and 15%) together with a set of higher prevalence scenarios (20, 30, and 40%) (42). There are currently no published quantitative estimates of transmission rates from LMICs, hence for this model population we use a

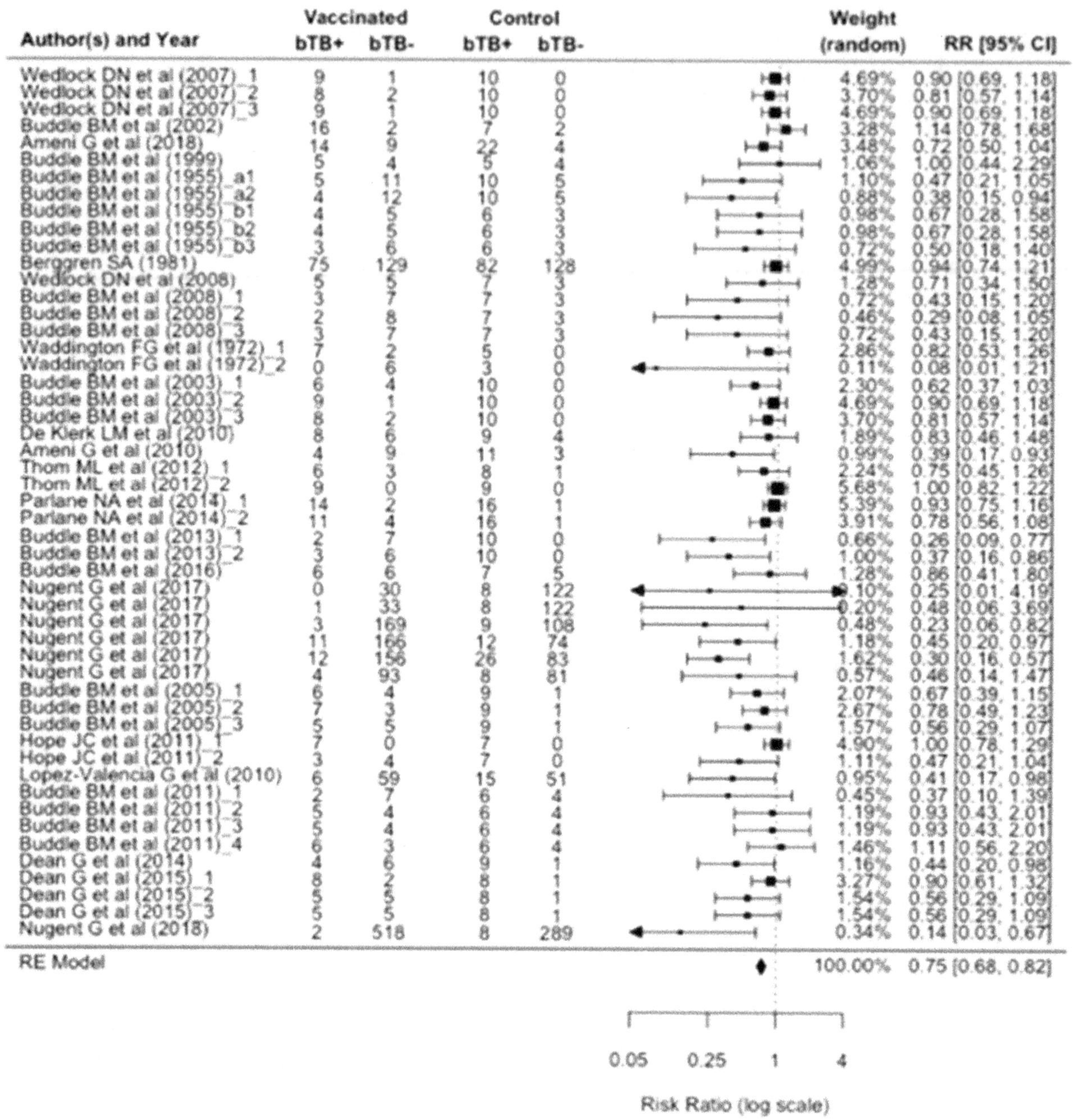

FIGURE 3 | Forest plot visualizing the relative risk ratio calculated for each included publication in the meta-analysis. The weight given to each included publication per the RE model is shown. "bTB+" refers to the number of animals reported to have infection and/or pathology (per culture and/or postmortem examination). And "bTB-" refers to the number of animals not reported to have infection and/or pathology.

density dependent transmission function estimated from herds in Great Britain (11).

In the absence of estimates of indirect BCG effects based on empirical trials, we used data from long-term natural challenge models to estimate the relative contribution of indirect effects when force of infection is low (representative of field setting). Overall efficacy in those recent field trials included in this meta-analysis [excluding the older Berggren (13) study] was estimated to be of 61% (95% CI: 40, 74) for natural transmission compared to 18% (95% CI: 11, 24) for experimental challenge studies (**Table 3**). The key distinction between experimental challenge and natural transmission studies—beyond being more representative of a field setting—is that the latter measures the total effect of vaccination (**Figure 5**). The total effect

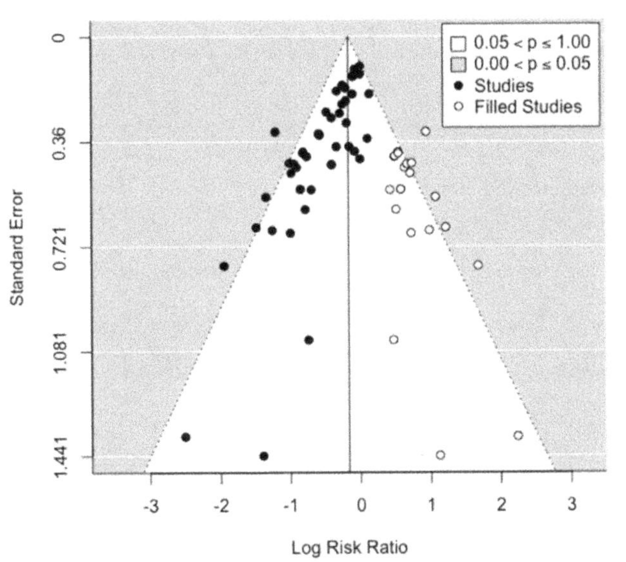

FIGURE 4 | Funnel plot showing the 21 studies (open circles, on the right side) imputed by the trim-and-fill method to carry out a sensitivity analysis for publication bias.

TABLE 2 | Multivariable meta-regression of the selected predictors on BCG efficacy ($R^2 = 49.10\%$, $n = 49$).

Moderators	Categories	RR (95% CI)	*p*-value (RE)
Revaccination	No	Reference	
	Yes	1.04 (0.79, 1.38)	0.77
BCG route	Endobronchial	Reference	
	Intramuscular	2.16 (0.55, 8.50)	0.27
	Intratracheal	1.01 (0.28, 3.67)	0.99
	Oral	2.04 (0.75, 5.53)	0.16
	Subcutaneous	1.46 (0.71, 3.00)	0.3
	Subcutaneous and Endobronchial	1 (0.38, 2.66)	1.00
Challenge method	Natural	Reference	
	Experimental	0.83 (0.40, 1.70)	0.61
BCG source	Danish 1331	Reference	
	Danish freeze-dried	1.14 (0.77, 1.68)	0.51
	Glaxo	12.14 (1.52, 97.09)	0.02
	Pasteur 1173P2	0.98 (0.77, 1.23)	0.84
BCG Dose		0.68 (0.31, 1.51)	0.35
Time from vaccination to challenge		1.00 (0.99, 1.001)	0.5
Length of exposure to challenge		0.998 (0.997, 1)	0.06

of vaccination will be greater than the direct protection of individuals (ε_s) due to the reduction in transmission from herd immunity effects, along with any additional protection from reduction in infectiousness (ε_I) of vaccinated individuals.

In the absence of control, the null model predicts a gradual increase in prevalence with herd size saturating around ~70% for all initial conditions (**Figure 6**). We considered a vaccine efficacy to reduce infectiousness (ε_I) at two hypothetical thresholds: (i) ~36%, approximating the difference between average overall efficacy in the natural transmission studies (0.61) and the overall direct efficacy as revealed by the meta-analyses of 0.25; and (ii) ~49%—representing the difference between the upper bound of efficacy in the natural transmission studies (0.74) and overall direct efficacy as revealed by the meta-analyses of 0.25.

Our model scenarios illustrate the benefits of early intervention. Even with only a modest efficacy (ε_S) of 25%, a window of up to 25 years of slightly lower than the current disease prevalence levels may be achieved (**Figure 6A**), should BCG be implemented immediately in the low to moderate prevalence scenario (5, 10, 15%). With an additional reduction in infectiousness (ε_I) of vaccinates (49%), disease prevalence could be driven down close to Officially TB Free (OTF) status (<0.1% per the European Union) if BCG were introduced in the next 10-year time period in low to moderate prevalence settings. Immediate implementation, but with a lower ε_I of 36%, prevalence may start to rise again in 30–40-years, driven by increased herd size, suggesting that other strategies will also be required.

These scenarios predict considerable benefits in terms of reducing cumulative cases if BCG is implemented now. With an impact of vaccination on infectiousness, between ~80 and 100% of cases can be saved in 50 years, driven by the strength of indirect effects on transmission (**Figure 6B**). Encouragingly, this model also predicts that from ~50 to 95% of cumulative cases can be averted in higher disease burden settings (>15%) if acted upon now (**Figure 6**).

DISCUSSION

Following promising initial studies conducted by Calmette, Guérin and others that showed both safety of BCG and BCG-induced protection of cattle against both natural and experimental challenge with *M. bovis*, several trials were carried out through the early and mid 20th century in many different countries to better assess and define the efficacy of ancestral variants of BCG in cattle and showed varying levels of protection (3, 44) (**Supplementary Table 1**). While BCG went on to become the most widely used of all human vaccines (and the only available vaccine against human TB), it has not been considered for routine use in domestic livestock despite early promise. This is primarily because of the fact that BCG sensitizes animals to the widely used and OIE-recommended PPD based skin tests, which precludes its use where skin test-based control is being actively pursued (5), and it is with this context that an Expert Committee of the WHO/FAO Expert Committee on Zoonoses (45) stated that: "generally speaking, vaccination has no place in the eradication of tuberculosis in cattle."

The early proof-of-concept experiments conducted by Calmette and Guérin in the early 1900s to demonstrate safety of BCG and protection against progressive TB in cattle were replicated and refined by several other investigators in both Europe and the Americas (44, 46–53). Their findings led to considerable international interest in exploring the possibility

TABLE 3 | Natural transmission studies included in the meta-analysis.

Database #	Authors	Location	BCG source	BCG route	BCG dose	Controls_n	Vaccinates_n	Reported efficacy
579	Ameni et al. (35)	Ethiopia	BCG Danish 1331	Subcutaneous	1–4 × 10^6 CFU	26	23	30%
1266	Ameni et al. (23)	Ethiopia	BCG Danish 1331	Subcutaneous	1 × 10^6 CFU	14	13	60%
1358	Nugent et al. (34)	New Zealand	BCG Danish 1331	Oral and Subcutaneous	1 × 10^8 CFU	531	644	67%
1373	Lopez-Valencia et al. (25)	Mexico	BCG Tokyo	Subcutaneous	1 × 10^6 CFU	66	65	60%
1410	Nugent et al. (36)	New Zealand	BCG Danish 1331	Subcutaneous	3 × 10^5 CFU	297	520	85%

The studies conducted in Ethiopia by Ameni et al. (23, 35) used a reactor to sentinel ratio of >1. Nugent et al. (34) included 1,286 free-ranging cattle (676 vaccinates and 531 naïve controls) stocked at low densities, and challenged with a low force of infection, mimicking a more representative field setting. This was followed up with a subsequent field study (36) conducted in ~800 free-ranging cattle that were followed up for over 3 years and similarly showed a relatively high overall protective efficacy of ~85%. Lopez-Valencia et al. (25) did not conduct necropsy.

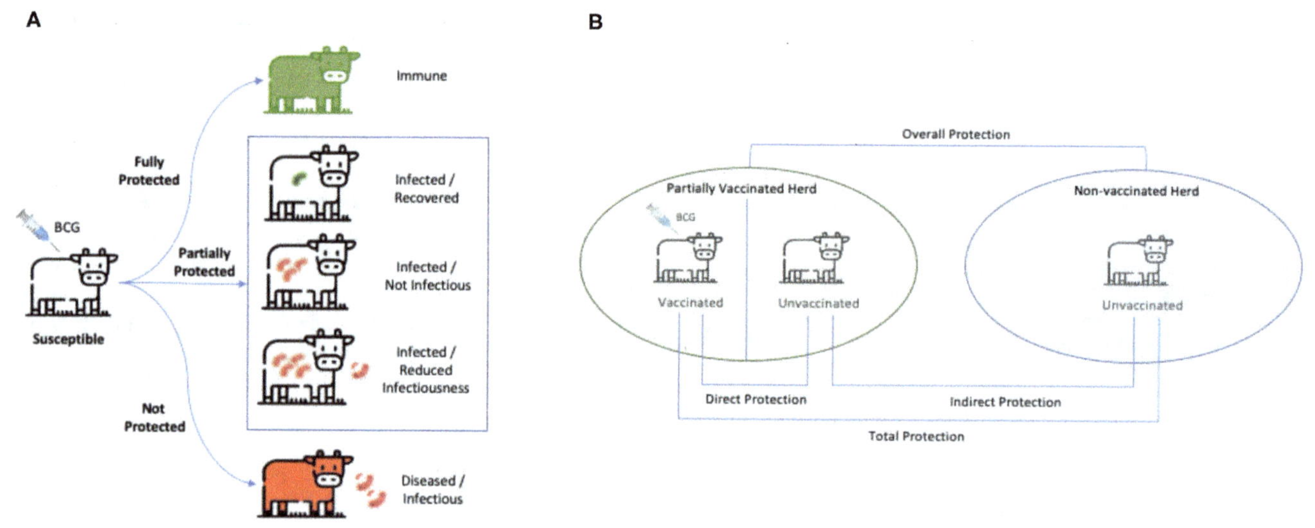

FIGURE 5 | Measures of vaccine-induced protection. **(A)** BCG vaccine confers a spectrum of protection ranging from complete (for a limited time period in certain population) to none. While completely protected individuals are immune, and unprotected ones succumb to infection and become heavily diseased, BCG can also be partially protective by reducing risk of disease transmission to unvaccinated individuals. **(B)** The green herd is partially vaccinated and the blue herd is unvaccinated. "Direct protection" is the reduction in susceptibility of vaccinated animals (as measured by ε_s). "Indirect protection" is a reduction in transmission due to any reduction in infectiousness of vaccinated individuals that become infected (as measured by ε_I) in addition to the reduction in transmission from herd immunity effects. "Total" protection is the risk of infection in vaccinated animals compared to that of unvaccinated animals. "Overall protection" is the reduction in rate of transmission in a population with vaccination program compared to that in a population with no vaccination program. This stems from both vaccinated and unvaccinated individuals and is used to evaluate the impact of a vaccination program at the population level. **(B)** Is adapted from Halloran et al. (43).

of eradicating bTB by vaccinating cattle with BCG as has been reviewed elsewhere (3, 10, 54–57). As part of the current systematic review, we extracted data from eight studies that were published between 1930 and 1972 (**Supplementary Table 1**). However, given that these studies used ancestral strains of BCG and doses that are not possible to accurately estimate, these studies were excluded from the formal analyses. However, it is noteworthy that these studies provided key foundational evidence that highlighted both the variable protection afforded by BCG in experimental and natural challenge, as well as showed that BCG vaccination sensitizes animals to tuberculins and hence would confound ongoing test and slaughter tuberculosis eradication programs. However, recent attempts to develop BCG-compatible diagnostic tests have shown great promise and paved the way for implementation of BCG-based control programs in LMICs and other endemic regions (7–9). Thus, there is renewed interest in exploring the use of BCG vaccination as a component of national control programs, particularly where test and slaughter is unfeasible (58, 59).

We systematically reviewed the literature to obtain estimates of the efficacy of BCG against bTB and assessed its potential utility in future control programs. The analyses suggest an overall vaccine efficacy of 25% (95% CI: 18, 32) as measured by the presence of visible lesions and/or culture. The potential contribution of vaccine strain as a confounder or predictor of BCG efficacy is intriguing. This is relevant since a majority of the studies that were included in the current review used either BCG Pasteur 1173P2

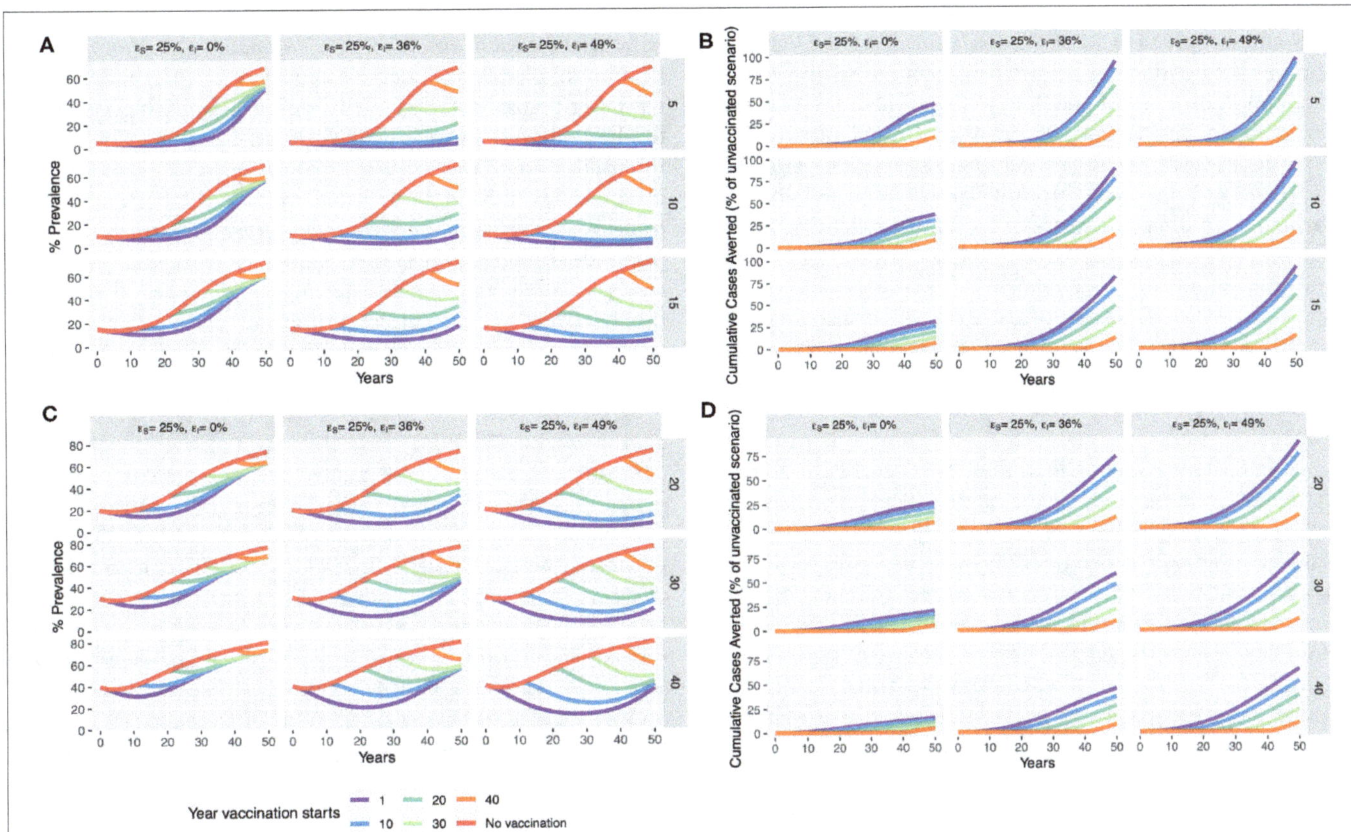

FIGURE 6 | Scenario analysis for impact of BCG vaccination in an expanding dairy herd. We compare a baseline "control" scenario (with no vaccination) to the introduction of whole-herd vaccination at 1, 10, 20, 30, and 40 years which only provides direct protection (ε_S of 25%), and one with an additional reduction in infectiousness of vaccinates (ε_I of 36 and 49%). We compare the effect of vaccination in terms of % prevalence and cumulative cases averted with assumed initial **(A,B)** moderate prevalence of 5, 10, and 15% (rows), and **(C,D)** high prevalence of 20, 30, and 40%.

(9 out of 24 studies) or BCG Danish 1331 (10 out of 24 studies). The meta-regression model suggests that neither of these strains had any significant effect on the observed heterogeneity. However, given the small sample size, further investigations may be warranted to assess the robustness of these inferences.

Given the large variability in the age at which animals were vaccinated in the included studies, the ideal timing for vaccination could not be subjected to rigorous analysis. While there is evidence in the published literature showing that BCG vaccination within a few days of birth (<1 month of age) can induce high levels of protective immunity (18, 60), there is a need for more studies in relevant settings, such as in bTB-endemic regions where high burden of environmental mycobacteria has been reported (61). In these settings, some studies suggest prior sensitization with environmental mycobacteria prevent induction of protection in calves, while others report that exposure to *M. avium* helps induce protection against *M. bovis* (17, 62). It is plausible that these seemingly contradictory results could be because exposure to different environmental mycobacteria could either enhance or reduce BCG's efficacy, and hence, future studies are needed to help clarify the role of these confounders to vaccine efficacy. Curiously, despite the early recognition by Calmette and Guerin and other investigators of the need for revaccination (at annual or 18 month intervals) in order to maintain protection (3), only a total of five studies performed revaccination, highlighting the scarcity of reliable data available on duration of immunity and revaccination intervals to formulate evidence-based approaches to control bTB (13, 16, 18, 24, 31). Thus, it is important to assess the true duration of immunity and role, if any, of revaccination to obtain better estimates of the efficacy of BCG and inform the parameterization of robust transmission dynamics and econometric models that may be used to guide development and implementation of future cost-effective vaccine-based intervention strategies (18, 31).

The roles of dose and type of challenge (experimental challenge or natural infection) were also investigated. A total of 17 studies that are part of this meta-analysis performed experimental challenge of their animals to infection. These studies call for high dose infection protocols in order to generate high levels of infection in control animals, which do not reflect the reality in natural conditions where animals most likely are not exposed to such high numbers of virulent bacteria as a single bolus. Such experimental challenge models with high infection doses do not allow BCG protection to be revealed. One reason for this may be that these models are often used for the development of novel vaccines aimed at improving BCG efficacy and not *per se* to study BCG efficacy. This highlights the importance of conducting robust natural transmission studies in field conditions and in endemic settings where the real need for vaccination lies. It is noteworthy that most experimental trials have used *M. bovis* as the challenge strain. However, *M. bovis* is not the only causative agent of bTB since *M. tuberculosis* and other members of the *M. tuberculosis* complex are frequently isolated from cattle samples, and certain species of non-tuberculous mycobacteria (NTM) that contain virulence factors encoded in the Region of Difference-1 are also known to cause TB-like lesions (63, 64). Hence, future studies are needed to better estimate efficacy of BCG vaccine-induced protection with locally relevant bTB causing mycobacteria other than *M. bovis*.

It is important to note that there are several limitations to systematic reviews and meta-analyses. They can provide a summary of published evidence about a specific question, but our ability to answer it is limited by variation in experimental design and the consistency and completeness of reporting. This systematic review was limited to studies in English indexed in the four databases screened, and hence may have missed relevant investigations. Studies that did not report essential details were excluded. It is not surprising that systematic biases in the fit of the meta-analysis models suggest existence of publication bias and the potential to inflate or underestimate estimates of direct vaccine efficacy. One of the primary limitations of the included studies is that the reported measures of protection, evidence of lesions at necropsy and culture, together with immune reactions, are the current "gold standards," but have variable sensitivity and specificity (65). In order to address any potential bias in measurement of the outcome, we focused on studies which reported culture or necropsy data for calculation of RR estimation and further analyses. An exception was made however for the Lopez-Valencia et al. (25) study since it was one of only five estimates from a recent natural transmission study. This study considered an animal to be infected if there were positive reactions to the tuberculin skin test and the IFNγ release assay upon stimulation with PPD-B and recombinant ESAT6-CFP10 (25). While many studies followed a simple or stratified sampling strategy for randomization, two studies (13, 25) used a more systematic approach of vaccinating every alternate calf in the herd which may have introduced potential biases from the randomization process (**Table 1**). However, a rigorous assessment of other risks of bias due to deviations from intended interventions, missing outcome data and selection of reported result could not be performed due to lack of access to the complete data or detailed experimental protocols from these studies. Another limitation is that only the direct effect of vaccination (reduction in susceptibility, ε_S) could be estimated from the experimental challenge experiments (66). This is important, in particular, given our scenario analyses which demonstrate the transformative effect an additional reduction in infectiousness of vaccinates (ε_I) could have (67, 68). Thus, studies to assess the impact of BCG on infectiousness of vaccinates through natural transmission experiments or field trials are urgently needed (67).

Herd-size is perhaps the most important risk factor associated with transmission of bTB (69), leading to the common assumption that transmission is density dependent and increases with herd size (70, 71). This poses a particular challenge for bTB control in emerging dairy markets in LMICs where intensification of the dairy sector may make achieving control increasingly difficult over time. We developed herd level transmission dynamic models and performed scenario analyses using deterministic models to illustrate this challenge. The results of these analyses are striking—and suggest that despite the relatively modest direct protection afforded by BCG, a strong case may be made for implementing vaccination for bTB control sooner rather than later, with overall benefits reducing progressively over time to intervention (72) (**Figure 6**). Overall, a leaky vaccine like BCG could still play a pivotal role in disease control, particularly if implemented sooner than later in the face of dairy intensification efforts in bTB endemic countries.

Finally, even while scenario analyses are for illustrative purposes, there are several limitations to these analyses that we recognize and should be addressed in future investigations. To begin with, in the absence of surveillance programs in LMICs, transmission estimates are lacking and should be determined to accurately assess risk. Given that recent studies show increasing prevalence in intensifying cattle herds in endemic settings (69), these observations have major implications for informing and implementing disease control policy and suggest a potential role for BCG vaccination that has hitherto remained unexplored. Next, in order to realize herd-level benefits of vaccination, estimating the reduction in the risk of transmission from vaccinated individuals (ε_I) is crucial. Animal trials in relevant endemic settings are urgently needed to evaluate the potential of BCG to reduce onward transmission in the field (11).

It is important to note that in addition to cattle, tuberculosis affects a wide variety of livestock and both free-living and captive wildlife species including goats, sheep, pigs, cervids, wild boars, badgers, brushtail possums, and ferrets, many of which are recognized as potential reservoir hosts. Indeed, experimental and field trials to study the response to BCG vaccination of some these species suggests that, while vaccination confers incomplete protection, it's use in domestic and captive or free-living wildlife species should be seriously considered to reduce risk of cross-species spillover (73). Alternative approaches to control bTB, such as test-and-segregate and treatment with anti-mycobacterial agents including isoniazid have also been explored (74, 75). Treatment with isoniazid is uneconomical and not advised given the long duration of treatment needed and the need to withdraw milk together with reports that bacterial shedding may resume as soon as isoniazid is withdrawn (76). Moreover, use of a first line antimycobacterial agent in food animals is of major concern due to potential for contribution to the spread of drug resistant tuberculosis (77). Over the past decade, research in the field has also focused on improving TB vaccination using alternative approaches including the heterologous prime-boost strategy, introducing genetic modifications in BCG strains to increase immunogenicity, and also completely replacing BCG with attenuated *M. bovis* strains (78–82). Heat-inactivated *M. bovis* vaccines have also recently shown promise in wild boars, pigs, red deer, badgers, and goats (73, 83–88). However, despite significant efforts and promising results in preclinical studies, there is only limited evidence from clinical and field trials for significant gains in efficacy of these newer generation or modified BCG vaccines. Interestingly, both heat-inactivated and attenuated vaccines for another major mycobacterial disease, paratuberculosis (Johne's disease), have been licensed and tested extensively for use in cattle and small ruminants, but their use is limited in countries because of potential for interference with tuberculin testing and diagnostic tools currently used in bTB eradication and control programs (89, 90).

In conclusion, in the short-term, in endemic regions where test and slaughter approaches to bTB control have not been shown to be effective or, BCG vaccination alongside a DIVA diagnostic test appears to be the most promising option in the near future. However, it is important to continue to develop and assess next generation vaccines as well as complementary strategies of disease control alongside that of BCG. For instance, the assessment of routine testing and segregation of reactor animals, mandatory pasteurization of milk fed to calves and sold for human consumption, enhanced husbandry practices, such as segregation of reactor or likely infected animals, herd certification policies for recruitment of disease-free animals, slaughterhouse surveillance, regulating movement and trade of reactor animals, etc., in conjunction with or as alternatives to BCG need to be rigorously evaluated in different production settings and epidemiological contexts. Together, our studies highlight an urgent need as well to perform sensitivity analyses and build econometric frameworks to assess the cost-benefit impacts of implementing vaccine-based control strategies to establish the business case for (or against) implementation of BCG vaccination as a component of a national bovine TB control program.

CONCLUSION

This systematic review and meta-analysis of the efficacy of BCG vaccination in cattle together with transmission dynamic model-based scenario analyses provides strong evidence for the consideration of implementation of BCG vaccine-based bTB control strategies, particularly in LMICs and other high burden settings. Despite a relatively small but positive protective effect, conservative transmission models suggest an important role for BCG in limiting spread of the disease and buying time for improvement of vaccine efficacy or the development of alternative approaches to disease control. Taken together with the predicted increase in prevalence associated with intensification of dairy production, our investigations suggest that BCG vaccination may indeed be simply good (enough) to accelerate control of bTB in endemic settings.

METHODS

Literature Search Strategy

A systematic search was performed for published articles reporting the effect of BCG against bTB in cattle as of February 24, 2020. Various combinations of Boolean operators and MeSH terms common to known articles of interest were evaluated before the following search terms were finalized: (BCG AND (("mycobacterium bovis" OR tuberculosis) AND (cows OR cattle OR bovine) AND (protect* OR effica* OR lesion* OR immune* OR vaccin*))). In order to minimize publication bias, search terms were kept uniform across the four databases (PubMed, CAB, Biological Abstracts, and Web of Science), which were selected for their inclusion of major and minor international journals. No limits were placed on publication date, and only published studies were considered. EndNote X8, a citation software program, was used to organize the articles generated by the four databases as well as remove duplicate publications. The study conforms to Preferred Reporting Items for Systematic Reviews and Meta-analyses (PRISMA) guidelines (91).

TABLE 4 | Study inclusion/exclusion criteria.

Inclusion	Exclusion
Bovine TB	Wrong disease
Cattle or buffalo	Wrong species
Used BCG to vaccinate (and specified the strain used)	Wrong vaccine
Evaluated efficacy of BCG vaccination	Wrong type of study
English	Language limitation: not in English
Full text of publication obtanied	Full-text unavailable
	Other

Study Inclusion Criteria

Inclusion and exclusion criteria are detailed in **Table 4**. All included studies compared the potentially protective effects induced by a BCG variant against natural or experimental challenge with bTB in a vaccinated group of cattle and a control group of unvaccinated cattle. Studies with no control group, such as surveys evaluating the effectiveness of vaccination campaigns, were excluded. Additionally, articles that failed to report the BCG vaccine strain tested were excluded (summarized in **Supplementary Table 1**). While efforts were made to identify articles manually, all final included articles were represented in the formal database search. Primary studies were included when available. However, review articles were included when the primary article was inaccessible and adequate information on BCG strain, bTB challenge, and protection was detailed for vaccinate and control groups.

Data Extraction

A uniform data extraction form was developed based on information of interest from pre-identified articles and used by each of the extractors. Study identifiers included author, publication date, title, journal, study location, and study time period. Headings for study design included control and vaccinate group sizes; BCG strain (Danish 1331, Danish freeze-dried, Glaxo, Pasteur 1173P2, Tokyo); BCG dose; and BCG administration route (subcutaneous, endobronchial, intratracheal, intramuscular, oral); cattle age at time of vaccination; revaccination timing, frequency, and dose (if applicable); animal breed; and time from vaccination to

TABLE 5 | A summary of all studies included in the meta-analysis.

		Infection	
		Yes	**No**
Vaccination	Yes	362	1,540
	No	530	1,137

Out of a total of 1,902 BCG vaccinated animals, 356 were found to be positive (either by culture and/or presence of visible lesions) for bTB while 1,502 remained negative. Similarly, out of 1,667 control animals, 520 were infected while 1,104 animals neither had lesions nor any growth in culture.

challenge. Headings detailing bTB challenge methods included challenge type (natural or experimental) and duration (from challenge to slaughter or end of study period); as well as challenge strain, route (intratracheal, subcutaneous, oral, endobronchial) and dose if challenge type was experimental. Headings for protection included the infection measurement method (post-mortem, culture), number of vaccinates and controls affected, and the protection percentage reported. Vaccine efficacy was measured based on culture growth, and in the absence of culture data, presence or absence of visible lung or lymph node lesions in the control and treatment groups was used.

Prior to the formal review of all articles in the pool, data extractors (SS, LE, and CH) conducted a pilot run of 20 random articles in order to test inclusion/exclusion criteria and finalize the data extraction form. SS, LE, and CH independently performed the formal review of all articles, which comprised an initial screening of article titles and abstracts for inclusion or exclusion. Full-text review for data extraction from included studies was performed by SS and LE. When discrepancies arose in study inclusion/exclusion or extracted data between reviewers, studies were collectively revisited and discussed in order to reach a final decision.

Included studies used common protection measurement methods, primarily post-mortem examination (PM) and/or culture. In the case that a study used both PM and culture to measure protection, preference was given to culture (65); in the case that lung and lymph node lesions were reported, we considered positivity per lung lesions for effect measure. We only included studies that specified the challenge strain. A majority of the included publications performed experimental (17/24) challenge and did not revaccinate animals (18/24). A complete list of all included and excluded studies is publicly available at https://doi.org/10.26208/pykx-8s25.

Statistical Analysis

All statistical analyses were performed in R (version 3.5.0) using RStudio (version 1.1.442). Full source codes used for the statistical analyses are publicly available with this publication at https://doi.org/10.26208/pykx-8s25. Random effects (RE) (4) and fixed effects (FE) meta-analysis models were estimated using the "rma" function of the "metaphor" package and analyzed using additional functions from the "meta" package (92, 93). Funnel plots were constructed to assess for systematic bias in the fitted models. Cochran's Q statistic was computed to test for unexplained heterogeneity, and Higgin's statistic helped describe the inconsistencies in studies' results (94, 95). Key parameters used to define protocols for BCG vaccination trials that were judged on biological grounds to be important were assessed as moderators in a multivariate meta-regression model, estimated using the rma function of the metafor package.

Due to the variability between reporting of pathology between different studies, vaccine efficacy was measured as a binary dichotomous variable based on the presence or absence of culture growth, or visible lesions in the control and treatment groups. Vaccine efficacy is most commonly measured using the relative risk or risk ratio (RR) (4), defined as the ratio of attack rate in the vaccinated and control groups. As well as being more easily interpretable than other measures (such as odds ratios and risk differences), RR can be used to define vaccine efficacy (1-RR) and was estimated here per the RE model. The 2 × 2 contingency table below provides a summary of included sample size (**Table 5**).

Scenario Analysis

Thus far, no study on BCG efficacy has attempted to estimate the efficacy of BCG to reduce the infectiousness of vaccinates who subsequently become infected. In the absence of empirical data, the reduction in lesions in vaccinated animals estimated from natural transmission studies may be considered as a proxy for reduction in infectiousness. While how the extent of lesions directly relates to a reduction in infectiousness and thus transmission risk was not quantified, this significant reduction in lesion severity following BCG vaccination likely contributes to reduction in risk of transmission from vaccinates to susceptible cattle. Here, we conducted scenario analyses to explore the potential implications for disease control and the importance of estimating this neglected—but critical—aspect of BCG efficacy. We consider this proportionate reduction in lesions as a plausible upper bound for the total vaccine-induced protection.

For a well-mixed population, the critical vaccination threshold (V_c) for elimination of a disease can be calculated from the basic reproduction number (R_0) using the formula $V_c = (1 - 1/R_0)/E$, where E is the relative (combined direct and indirect) efficacy of the vaccine (96). For domesticated livestock species in organized settings, routine vaccinations are often performed for all animals, hence we can reframe the critical threshold in terms of the critical efficacy $E_c = (1 - 1/R_0)$. Thus, with a direct vaccine efficacy of 25% (95% CI: 18, 32), BCG could be expected to successfully eliminate infection from fully vaccinated herds when the within-herd R_0 is 1.32 (95% CI, 1.20–1.45) or lower.

A simple deterministic model for the within-herd transmission of bTB was used to explore the potential impact of BCG vaccination in an expanding dairy sector. The model assumes a well-mixed herd with animals stratified into four epidemiological compartments. In an unvaccinated population, animals are either susceptible (S) or infected and potentially infectious (I). Vaccinated individuals (V) have a reduced risk of becoming infected and we add a final infected after vaccination compartment to model a reduced infectiousness for these animals (I_V). Density dependence in transmission is modeled using the non-linear relationship estimated from herds in Great Britain (GB) using the so-called SOR model (71). The SOR model subdivides the infectious class into an occult (O) and reactive (R) groups that differ in their reaction to the tuberculin skin test, but also assumes infected animals are potentially infectious immediately and is thus structurally equivalent to the $SI(VI_V)$ model used here.

The full model equations are:

$$\frac{dS}{dt} = (1-p)\,\mu N - \frac{\beta}{(N/N_m)^q}(I + (1-\varepsilon_I)\ I_V)\,S - \nu S$$

$$\frac{dI}{dt} = \frac{\beta}{(N/N_m)^q}(I + (1-\varepsilon_I)\ I_V)\,S - \nu I$$

$$\frac{dV}{dt} = p\mu N - (1-\varepsilon_s)\,\frac{\beta}{(N/N_m)^q}(I + (1-\varepsilon_I)\ I_V)\,V - \nu V$$

$$\frac{dI_V}{dt} = (1-\varepsilon_s)\,\frac{\beta}{(N/N_m)^q}(I + (1-\varepsilon_I)\ I_V)\,V - \nu I_V$$

$$\frac{dC}{dt} = \frac{\beta}{(N/N_m)^q}\,(I + (1-\varepsilon_I)\ I_V)\,S + (1-\varepsilon_s)\,\frac{\beta}{(N/N_m)^q}(I + (1-\varepsilon_I)\ I_V)\,V$$

$$\frac{dN}{dt} = (\mu - \nu)N$$

where ε_s is the efficacy of vaccination to protect against infection (reduction in susceptibility), ε_I is the efficacy of vaccination with respect to reducing the infectiousness of vaccinates that subsequently become infected and N_m is a constant centering parameter (=165) used for the estimation of q in the original GB model. β is a transmission parameter which we fix using the assumed initial prevalence (I_0) and initial herd size (N_0) for each scenario and q measures the strength of density dependence of transmission with $q = 0$ corresponding to density dependence and $q = 1$ frequency dependence. For the default scenario we use the point estimate from Conlan et al. (71) of $q = 0.15$ and present an alternative weaker density dependent scenario ($q = 0.71$, upper bound of approximate posterior distribution) in **Supplementary Material**.

For illustration we consider a herd with initial size $N_0 = 30$, a 20% per annum replacement rate ($\nu = 0.2$ per year) and per capita birth rate $\mu = 1.15\ \nu$ to give a population growth rate of 15% per year ($N = N_0 e^{-(\mu-\upsilon)t}$).

The basic reproduction ratio for this model (for fixed herd size N_0) can be calculated (next generation method) as:

$$R_0 = \frac{\beta}{\upsilon} N_0\,(N_0/N_m)^{-q}$$

We set the (97) value of β for each scenario by assuming that the initial population is at the equilibrium point of the constant population model. Thus, at $t = 0$, we assume that:

$$R_0 = 1/(1 - I_0/N_0)$$

and thus set:

$$\beta = \frac{\nu R_0\,(N_0/N_m)^q}{N_0}$$

Full source codes used for the statistical analyses are publicly available with this publication at https://doi.org/10.26208/pykx-8s25.

AUTHOR CONTRIBUTIONS

SS, LE, and VK designed the study. SS, LE, and CH performed data extraction. SS and AC compiled the final data and analyzed the data. SS drafted the paper. SS, AC, PD, MVe, GA, GR, JW, NJ, DB, MVo, and VK contributed to the writing. All authors contributed to the article and approved the submitted version.

FUNDING

This study was supported by a grant (OPP1176950) from the Bill & Melinda Gates Foundation and the U.K. Department for International Development.

REFERENCES

1. Cousins DV. *Mycobacterium bovis* infection and control in domestic livestock. *Rev Sci Tech.* (2001) 20:71–85. doi: 10.20506/rst.20.1.1263
2. Doyle TM, Stuart P. Vaccination of Cattle with B.C.G. *Br Vet J.* (1958) 114:3–10. doi: 10.1016/S0007-1935(17)45652-1
3. Haring CM, Traum J, Hayes FM, Henry BS. Vaccination of calves against tuberculosis with Calmette-Guérin Culture, BCG. *Hilgardia J Agric Sci.* (1930) 4:307–94. doi: 10.3733/hilg.v04n12p307
4. Vordermeier HM, Jones GJ, Buddle BM, Hewinson RG, Villarreal-Ramos B. Bovine tuberculosis in cattle: vaccines, DIVA tests, and host biomarker discovery. *Annu Rev Anim Biosci.* (2016) 4:87–109. doi: 10.1146/annurev-animal-021815-111311
5. Olmstead AL, Rhode PW. An impossible undertaking: the eradication of bovine tuberculosis in the United States. *J Econ Hist.* (2004) 64:734–72. doi: 10.1017/S0022050704002955
6. Sidders B, Pirson C, Hogarth PJ, Hewinson RG, Stoker NG, Vordermeier HM, et al. Screening of highly expressed mycobacterial genes identifies Rv3615c as a useful differential diagnostic antigen for the *Mycobacterium tuberculosis* complex. *Infect Immun.* (2008) 76:3932–9. doi: 10.1128/IAI.00150-08
7. Whelan AO, Clifford D, Upadhyay B, Breadon EL, Mcnair J, Hewinson GR, et al. Development of a skin test for bovine tuberculosis for differentiating infected from vaccinated animals. *J Clin Microbiol.* (2010) 48:3176–81. doi: 10.1128/JCM.00420-10

8. Srinivasan S, Jones G, Veerasami M, Steinbach S, Holder T, Zewude A, et al. A defined antigen skin test for the diagnosis of bovine tuberculosis. *Sci Adv.* (2019) 5:eaax4899. doi: 10.1126/sciadv.aax4899
9. Srinivasan S, Subramanian S, Shankar Balakrishnan S, Ramaiyan Selvaraju K, Manomohan V, Selladurai S, et al. A defined antigen skin test that enables implementation of BCG vaccination for control of bovine tuberculosis: proof of concept. *Front Vet Sci.* (2020) 7:391–391. doi: 10.3389/fvets.2020.00391
10. Buddle BM, Vordermeier HM, Chambers MA, De Klerk-Lorist LM. Efficacy and safety of BCG vaccine for control of tuberculosis in domestic livestock and wildlife. *Front Vet Sci.* (2018) 5:259–259. doi: 10.3389/fvets.2018.00259
11. Conlan AJK, Vordermeier M, De Jong MCM, Wood JLN. The intractable challenge of evaluating cattle vaccination as a control for bovine tuberculosis. *eLife.* (2018) 7:e27694. doi: 10.7554/eLife.27694
12. Waddington FG, Ellwood DC. An experiment to challenge the resistance to tuberculosis in B.C.G. vaccinated cattle in Malawi. *Br Vet J.* (1972) 128:541–52. doi: 10.1016/S0007-1935(17)36683-6
13. Berggren SA. Field experiment with BCG vaccine in Malawi. *Br Vet J.* (1981) 137:88–96. doi: 10.1016/S0007-1935(17)31792-X
14. Buddle BM, De Lisle GW, Pfeffer A, Aldwell FE. Immunological responses and protection against *Mycobacterium bovis* in calves vaccinated with a low dose of BCG. *Vaccine.* (1995) 13:1123–30. doi: 10.1016/0264-410X(94)00055-R
15. Buddle BM, Keen D, Thomson A, Jowett G, Mccarthy AR, Heslop J, et al. Protection of cattle from bovine tuberculosis by vaccination with BCG by the respiratory or subcutaneous route, but not by vaccination with killed *Mycobacterium vaccae. Res Vet Sci.* (1995) 59:10–6. doi: 10.1016/0034-5288(95)90023-3
16. Buddle BM, Parlane NA, Keen DL, Aldwell FE, Pollock JM, Lightbody K, et al. Differentiation between *Mycobacterium bovis* BCG-vaccinated and *M. bovis*-infected cattle by using recombinant mycobacterial antigens. *Clin Diagn Lab Immunol.* (1999) 6:1–5. doi: 10.1128/CDLI.6.1.1-5.1999
17. Buddle BM, Wards BJ, Aldwell FE, Collins DM, De Lisle GW. Influence of sensitisation to environmental mycobacteria on subsequent vaccination against bovine tuberculosis. *Vaccine.* (2002) 20:1126–33. doi: 10.1016/S0264-410X(01)00436-4
18. Buddle BM, Wedlock DN, Parlane NA, Corner LA, De Lisle GW, Skinner MA. Revaccination of neonatal calves with *Mycobacterium bovis* BCG reduces the level of protection against bovine tuberculosis induced by a single vaccination. *Infect Immun.* (2003) 71:6411–9. doi: 10.1128/IAI.71.11.6411-6419.2003
19. Buddle BM, Aldwell FE, Skinner MA, De Lisle GW, Denis M, Vordermeier HM, et al. Effect of oral vaccination of cattle with lipid-formulated BCG on immune responses and protection against bovine tuberculosis. *Vaccine.* (2005) 23:3581–9. doi: 10.1016/j.vaccine.2005.01.150
20. Wedlock DN, Denis M, Vordermeier HM, Hewinson RG, Buddle BM. Vaccination of cattle with Danish and Pasteur strains of *Mycobacterium bovis* BCG induce different levels of IFNgamma post-vaccination, but induce similar levels of protection against bovine tuberculosis. *Vet Immunol Immunopathol.* (2007) 118:50–8. doi: 10.1016/j.vetimm.2007.04.005
21. Buddle BM, Denis M, Aldwell FE, Martin Vordermeier H, Glyn Hewinson R, Neil Wedlock D. Vaccination of cattle with *Mycobacterium bovis* BCG by a combination of systemic and oral routes. *Tuberculosis (Edinb).* (2008) 88:595–600. doi: 10.1016/j.tube.2008.01.005
22. Wedlock DN, Denis M, Painter GF, Ainge GD, Vordermeier HM, Hewinson RG, et al. Enhanced protection against bovine tuberculosis after coadministration of *Mycobacterium bovis* BCG with a Mycobacterial protein vaccine-adjuvant combination but not after coadministration of adjuvant alone. *Clin Vaccine Immunol.* (2008) 15:765–72. doi: 10.1128/CVI.00034-08
23. Ameni G, Vordermeier M, Aseffa A, Young DB, Hewinson RG. Field evaluation of the efficacy of *Mycobacterium bovis* bacillus Calmette-Guerin against bovine tuberculosis in neonatal calves in Ethiopia. *Clin Vaccine Immunol.* (2010) 17:1533–8. doi: 10.1128/CVI.00222-10
24. De Klerk LM, Michel AL, Bengis RG, Kriek NP, Godfroid J. BCG vaccination failed to protect yearling African buffaloes (*Syncerus caffer*) against experimental intratonsilar challenge with *Mycobacterium bovis. Vet Immunol Immunopathol.* (2010) 137:84–92. doi: 10.1016/j.vetimm.2010.04.013
25. Lopez-Valencia G, Renteria-Evangelista T, Williams JEJ, Licea-Navarro A, Mora-Valle AEL, Medina-Basulto G. Field evaluation of the protective efficacy of *Mycobacterium bovis* BCG vaccine against bovine tuberculosis. *Res Vet Sci.* (2010) 88:44–9. doi: 10.1016/j.rvsc.2009.05.022
26. Buddle BM, Aldwell FE, De Lisle GW, Vordermeier HM, Hewinson RG, Wedlock DN. Low oral BCG doses fail to protect cattle against an experimental challenge with *Mycobacterium bovis. Tuberculosis (Edinb).* (2011) 91:400–5. doi: 10.1016/j.tube.2011.07.001
27. Hope JC, Thom ML, Mcaulay M, Mead E, Vordermeier HM, Clifford D, et al. Identification of surrogates and correlates of protection in protective immunity against *Mycobacterium bovis* infection induced in neonatal calves by vaccination with *M. bovis* BCG Pasteur and *M. bovis* BCG Danish *Clin Vaccine Immunol.* (2011) 18:373–9. doi: 10.1128/CVI.00543-10
28. Thom ML, Mcaulay M, Vordermeier HM, Clifford D, Hewinson RG, Villarreal-Ramos B, et al. Duration of immunity against *Mycobacterium bovis* following neonatal vaccination with bacillus Calmette-Guérin Danish: significant protection against infection at 12, but not 24, months. *Clin Vaccine Immunol.* (2012) 19:1254–60. doi: 10.1128/CVI.00301-12
29. Buddle BM, Hewinson RG, Vordermeier HM, Wedlock DN. Subcutaneous administration of a 10-fold-lower dose of a commercial human tuberculosis vaccine, *Mycobacterium bovis* bacillus Calmette-Guerin Danish, induced levels of protection against bovine tuberculosis and responses in the tuberculin intradermal test similar to those induced by a standard cattle dose. *Clin Vaccine Immunol.* (2013) 20:1559–62. doi: 10.1128/CVI.00435-13
30. Dean G, Whelan A, Clifford D, Salguero FJ, Xing Z, Gilbert S, et al. Comparison of the immunogenicity and protection against bovine tuberculosis following immunization by BCG-priming and boosting with adenovirus or protein based vaccines. *Vaccine.* (2014) 32:1304–10. doi: 10.1016/j.vaccine.2013.11.045
31. Parlane NA, Shu D, Subharat S, Wedlock DN, Rehm BH, De Lisle GW, et al. Revaccination of cattle with bacille Calmette-Guérin two years after first vaccination when immunity has waned, boosted protection against challenge with *Mycobacterium bovis. PLoS ONE.* (2014) 9:e106519. doi: 10.1371/journal.pone.0106519
32. Dean GS, Clifford D, Whelan AO, Tchilian EZ, Beverley PC, Salguero FJ, et al. Protection induced by simultaneous subcutaneous and endobronchial vaccination with BCG/BCG and BCG/adenovirus expressing antigen 85A against *Mycobacterium bovis* in cattle. *PLoS ONE.* (2015) 10:e0142270. doi: 10.1371/journal.pone.0142270
33. Buddle BM, Shu D, Parlane NA, Subharat S, Heiser A, Hewinson RG, et al. Vaccination of cattle with a high dose of BCG vaccine 3 weeks after experimental infection with *Mycobacterium bovis* increased the inflammatory response, but not tuberculous pathology. *Tuberculosis (Edinb).* (2016) 99:120–7. doi: 10.1016/j.tube.2016.05.004
34. Nugent G, Yockney IJ, Whitford J, Aldwell FE, Buddle BM. Efficacy of oral BCG vaccination in protecting free-ranging cattle from natural infection by *Mycobacterium bovis. Vet Microbiol.* (2017) 208:181–9. doi: 10.1016/j.vetmic.2017.07.029
35. Ameni G, Tafess K, Zewde A, Eguale T, Tilahun M, Hailu T, et al. Vaccination of calves with *Mycobacterium bovis* Bacillus Calmette-Guerin reduces the frequency and severity of lesions of bovine tuberculosis under a natural transmission setting in Ethiopia. *Transbound Emerg Dis.* (2018) 65:96–104. doi: 10.1111/tbed.12618
36. Nugent G, Yockney IJ, Cross ML, Buddle BM. Low-dose BCG vaccination protects free-ranging cattle against naturally-acquired bovine tuberculosis. *Vaccine.* (2018) 36:7338–44. doi: 10.1016/j.vaccine.2018.10.025
37. Viechtbauer W. Accounting for heterogeneity via random-effects models and moderator analyses in meta-analysis. *J Psychol.* (2007) 215:104–21. doi: 10.1027/0044-3409.215.2.104
38. Mavridis D, Salanti G. How to assess publication bias: funnel plot, trim-and-fill method and selection models. *Evid Based Mental Health.* (2014) 17:30. doi: 10.1136/eb-2013-101699
39. Duval S, Tweedie R. Trim and fill: a simple funnel-plot-based method of testing and adjusting for publication bias in meta-analysis. *Biometrics.* (2000) 56:455–63. doi: 10.1111/j.0006-341X.2000.00455.x
40. Remlinger P, Bailly J. Nasal immunization against tuberculosis. *Compt Rend Soc Biol.* (1928) 99:1556–7.
41. Conlan AJK, Wood JLN. *The Epidemiology of Mycobacterium bovis Infection in Cattle, Chapter 4, Bovine Tuberculosis* (2018). Available online at: https://www.cabi.org/vetmedresource/ebook/20183117961
42. Srinivasan S, Easterling L, Rimal B, Niu XM, Conlan AJK, Dudas P, et al. Prevalence of bovine tuberculosis in India: a systematic review and

meta-analysis. *Transbound Emerg Dis.* (2018) 65:1627–40. doi: 10.1111/tbed.12915
43. Halloran ME, Struchiner CJ, Longini IM Jr. Study designs for evaluating different efficacy and effectiveness aspects of vaccines. *Am J Epidemiol.* (1997) 146:789–803.
44. Watson E. Studies on bacillus Calmette-Guérin (BCG) and vaccination against tuberculosis. *Can J Res.* (1933) 9:128–36. doi: 10.1139/cjr33-073
45. WHO/FAO Expert Committee on Zoonoses. *Second Report. World Health Organisation Technical Report Series No 169.* (1959)
46. Various papers on Calmette's BCG. *Ann Inst Pasteur.* (1927) 41:201–368.
47. Gerlach F. Preventive inoculation against tuberculosis with Calmette's BCG. *Z Immun U Exp Therap.* (1927) 51:256–75.
48. Watson EA. *Report of the Pathological Division, Health of Animals Branch, Department of Agriculture, for the year ending March 81st, 1930.* Ottawa, ON: F. A. Acland (1930).
49. Calmette A. Preventive vaccination against tuberculosis with BCG. *Proc R Soc Med.* (1931) 24:1481–90. doi: 10.1177/003591573102401109
50. Gerlach F. *Vaccination Against Tuberculosis* (1931). Available online at: https://www.cabdirect.org/cabdirect/abstract/19322200716
51. Gloyne SR. *BCG Vaccine–A Review of Its Uses* (1931).
52. Griffith AS, Buxton JB, Glover RE. *Further Results of Immunity Experiments on Calves With the BCG Vaccine.* Cambridge: University of Cambridge (1931).
53. Gerlach F. Results of BCG vaccination on cattle in Austria. *Wien Tierarztl Monatssch.* (1932) 19:353–66.
54. Young JA, Paterson JS. Studies on the vaccination of cattle as a measure against infection with tuberculosis with the living vole acid-fast bacillus. *J Hyg. (London).* (1949) 4:39–78.
55. Young JA. B.C.G. vaccination. *Lancet.* (1949) 254:1055–6. doi: 10.1016/S0140-6736(49)91629-3
56. Ellwood DC, Waddington FG. A second experiment to challenge the resistance to tuberculosis in B.C.G. vaccinated cattle in Malawi. *Br Vet J.* (1972) 128:619–26. doi: 10.1016/S0007-1935(17)36634-4
57. Ellwood DC. First results of the field use of BCG vaccine to control bovine tuberculosis in Malawi. *Br Vet J.* (1975) 131:186–9. doi: 10.1016/S0007-1935(17)35339-3
58. Waters WR, Palmer MV, Buddle BM, Vordermeier HM. Bovine tuberculosis vaccine research: historical perspectives and recent advances. *Vaccine.* (2012) 30:2611–22. doi: 10.1016/j.vaccine.2012.02.018
59. Olea-Popelka F, Muwonge A, Perera A, Dean AS, Mumford E, Erlacher-Vindel E, et al. Zoonotic tuberculosis in human beings caused by *Mycobacterium bovis*-a call for action. *Lancet Infect Dis.* (2017) 17:e21–5. doi: 10.1016/S1473-3099(16)30139-6
60. Hope JC, Thom ML, Villarreal-Ramos B, Vordermeier HM, Hewinson RG, Howard CJ. Vaccination of neonatal calves with *Mycobacterium bovis* BCG induces protection against intranasal challenge with virulent *M. bovis. Clin Exp Immunol.* (2005) 139:48–56. doi: 10.1111/j.1365-2249.2005.02668.x
61. Gopinath K, Singh S. Non-tuberculous mycobacteria in TB-endemic countries: are we neglecting the danger? *PLoS Negl Trop Dis.* (2010) 4:e615. doi: 10.1371/journal.pntd.0000615
62. Hope JC, Thom ML, Villarreal-Ramos B, Vordermeier HM, Hewinson RG, Howard CJ. Exposure to *Mycobacterium avium* induces low-level protection from *Mycobacterium bovis* infection but compromises diagnosis of disease in cattle. *Clin Exp Immunol.* (2005) 141:432–9. doi: 10.1111/j.1365-2249.2005.02882.x
63. Nuru A, Zewude A, Mohammed T, Wondale B, Teshome L, Getahun M, et al. Nontuberculosis mycobacteria are the major causes of tuberculosis like lesions in cattle slaughtered at Bahir Dar Abattoir, northwestern Ethiopia. *BMC Vet Res.* (2017) 13:237. doi: 10.1186/s12917-017-1168-3
64. Sweetline Anne N, Ronald BSM, Kumar TMS, Kannan P, Thangavelu A. Molecular identification of *Mycobacterium tuberculosis* in cattle. *Vet Microbiol.* (2017) 198:81–7. doi: 10.1016/j.vetmic.2016.12.013
65. De La Rua-Domenech R, Goodchild AT, Vordermeier HM, Hewinson RG, Christiansen KH, Clifton-Hadley RS. Ante mortem diagnosis of tuberculosis in cattle: a review of the tuberculin tests, gamma-interferon assay and other ancillary diagnostic techniques. *Res Vet Sci.* (2006) 81:190–210. doi: 10.1016/j.rvsc.2005.11.005
66. Shim E, Galvani AP. Distinguishing vaccine efficacy and effectiveness. *Vaccine.* (2012) 30:6700–5. doi: 10.1016/j.vaccine.2012.08.045
67. Halloran ME, Haber M, Longini IM Jr., Struchiner CJ. Direct and indirect effects in vaccine efficacy and effectiveness. *Am J Epidemiol.* (1991) 133:323–31. doi: 10.1093/oxfordjournals.aje.a115884
68. Carter SP, Chambers MA, Rushton SP, Shirley MDF, Schuchert P, Pietravalle S, et al. BCG vaccination reduces risk of tuberculosis infection in vaccinated badgers and unvaccinated Badger Cubs. *PLoS ONE.* (2012) 7:e49833. doi: 10.1371/journal.pone.0049833
69. Skuce RA, Allen AR, Mcdowell SW. Herd-level risk factors for bovine tuberculosis: a literature review. *Vet Med Int.* (2012) 2012:621210. doi: 10.1155/2012/621210
70. Barlow ND, Kean JM, Hickling G, Livingstone PG, Robson AB. A simulation model for the spread of bovine tuberculosis within New Zealand cattle herds. *Prev Vet Med.* (1997) 32:57–75. doi: 10.1016/S0167-5877(97)00002-0
71. Conlan AJK, Mckinley TJ, Karolemeas K, Pollock EB, Goodchild AV, Mitchell AP, et al. Estimating the hidden burden of bovine tuberculosis in Great Britain. *PLoS Comput Biol.* (2012) 8:e1002730. doi: 10.1371/journal.pcbi.1002730
72. Mekonnen GA, Conlan AJK, Berg S, Ayele BT, Alemu A, Guta S, et al. Prevalence of bovine tuberculosis and its associated risk factors in the emerging dairy belts of regional cities in Ethiopia. *Prev Vet Med.* (2019) 168:81–9. doi: 10.1016/j.prevetmed.2019.04.010
73. Balseiro A, Prieto JM, Álvarez V, Lesellier S, Davé D, Salguero FJ, et al. Protective effect of oral BCG and inactivated *Mycobacterium bovis* vaccines in European Badgers (*Meles meles*) experimentally infected with *M. bovis. Front Vet Sci.* (2020) 7:41. doi: 10.3389/fvets.2020.00041
74. Ameni G, Aseffa A, Sirak A, Engers H, Young DB, Hewinson RG, et al. Effect of skin testing and segregation on the prevalence of bovine tuberculosis, and molecular typing of *Mycobacterium bovis*, in Ethiopia. *Vet Rec.* (2007) 161:782–6.
75. Dean GS, Rhodes SG, Coad M, Whelan AO, Wheeler P, Villareal-Ramos B, et al. Isoniazid treatment of *Mycobacterium bovis* in cattle as a model for human tuberculosis. *Tuberculosis.* (2008) 88:586–94. doi: 10.1016/j.tube.2008.01.004
76. Thoen CO, Steele JH, Gilsdorf MJ. *Mycobacterium bovis Infection in Animals and Humans.* Ames, IA: Blackwell Publishing (2008). p. 329.
77. McLaughlin AM, Gibbons N, Fitzgibbon M, Power JT, Foley SC, Hayes JP, et al. Primary isoniazid resistance in *Mycobacterium bovis* disease: a prospect of concern. *Am J Respir Crit Care Med.* (2012) 186:110–1. doi: 10.1164/ajrccm.186.1.110
78. Skinner MA, Ramsay AJ, Buchan GS, Keen DL, Ranasinghe C, Slobbe L, et al. A DNA prime-live vaccine boost strategy in mice can augment IFN-γ responses to mycobacterial antigens but does not increase the protective efficacy of two attenuated strains of *Mycobacterium bovis* against bovine tuberculosis. *Immunology.* (2003) 108:548–55. doi: 10.1046/j.1365-2567.2003.01589.x
79. Vordermeier HM, Rhodes SG, Dean G, Goonetilleke N, Huygen K, Hill AVS, et al. Cellular immune responses induced in cattle by heterologous prime-boost vaccination using recombinant viruses and bacille Calmette-Guérin. *Immunology.* (2004) 112:461–70. doi: 10.1111/j.1365-2567.2004.01903.x
80. Skinner MA, Wedlock DN, De Lisle GW, Cooke MM, Tascon RE, Ferraz JC, et al. The order of prime-boost vaccination of neonatal calves with *Mycobacterium bovis* BCG and a DNA vaccine encoding mycobacterial proteins Hsp65, Hsp70, and Apa is not critical for enhancing protection against bovine tuberculosis. *Infect Immun.* (2005) 73:4441–4. doi: 10.1128/IAI.73.7.4441-4444.2005
81. Vordermeier HM, Huygen K, Singh M, Hewinson RG, Xing Z. Immune responses induced in cattle by vaccination with a recombinant adenovirus expressing mycobacterial antigen 85A and Mycobacterium bovis BCG. *Infect Immun.* (2006) 74:1416–8. doi: 10.1128/IAI.74.2.1416-1418.2006
82. Maue AC, Waters WR, Palmer MV, Nonnecke BJ, Minion EC, Browne WC, et al. An ESAT-6 : CFP10 DNA vaccine administered in conjunction with *Mycobacterium bovis* BCG confers protection to cattle challenged with virulent *M. bovis. Vaccine.* (2007) 25:4735–46. doi: 10.1016/j.vaccine.2007.03.052
83. Garrido JM, Sevilla IA, Beltrán-Beck B, Minguijón E, Ballesteros C, Galindo RC, et al. Protection against tuberculosis in Eurasian wild boar vaccinated

with heat-inactivated *Mycobacterium bovis*. *PLoS ONE.* (2011) 6:e24905. doi: 10.1371/journal.pone.0024905
84. Beltrán-Beck B, Romero B, Boadella M, Casal C, Bezos J, Mazariegos M, et al. Tonsils of the soft palate do not mediate the response of pigs to oral vaccination with heat-inactivated *Mycobacterium bovis*. *Clin Vaccine Immunol.* (2014) 21:1128–36. doi: 10.1128/CVI.00221-14
85. Thomas J, Risalde M, Serrano M, Sevilla I, Geijo M, Ortíz JA, et al. The response of red deer to oral administration of heat-inactivated *Mycobacterium bovis* and challenge with a field strain. *Vet Microbiol.* (2017) 208:195–202. doi: 10.1016/j.vetmic.2017.08.007
86. Díez-Delgado I, Sevilla IA, Romero B, Tanner E, Barasona JA, White AR, et al. Impact of piglet oral vaccination against tuberculosis in endemic free-ranging wild boar populations. *Prev Vet Med.* (2018) 155:11–20. doi: 10.1016/j.prevetmed.2018.04.002
87. Risalde MA, López V, Contreras M, Mateos-Hernández L, Gortázar C, De La Fuente J. Control of mycobacteriosis in zebrafish (*Danio rerio*) mucosally vaccinated with heat-inactivated *Mycobacterium bovis*. *Vaccine.* (2018) 36:4447–53. doi: 10.1016/j.vaccine.2018.06.042
88. Roy Á, Risalde MA, Bezos J, Casal C, Romero B, Sevilla I, et al. Response of goats to intramuscular vaccination with heat-killed *Mycobacterium bovis* and natural challenge. *Comp Immunol Microbiol Infect Dis.* (2018) 60:28–34. doi: 10.1016/j.cimid.2018.09.006
89. Serrano M, Elguezabal N, Sevilla IA, Geijo MV, Molina E, Arrazuria R, et al. Tuberculosis detection in paratuberculosis vaccinated calves: new alternatives against interference. *PLoS ONE.* (2017) 12:e0169735. doi: 10.1371/journal.pone.0169735
90. Serrano M, Elguezabal N, Sevilla IA, Geijo MV, Molina E, Juste RA, et al. Preliminary results indicate that inactivated vaccine against paratuberculosis could modify the course of experimental *Mycobacterium bovis* infection in calves. *Front Vet Sci.* (2017) 4:175–175. doi: 10.3389/fvets.2017.00175
91. Liberati A, Altman DG, Tetzlaff J, Mulrow C, Gotzsche PC, Ioannidis JP, et al. The PRISMA statement for reporting systematic reviews and meta-analyses of studies that evaluate health care interventions: explanation and elaboration. *PLoS Med.* (2009) 6:e1000100. doi: 10.1371/journal.pmed.1000100
92. Schwarzer G. meta: An R package for meta-analysis. *R News.* (2007) 7:40–5.
93. Viechtbauer W. Conducting meta-analyses in R with the metafor package. *J Stat Softw.* (2010) 36:48. doi: 10.18637/jss.v036.i03
94. Cochran WG. The combination of estimates from different experiments. *Biometrics.* (1954) 10:101–29. doi: 10.2307/3001666
95. Higgins JP, Thompson SG, Deeks JJ, Altman DG. Measuring inconsistency in meta-analyses. *BMJ.* (2003) 327:557–60. doi: 10.1136/bmj.327.7414.557
96. Anderson RM. Infectious diseases of humans: dynamics and control. *Epidemiol Infect.* (1991) 108:211.
97. Pires D, Valente E, Simoes MF, Carmo N, Testa B, Constantino L, et al. Esters of pyrazinoic acid are active against pyrazinamide-resistant strains of *Mycobacterium tuberculosis* and other naturally resistant mycobacteria *in vitro* and *ex vivo* within macrophages. *Antimicrob Agents Chemother.* (2015) 59:7693–9. doi: 10.1128/AAC.00936-15

17

Bovine Tuberculosis: The Emergence of a New Wildlife Maintenance Host

David J. Kelly[1*]*, Enda Mullen*[2] *and Margaret Good*[1,3]

[1] *Discipline of Zoology, School of Natural Sciences, Trinity College Dublin, The University of Dublin, Dublin, Ireland,* [2] *National Parks and Wildlife Service, Department of Housing, Local Government and Heritage, Dublin, Ireland,* [3] *Independent Researcher and Private Consultant, Dun Laoghaire, Co. Dublin, Ireland*

***Correspondence:**
David J. Kelly
djkelly@tcd.ie

Despite advances in herd management, tuberculosis (TB) continues to affect ~0. 5% of Ireland's national cattle herd annually. It is clear that any "final" eradication of TB in cattle will need to address all TB maintenance hosts in the same environment. In Ireland and the UK, European Badgers (Meles meles) are a known TB maintenance host, while deer are recognised as spillover hosts. However, deer have been identified as maintenance hosts in other countries and Sika deer, specifically, have been identified with TB in Ireland. We examined the power of cattle, badger and Sika deer densities (at the county level) to predict cattle TB-breakdowns in Ireland, at both the herd and the individual level, using data collected between 2000 and 2018. Our hypothesis was that any positive correlations between deer density and cattle TB-breakdowns would implicate deer as TB maintenance hosts. Using linear multiple regressions, we found positive correlations between deer density and cattle TB-breakdowns at both the herd and individual levels. Since Sika deer in County Wicklow are known to have TB, we ran further regressions against subsets of data which excluded individual Irish counties. Analyses excluding Wicklow data showed much weaker correlations between Sika deer density and cattle TB-breakdowns at both the herd and individual levels, suggesting that these correlations are strongest in County Wicklow. A similar effect for badger density was seen in County Leitrim. While locally high densities of Sika deer persist in Irish counties, we believe they should be considered an integral part of any TB-control programme for those areas.

Keywords: Sika deer, Cervus nippon, tuberculosis, TB, cattle, European badger, maintenance host, Ireland

INTRODUCTION

Tuberculosis (TB), an infectious disease caused by members of the *Mycobacterium tuberculosis* (*M. tuberculosis*) complex (MTBC) (1), is one of the leading causes of infectious disease mortality worldwide. As a zoonotic disease TB affects humans and multiple animal species and has been recognised as a major health risk to humans and animals for more than a century (2). In 2019, 1.4 million people died of tuberculosis (1). Bovine tuberculosis (bTB) is a chronic disease of cattle caused by members of the MTBC, primarily by *M. bovis*, but also *M. caprae* and, to a lesser extent, *M. tuberculosis* (3). In addition to infecting cattle and humans, the same Mycobacteria also infect other domestic animals and wildlife populations (4), causing general illness, pneumonia, weight loss and deaths. In countries where bTB is still common, and particularly where pasteurization of milk is not practiced, an estimated 10–15% of human cases of TB are caused by *M. bovis*.

Host density is a key driver of tuberculosis transmission rates and the aggregation of hosts (e.g., in large social groups) can create, or increase, opportunities for intra- or interspecific disease transmission (5). In Ireland bTB is most frequently caused by *M. bovis* (6). In cattle, TB transmission is most likely when stocking density is high (7). Depending on the infection dynamics of populations, infected wild animals are described as either maintenance or spillover hosts (8). In maintenance hosts, infection persists by intra-species transmission. By contrast, in spillover hosts, infection will not persist indefinitely, unless there is re-infection from another species.

The social structure of European Badgers (*Meles meles*) and their longevity, when infected, make them an ideal maintenance host for *M. bovis* (9). Indeed, badgers are recognised as wildlife reservoirs of *M. bovis* in the UK and Ireland (10). Other species are recognised as TB maintenance hosts in other countries; wild boar (*Sus scrofa*) in Iberia (11), African buffalo (*Syncerus caffer*) and Marsh antelope (*Kobus leche*) in Africa (12), Brushtail Possum (*Trichosurus vulpecula*) in New Zealand (13) and White-tailed Deer (*Odocoileus virginianus*) in the USA (14). In all cases, consideration of *M. bovis* (or other MTBC members) within these maintenance host populations is essential for bTB control programmes (15–19).

In general terms, disease emergence, or increased disease risk, is a frequent consequence of high density, close association and/or ungulate overabundance (20, 21). Red Deer (*Cervus elaphus*) and Fallow Deer (*Dama dama*), social species that naturally aggregate into groups, are considered TB spillover hosts in Spain (22), but recent work has shown that Red Deer, in Austria, Germany, and Italy, can also act as maintenance hosts for both *M. bovis* and *M. caprae* (another MTBC member) when they reach high densities (23–25). While regional density estimates appeared relatively low (e.g., 5.6 animals/km^2), aggregation behaviour of Red Deer was shown to increase local densities by an order of magnitude (up to 46.2 animals/km^2) at sites where supplementary winter feeding was provided (23). In the USA, White-tailed Deer numbers fluctuate from year to year in Michigan. In 1995 the population was estimated to be 2.2 million (26). Since that time the Michigan Department of Natural Resources (MDNR) have restricted supplementary winter feeding (27) and have attempted to reduce the state population to one million deer (in the spring herd). The MDNR have not been issuing estimates of deer populations for many years, but as the number of hunters and the deer harvest have both been on general declines since 1998 (28), we believe the White-tailed Deer population in Michigan is currently increasing. State-wide estimates of White-tailed Deer range from 4.5 to 8.8 animals/km^2, using population estimates from 1937 to 1995, respectively (26). Yet the density of White-tailed Deer at DeSoto National Wildlife Refuge, Michigan, USA has been recorded between 36.5 and 50.6 animals/km^2 (29). It is clear that aggregation behaviour in White-tailed Deer produces dramatic increases in local population density, in comparison to regional density estimates.

Estimates of Sika Deer (*Cervus nippon*) density for County Wicklow have risen from 7.8 animals/km^2 in 2000 to 31.4 animals/km^2 in 2018 (based on Sika Deer harvest or "bag" numbers published by the National Parks and Wildlife Service – NPWS–**Supplementary Table 1**). Although density calculations based on "bag" numbers are likely to be underestimates, as not all deer deaths (e.g., road deaths and natural causes) are reported in any given year, the technique has proved to be a good predictor of deer populations (30). The most recent estimate (31.4 animals/km^2 in 2018) for Sika in County Wicklow provides a regional density far greater than that of both Red Deer in an Austrian bTB hotspot (23) and that of state-wide estimates for White-tailed Deer in Michigan (26). If Sika Deer exhibit aggregation behaviour similar to Red and White-tailed Deer, it is likely that they have reached a threshold density in County Wicklow and are now acting as maintenance hosts for TB, rather than spillover hosts.

TB has been recorded in both farmed and wild deer in Ireland (31), but records from the Irish Department of Agriculture, Food and the Marine (DAFM) show that Wicklow is the only county in Ireland where TB has been confirmed in multiple hunted deer over many years (6). In 2007/08, within Wicklow, 80 Sika deer were culled and their entire carcases examined for the presence of typical TB lesions. Incidence of TB was 5% and the strains of TB in the deer were also found to be present in local badger and cattle populations (6). In 2014/15 a more thorough TB detection protocol identified 17% prevalence (23 of 133 deer) (6). Unfortunately, it is unclear whether the difference in prevalence between these two studies represents a rise in TB infection in Wicklow's Sika Deer, as detection protocols varied between years. Despite that uncertainty, it is clear that TB has persisted in Wicklow's Sika deer for at least the last decade. A recent study (32) has identified a high level of diversity of TB strains in Sika deer in County Wicklow. The same study also found that the TB strains in the deer were shared between badgers and cattle (32). This indicates that deer are sharing TB with other TB hosts in their environment and may, therefore, be acting as a source of infection for local cattle populations. Thus, we investigated whether Sika deer met the characteristics of a wildlife reservoir host for *M. bovis* (15, 19).

MATERIALS AND METHODS

We conducted two multiple linear regression analyses. The first analysis (herd-level analysis) used the density of cattle herds in each Irish county experiencing bTB breakdowns as the dependent variable and densities of cattle herds, Sika deer and badgers in each Irish county, as well as the year of recording (2000–2018), as predictive variables. The second analysis (individual-level analysis) used the density of cattle which were removed under the bTB eradication programme (i.e., number of "reactors") in each Irish county as the dependent variable, and densities of cattle, Sika deer, and badgers in each Irish county, as well as the year of recording, as predictive variables. The way in which the values for the dependent and predictive variables were determined is explained below.

Estimations of Deer Populations From Hunting Bags

A study of Sika Deer in the Wicklow Mountains National Park (WMNP) (33) identified a nett annual productivity of about

25% (including estimations of female productivity, double births, calf survival, and adult survival). Another estimate (34) puts the nett annual productivity of Sika Deer in County Wicklow at 28%. This means that in order to maintain stable numbers, the maximum sustainable yield of local Sika Deer would be 28% of the population.

Using hunting bag data from the NPWS (www.npws.ie), we considered any increases in county bag numbers in consecutive years as an indication of population increase, i.e., more deer were being born than being removed. In those circumstances, bag totals were considered to be 25% of the population. When consecutive years showed slight decreases in hunting bags, those bag numbers were considered to indicate more deer were being removed than being born. We assumed those bags to represent 33% of the deer population. While bag numbers appear to offer a relatively crude method of assessing deer populations (35, 36), they can provide good estimates of county-level populations (30) (**Supplementary Table 2**). A variety of Sika density estimates were produced for each county by dividing population estimates of each deer species by habitat areas derived from CORINE 2012 (37) (**Supplementary Table 3**). This technique provided a way of allowing for deer aggregations in preferred habitats (e.g., pasture and woodland). The Sika density estimates which best explained variation in the herd-level (**Supplementary Table 4**) and individual-level (**Supplementary Table 5**) breakdown data for cattle were selected for those models, respectively, although all Sika density estimates gave similar results (**Supplementary Tables 4, 5**).

Badger Population Estimates

A survey of badger main setts in Ireland (38) was used to provide a baseline for badger densities across Ireland. Despite attempts at modelling fluctuations in badger populations using occupancy rates (39), nett productivity estimates (40) and removals over the study period, we were unable to produce credible population estimates. In County Wicklow, a seven-year study of badgers in an unculled population, found that the local density remained stable between 2010 and 2016, despite numerous badgers dying on roads in the study area (41). Indeed, this population showed a nett migration into surrounding areas, where DAFM culling was in operation. If such a pattern were repeated across the country, it seems likely that culled areas would show only temporary reductions in local population density. Bearing this in mind, we assumed that badger populations, at the county level, remained constant over the study period (**Supplementary Table 6**). This assumption tallies with anecdotal data.

A variety of badger density estimates were produced for each county by dividing estimates of badger numbers by habitat areas derived from CORINE 2012 (37). The badger density estimates which best explained variation in the herd-level (**Supplementary Table 7**) and individual level (**Supplementary Table 8**) breakdown data for cattle were selected for those models, respectively. As the badger populations in all counties were assumed to be stable, badger density values for individual counties were constant across the study period (2000–2018) in both the herd-level and individual-level models.

Cattle Population Densities

We used data from DAFM to identify the number of herds registered in each county (**Supplementary Table 9**), the number of infected herds within each county (**Supplementary Table 10**), the number of cattle removed as reactors in each county (**Supplementary Table 11**) and the number of individual cattle in each county (**Supplementary Table 12**), for each year of the study period (42).

Density estimates of herds, or individuals, were produced by dividing cattle numbers for each county by pasture areas derived from CORINE 2012 (37) (**Supplementary Table 3**).

Statistical Analysis

Analyses were performed in R (43) we used the *lmer* function from the **lme4** package (44) to perform Generalised Linear Models (GLMs). Data were centred and scaled, to remove any numeric bias from individual predictive variables, using the *standardize* function from the **arm** package (45). County cattle density, county badger density, county deer density, year and all two-way interactions of animal densities with year, were included in full models for herd-level and individual-level analyses. The R code for these models is included for the reference of readers (**Supplementary Figure 1**).

RESULTS

Herd-level Analysis

This analysis used the density of cattle herds, Sika deer and badgers to explain the variation in herds with breakdowns at the county level between 2000 and 2018. Cattle herd densities were calculated per square kilometre of pasture. Following a comparison of density alternatives which best explained the variation in herd TB-breakdown density (**Supplementary Table 4**), Sika deer densities were calculated per combined square kilometre of pasture and forestry. A similar comparison for badgers (**Supplementary Table 7**), identified densities calculated per square kilometre of pasture as most appropriate.

The GLM provided several details about the trends in herd breakdown density (**Table 1**). Over the period of the study (2000–2018), the number of herd breakdowns fell (Year; estimate = −0.547431, $t = -19.93$, $P < 0.001$). The density of cattle herds was strongly and positively correlated with herd breakdown density (Cattle Herds; estimate = 0.319594, $t = 6.877$, $P < 0.001$), and this correlation showed a slight (but statistically insignificant) weakening over the course of the study (Cattle:Year interaction; estimate = −0.114097, $t = -1.259$, $P > 0.05$). The density of badgers was also strongly and positively correlated with the herd breakdown density (Badgers; estimate = 0.234398, $t = 5.201$, $P < 0.001$), and this correlation also weakened over the course of the study (Badger:Year interaction; estimate = −0.222166, $t = -2.487$, $P = 0.0132$). The density of Sika deer was weakly (lacking statistical significance) positively correlated with herd breakdown density (Deer; estimate = 0.05551, $t = 1.674$, $P > 0.05$), but the strength of this correlation increased over the course of the study (Deer:Year interaction; estimate = 0.139537, $t = 2.134$, $P = 0.0334$).

TABLE 1 | Output from the GLM of herd-level analysis.

	Estimate	Std. Error	*t*-value	Pr(>|t|)	Significance
(Intercept)	−0.005468	0.01371	−0.399	0.6902	
Cattle (herd) density	0.319594	0.046474	6.877	<0.001	***
Badger density	0.234398	0.045066	5.201	<0.001	***
Deer density	0.05551	0.033163	1.674	0.0948	
Year	−0.547431	0.027464	−19.93	<0.001	***
Cattle: Year	−0.114097	0.090601	−1.259	0.2085	
Badger: Year	−0.222166	0.089342	−2.487	0.0132	*
Deer: Year	0.139537	0.065393	2.134	0.0334	*

*The nature of the correlations between explanatory variables and the dependent variable (cattle herd breakdown density) are indicated by the values in the Estimate column; positive values indicate a positive correlation and negative values indicate a negative correlation. The P-values of correlations are given in the Pr(>|t|) column, and the starred rating of these correlations is given in the significance column; *p < 0.05, **p < 0.01, ***p < 0.001.*

Individual-level Analysis

This analysis used the density of cattle, Sika deer and badgers to explain the variation in the density of "reactor" cattle from herds with breakdowns, at the county level, between 2000 and 2018. Cattle densities were calculated per square kilometre of pasture. Following a comparison of density alternatives which best explained the variation in "reactor" density (**Supplementary Table 5**), Sika deer densities were calculated per square kilometre of agricultural land. A similar comparison for badgers (**Supplementary Table 8**), identified densities calculated per square kilometre of pasture as most appropriate.

The GLM provided several details about the trends in "reactor" cattle density (**Table 2**). Over the period of the study (2000–2018), the number of "reactors" fell (Year; estimate = −0.43572, $t = -12.582$, $P < 0.001$). The density of cattle was strongly and positively correlated with "reactor" density (Cattle; estimate = 0.2498, $t = 4.831$, $P < 0.001$), but the strength of this correlation showed a dramatic reduction over the course of the study (Cattle:Year interaction; estimate = −0.39112, $t = -4.095$, $P < 0.001$). The density of badgers was positively correlated with "reactor" breakdown density (Badgers; estimate = 0.15049, $t = 2.983$, $P = 0.03$), but this correlation did not change over the course of the study (Badger:Year interaction; estimate = 0.03452, $t = 2.983$, $P > 0.05$). The density of Sika deer was strongly and positively correlated with "reactor" density (Deer; estimate = 0.18767, $t = 4.461$, $P < 0.001$). While the strength of this correlation increased over the course of the study, that change did not reach statistical significance (Deer:Year interaction; estimate = 0.13961, $t = 1.712$, $P = 0.0876$).

General Findings

Although there were differences between the two analyses, some general effects can be seen. Principally, the incidence of TB in cattle reduced dramatically during the study period. Despite this reduction, the local density of cattle, badgers, and Sika deer were all positively correlated with local TB density. While the correlation between local cattle density and local TB incidence, along with the correlation between local badger density with local TB incidence have been decreasing over time, the correlation between local deer density and local TB incidence has been increasing.

Having established that local Sika deer density was a useful predictor of local TB incidence, we investigated whether there were any regional aspects to this relationship. We ran further iterations of the herd-level and individual level analyses with subsets of the national data, excluding individual counties.

When Wicklow data were removed from the herd-level dataset (**Supplementary Table 13**), the resultant model no longer identified Sika deer density as an important predictor of TB breakdowns (Deer:Year interaction; estimate = 0.030361, $t = 0.431$, $P = 0.6665$). The same trend was seen when Westmeath data were removed from the herd-level dataset (**Supplementary Table 13**) (Deer:Year interaction; estimate = 0.130046, $t = 1.955$, $P = 0.0512$).

When Wicklow data were removed from the individual-level dataset (**Supplementary Table 14**), the resultant model no longer identified Sika deer density as an important predictor of TB reactors (Deer; estimate = −0.05224, $t = -1.258$, $P = 0.20896$). County Wicklow was the only county which affected the individual-level analysis in this way.

Curiously, when Leitrim data were removed from the herd-level dataset (**Supplementary Table 13**), the resultant model no longer identified badger density as an important predictor of TB breakdowns (Badgers; estimate = 0.040442, $t = 1.203$, $P = 0.2295$). The same trend was seen when Leitrim data were removed from the individual-level dataset (**Supplementary Table 14**) (Badgers; estimate = 0.05352, $t = 1.316$, $P = 0.1887$).

DISCUSSION

Herd-level Analysis

Higher local cattle densities and higher local badger densities correlate with higher local cattle herd TB-breakdown densities (**Table 1**). Such correlations are expected, since cattle and badgers are known maintenance hosts of TB in Ireland (46). The herd-level model shows the correlation between local badger density and local cattle herd TB-breakdown density has been decreasing over the last 19 years. This suggests that the national bTB

TABLE 2 | Output from the GLM of individual-level analysis.

	Estimate	Std. Error	*t*-value	Pr(>|t|)	Significance
(Intercept)	−0.01777	0.01719	−1.034	0.3016	
Cattle ("reactor") density	0.24980	0.05170	4.831	1.82 e−06	***
Badger density	0.15049	0.05045	2.983	0.0030	**
Deer density	0.18767	0.04207	4.461	1.01 e−05	***
Year	−0.43572	0.03463	−12.582	2.00 e−16	***
Cattle: Year	−0.39112	0.09552	−4.095	4.95 e−05	***
Badger: Year	0.03452	0.09598	0.360	0.7193	
Deer: Year	0.13961	0.8157	1.712	0.0876	

*The nature of the correlations between explanatory variables and the dependent variable (cattle "reactor" density) are indicated by the values in the Estimate column; positive values indicate a positive correlation and negative values indicate a negative correlation. The P-values of correlations are given in the Pr(>|t|) column, and the starred rating of these correlations is given in the significance column; *p < 0.05, **p < 0.01, ***p < 0.001.*

eradication policy in Ireland (47, 48), and in particular the control of TB in the badger population, has been achieving success. Indeed, recent monitoring of TB in culled badgers has shown a reduction in infection rate from 26% in 2007 to 11% in 2011 (49). Such progress may encourage a progressive shift from culling towards badger vaccination (50). However, the correlation between local cattle herd density and local cattle herd TB-breakdown density has remained static. This indicates that whatever controls on herds are currently in place have been insufficient to make significant reductions in herd-level TB infection over the last 19 years. A recent study has suggested that high risk herds should be monitored even more closely (50).

While the management of cattle and badgers appears to have reduced local rates of TB breakdowns in cattle herds, Sika populations do not appear to have been under management. Increases in local Sika deer densities were correlated with an increase in local rates of TB breakdowns in cattle herds (**Table 1**). From further analyses it appears that the data from Counties Wicklow and Westmeath were driving this correlation (**Supplementary Table 13**). These counties show the highest correlations of Sika deer density with TB levels in cattle. It is here that we believe Sika deer, as maintenance hosts of TB, pose the greatest threat to cattle.

Individual-level Analysis

Higher local cattle densities and higher local badger densities correlate with higher numbers of "reactor" cattle at test (**Table 2**). This is to be expected, as cattle and badgers are known maintenance hosts of TB in Ireland (46). Our individual-level model identifies the correlation between local cattle density and local "reactor" density has decreased over the study period. This suggests that herd management and monitoring practices have improved over the last 19 years. Potentially, it is these improvements which have prevented the influence of TB wildlife vectors (i.e., badgers or deer) changing over the course of the study. However, the local density of Sika deer was strongly positively correlated with the density of "reactor" cattle. It appears that data from County Wicklow were driving this correlation (**Supplementary Table 14**).

Sika Deer as Maintenance Hosts of *M. bovis*

While a growing body of evidence (6, 32) has identified TB in Sika deer in Wicklow, it has been difficult to identify Sika deer as maintenance hosts of TB. Several unique strains of *M. bovis* have been found in Sika deer within Wicklow (32), which suggests they act as wildlife reservoirs of TB. The data presented here provides clear evidence that higher levels of TB in cattle are associated with higher local densities of Sika deer. While this does not demonstrate Sika deer act as maintenance hosts of TB in Ireland, it adds further weight to the argument.

Sika deer in Wicklow now have regional densities comparable to other deer populations where TB maintenance has been demonstrated (23, 51). While no other deer species are implicated in our findings, Roe deer (*Capreolus capreolus*) are known to act as spillover hosts (52), and both Red deer (10, 23) and Fallow deer (53, 54) have been found to act as TB maintenance hosts at higher densities. So, while we would encourage active management of Sika Deer in Wicklow, we would also encourage the monitoring of Sika, Red and Fallow deer numbers in other counties. Such monitoring should be of particular interest to those who harbour the ambition of making Ireland TB-free by 2030 (48), or England TB-free by 2038 (55), as well as stakeholders in countries where the management of bovine TB continues to cost tax-payers eye-watering sums (48, 55).

It is difficult to offer clear guidelines regarding a "safe" Sika deer population density within Wicklow. Sika are not distributed evenly across the county (Wesley Atkinson *pers. comm.*), so assessment of density may require calculation at a finer scale (e.g., electoral district). Normal aggregation behaviour by deer means that local population densities may be an order of magnitude higher than the overall regional population densities (23). While we are unaware of a tradition of supplementary feeding of wild deer in Ireland, White-tailed deer in the United States (56) and Red deer in the Tyrol (23) may be encouraged to aggregate when they receive supplementary winter feed. The practice of providing supplementary feeding at pasture to farmed livestock grazing, in the vicinity of Sika habitat, may offer unintended supplementary feed for deer. This could promote aggregation behaviour and bring deer and cattle into contact at high density. Allowing cattle access to woodland, or higher rough-grazing areas, would also increase cattle-deer interaction opportunities, as well as potentially increasing MTBC contamination in the environment where persistence of these diseases and exposure to susceptible species is a concern (4). Interspecies transmission of MTBC has been reported at interface areas between species (57–59).

Our findings serve as a timely reminder that the final eradication of TB in any national cattle herd, is likely to prove problematic unless all MTBC diseases are addressed in all livestock (60) and wildlife reservoirs (4, 16–19, 61).

ETHICS STATEMENT

Ethical review and approval was not required for the animal study because while the species considered in this study were vertebrates, we were not required to conduct any experiments with them. We relied on data which had already been collected and was freely available in the public domain.

AUTHOR CONTRIBUTIONS

DK formulated the idea, which was then developed by DK, MG, and EM. MG and EM sourced the data. DK developed the models to analyse the data and drafted the manuscript. MG fleshed out the outline. All authors continually reviewed and edited the manuscript, in order to produce the submitted draft.

ACKNOWLEDGMENTS

We are grateful to Dr. Ruth Kelly for assistance in extracting data from the GIS layers of the CORINE maps, and to NPWS for the provision of annual hunting returns.

REFERENCES

1. WHO. *Global Tuberculosis Report*. Geneva: World Health Organisation (2020).
2. Olea-Popelka F, Muwonge A, Perera A, Dean AS, Mumford E, Erlacher-Vindel E, et al. Zoonotic tuberculosis in human beings caused by Mycobacterium bovis-a call for action. *Lancet Infect Dis.* (2017) 17:E21–5. doi: 10.1016/S1473-3099(16)30139-6
3. OIE. *Terrestrial Animal Health Code Chapter 8.11*. P: Office International des Epizooties(2019).
4. Kanipe C, Palmer MV. *Mycobacterium bovis* and you: a comprehensive look at the bacteria, its similarities to *Mycobacterium tuberculosis*, and its relationship with human disease. *Tuberculosis.* (2020) 125:102006. doi: 10.1016/j.tube.2020.102006
5. Estrada-Pena A, Ostfeld RS, Peterson AT, Poulin R, de la Fuente J. Effects of environmental change on zoonotic disease risk: an ecological primer. *Trends Parasitol.* (2014) 30:205–14. doi: 10.1016/j.pt.2014.02.003
6. Good M, Duignan A. *Veterinary handbook for herd management in the bovine TB eradication programme*. Department of Agriculture, Food and the Marine, Dublin, Ireland (2017).
7. Neill SD, Hanna J, Obrien JJ, McCracken RM. Transmission of tuberculosis from experimentally infected cattle to in-contact calves. *Vet Rec.* (1989) 124:269–71. doi: 10.1136/vr.124.11.269
8. Morris RS, Pfeiffer DU. Directions and issues in bovine tuberculosis epidemiology and control in New Zealand. *N Z Vet J.* (1995) 43:256–65. doi: 10.1080/00480169./1995.35904
9. Gormley E, Corner LAL. Pathogenesis of *Mycobacterium bovis* infection: the badger model as a paradigm for understanding tuberculosis in animals. *Front Vet Sci.* (2018) 4:247. doi: 10.3389/fvets.2017.00247
10. Gortázar C, Delahay RJ, McDonald RA, Boadella M, Wilson GJ, Gavier-Widén D, et al. The status of tuberculosis in European wild mammals. *Mammal Rev.* (2012) 42:193–206. doi: 10.1111/j.1365-2907.2011.00191.x
11. Muñoz-Mendoza M, Marreros N, Boadella M, Gortázar C, Menéndez S, de Juan L, et al. Wild boar tuberculosis in Iberian Atlantic Spain: a different picture from Mediterranean habitats. *BMC Vet Res.* (2013) 9:176. doi: 10.1186/1746-6148-9-176
12. Renwick AR, White PCL, Bengis RG. Bovine tuberculosis in southern African wildlife: a multi-species host-pathogen system. *Epidemiol Infect.* (2007) 135:529–40. doi: 10.1017/S0950268806007205
13. Nugent G, Buddle BM, Knowles G. Epidemiology and control of *Mycobacterium bovis* infection in brushtail possums (*Trichosurus vulpecula*), the primary wildlife host of bovine tuberculosis in New Zealand. *N Z Vet J.* (2015) 63:28–41. doi: 10.1080/00480169.2014.963791
14. VerCauteren KC, Lavelle MJ, Campa H. Persistent spillback of bovine tuberculosis from white-tailed deer to cattle in Michigan, USA: Status, strategies, and needs. *Front Vet Sci.* (2018) 5:301. doi: 10.3389/fvets.2018.00301
15. Corner LAL. The role of wild animal populations in the epidemiology of tuberculosis in domestic animals: how to assess the risk. *Vet Microbiol.* (2006) 112:303–12. doi: 10.1016/j.vetmic.2005.11.015
16. Francis J. *Tuberculosis in Animals and Man: a Study in Comparative Pathology*. London: Cassell & Co. Ltd (1958).
17. Good M, Bakker D, Duignan A, Collins DM. The history of *in vivo* tuberculin testing in bovines: tuberculosis, a "One Health" issue. *Front Vet Sci.* (2018) 5:59. doi: 10.3389/fvets.2018.00059
18. Martinez-Guijosa J, Romero B, Infantes-Lorenzo JA, Diez E, Boadella M, Balseiro A, et al. Environmental DNA: a promising factor for tuberculosis risk assessment in multi-host settings. *PLoS ONE.* (2020) 15:e0233837. doi: 10.1371/journal.pone.0233837
19. Palmer MV. *Mycobacterium bovis*: characteristics of wildlife reservoir hosts. *Transbound Emerg Dis.* (2013) 60:1–13. doi: 10.1111/tbed.12115
20. Gortázar C, Acevedo P, Ruiz-Fons F, Vicente J. Disease risks and overabundance of game species. *Eur J Wildl Res.* (2006) 52:81–7. doi: 10.1007/s10344-005-0022-2
21. Ryan TJ, Livingstone PG, Ramsey DSL, de Lisle GW, Nugent G, Collins DM, et al. Advances in understanding disease epidemiology and implications for control and eradication of tuberculosis in livestock: the experience from New Zealand. *Vet Microbiol.* (2006) 112:211–9. doi: 10.1016/j.vetmic.2005.11.025
22. Aranaz A, de Juan L, Montero N, Sanchez C, Galka M, Delso C, et al. Bovine tuberculosis (*Mycobacterium bovis*) in wildlife in Spain. *J Clin Microbiol.* (2004) 42:2602–8. doi: 10.1128/JCM.42.6.2602-2608.2004
23. Fink M, Schleicher C, Gonano M, Prodinger WM, Pacciarini M, Glawischnig W, Ryser-Degiorgis MP, et al. Red deer as maintenance host for bovine tuberculosis, Alpine Region. *Emerg Infect Dis.* (2015) 21:464–7. doi: 10.3201/eid2103.141119
24. Kohl TA, Utpatel C, Nieman S, Moser I. Mycobacterium bovis persistence in two different captive wild animal populations in Germany: a longitudinal molecular epidemiological study revealing pathogen transmission by whole-genome sequencing. *J Clin Microbiol.* (2018) 56:e00302–18. doi: 10.1128/JCM.00302-18
25. Schoepf K, Prodinger WM, Glawischnig W, Hofer E, Revilla-Fernandez S, Hofrichter J, et al. A two-years' survey on the prevalence of tuberculosis caused by *Mycobacterium caprae* in red deer (*Cervus elaphus*) in the Tyrol, Austria. *ISRN Vet Sci.* (2012) 2012:245138. doi: 10.5402/2012/245138
26. MDNR. *Michigan deer management plan*. Michigan Department of Natural Resources, Lansing, Michigan, USA (2016).

27. Cosgrove MK, O'Brien DJ, Ramsey DSL. Baiting and feeding revisited: Modeling factors influencing transmission of tuberculosis among deer and to cattle. *Front Vet Sci.* (2018) 5:306. doi: 10.3389/fvets.2018.00306
28. Frawley BJ. *Michigan Deer Harvest Survey Report 2018 Seasons.* Michigan Department of Natural Resources (2019).
29. Hefley TJ, Hygnstrom SE, Gilsdorf JM, Clements GM, Clements MJ, Tyre AJ, et al. Effects of deer density and land use on mass of white-tailed deer. *J Fish Wildl Manag.* (2013) 4:20–32. doi: 10.3996/022012-JFWM-015
30. Adams HL, Kissell RE, Ratajczak D, Warr EL, Applegate RD, Barrett L, et al. Relationships among white-tailed deer density, harvest, and landscape metrics in TN, USA. *Eur J Wildl Res.* (2020) 66:19. doi: 10.1007/s10344-019-1353-8
31. Quigley FC, Costello E, Flynn O, Gogarty A, McGuirk J, Murphy A, et al. Isolation of mycobacteria from lymph node lesions in deer. *Vet Rec.* (1997) 141:516–8. doi: 10.1136/vr.141.20.516
32. Crispell J, Cassidy S, Kenny K, McGrath G, Warde S, Cameron H, et al. *Mycobacterium bovis* genomics reveals transmission of infection between cattle and deer in Ireland. *Microb Genomics.* (2020) 6:mgen000388. doi: 10.1099/mgen.0.000388
33. Atkinson W. *To Assess the Productivity, Condition, and Reproductive Success of Deer in the Wicklow Mountains National Park From Post-Mortem Cull Data Between 1995 and 1998.* Diploma in Field Ecology, University College Cork (1998).
34. O'Brien D, Rooney SM, Hayden TJ. Reproduction and potential rate of increase of the sika deer herd in County Wicklow. *Ir For.* (2007) 64:32–43.
35. Borchers DL, Buckland ST, Zucchini W. *Estimating Animal Abundance.* London: Springer (2002). doi: 10.1007/978-1-4471-3708-5
36. Morellet N, Klein F, Solberg E, Andersen R The census and management of populations of ungulates in Europe. In: Putman RJ, Apollonio M, Andersen R, editors. *Ungulate Management in Europe-Problems and Practices.* Cambridge: Cambridge University Press (2011). p. 106–43. doi: 10.1017/CBO9780511974137.006
37. Lydon K, Smith G. *CORINE landcover 2012 Ireland-Final Report.* Environmental Protection Agency, Johnstown Castle, County Wexford, Ireland (2014)
38. Smal C. *A badger and habitat survey of Ireland.* The Stationary Office, Dublin, Ireland (1995).
39. Sleeman DP, Davenport J, More SJ, Clegg TA, Collins JD, Martin SW, et al. How many Eurasian badgers *Meles meles* L. are there in the Republic of Ireland? *Eur J Wildl Res.* (2009) 55:333–44. doi: 10.1007/s10344-008-0244-1
40. Anderson RM, and Trewhella W. Population-dynamics of the badger (*Meles meles*) and the epidemiology of bovine tuberculosis (*Mycobacterium bovis*). *Philos Trans R Soc London Ser B.* (1985) 310:327–81. doi: 10.1098/rstb.1985.0123
41. Gaughran A, Kelly DJ, MacWhite T, Mullen E, Maher P, Good M, et al. Super-ranging. A new ranging strategy in European badgers. *PLoS ONE.* (2018) 13:e0191818. doi: 10.1371/journal.pone.0191818
42. DAFM. *Bovine Tuberculosis by Regional Veterinary Offices, Year and Statistical Indicator.* Central Statistics Office (2020).
43. R Core Team, R. *A Language and Environment for Statistical Computing.* Vienna: R Foundation for Statistical Computing (2020).
44. Bates D, Maechler M, Bolker B, Walker S. Fitting linear mixed-effects models using lme4. *J Stat Softw.* (2015) 67:1–48. doi: 10.18637/jss.v067.i01
45. Gelman A, Su Y-S. arm: Data analysis using regression and multilevel/hierarchical models (2020). Available online at: https://CRAN.R-project.org/package=arm
46. More SJ. Can bovine TB be eradicated from the Republic of Ireland? Could this be achieved by 2030? *Ir Vet J.* (2019) 72:3. doi: 10.1186/s13620-019-0140-x
47. DAFM. *National farmed animal health strategy.* Department of Agriculture, Food and the Marine, Dublin, Ireland (2017)
48. DAFM. *Bovine TB stakeholder forum.* Department of Agriculture, Food and the Marine, Dublin, Ireland (2018)
49. Byrne AW, Kenny K, Fogarty U, O'Keeffe JJ, More SJ, McGrath G, et al. Spatial and temporal analyses of metrics of tuberculosis infection in badgers (Meles meles) from the Republic of Ireland: Trends in apparent prevalence. *Prev Vet Med.* (2015) 122:345–54. doi: 10.1016/j.prevetmed.2015.10.013
50. Houtsma E, Clegg TA, Good M, More SJ. Further improvement in the control of bovine tuberculosis recurrence in Ireland. *Vet Rec.* (2018) 183:622. doi: 10.1136/vr.104642
51. Palmer MV, Thacker TC, Waters WR, Robbe-Austerman S. Oral vaccination of white-tailed deer (*Odocoileus virginianus*) with *Mycobacterium bovis* Bacillus Calmette-Guerin (BCG). *PLoS ONE.* (2014) 9:e97031. doi: 10.1371/journal.pone.0097031
52. Lambert S, Hars J, Reveillaud E, Moyen JL, Gares H, Rambaud T, et al. Host status of wild roe deer in bovine tuberculosis endemic areas. *Eur J Wildl Res.* (2017) 63:15. doi: 10.1007/s10344-016-1071-4
53. Griffin JFT, Chinn DN, Rodgers CR. Diagnostic strategies and outcomes on three New Zealand deer farms with severe outbreaks of bovine tuberculosis. *Tuberculosis.* (2004) 84:293–302. doi: 10.1016/j.tube.2003.11.001
54. Robinson RC, Phillips PH, Stevens G, Storm PA. An outbreak of *Mycobacterium bovis* infection in fallow deer (*Dama dama*). *Aust Vet J.* (1989) 66:195–7. doi: 10.1111/j.1751-0813.1989.tb09806.x
55. Defra. *The strategy for achieving officially bovine tuberculosis free status for England.* Department for Environment, Food and Rural Affairs, London, United Kingdom (2014). Available online at: www.gov.uk/defra
56. Bowman B, Belant JL, Beyer DE, Martel D. Characterizing nontarget species use at bait sites for white-tailed deer. *Human Wildlife Interact.* (2015) 9:110–8.
57. Katale BZ, Mbugi EV, Siame KK, Keyyu JD, Kendall S, Kazwala RR, et al. Isolation and potential for transmission of *Mycobacterium bovis* at human-livestock-wildlife interface of the Serengeti Ecosystem, Northern Tanzania. *Transbound Emerg Dis.* (2017) 64:815–25. doi: 10.1111/tbed.12445
58. LaHue NP, Banos JV, Acevedo P, Gortazar C, Martinez-Lopez B. Spatially explicit modeling of animal tuberculosis at the wildlife-livestock interface in Ciudad Real province, Spain. *Prev Vet Med.* (2016) 128:101–11. doi: 10.1016/j.prevetmed.2016.04.011
59. Sichewo PR, Hlokwe TM, Etter EMC, Michel AL. Tracing cross species transmission of *Mycobacterium bovis* at the wildlife/livestock interface in South Africa. *BMC Microbiol.* (2020) 20:49. doi: 10.1186/s12866-020-01736-4
60. Kean JM, Barlow ND, Hickling GJ. Evaluating potential sources of bovine tuberculosis infection in a New Zealand cattle herd. *New Zeal J Agr Res.* (1999) 42:101–6. doi: 10.1080/00288233.1999.9513358
61. Balseiro A, Thomas J, Gortázar C, Risalde MA. Development and Challenges in Animal Tuberculosis Vaccination. *Pathogens.* (2020) 9:472. doi: 10.3390/pathogens9060472

18

Multispacer Sequence Typing for *Mycobacterium bovis* Genotyping

Érica Bravo Sales [1], Antônio Augusto Fonseca Jr [1], Cristina Magalhães Gonçalves [1], Andrey Pereira Lage [2], Giovanna Ivo Andrade [2], Philip Noel Suffys [3], Harrison Magdinier Gomes [3], Natanael Lamas Dias [1], José Soares Ferreira Neto [4], Ana Marcia de Sá Guimarães [4] and Marcos Bryan Heinemann [4]*

[1] Laboratório Federal de Defesa Agropecuária de Minas Gerais, Pedro Leopoldo, Minas Gerais, Brazil, [2] Escola de Veterinária, Universidade Federal de Minas Gerais, Belo Horizonte, Minas Gerais, Brazil, [3] FioCruz, Rio de Janeiro, Rio de Janeiro, Brazil, [4] Universidade de São Paulo, São Paulo, São Paulo, Brazil

***Correspondence:**
Marcos Bryan Heinemann
marcosbryan@usp.br*

The molecular typing of *Mycobacterium bovis*, which causes bovine tuberculosis, can be accomplished by combining different polymorphic markers, contributing to its epidemiological investigation. Multispacer sequence typing (MST) is a sequencing-based method that employs intergenic regions susceptible to higher mutation rates given the low selection pressure. It has been applied to *M. tuberculosis*, but not to *M. bovis*. The aim of this study was to evaluate a MST for *M. bovis*. A total of 58 strains isolated from tissues with lesions suggestive of bovine tuberculosis, coming from cattle herds in six Brazilian states and four standard samples of *M. bovis* were typified employing the MST technique. Fourteen intergenic regions were used, and four types of genetic events were reported: single nucleotide mutation (SNP), insertion, deletion, and tandem repeat (TR). Seven loci were chosen for typing. Twenty-eight type sequences (ST) were identified, indicating type sequences (ST) were identified, indicating a 92.9% HGDI (Hunter Gaston Discriminatory Index). The data were used to analyze the evolutionary patterns of these isolates and correlate them to phylogeographic lineages based on the formation of clonal complexes generated from eBURST software. Later, we associated the MST with spoligotyping technique, currently considered the gold standard for classification of *M. bovis*. The results support the MST as an alternative method for genotyping of *M. bovis*. The method has the advantage of sequencing and the availability of sequences analyzed in public databases, which can be used by professionals around the world as a tool for further analysis. This was the first study to identify the variability of isolates of *M. bovis* by the MST method.

Keywords: *Mycobactereium bovis*, bovine tuberculosis, genotype, epidemiology, MST

INTRODUCTION

Mycobacterium bovis is the main pathogen of bovine tuberculosis (TB), an important disease of domestic cattle, which can also be associated with an underestimated number of human TB cases (zoonotic TB) and serious threats to wildlife conservation (1–4). Bovine TB is a disease of high health and economic relevance for livestock and is part of the group of notifiable diseases listed by the World Organization for Animal Health (OIE) (5). Infection routes in the cattle are influenced by factors such as age, environment, and hygiene practices, as the bacterium can be eliminated via various routes, such as respiratory droplets and aerosol, milk, feces, urine, vaginal secretions and/or semen (6). The presence of wildlife reservoirs in certain regions also hampers the control of the disease in livestock and translate into serious consequences for the preservation of wildlife species in multi-host systems (7). The disease directly affects livestock productivity, influencing international trade of animal products and, due to its zoonotic potential, is also of public health concern (8, 9).

Mycobacterium bovis belongs to the *Mycobacterium tuberculosis* complex (MTBC), a clonal group of mycobacterium species, lineages and/or ecotypes that cause similar diseases in a variety of mammalian hosts (10–12). Genomes of MTBC members are highly similar, with >99.9% identity over homologous regions, including the 16S rRNA gene, and absent remodeling through horizontal gene transfer or DNA recombination (10, 13, 14). This bacterial complex evolves only through SNPs (single nucleotide polymorphisms), short indels, large deletions, transposition of insertion sequence (IS) elements, and duplication of few paralogous gene families (10, 15, 16). Despite this high genetic similarity, species and lineages of the MTBC present variable phenotypes of host tropism and virulence (10–14).

Over the years, molecular genotyping techniques have significantly contributed to epidemiological studies of bovine TB, facilitating the knowledge of the spatial and temporal distribution of *M. bovis* strains, from populational structure to outbreak investigations (17, 18). Given the clonal nature of the MTBC, these techniques are based on few highly polymorphic regions of their genomes, including tandem repeats, a CRISPR locus, PGRS genes, and IS elements (17–21). The IS*6110*-based RFLP is a technique commonly used in *M. tuberculosis* genotyping, but of little application for *M. bovis* strains, as they carry only few IS*6110* copies in their genomes (22). Among the remaining techniques, spacer oligonucleotide typing (spoligotyping; based on the CRISPR locus) and variable number tandem repeat- mycobacterial interspersed repetitive units (MIRU-VNTR) have been the preferred combination for typing isolates of *M. bovis* in several countries (17–21). However, both techniques have limitations. Spoligotyping does not provide good resolution at the region or farm level, which limits its use for pathogen's transmission detection (17, 18). Spoligotyping is also sensitive to homoplasy, i.e., unrelated lineages presenting identical spoligotypes (23). This happens because the loss of a spacer region at the spoligotyping locus is a common event that can occur in strains that are not phylogenetically related (23, 24). While MIRU-VNTR has been reported to better discriminate among isolates at the farm level, there are 24 loci to choose from, and laboratories must frequently test which loci would better fit their reality for better discriminatory power (25). MIRU-VNTR is also influenced by homoplasy (24) and depending on the laboratory infrastructure, a 24 loci evaluation of *M. bovis* isolates to avoid homoplasy bias can be very laborious and time consuming (17).

Recently, *M. bovis* whole-genome sequencing (WGS) using next-generation sequencing platforms has been suggested to replace these genotyping assays (17, 18). However, WGS still faces many challenges related to its financial burden and requirement of specialized personnel, particularly in low and middle-income countries in which bovine TB is highly endemic. Most reported *M. bovis* WGS studies have been conducted in developed countries or in developing countries by researchers from high-income nations (26–32). Thus, albeit likely ideal, WGS use is still unreachable to many programs of bovine TB control and eradication around the world. Thus, there is a need for the continuous development of genotyping techniques with high resolution power. Accordingly, a multispacer sequence typing (MST) scheme for *M. tuberculosis* based on the Sanger sequencing of eight PCR-amplified intergenic regions, including four regions previously reported as VNTR regions, has been proposed (33). The aim of this study was to investigate the usefulness of this MST scheme to genotype 58 *M. bovis* isolates obtained from different Brazilian states.

MATERIALS AND METHODS

Bacterial Isolates

A total of 58 cultured isolates of *M. bovis*, deposited in the sample bank of the National Agricultural Laboratory of Minas Gerais (Lanagro/MG), Brazil, were selected. These isolates were obtained from cattle herds located in six Brazilian states [Minas Gerais ($n = 48$), Goiás ($n = 3$), Mato Grosso-MT ($n = 1$), Rio Grande do Sul-RS ($n = 1$), Paraná-PR ($n = 1$) and São Paulo ($n = 4$)] between the years 2006 and 2010. First isolation of these *M. bovis* from clinical samples were performed in Lanagro/MG according to previous publications (34). Isolated strains were identified as *M. bovis* by using a PCR assay described by Sales et al. (35). Four additional laboratory strains [*M. bovis* CR01; *M. bovis* AN5 (36); *M. bovis* BCG CR13; *M. bovis* México CR36] were also selected. All procedures were performed in a Biosafety Level 3+ Laboratory (BSL-3+) located at the Farming National Laboratory (LANAGRO) Minas Gerais, Ministry of Agriculture, Livestock and Supply, Brazil. Tubes containing DNA were properly disinfected, removed from BSL3+ and stored at −20°C until further analysis.

DNA Extraction and PCR Assays

A loop of each bacterial strain cultured in Stonebrink medium was subjected to a phenol-chloroform DNA extraction as previously described (37). Extracted DNA was subjected to conventional PCR assays of 14 intergenic spacer regions using previously described primer sequences (33). Each PCR assay was performed in a PX2 Thermal Cycler thermocycler (Milford, MA, USA). Briefly, 20 μL were prepared with the following concentrations of reagents: 10 pmol of each primer, 1.5 mM $MgCl_2$, 10 mM dNTPs (Invitrogen, USA), 1 U Jump Start®Taq DNA Polymerase (Sigma, USA) and 1 X GoTaq Green® buffer (Promega, USA). DNA sample concentration added in each reaction was 100 ng/μL. As positive controls, we used DNA extracted from *M. bovis* strain AN5 (38), while negative controls consisted of ultrapure water. The conditions of the PCR assays determined for each pair of primers are shown in **Supplementary Table 1**. Amplification products were detected by gel visualization following electrophoresis.

Sequencing and Data Analysis

The PCR products were purified using the PureLink® PCR Purification Kit (Invitrogen, USA) and sequenced using Big Dye® Terminator V.3.1 Cycle Sequencing Kit (Applied Biosystems, USA) according to the manufacturer's recommendations. Sequencing was performed in both directions in the 3130 Genetic Analyzer (Applied Biosystems, USA) equipment.

Sequence assemblies were performed with CAP3 program (39) using nucleotide data with quality higher than PHRED 20. Sequences were edited in Bioedit v.7.2.5 program (40). Subsequently, all sequences obtained for each primer pair were subjected to a multiple sequence alignment using Clustal Omega (https://www.ebi.ac.uk/Tools/msa/clustalo/) to verify the degree of identity between two or more sequences and the allelic diversity present in each spacer region. Each allele detected was assigned an identification number. For each individual DNA sample, the set of loci and their respective allele defined an allelic profile or sequence type (ST), which identified a clone. Bacterial isolates analyzed in this study were identified by numbers 1–58. The laboratory strains *M. bovis* CR01, AN5, CR13, CR36, and AF2122/97 (Genbank: NC002945.3) included in the analyses were represented by the numbers 59–63, respectively.

Spoligotyping

The spoligotyping was performed as described by Kamerbeek (41) using spolygotyping kit by Ocimum Biosolutions. The identification of individual spoligotypes and the appointment of unpublished patterns were made using Mbovis.org website (www.mbovis.org) (42).

Analysis of Genetic Relationship Among the Isolates

An evolutionary descent analysis of *M. bovis* isolates was performed using eBURST algorithm (43), available in Phyloviz software (44). Clonal complexes (CC) as defined by eBURST were identified and organized in dendrograms based on the comparison of the obtained allelic profiles of the tested *M. bovis* isolates. Briefly, CCs were determined by a simple model of clonal expansion and diversification based on the differences between these allelic profiles. Each CC was assigned a founder genotype that displays a more likely hypothetical pattern of evolutionary descent among the STs that make up this complex. The STs were organized into complexes by comparing the variation that exists among the loci of each founder genotype loci compared to other isolates (43). Accordingly, genotypic variations found in only one locus are called single locus variants (SLV), in two loci are called double locus variants (DLV), and in three loci are called triple locus variants (TLV) (43, 44). Confidence values for each SLV, DLV and TLV detected in each ST founder in a CC were assessed by bootstrapping (43). The geographic location and year of isolation of the strains were also included in the analysis.

Phylogenetic Analysis

The phylogenetic reconstruction of *M. bovis* isolates was performed by PubMLST program (http://pubmlst.org/) using the Neighbor-Joining model. The program uses PHILIP package to create Neighbor-Joining and UPGMA trees based on allelic profiles determined in the study.

Calculation of Allelic Diversity

The discrimination index (D) previously described by Hunter-Gaston (45) was used to calculate the allelic diversity at each locus and to assess genotypic diversity for each method employed (MST and spoligotyping).

RESULTS

Multispacer Sequence Typing (MST)

Fourteen intergenic spacer regions were analyzed in the selected *M. bovis* isolates. Regions MST1, MST2, MST3, MST6, and MST8 showed no sequence variation in an initial evaluation of 15 randomly chosen *M. bovis* isolates of the collection and were then excluded from the study. In addition, after multiple attempts, the PCR assay of the MST10 region failed to amplify appropriate PCR products, and this region was also excluded from the study. For the MST14 region, Sanger sequencing was not able to cover the whole extent of the region, hampering the identification of possible polymorphic positions for some of the samples and was also excluded from further evaluation. Finally, the remaining regions MST4, MST5, MST7, MST9, MST11, MST12, and MST13 proved quite variable, with a total of 28 mutational events, including single nucleotide polymorphisms (SNP), insertions, deletions, and tandem repeats. **Figure 1** shows the alleles identified for each of the seven evaluated spacer regions.

Definition of Genetic Profiles

Multiple sequence alignment of the DNA sequences of all *M. bovis* isolates for each locus allowed the identification of up to 8 different alleles which received individual identifier numbers (**Figure 1**). The grouping of all loci for each individual defined an allelic profile that was represented by a sequence type (ST). For the 63 isolates of *M. bovis* studied, 28 STs were found, where eight were represented by more than one *M. bovis* isolate, and 20 were described as orphan STs, as shown in **Table 1**.

Evolutionary Descent Analysis

The STs detected in the study were used to determine the genetic relationship of *M. bovis* isolates. A total of five CCs (ST6, ST10, ST11, ST17, and ST59) were detected (**Figure 2**). ST17, consisting of nine *M. bovis* isolates, being eight from Minas Gerais state and one from São Paulo state, was appointed as the founder CC of the whole group, as it had the highest number of SLVs (ST4, ST6, ST10, ST14, ST19, ST39, ST45, and ST54, including 24 *M. bovis* isolates from Minas Gerais, two from São Paulo and one from Mato Grosso) with diverging genotypes in only one of seven loci. ST6 was appointed the largest CC and presented the highest frequency of isolates with the same genotypic profile from different geographical locations: 10 *M. bovis* isolates from Minas Gerais, two from São Paulo, and one from Mato Grosso. This complex presented six SLVs, which expressed close relationship to ST1, ST11, ST12, ST17, ST25, and ST55, with 22 *M. bovis* isolates from the states of Minas Gerais ($n = 19$), São Paulo (n

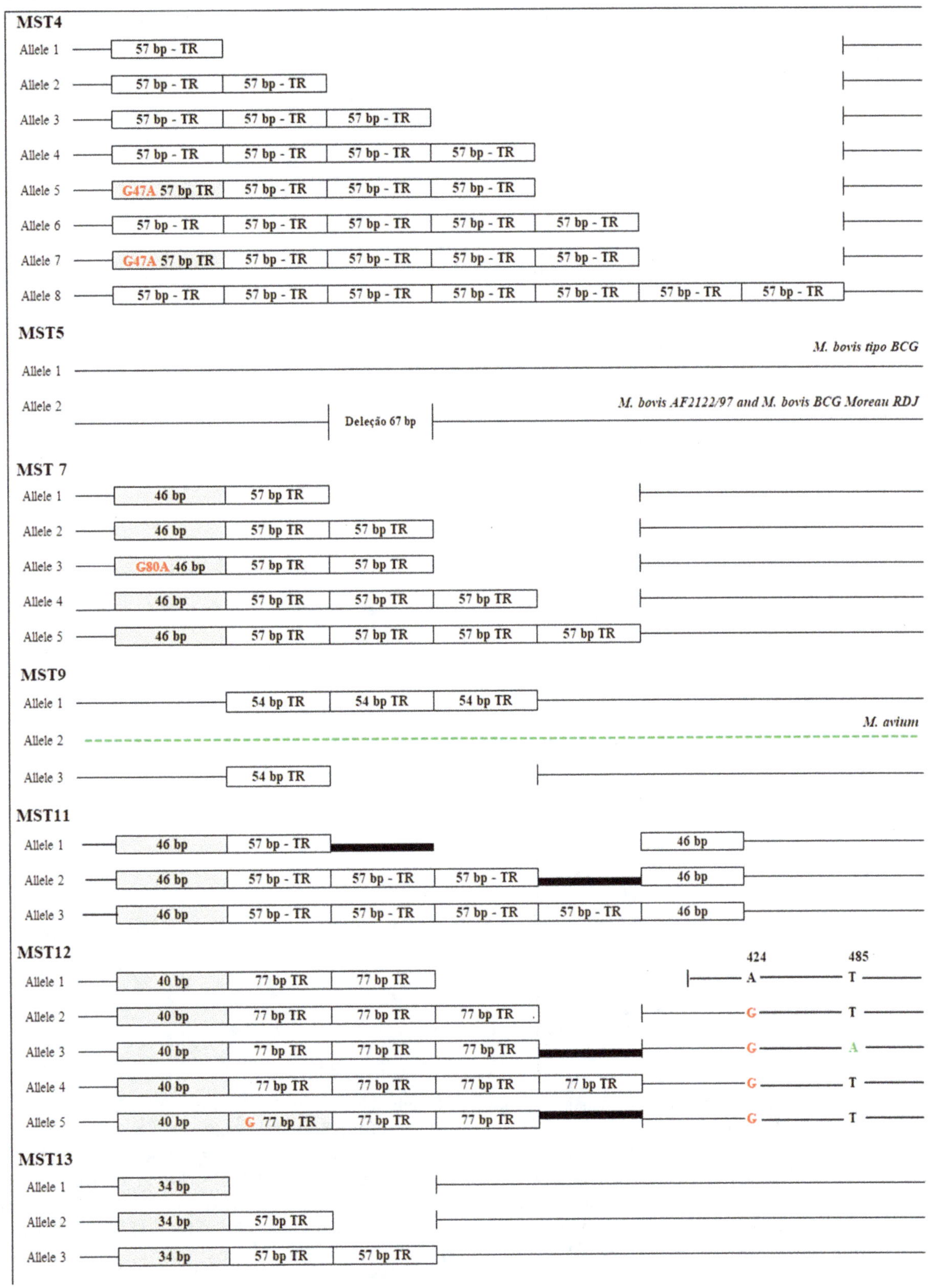

FIGURE 1 | Alleles identified in seven intergenic spacers in *Mycobacterium bovis*. MST4 (ETR-B): eight alleles containing 1, 2, 3, 4, 5, and 7 copies of the 57 bp tandem repeat sequence (TR) and the presence of a SNP G47A (alleles 5 and 7). MST5: deletion of 67 bp. MST7: Five alleles containing from 2, 3, 4 and 5 copies

(Continued)

FIGURE 1 | of the 57 bp tandem repeat, a deletion of the first 11 bp repeat for all samples and a SNP G80A in allele 3. MST9: two alleles containing one and three repeat tandem copies of 54 bp, and a sequence represented by some polymorphisms in the genome of *M. bovis*, characterized by a different allele of a repeated region also present in the genome of *M. avium*. MST11: three alleles containing 3, 5, and 6 tandem repeats of 57 bp, the first and last repetition characterized by a deletion of 11 bp in all isolates. MST12: five alleles containing 3–5 repeat tandem copies of 77 bp with the first repetition characterized by a deletion of 37 bp in all isolates, the presence of a G76 base (allele 5), A424G SNP (allele 2–5), T485A SNP (allele 3) and a deletion of 18 bp after the last repeat (allele 1). MST13: three alleles containing from 1 to 3 copies of the 57 bp and a 23 bp deletion in the first repetition in all isolates.

TABLE 1 | Twenty-eight (28) ST identified by the comparison of genotypic profiles of 63 isolates of *M. bovis*.

ST	Number of *M. bovis* isolates	Allelic profile							%
		MST4	MST5	MST7	MST9	MST11	MST12	MST13	
6	12	4	2	4	1	2	2	3	19.05
17	9	4	2	4	1	1	2	3	14.29
1	5	3	2	4	1	2	2	3	7.94
10	5	4	2	4	1	1	2	2	7.94
19	4	4	2	4	1	1	5	3	6.35
11	4	6	2	4	1	2	2	3	6.35
14	2	4	2	4	1	1	3	3	3.17
25	2	4	2	4	1	2	5	3	3.17
45	1	1	2	4	1	1	2	3	1.59
30	1	2	2	4	1	1	2	2	1.59
61	1	3	2	1	1	2	2	1	1.59
54	1	3	2	4	1	1	2	3	1.59
31	1	4	1	4	1	2	2	1	1.59
5	1	4	2	2	2	2	2	3	1.59
39	1	4	2	4	1	1	2	1	1.59
9	1	4	2	4	1	3	4	3	1.59
4	1	4	2	4	2	1	2	3	1.59
13	1	5	1	4	1	1	2	2	1.59
12	1	5	2	4	1	2	2	3	1.59
52	1	6	1	4	1	2	2	3	1.59
63	1	6	1	4	1	2	4	3	1.59
29	1	6	2	4	1	1	2	2	1.59
62	1	6	2	4	1	2	1	2	1.59
59	1	6	2	4	1	2	2	2	1.59
60	1	6	2	4	1	2	4	2	1.59
58	1	7	2	3	3	2	2	3	1.59
55	1	7	2	4	1	2	2	3	1.59
34	1	8	2	4	1	2	2	1	1.59

ST identifies the sequence type featuring a genotypic profile (or allelic).
**Displays standard strains of M. bovis without source information. % Percentage of M. bovis isolates with corresponding ST.*

= 1), Goiás ($n = 1$), and Paraná ($n = 1$). ST11, consisting of four strains, coming from Minas Gerais and Goiás, is one of the SLVs of ST6 that has diversified producing their own SLV, characterized by members with unique genotypic profiles. Interestingly, the single *M. bovis* isolate from Rio Grande do Sul, the only state not bordering any of the states evaluated herein, having unique genotype (ST13) without associated SLVs, DLVs or TLVs.

Spoligotyping and MST

Spoligotyping was performed for 55 of the 63 *M. bovis* isolates that composed the study. A total of 22 spoligotypes were detected, 19 of which were already mentioned in the literature. A total of eight clusters (G1–G8) were formed, representing 74.54% (41/55) of the *M. bovis* isolates. The remaining 14 (24.45%) *M. bovis* isolates had the spoligotype described as orphans (**Table 2**). SB2211, SB2212, and SB2213, found in samples from Minas Gerais, São Paulo, and Mato Grosso, respectively, have never been described prior to this study. SB1135 was the most frequent spoligotype (n = 12), followed by SB0121 ($n = 9$), SB0295 ($n = 6$), and SB0881 ($n = 5$). SB1135 had samples only from Minas Gerais, while SB0121 and SB0295 were represented by Minas Gerais and São Paulo; and SB0881 by Minas Gerais and Goiás.

A separate analysis contrasting MST and Spoligotyping was also performed using samples from Minas Gerais only, which

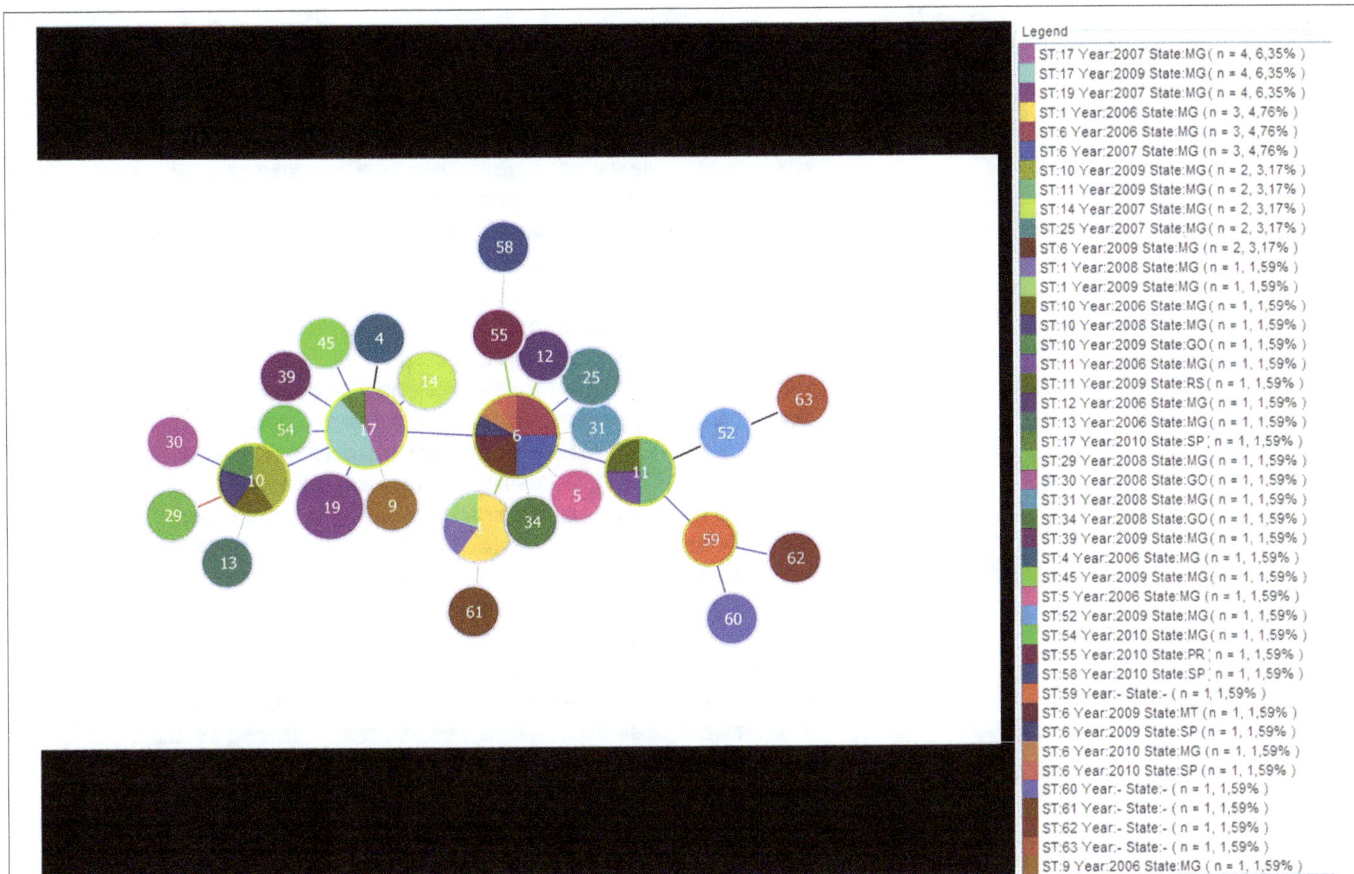

FIGURE 2 | Minimum spanning tree exhibiting the formation of clonal complexes according to genotypic profiles obtained by the multi sequence typing of *Mycobacterium bovis*. Distribution of 58 samples of *M. bovis* isolated from the years 2006 to 2010, four standard samples of *M. bovis* (CR01, CR02, CR13, and CR36) and the strain *M. bovis* (AF2122/97). The dendrogram reveals the formation of five clonal complexes ST6, ST10, ST11, ST17, and ST59 that formed from the comparison of 28 ST. In the subtitle "N" figure indicates the number of isolates with the same genotypic profile, as well as the size of the circles (the larger the circle, the larger the population represented). Circles with more than one color profile indicate the same genotype isolated from different regions and year of isolation of the pathogen.

corresponded to 43 of the 58 *M. bovis*. These samples came from 22 different towns and were isolated between 2006 and 2010. A total of 19 STs and 17 spoligotypes were identified. The eBURST displayed ST6 as the main clonal complex, showing for this CC three SLVs (ST17, ST11, and ST1). ST6 reported eight samples from seven different cities, and four spoligotypes (SB0295, SB0121, SB1135, and SB0333); ST17 reported seven samples from three different cities, and four spoligotypes (SB1135, SB0295, SB0333, and SB0881); ST1 composed five *M. bovis* isolates, from three cities, and three spoligotypes (SB1033, SB1050, and SB2212); and ST11, which depicted three samples, each one from a different city and showed orphans spoligotypes (SB0267, SB0849, and SB1802). The three most frequent spoligotypes were SB1135, represented by 12 samples isolated in 2007, all of them from a same town; SB0121 which was reported in eight samples, from seven cities and isolated in 2006, 2007, 2009, and 2010; and SB0295 reported in five samples, from four cities and isolated in 2008 and 2009 (**Figure 3**).

Phylogenetic Analysis

The phylogenetic tree was generated from 28 STs constituting a cladogram where each ST was represented by its number (**Figure 4**). Overall, *M. bovis* isolates were similarly clustered in the same groups formed by eBURST. It was observed that ST1, ST6, and ST12 were closely located in the center of the tree. When comparing this phylogenetic tree with the genotypic profiles of each ST, the genetic variation was limited by the difference in a single locus, admitting the close relationship between these isolates, which coincide with data observed previously by eBURST. The formation of five clades distributed in the tree edges was observed and the relationship between these clades was generated by variation of three or more loci identified by MST. Clade A was represented by the sequence type coming from Minas Gerais, São Paulo, and Paraná. Clade B was formed only by isolates from Minas Gerais. Clade C was represented by members of Minas Gerais and Goiás. And finally, clade D was represented by a single sample from Goiás and *M. bovis* BCG CR13, while

TABLE 2 | Spoligotypes of 55 *Mycobacterium bovis* isolates.

	Spoligotypes	# *M. bovis* isolates	Clustering	Orphan profiles	Patterns description	State
1	SB0120	2	G1	–	■■□■■■■■□■■■■■■□■■■■■■■■■■■■■■■■■■■■■■□□□□□	GO/*
2	SB0121	9	G2	–	■■□■■■■■□■■■■■■□■■■■□■■■■■■■■■■■■■■■■□□□□□	MG/SP
3	SB0295	6	G3	–	■■□■■■■■□■■■■■■□■■■■□■■■■■■■■■■■■■■■□■□□□□□	MG/SP
4	SB0333	2	G4	–	■■□■■□■■□■■■■□□□■■■■□■■■■■■■■■■■■■■■■■□□□□□	MG
5	SB0881	5	G5	–	■■□■■■■■□■■■■■■□■■■■□■■■■□□□□□□■■■■■■■□□□□□	MG/GO
6	SB1033	3	G6	–	■■□■■□■□□□□□■■■□■■■■■■■■■■■■■■■■■□■■■■□□□□□	MG
7	SB1135	12	G7	–	■■□■■■■□□■■■■■■□■■■■□■■■■■■■■■■■■■■■□■□□□□□	MG
8	SB1139	2	G8	–	■■□■■■■■□■■■■■■□■■■■■■■■□□□□□□□□□□■■■■□□□□□	MG/SP
9	SB0140	1		9	■■□■■□■□□□□□■■■□■■■■■■■■■■■■■■■■■■■■■■□□□□□	MG
10	SB0267	1		10	■■□■□■■■□■□■■■■□■■□■■■■■■■■■■■■■■■■■■■□□□□□	MG
11	SB0268	1		11	■■□■□■■■□■□□■■■□■■■■■□■■■■■■■■■■■■■■■■□□□□□	**
12	SB0486	1		12	■■□■■□■□□□□□□□■□■■■■■■■■■■■■■■■■■■■■■■□□□□□	RS
13	SB0849	1		13	■■□■□■■■□■■■■■■□■■■■■■■■■■■■■■■■■■■■■■□□□□□	MG
14	SB1050	1		14	■■□■■■■■□■■■■■■□■■■■□■■■■■■■■□□□□□■■■■□□□□□	MG
15	SB1093	1		15	■■□□■■■■□■■■■■■□■■■■□■■■■■■■■■■■■■■■■■□□□□□	MG
16	SB1136	1		16	□□□□□□□□□□□■■■■□■■■■■■■■■■■■■■■■■■■■■■□□□□□	MG
17	SB1145	1		17	■■□□□□□■□■■■■■■□■■■■□■■■■□□□□■■■■■■■■■□□□□□	GO
18	SB1369	1		18	■■□■■■■■□■■■■■■□■■■■□■■■■■■■■■□□□□■■■■□□□□□	PR
19	SB1802	1		19	■■□■□■■■□■□■■■■□■□■■■■■■■■■■■■■■■■■■■■□□□□□	MG
20	SB2211	1		20	■■□■■■■■□■■■■■■□■■■■□■■■■■■■■□□■■■■■■■□□□□□	SP
21	SB2212	1		21	■■□■■■■■□□■■■■■□■■■■□■■■■■■■■□□□□□■■■■□□□□□	MG
22	SB2213	1		22	■■□□■■■■□□■■■■■□■■■■□■■■■■■■■■■■■■■■■■□□□□□	MT

**Laboratory strain M. bovis BCG CR13 **Laboratory strain M. bovis Mexico CR36. GO, Goiás; MG, Minas Gerais; RS, Rio Grande do Sul; SP, São Paulo; MT, Mato Grosso.*

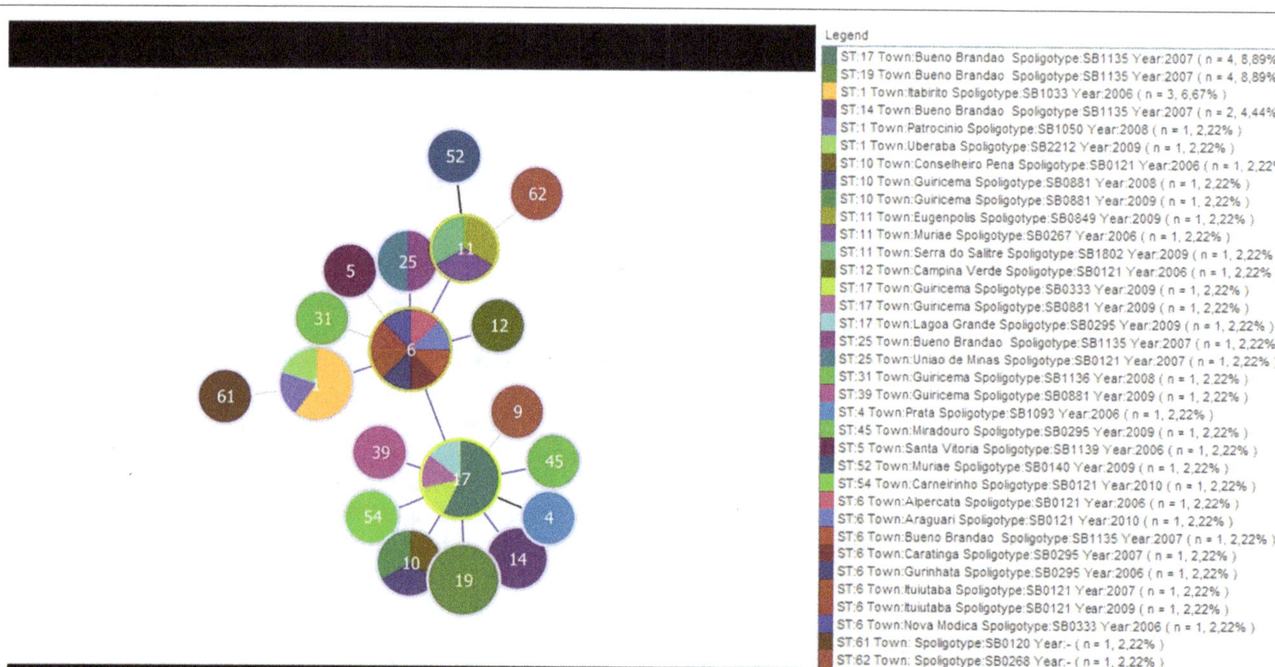

FIGURE 3 | Minimum spanning tree displaying the distribution of 19 type sequences and 17 spoligotypes determined by the MST and Spoligotyping, respectively. The data were obtained from 43 isolates of *M. bovis* from 22 municipalities in MG and isolates between the years 2006 and 2010. The colors represent the different spolitypes and '*n*' indicates the number of isolates with the same genotype profile.

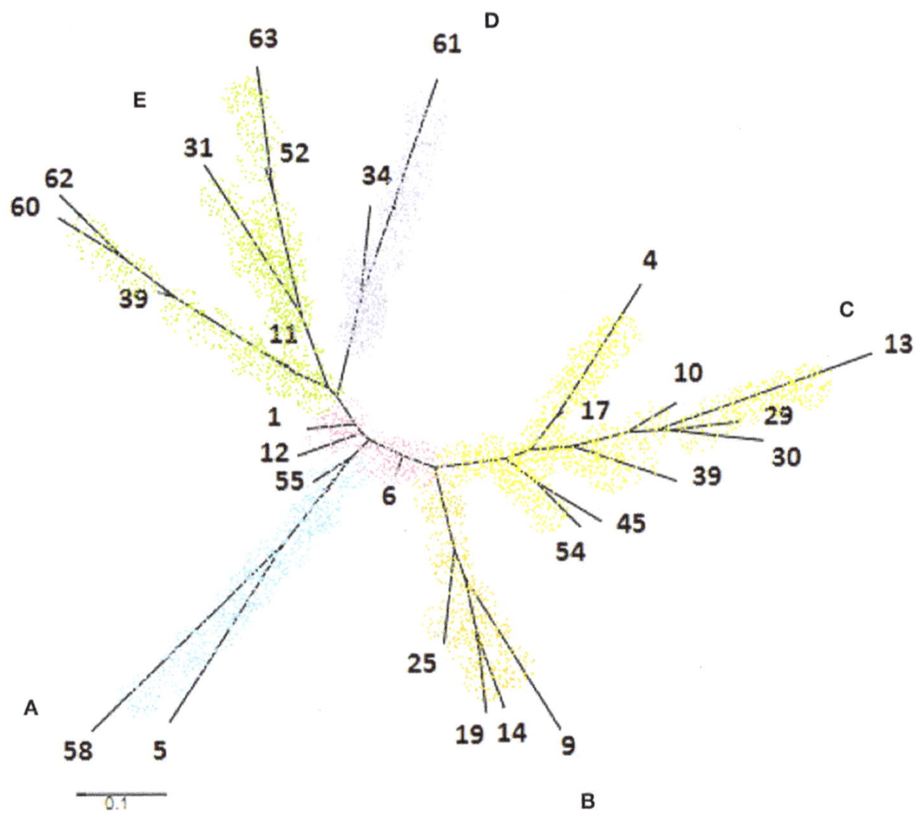

FIGURE 4 | Phylogenetic tree generated by PubMLST program based on 28 sequence types of *Mycobacterium bovis* obtained in the study. It was observed the formation of five clades identified by letters and colors as follows: clade **A** (blue), clade **B** (orange), clade **C** (yellow), clade **D** (purple), and clade **E** (green).

clade E was formed by laboratory strains *M. bovis* CR01, CR02, AN5, CR36, and AF2122/97.

The clade A, marked by the ST5 and ST58, showed the same pattern of spoligotype (SB1139), so as clade D, composed of ST34 and ST61 of spoligotype SB0120. The clade B, formed by ST9, ST14, ST19, and ST25, is composed of spoligotypes SB0295 and SB1135. These two spoligotypes differ only by the absence of the spacer eight in SB1135 compared to SB0295. Clade C includes eight different ST and four spoligotypes. The three ST located in the base of the tree were well-diversified in terms of spoligotypes patterns, corresponding to the high diversity of the ST6. Interestingly, although highly diverse in terms of ST types, these isolates differ only by SLVs. Clade E presented high diversity both of spoligotypes and of genotypic profiles described for ST (**Figure 4**).

Calculation Hunter and Gaston

The discriminatory power of MST and spoligotyping techniques were calculated according to the Hunter-Gaston discrimination index (45). The determination was based on the number of genotypic profiles defined during the test and the relative frequencies of each profile. For MST, the calculations were made for the 63 strains of *M. bovis* and 28 ST resulting in a 92.9% HGDI. Yet for spoligotype, reducing to 55 the number of isolates and to 22 the number of patterns, the index lowered to 91%.

DISCUSSION

The 14 spacer regions analyzed in this study for isolates of *M. bovis* were first described by Djelouadji et al. (33) to characterize *M. tuberculosis* isolates. The decision of analyzing them was taken based on the genetic similarity corresponding to 99.95% between these two species. The markers used are from intergenic regions susceptible to higher mutation rates given the low selection pressure. As the bovine bacillus has a broad host range compared to human germ and evolution occur under various conditions for both, we studied the 14 regions to find the most variable in *M. bovis*.

Genotyping by the MST included the evaluation of 14 intergenic spacer regions, 58 representative samples of *M. bovis*, four standard samples and AF2122/97 strain obtained from GenBank. A total of seven spacers showed genetic variability for the analyzed isolates. Four of them were previously described as Exact Tandem Repeat (ETR) defining ETR-B (MST4), ETR-C (MST11), ETR-D also called MIRU4 (MST12) (46, 47) and Mtub21 (MST13) (48). The other three spacers used were MST5, MST7, and MST9. The results showed the occurrence of 28 genetic events, distributed among deletions, insertions, variation in the number of tandem repeats and point mutations. Sequencing shows the exact number of tandem repeats present in each sequence, and also determines stable markers within them such as SNPs (49) considered very important for studies of genetic events such as phylogeny.

Drancourt et al. (50) used ETR D-region (MST12) to differentiate eight *M. tuberculosis* complex members by sequencing. The region MST12 (ERT-D) in this study revealed the presence of five alleles characterized by a 40 bp sequence in all isolates, followed by 2–4 copies of the tandem repeat of 77 bp. It was also revealed G76 insertion of a base, an SNP A424G, an SNP T485A and a deletion of 18 bp after the last repetition of the first allele. These events were detected by comparison with the genome of the strain AF2122/97 analyzed *in silico* (**Figure 1**). These data, when compared to sequences characterized by (50) available in Genbank (EU180228- EU180234), showed that profiles found for *M. bovis* in this study were different from the profiles described by the author for the number of repetitions and for SNP.

MST performed for isolates of *M. tuberculosis* defined eight of 14 loci analyzed as variables (MST1, MST2, MST3, MST4, MST8, MST11, MST12, and MST13). In our study, four of these (MST1, MST2, MST3, and MST8) were excluded from our study due to low variability in the isolates of *M. bovis*. Djelouadji et al. (33) identified thirteen alleles in these regions that constituted genetic events of deletions and nucleotide substitutions. The other four spacers (MST4, MST11, MST12, and MST13) were characterized mainly by tandem repeats and showed a different profile found for *M. bovis*. A frequently observed event was the presence of a point mutation at the first base of many of the repetitions, which did not occur in any of the isolates of *M. bovis* studied in this work. MST12 and MST13 had a larger number of alleles for *M. tuberculosis*, while MST4 and MST12 were more variable for *M. bovis*.

The low genetic variability observed in the excluded MST may be related to the sampling bias in samples from Minas Gerais in relation to other states. The existing allelic diversity among *M. bovis* and *M. tuberculosis* may be due to the wide range of hosts of the bacillus of bovine, evolving in different environments and under different conditions (51). The population size and genetic diversity found in *M. tuberculosis* strains in relation to *M. bovis* can also be representative of these differences.

The most common spoligotypes in our study were SB1135 (21.8%), SB0121 (16.36%), SB0295 (10.9%) and SB0881 (9%) (**Table 2**). Of these, SB1135 has been described so far only in Brazil (Mbovis.org). Except for SB1135, the other three SB were also reported by Parreiras et al. (52), as well as SB0120, SB1802, SB1145, SB1033, and SB0267 described as an orphan or less frequent. Corroborating our findings, Rodriguez et al. (53) described SB0295 and SB0121 as the majority SB in a study conducted on a national level, as well as (38) which also recorded the occurrence of SB0295 spoligotype in the country. There have been reports of both in many Brazilian isolates and other Latin American countries (54). SB0881 was described previously in Brazil (55), France (56) and Spain (57). Haddad et al. (56) described the SB0295 and SB0121 in Holland in Belgium. SB0120 and SB0295 were also reported among animal wildlife and domestic species, in southern Spain (58), while SB0121 was identified in cattle and wild fauna in the Iberian Peninsula (59) and had also occurred in Mexico and Venezuela (54).

On the less frequent spoligotypes or orphans, SB0140 was described by Smith et al. (60, 61) as one of the most frequent patterns found throughout the world, particularly in Europe and the British Isles; however, the pattern was observed only in a single isolate in our study. SB0140 was also the most frequent pattern according to a study by (54) using isolates from Latin America. SB1145 and SB1802 were only isolated in Brazil, previously reported in Minas Gerais, also with low frequency (52).

CCs were formed and organized from the association of seven genetic regions. The use of clonal complexes as a tool for population analysis is important because it allows us to recognize specific subpopulations or clones that have unique genetic characteristics. Epidemiologically related isolates are derived from the clonal expansion of a single cell, resulting in common characteristics (62). By analyzing MST in association with spoligotyping we observed that some isolates were closely related with exclusive MST profiles and spoligotypes while others, coming from the same region and year, showed different profiles and patterns. The results identified 15 orphans' profiles for MST, 14 orphan spoligotypes and eight groups represented by more than one isolate with equal genotypes in both techniques (**Figure 2**). Similar results were obtained by Parreiras et al. (52) by associating spoligotyping and MIRU-VNTR. The procedure used for this kind of occurrence typed by VNTR in association with spoligotyping is to rearrange the isolates identified by the same VNTR profiles groups geographically located at spoligotyping (60), thereby obtaining more data on the phylogeny of the bovine bacillus.

The importance of finding an alternative method for genotyping *M. bovis* is a result of the occurrence of remarkably diverse populations in different countries, making it difficult to determine a set of useful markers that meets all regions (59). Regional differences in the discriminatory power of genetic markers make it necessary to define an optimal combination of markers that can be used in a particular region or country (63). The different patterns obtained indicate the variety of strains that infect cattle from different geographical areas.

In this study, seven polymorphic loci MST were characterized as variables for *M. bovis*. The observed molecular variation was explored to determine the evolutionary relationships of this pathogen. The results showed that the tested regions can be a promising tool in epidemiological studies. IS*6110* RFLP techniques, spoligotyping, and VNTR have been used as a reference for studying the diversity of species of the *M. tuberculosis* complex (55). However, these methods do not recognize the genetic diversity of strains analyzed as sequencing-based methods capable of identifying all the genetic events present in the molecular marker. The MST method proposed offers the advantage of sequencing, which allows for the detection of different genetic events observed in one sequence. The typing methods performed based on sequencing provide important data on evolutionary forces that shape bacterial populations (64). Bing et al. (65) determined that a methodology based on sequencing of non-constotive genes (MLSA) can be used for molecular typing, in addition to being an excellent method for use in phylogenetic analyzes, for epidemiological and surveillance studies.

Our results demonstrate that the number of samples needs to be increased to provide additional data to monitor the formation and expansion of clonal complexes according to geographic location and year of isolation. This was the first study to identify the variability of isolates of *M. bovis* by the MST method. The results indicated that the method works to typify differentiate isolates of *M. bovis* using fewer than those used in VNTR or special reagents like the membranes used in spoligotyping.

CONCLUSIONS

Genotyping by MST can contribute to epidemiological studies of *M. bovis*. The method was efficient to detect the genetic variability present in the sequences analyzed and to infer evolutionary relationships in the short term. The method was also suitable to correlate geographical location and phylogenetic data of *M. bovis* isolates used in this study.

AUTHOR CONTRIBUTIONS

ES, CG, GA, HG, ND, and PS performed the all-laboratory tests. ES, AF, and AL performed the interpretation of DNA sequencing results. AF, MH, and AL wrote the manuscript and AG did the translation. MH, AG, PS, and JF accurately reviewed the manuscript. All authors have read and approved the final version of the manuscript.

ACKNOWLEDGMENTS

MH, AL, JF are grateful to CNPq (Conselho Nacional de Desenvolvimento Científico e Tecnológico) the fellowship. ES would like to thank CAPES (Coordenação de Aperfeiçoamento de Pessoal de Nível Superior) for the scholarship.

REFERENCES

1. Olea-Popelka F, Muwonge A, Perera A, Dean A, Mumford E, Erlacher-Vindel E, et al. Zoonotic tuberculosis in human beings caused by Mycobacterium bovis - a call for action. *Lancet Infect Dis.* (2017) 17:e21-5. doi: 10.1016/S1473-3099(16)30139-6
2. Miller RS, Sweeney SJ. Mycobacterium bovis (bovine tuberculosis) infection in North American wildlife: current status and opportunities for mitigation of risks of further infection in wildlife populations. *Epidemiol Infect.* (2013) 141:1357–70. doi: 10.1017/S0950268813000976
3. De Kantor IN, Ritacco V. An update on bovine tuberculosis programs in Latin American and Caribbean countries. *Vet. Microbiol.* (2006) 112:111-8. doi: 10.1016/j.vetmic.2005.11.033
4. Godfray HCJ, Donnelly CA, Kao RR, Macdonald DW, McDonald RA, Petrokofsky G, et al. A restatement of the natural science evidence base relevant to the control of bovine tuberculosis in Great Britain. *Proc R Soc B Biol Sci.* (2013) 280:20131634. doi: 10.1098/rspb.2013.1634
5. World Organizatio for Animal Health. Bovine Tuberculosis Chapter 3.4.6. In: *Terrestrial Manual p1058-1074.* 8th ed. (2018).
6. Domingo M, Vidal E, Marco A. Pathology of bovine tuberculosis. *Res Vet Sci.* (2014) 97:S20–9. doi: 10.1016/j.rvsc.2014.03.017
7. Hardstaff JL, Marion G, Hutchings MR, White PCL. Evaluating the tuberculosis hazard posed to cattle from wildlife across Europe. *Res Vet Sci.* (2014) 97:S86–93. doi: 10.1016/j.rvsc.2013.12.002
8. Acha PN, Szyfres B. *Zoonosis y enfermidades transmisibles comunes al hombre y a los animales. Bacteriosis y micosis.* Washington: OPAS. (2001). p. 416. doi: 10.1590/S1135-57272001000300009
9. Cosivi O, Grange JM, Daborn CJ, Raviglione MC, Fujikura T, Cousins, D, et al. Zoonotic tuberculosis due to *Mycobacterium bovis* in developing countries. *Emerg Infect Dis.* (1998) 4:59–70. doi: 10.3201/eid0401.980108
10. Galagan JE. Genomic insights into tuberculosis. *Nat Rev Genet.* (2014) 15:307–20. doi: 10.1038/nrg3664
11. Gagneux S. Strain variation in the *Mycobacterium tuberculosis* complex: its role in biology, epidemiology and control. *Adv Exp Med Biol.* (2017) 1019:307. doi: 10.1007/978-3-319-6 4371-7
12. Brites D, Loiseau C, Menardo F, Borrell S, Boniotti MB, Warren R, et al. A new phylogenetic framework for the animal-adapted Mycobacterium tuberculosis complex. *Front Microbiol.* (2018) 9:2820. doi: 10.3389/fmicb.2018. 02820
13. Hirsh AE, Tsolaki AG, DeRiemer K, Feldman MW, Small PM. Stable association between strains of Mycobacterium tuberculosis and their human host populations. *Proc Natl Acad Sci.* (2004) 101:4871-6. doi: 10.1073/pnas.0305627101
14. Gagneux S, Small PM. Global phylogeography of *Mycobacterium tuberculosis* and implications for tuberculosis product development. *Lancet Infect Dis.* (2007) 7:328–37. doi: 10.1016/S1473-3099(07)70108-1
15. Mulholland CV, Shockey AC, Aung HL, Cursons RT, O'Toole RF, Gautam SS, et al. Dispersal of *Mycobacterium tuberculosis* driven by historical European trade in the South Pacific. *Front Microbiol.* (2019) 4:2778. doi: 10.3389/fmicb.2019.02778
16. Brosch R, Gordon SV, Marmiesse M, Brodin P, Buchrieser C, Eiglmeier K, et al. A new evolutionary scenario for the Mycobacterium tuberculosis complex. *Proc Natl Acad Sci.* (2002): 99:3684–9. doi: 10.1073/pnas.0525 48299
17. Guimaraes AMS, Zimpel CK. *Mycobacterium bovis*: From genotyping to genome sequencing. *Microorganisms.* (2020) 8:667. doi: 10.3390/microorganisms8050667
18. Kao RR, Price-Carter M, Robbe-Austerman S. Use of genomics to track bovine tuberculosis transmission. *Rev Sci Tech.* (2016) 35:241–58. doi: 10.20506/rst.35.1.2430
19. Ramos DF, Tavares L, da Silva PEA, Dellagostin OA. Molecular typing of *Mycobacterium bovis* isolates: a review. *Braz J Microbiol.* (2014) 45:365–72. doi: 10.1590/S1517-83822014005000045
20. Haddad N, Masselot M, Durand B. Molecular differentiation of *Mycobacterium bovis* isolates. Review of main techniques and applications. *Res Vet Sci.* (2004) 76:1–18. doi: 10.1016/S0034-5288(03)00078-X
21. Merker M, Kohl TA, Niemann S, Supply P. The evolution of strain typing in the Mycobacterium tuberculosis complex. *Adv Exp Med Biol.* (2017) 1019:79–93. doi: 10.1007/978-3-319-64371-7_3
22. Gonzalo-Asensio J, Pérez I, Aguiló N, Uranga S, Picó A, Lampreave C, et al. New insights into the transposition mechanisms of IS6110 and its dynamic distribution between Mycobacterium tuberculosis Complex lineages. *PLoS Genet.* (2018) 14:e1007282. doi: 10.1371/journal.pgen.1007282
23. Warren RM, Streicher EM, Sampson SL, van der Spuy GD, Richardson M, Nguyen D, et al. Microevolution of the direct repeat region of *Mycobacterium tuberculosis*: Implications for interpretation of spoligotyping data. *J Clin Microbiol.* (2002) 40:4457–65. doi: 10.1128/JCM.40.12.4457-4465.2002

24. Reyes JF, Chan CHS, Tanaka MM. Impact of homoplasy on variable numbers of tandem repeats and spoligotypes in *Mycobacterium tuberculosis*. *Infect Genet Evol.* (2012) 12:811–8. doi: 10.1016/j.meegid.2011.05.018
25. Hauer A, Michelet L, De Cruz K, Cochard T, Branger M, Karoui C, et al. MIRU-VNTR allelic variability depends on *Mycobacterium bovis* clonal group identity. *Infect Genet Evol.* (2016) 45:165–9. doi: 10.1016/j.meegid.2016.08.038
26. Biek R, O'Hare A, Wright D, Mallon T, McCormick C, Orton RJ, et al. Whole genome sequencing reveals local transmission patterns of *Mycobacterium bovis* in sympatric cattle and badger populations. *PLoS Pathog.* (2012) 8: e1003008. doi: 10.1371/journal.ppat.1003008
27. Trewby H, Wright D, Breadon EL, Lycett SJ, Mallon TR, McCormick C, et al. Use of bacterial whole-genome sequencing to investigate local persistence and spread in bovine tuberculosis. *Epidemics.* (2016) 14:26–35. doi: 10.1016/j.epidem.2015.08.003
28. Ghebremariam MK, Hlokwe T, Rutten VPMG, Allepuz A, Cadmus S, Muwonge A, et al. Genetic profiling of *Mycobacterium bovis* strains from slaughtered cattle in Eritrea. *PLoS Negl Trop Dis.* (2018) 12:e0006406. doi: 10.1371/journal.pntd.0006406
29. Zimpel CK, Patané JSL, Guedes ACP, Souza RF, Pereira-Silva TT, Soler Camargo NC, et al. Global distribution and evolution of Mycobacterium bovis. *Front Microbiol.* (2020) 11:843. doi: 10.3389/fmicb.2020.00843
30. Otchere ID, van Tonder AJ, Asante-Poku A, Sánchez-Busó L, Coscollá M, Osei-Wusu S, et al. Molecular epidemiology and whole genome sequencing analysis of clinical *Mycobacterium bovis* from Ghana. *PLoS ONE.* (2019) 14:e0209395. doi: 10.1371/journal.pone.0209395
31. Salvador LCM, O'Brien DJ, Cosgrove MK, Stuber TP, Schooley AM, Crispell J, et al. Disease management at the wildlife-livestock interface: Using whole-genome sequencing to study the role of elk in *Mycobacterium bovis* transmission in Michigan, USA. *Mol Ecol.* (2019) 28:2192–205. doi: 10.1111/mec.15061
32. Zimpel CK, Brandão PE, Souza Filho AF, De Souza RF, Ykuta CY, Ferreira Neto JS, et al. Complete genome sequencing of *Mycobacterium bovis* SP38 and comparative genomics of *Mycobacterium bovis* and *M. tuberculosis* strains. *Front Microbiol.* (2017) 8:2389. doi: 10.3389/fmicb.2017.02389
33. Djelouadji Z, Arnold C, Gharbia S, Raoult D, Drancourt M. Multispacer sequence typing for *Mycobacterium tuberculosis* genotyping. *PLoS ONE.* (2008) 3:e2433. doi: 10.1371/journal.pone.0002433
34. De Azevedo Issa M, Martins Filho OS, Fonseca Júnior AA, Arrais MH, Santos LS, Reis JKP, et al. Comparative study of *Mycobacterium bovis* primary isolation methods. *Braz J Microbiol.* (2017) 48:139–44. doi: 10.1016/j.bjm.2016.07.026
35. Sales ML, Fonseca AA, Jr, Orzil L, Alencar AP, Hodon MA, Issa MA, et al. Validation of two real-time PCRs targeting the PE-PGRS 20 gene and the region of difference 4 for the characterization of *Mycobacterium bovis* isolates. *Genet Mol Res.* (2014) 13:4607–16. doi: 10.4238/2014.June.18.3
36. Canevari Castelão AB, Nishibe C, Moura A, de Alencar AP, Issa MA, Hodon MA, et al. Draft genome sequence of Mycobacterium bovis strain AN5, used for production of purified protein derivative. *Genome Announc.* (2014) 2:e00277. doi: 10.1128/genomeA.00277-14
37. Sambrook J, Fritcsh EF, Maniatis T. *Molecular Cloning: A Laboratory Manual.* 2nd ed. New York, NY: Cold Spring Harbor Laboratory (1989). p. 3104.
38. Zanini MS, Moreira EC, Lopes MTP, Oliveira RS, Leão SC, Fioravanti RL, et al. *Mycobacterium bovis*: polymerase chain reaction identification in bovine lymph node biopsies and genotyping in isolates from Southeast Brazil by spoligotyping and restriction fragment length polymorphism. *Mem Inst Oswaldo Cruz.* (2001) 96:809–13. doi: 10.1590/S0074-02762001000600012
39. Huang X, Madan A. CAP3: A DNA sequence assembly program resource genome research. *Genome Res.* (1999) 9:868–77. doi: 10.1101/gr.9.9.868
40. Hall T. BioEdit: a user-friendly biological sequence alignment editor and analysis program for Windows 95/98/NT. *Nucleic Acids Symp Ser.* (1999) 41:95–98.
41. Kamerbeek J, Schouls LEO, Kolk A, Kuijper S, Bunschoten A, Molhuizen H, et al. Simultaneous detection and strain differentiation of *Mycobacterium tuberculosis* for diagnosis and epidemiology. *J Clin Microbiol.* (1997) 35:907–14. doi: 10.1128/JCM.35.4.907-914.1997
42. Smith NH, Upton P. Naming spoligotype patterns for the RD9-deleted lineage of the Mycobacterium tuberculosis complex; www.Mbovis.org. *Infect Genet Evol.* (2012) 12:873–6. doi: 10.1016/j.meegid.2011.08.002
43. Feil EJ, Li BC, Aanensen DM, Hanage WP, Spratt BG. eBURST: inferring patterns of evolutionary descent among clusters of related bacterial genotypes from multilocus sequence typing data. *J Bacteriol.* (2004) 186:1518–30. doi: 10.1128/JB.186.5.1518-1530.2004
44. Francisco AP, Bugalho M, Ramirez M, Carriço JÁ. Global optimal eBURST analysis of multilocus typing data using a graphic matroid approach. *BMC Bioinform.* (2009) 10:152. doi: 10.1186/1471-2105-10-152
45. Hunter PR, Gaston MA. Numerical index of the discriminatory ability of typing systems: an application of Simpson's index of diversity. *J Clin Microbiol.* (1988) 26:2465–6. doi: 10.1128/JCM.26.11.2465-2466.1988
46. Supply P, Magdalena J, Himpens S, Locht C. Identification of novel intergenic repetitive units in a mycobacterial two-component system operon. *Mol Microbiol.* (1997) 26:991–1003. doi: 10.1046/j.1365-2958.1997.6361999.x
47. Frothingham R, Meeker-O'Connell WA. Genetic diversity in the Mycobacterium tuberculosis complex based on variable numbers of tandem DNA repeats. *Microbiol.* (1998) 144:1189–96. doi: 10.1099/00221287-144-5-1189
48. Le Flèche P, Fabre M, Denoeud F, Vergnaud G. High resolution, on-line identification of strains from Mycobacterium tuberculosis complex based on tandem repeat typing. *BMC Microbiol.* (2002) 2:37–48. doi: 10.1186/1471-2180-2-37
49. Gutacker MM, Mathema B, Soini HM, Shashkina E, Kreiswirth BN, Graviss EA, et al. Single-nucleotide polymorphism-based population genetic analysis of *Mycobacterium tuberculosis* strains from 4 geographic sites. *J Infect Dis.* (2006) 193:121–8. doi: 10.1086/498574
50. Djelouadji Z, Raoult D, Drancourt MA. Single-step sequencing method for the identification of Mycobacterium tuberculosis complex species. *Plos Negl Trop Dis.* (2008) 2:e253. doi: 10.1371/journal.pntd.0000253
51. Riojas MA, McGough KJ, Rider-Riojas CJ, Rastogi N, Hazbón MH. Phylogenomic analysis of the species of the Mycobacterium tuberculosis complex demonstrates that *Mycobacterium africanum, Mycobacterium bovis, Mycobacterium caprae, Mycobacterium microti* and *Mycobacterium pinnipedii* are later heterotypic synonyms of *Mycobacterium tuberculosis*. *Int J Syst Evol Microbiol.* (2018) 68:324–32. doi: 10.1099/ijsem.0.002507
52. Parreiras PM, Andrade GI, Nascimento TF, Oelemann MC, Gomes HM, Alencar AP, et al. Spoligotyping and variable number tandem repeat analysis of *Mycobacterium bovis* isolates from cattle in Brazil. *Mem Inst Oswaldo Cruz.* (2012) 107:64–73. doi: 10.1590/S0074-02762012000100009
53. Rodriguez CAR, Zumárraga MJ, Oliveira EM, Cataldi AA, Romano MI, Otto HH, et al. Caracterização molecular de isolados de *Mycobacterium bovis* do Estado de São Paulo Brasil, utilizando a técnica de spoligotyping. *Arq Inst Biolog.* (2004) 71:277–82. Available online at: http://www.biologico.sp.gov.br/uploads/docs/arq/V71_3/rodriguez.PDF.
54. Zumárraga MJ, Arriaga C, Barandiaran S, Cobos-Marín L, de Waard J, Estrada-Garcia I, et al. Understanding the relationship between *Mycobacterium bovis* spoligotypes from cattle in Latin American countries. *Res Vet Sci.* (2013) 94:9–21. doi: 10.1016/j.rvsc.2012.07.012
55. Viana-Niero C, Rodriguez CAR, Bigi F, Zanini MS, Ferreira-Neto JS, Cataldi A, Leão SC. Identification of an IS6110 insertion site in plcD, the unique phospholipase C gene of *Mycobacterium bovis*. *J Med Microbiol.* (2006) 55:451–7. doi: 10.1099/jmm.0.46364-0
56. Haddad N, Ostyn A, Karoui C, Masselot M, Thorel MF, Hughes SL, et al. Spoligotype diversity of *Mycobacterium bovis* strains isolated in France from 1979 to 2000. *J Clin Microbiol.* (2001) 39:3623–32. doi: 10.1128/JCM.39.10.3623-3632.2001
57. Zanini MS, Moreira EC, Salas CE, Lopes MTP, Barouni AS, Roxo E, et al. Molecular typing of Mycobacterium bovis isolates from south-east Brazil by spoligotyping and RFLP. *J Vet Med B Infect Dis Vet Public Health.* (2005) 52:129–33. doi: 10.1111/j.1439-0450.2005.00835.x
58. García-Bocanegra I, Barranco I, Rodríguez-Gómez IM, Pérez B, Gómez-Laguna J, Rodríguez S, et al. Tuberculosis in alpacas (Lama pacos) caused by *Mycobacterium bovis*. *J Clin Microbiol.* (2010) 48:1960–4. doi: 10.1128/JCM.02518-09
59. Duarte EL, Domingos M, Amado A, Botelho A. Spoligotype diversity of *Mycobacterium bovis* and *Mycobacterium caprae* animal isolates. *Vet Microbiol.* (2008) 130:415–21. doi: 10.1016/j.vetmic.2008.02.012

60. Smith NH, Kremer K, Inwald J, Dale J, Driscoll JR, Gordon SV, et al. Ecotypes of the Mycobacterium tuberculosis complex. *J Theor Biol.* (2006) 239:220–5. doi: 10.1016/j.jtbi.2005.08.036
61. Smith NH. The global distribution and phylogeography of Mycobacterium bovis clonal complexes. *Infect Genet Evol.* (2012) 12:857–65. doi: 10.1016/j.meegid.2011.09.007
62. Milián-Suazo F, Banda-Ruíz V, Ramírez-Casillas C, Arriaga-Diaz C. Genotyping of *Mycobacterium bovis* by geographic location within Mexico. *Prev Vet Med.* (2002) 55:255–64. doi: 10.1016/S0167-5877(02)00015-6
63. Hilty M, Diguimbaye C, Schelling E, Baggi F, Tanner M, Zinsstag J. Evaluation of the discriminatory power of variable number tandem repeat (VNTR) typing of Mycobacterium bovis strains. *Vet Microbiol.* (2005) 109:217–22. doi: 10.1016/j.vetmic.2005.05.017
64. Comas I, Gagneux S. The past and future of tuberculosis research. *PLoS Pathogens.* (2009) 5:e1000600. doi: 10.1371/journal.ppat.1000600
65. Bing L, Yan DH, Qin ZX, Guang LZ, Can LH, Yaun ZY, et al. A new multilocus sequence analysis scheme for Mycobacterium tuberculosis. *Biomed Environ Sci.* (2012) 25:620–9. doi: 10.3967/0895-3988.2012.06.003

19

Real-Time PCR Validation for *Mycobacterium tuberculosis* Complex Detection Targeting IS*6110* Directly From Bovine Lymph Nodes

José María Sánchez-Carvajal[1*†§], *Ángela Galán-Relaño*[2*†], *Inés Ruedas-Torres*[1], *Francisco Jurado-Martos*[3], *Fernanda Larenas-Muñoz*[1], *Eduardo Vera*[1,2], *Lidia Gómez-Gascón*[2], *Fernando Cardoso-Toset*[3], *Irene Magdalena Rodríguez-Gómez*[1], *Alfonso Maldonado*[2], *Librado Carrasco*[1], *Carmen Tarradas*[2], *Jaime Gómez-Laguna*[1‡] and *Inmaculada Luque*[3‡]

[1] Department of Anatomy and Comparative Pathology and Toxicology, University of Córdoba, Córdoba, Spain, [2] Department of Animal Health, University of Córdoba, Córdoba, Spain, [3] CICAP—Food Research Centre, Córdoba, Spain

***Correspondence:**
José María Sánchez-Carvajal
v42sancj@uco.es
Ángela Galán-Relaño
agalanr12@gmail.com

†These authors have contributed equally to this work and share first authorship

‡These authors have contributed equally to this work and share senior authorship

§Present address:
José María Sánchez-Carvajal, Department of Anatomy and Comparative Pathology and Toxicology, Department of Animal Health, University of Córdoba, Córdoba, Spain

Rapid and accurate diagnostic tools, such as Real-Time PCR (qPCR), need to be implemented as a confirmatory test in the framework of bovine tuberculosis (bTB) surveillance and control programs, shortening the turnaround time to confirm bTB infection. The present study aimed to evaluate a direct qPCR from fresh tissue samples targeting the insertion sequence IS*6110* using individually homogenized bovine lymph nodes compared with microbiological culture. Retropharyngeal, tracheobronchial, and mesenteric lymph nodes fresh tissue samples (n = 687) were collected from 230 different cattle carcasses at the slaughterhouse. Only 23 of the 230 examined animals showed tuberculosis-like lesions, with 62 of 230 considered as positive. Among these 62 animals, 61 resulted as culture-positive, whereas 48 were qPCR-positive. Thus, this qPCR targeting IS*6110* showed an apparent diagnostic sensitivity and specificity values of 77.1% [95% confidence interval (CI): 66.5–87.6%] and 99.4% (95% CI: 98.3–100.6%), respectively, and a positive predictive value of 97.9% (95% CI: 93.9–102.0%) and negative predictive value of 92.3% (95% CI: 88.4–96.2%). Positive and negative likelihood ratios were 130.2 and 0.2, respectively, and the agreement between microbiological culture and this qPCR was almost perfect ($\kappa = 0.82$). These results highlight this qPCR targeting IS*6110* as a suitable complementary method to confirm bTB in animals with either tuberculosis-like lesions or non-tuberculosis-like lesions, decreasing the number of samples subjected to microbiological culture and, hence, its overall associated costs and the turnaround time (under 48 h) to confirm bTB infection. Besides, sampling mesenteric lymph node, which is uncommonly sampled, together with tracheobronchial and retropharyngeal ones, is advisable during postmortem inspection in bTB surveillance programs at the slaughterhouse, especially in areas with a low bTB prevalence scenario.

Keywords: bovine tuberculosis, fresh lymph node, IS*6110*, direct qPCR, *Mycobacterium tuberculosis* complex

INTRODUCTION

Bovine tuberculosis (bTB) is a chronic infectious disease caused by *Mycobacterium bovis* and other members of the *Mycobacterium tuberculosis* complex (MTC) (1, 2) that affects various species of mammals, including humans (3, 4). bTB is still one of the largely neglected zoonotic diseases, particularly in developing countries, as the control and surveillance programs for this disease are inadequate or are not carried out, and domestic and wild animals, which act as reservoirs, often share pasture areas. Thereby, it has been estimated that a quarter of the world's population has latent tuberculosis, requiring a global effort to develop new tools for the diagnostic and treatment of this disease (5). In the European Union (EU), bTB primarily affects livestock, which is of economic importance due to its impact on trade. Indeed, bTB is subjected to national eradication programs based on skin testing of all registered cattle herds, slaughtered policy, and abattoir surveillance (Council Directive 64/432/EEC). According to the EU legislation, the official diagnosis of bTB is based on the detection of the cellular immune response (single intradermal tuberculin testing) in reactor animals (skin test-positive animals), which is followed by slaughtering, histopathological examination of atypical or enlarged lymph nodes or parenchymatous organs with tuberculosis-like lesions (TBLs), and/or culture of MTC in primary isolation medium (6). Although a substantial economic expenditure is addressed to ensure efficient surveillance systems and control programs, the detection and confirmation of bTB infection in cattle herds should be more reliable and swifter (7).

Microbiological culture is considered the reference technique for bTB diagnosis with recovery rates ranging from 30 to 95% (8–10) and sensitivity (SE) and specificity (SP) values of 78.1 and 99.1%, respectively (7). It is reported that culture is an imperfect, laborious, and time-consuming technique that requires high biosecurity facilities and relatively high expertise (7, 8), whose performance can, moreover, be affected by several factors (8–11). A major drawback is the delayed culturing process (up to 2–3 months), making the time required to reach a final diagnosis longer (7, 11, 12).

In the current landscape, rapid, cost-effective, and accurate diagnostic tools could pave the way for managing and controlling bTB in cattle herds (13). Although enzyme-linked immunosorbent assay testing is useful to detect anergic tuberculous cattle as a complement to single intradermal tuberculin testing, this assay is not routinely applied in bTB control programs because of its reduced SE (14–16). By contrast, real-time PCR assays [so-called quantitative PCR (qPCR)] have been shown to directly detect MTC in fresh bovine tissue samples with moderate to high estimates of SE and SP (7, 11, 16). Direct qPCR can detect small amounts of MTC DNA independently of its viability with a turnaround time of 24–48 h, shortening the required time to reach confirmatory results (7, 15, 16).

IS*6110* is a target sequence with multiple copies only present in pathogens belonging to MTC, commonly used for MTC detection by PCR (7, 12, 17, 18). Besides IS*6110*, other targets have also been used for the same purpose, including IS*1081* (16, 19), hupB (20, 21), 16S-23S rRNA internally transcribed spacer (22), p34 gene (23), TbD1 (24), or mpb70 (11) with varying results.

In the light of the earlier mentioned, rapid and accurate diagnostic tools, such as qPCR, may be implemented as a confirmatory test in the framework of bTB surveillance and control programs at the slaughterhouse to shorten turnaround time and inform decision-makers on time. Therefore, the present study firstly aimed to evaluate the diagnostic performance of a direct qPCR from fresh tissue samples targeting IS*6110* using individually homogenized lymph nodes and, secondly, to validate the IS*6110* qPCR for the detection of MTC positive samples and animals in the framework of the bTB eradication campaign.

MATERIALS AND METHODS

Samples Selection and Processing

Fresh retropharyngeal, tracheobronchial, and mesenteric lymph node tissue samples ($n = 687$) were collected from 230 cattle carcasses at the slaughterhouse from 2018 to 2019. All samples were collected during routine postmortem veterinary examination within an official context and agreeing with national and European regulations. No purpose killing of animals was performed for this study, so no ethical or farmer's consent approval was required.

Every lymph node was independently sliced, and the presence of visible-TBL or non-tuberculosis-like lesions (NTBLs) was recorded. Individual homogenization was carried out to obtain a uniform mixture of every lymph node independently using a tissue homogenizer (Fisherbrand, Fisher Scientific, Madrid, Spain). Briefly, 4–7 g of each lymph node tissue was placed into a 15-ml Falcon™ tube (Corning, Madrid, Spain) with the same volume (w/v: 1/1) of 0.85% sterile sodium chloride and ground until a homogeneous mixture was obtained. Tissue homogenate was used for DNA isolation and selective bacterial culture.

Mycobacterium tuberculosis Complex Microbiological Culture

Selective bacterial culture was performed in the BSL3 facilities of the Production and Animal Health Laboratory of Córdoba (LPSACo, Regional Government of Andalusia). Briefly, the homogenate was decontaminated with an equal volume of 0.75% (w/v: 1/1) hexadecyl pyridinium chloride solution in agitation for 30 min (25). Samples were centrifuged for 30 min at 1,500×*g*. The pellets were collected with swabs and cultured in liquid media (MGIT™ 960, Becton Dickinson, Madrid, Spain) using an automatized BD Bacter™ MGIT™ System (Becton Dickinson). The culture was considered positive when isolates were confirmed as MTC by qPCR (26).

DNA Extraction From Homogenized Lymph Nodes

DNA extraction from homogenized tissue samples was performed using DNA Extract VK (Vacunek, Bizkaia, Spain) according to the manufacturer's guidelines with several modifications. In brief, a mix of 300 mg of homogenate, 250 µl of sterile distilled water, and 250 µl of sample lysis buffer

VK-SB were added in a 2-ml tube containing 300 mg of 0.5-mm glass beads and submitted to mechanical disruption at 30 Hz during 20 min. Then, the lysed tissue was centrifuged for 5 min at 7,000×g, transferring 200 μl of supernatant to a new 1.5-ml tube. Enzymatic digestion was carried out with 25 μl of 20 mg/ml proteinase K at 56°C for 3 h in a thermo-shaker at 750 rpm. After that, 200 μl of the lysis buffer VK-LB3 were added, and the mixture was incubated for 10 min at 70°C. Finally, 210-μl ethanol (96–100%) was added to the sample that was applied in a spin column following the manufacturer's guidelines. DNA elution was run using 100 μl of Tris/hydrochloride buffer supplied with the kit pre-heated at 70°C. Positive and negative extraction controls were also included. All the DNA extraction products were stored at −20°C until use.

Quantitative Real-Time PCR From Fresh Tissue Samples

The transposon IS*6110*, which is present in all species of the MTC, was the target of this qPCR. Specific primers (IS*6110*-forward: 5′-GGTAGCAGACCTCACCTATGTGT-3′; IS*6110*-reverse: 5′-AGGCGTCGGTGACAAAGG-3′) and a probe (IS*6110*- probe: 5′-FAM-CACGTAGGCGAACCC-MGBNFQ-3′) targeting a conserved region of IS*6110* transposon were used (27). The diagnostic performance of the qPCR was conducted using the QuantiFast® Pathogen PCR + IC Kit (QIAGEN, Hilden, Germany). Amplifications were run in duplicate for each sample in the MyiQ™2 Two-Color qPCR Detection System (Bio-Rad, Hercules, CA, USA) under the following cycling conditions: 95°C for 5 min followed by 45 cycles of 95°C for 15 s and 60°C for 30 s. Following the manufacturer's guidelines, an exogenous inhibition heterologous control [internal amplification control (IAC)] supplied with the kit was included. An inter-run calibrator with a known Ct value of 32 was introduced in each assay to self-control intra-assay repeatably and accuracy. Complete inhibition of amplification was considered when IAC did not amplify and partial inhibition when it showed a cycle threshold (Ct) > 33. When any inhibition was detected, samples were diluted up to a final concentration of 450 ng/μl, and qPCR was run again. Serial 10-fold dilution series of *M. bovis* genomic DNA with known quantities, ranging from 10^6 to 10^0, were used as standards to estimate the limit of detection (LOD) or analytical SE. The reactions were carried out in triplicate per dilution in three different assays, and LOD was determined as the lowest concentration in which 95% of replicates were positive according to the Clinical and Laboratory Standards Institute guidelines.

In the case of culture-positive and qPCR-negative samples, DNA extraction and qPCR were repeated to verify the results. Then, proteinase K digestion was increased up to 12 h (overnight incubation) at 56°C in a thermo-shaker at 750 rpm. Positive (MTC confirmed sample) and negative (MTC negative sample) controls were included, as well as an inter-run calibrator. The IS*6110* PCR product of culture-negative and PCR-positive samples were EtOH precipitated, purified using ExoSAP-ITTM (Thermo Fisher Scientific, Barcelona, Spain), and further analyzed by Sanger sequencing (performed at STABvida, Lisbon, Portugal). The obtained sequences were studied using the Bioedit software version 7.1.3.0. Samples confirmed by sequencing were considered as true positives and used to recalculate the diagnostic parameters of the qPCR targeting IS*6110*.

Validation of Diagnostic Tests

The results of qPCR targeting IS*6110* were compared with microbiological culture ones (*gold standard*) to estimate the diagnostic SE and SP, positive and negative predictive values (PPV and NPV, respectively), and positive and negative likelihood ratios (PLR and NLR, respectively) (WinEpi software 2.0, Faculty of Veterinary Medicine, University of Zaragoza, Spain). Moreover, an agreement between culture and qPCR results was assessed using Cohen's kappa coefficient (κ) (values ≤ 0 indicated no agreement and 0.01–0.20 as none to slight, 0.21–0.40 as fair, 0.41–0.60 as moderate, 0.61–0.80 as substantial, and 0.81–1.00 as almost perfect agreement) (WinEpi software 2.0).

RESULTS

Topographical Distribution of Tuberculosis-Like Lesion

A total of 687 retropharyngeal, tracheobronchial, and mesenteric lymph node samples belonging to 230 cattle carcasses were analyzed to serve as evidence of the presence of MTC using microbiological culture and qPCR directly from lymph nodes. Due to the logistic of the slaughterhouse and the timing of slaughtering, it was not always possible to collect the three lymph node samples from all 230 carcasses, lacking one retropharyngeal and two mesenteric lymph nodes. Before being analyzed, every single tissue sample was subjected to a visual inspection to disclose gross lesions, with 26 of 26/687 (3.8%) tissue samples belonging to 23 different cattle (23/230, 10.0%) showing TBL (**Table 1**). Most of the lesions were evidenced in only one lymph node (tracheobronchial = 11; retropharyngeal = 9), whereas in three animals, TBLs were observed in two lymph nodes (tracheobronchial–retropharyngeal = 1; tracheobronchial–mesenteric = 1; retropharyngeal–mesenteric = 1).

Mycobacterium tuberculosis Complex Microbiological Culture Results

Seventy-three of 687 tissue samples (10.6%) were positive to microbiological culture, whereas 614 were negative (89.4%). Bacteria were detected in tracheobronchial lymph nodes (42 of 73; 57.5%), followed by retropharyngeal (22 of 73; 30.1%), and mesenteric ones (9 of 73; 12.3%) (**Table 1**). An animal was considered culture-positive when MTC was detected by culture in at least one lymph node. Thus, 61 of 230 animals (26.5%) were positive to culture, whereas 169 were negative (73.5%). MTC was detected in most of the animals (50, 82.0%) in one lymph node (tracheobronchial = 31; retropharyngeal = 16; mesenteric = 3), whereas in 10 animals (16.4%), MTC was detected in two lymph nodes (retropharyngeal–tracheobronchial = 5; tracheobronchial–mesenteric = 5) and in one animal in the three lymph nodes.

TABLE 1 | Evaluation of the microbiological culture and direct qPCR targeting IS*6110* results obtained upon analyzing 687 lymph nodes, according to the presence or absence of tuberculosis-like lesions.

		TBL				NTBL			
		RF	**TB**	**MS**	**Total**	**RF**	**TB**	**MS**	**Total**
Culture	+	5	13	2	20	17	29	7	53
	–	6	0	0	6	201	188	219	608
qPCR	+	8	13	2	23	9 (10)	22 (24)	3	37
	–	3	0	0	3	209 (208)	195 (193)	223	624
Total		11	13	2	26	218	217	226	661

+, Positive; –, Negative; qPCR, real-time PCR; TBL, tuberculosis-like lesion; NTBL, non-tuberculosis-like lesion; RF, retropharyngeal lymph nodes (n = 229); TB, tracheobronchial lymph node (n = 230) s; MS, mesenteric lymph nodes (n = 228).
Culture-positive and qPCR-negative samples that were finally positive and/or negative to qPCR after DNA extraction was repeated (in brackets).

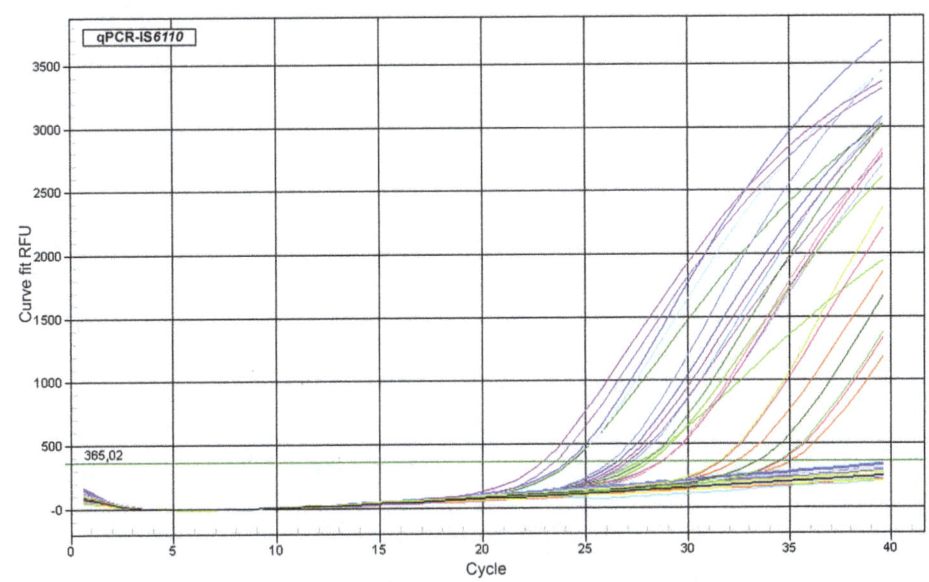

FIGURE 1 | Amplification plot of representative samples. qPCR targeting IS*6110* assay using representative fresh lymph node tissue samples belonging to different cattle. ΔRFU (Y axis) of the reaction was plotted against the Ct value (X axis). Samples with lowest DNA concentration could be detected ranging from 34 to 36 cycles roughly.

Quantitative Real-Time PCR Targeting IS*6110*

Fifty-seven of 687 tissue samples (8.3%) were detected as positive by means of qPCR targeting IS*6110*, with Ct values ranging from 24.2 to 37.5 (**Figure 1**). The IAC amplified in most of the samples without partial inhibition, showing complete inhibition in eight of the 687 samples due to the high yield of DNA (over 1,000 ng/μl). These samples were diluted up to a final concentration of 450 ng/μl and re-evaluated by qPCR, keeping a negative result for all of them for MTC but with IAC amplification. The LOD for this qPCR-IS*6110* was determined to be ranging from 10 to 100 genomic equivalents, and the cutoff was established to Ct < 38. Most of the qPCR-positive results were obtained from tracheobronchial lymph node (35 of 57; 61.4%), followed by retropharyngeal (17 of 57; 29.8%), and mesenteric (five of 57; 8.8%) lymph nodes, reflecting the same trend as observed in the microbiological culture (**Table 1**).

Following the same criterion used for the microbiological culture, an animal was considered PCR-positive when at least one of the examined lymph nodes yielded a positive result to the qPCR. Thus, 44 of 230 cattle (19.1%) were qPCR-positive, whereas 185 were negative (80.4%). Briefly, 36 of the 44 qPCR positive animals (81.8%) were detected in only one lymph node (tracheobronchial = 24; retropharyngeal = 11; mesenteric = 1), seven animals (15.9%) in two lymph nodes (retropharyngeal–tracheobronchial = 5; tracheobronchial—mesenteric = 2), and one animal (2.3%) in the three lymph nodes.

Diagnostic Performance of Quantitative Real-Time PCR Compared With Microbiological Culture

Fifty-three of the 73 lymph node samples positive to culture were also positive to qPCR targeting IS*6110*. Because extraction is a rate-limiting factor determining the success of downstream

TABLE 2 | Diagnostic performance of direct qPCR targeting IS*6110* compared with microbiological culture as gold standard analyzing 687 lymph nodes belonging to 230 cattle.

			True positives			Measures of diagnostic accuracy (95% CI)			
		Result	**+**	**–**	**Total**	**Sensitivity**	**Specificity**	**Reliability**	***k* value**
Lymph nodes	qPCR	+	56	4	60	76.7% (67–86.4%)	99.3% (98.7–100%)	96.9% (95.7–98.2%)	0.83
		–	17	610	627				
		Total	73	614	687				
Animals	qPCR	+	47	1	48	77.1% (66.5-87.6%)	99.4% (98.3%-100.6%)	93.5% (90.3–96.7%)	0.82
		–	14	168	182				
		Total	61	169	230				

+, Positive; –, Negative; qPCR, real-time PCR; 95% CI, 95% confidence level.

TABLE 3 | Validation of direct qPCR targeting IS*6110* for the detection of MTC analyzing 687 lymph nodes belonging to 230 cattle.

		MTC corrected positive results Culture/Sanger sequencing				Measures of diagnostic accuracy (95% CI)			
		Result	**+**	**-**	**Total**	**Sensitivity**	**Specificity**	**Reliability**	***k* value**
Lymph nodes	qPCR	+	60	0	60	77.9% (68.7–87.2%)	100% (100%)	97.5% (96.4–98.7%)	0.86
		–	17	610	627				
		Total	77	610	687				
Animals	qPCR	+	48	0	48	77.4% (67.0–87.8%)	100% (100%)	94% (90.8–97.0%)	0.83
		–	14	168	182				
		Total	62	168	230				

+, Positive; –, Negative; qPCR, real-time PCR; 95% CI, 95% confidence level.
MTC-corrected positive results: (i) samples positive to culture and (ii) culture-negative samples and PCR-positive after Sanger sequencing.

bTB detection by PCR, this step was repeated in those culture-positive and qPCR-negative samples (20/73 samples, 27.4%) to verify the results. Thereby, previous extraction conditions were changed by a proteinase K digestion up to 12 h at 56°C in a thermo-shaker at 750 rpm (overnight incubation), obtaining this time three positive samples of the 20 and remaining the rest ($n = 17$) negative to qPCR. Hence, an apparent SE of 76.7% (95% CI: 67–86.4%) was found. On the other hand, only four of the 614 samples negative to culture were positive to qPCR, with the remaining samples also giving a negative result to qPCR, with an apparent SP value of 99.3% (95% CI: 98.7–100%). The PPV and NPV values were 93.3% (95% CI: 87.0–99.6%) and 97.3% (95% CI: 96.0–98.6%), respectively. In addition, the PLR and NLR were 117.8 and 0.23, respectively. Finally, the concordance or level of agreement between both diagnostic assays for tissue samples was substantial ($\kappa = 0.83$) (**Tables 1, 2**).

Considering this re-run of the extraction step, 47 of 61 MTC culture-positive animals were also positive for qPCR targeting IS*6110*, resulting in an apparent SE of 77.0% (95% CI: 66.5–87.6%). Only one of the 169 MTC culture-negative animals was positive to qPCR, finding an apparent SP of 99.4% (95% CI: 98.3–100.6%). The measures of PPV and NPV were 97.9% (95% CI: 93.9–102.0%) and 92.3% (95% CI: 88.4–96.2%), respectively. The PLR and NLR were 130.2 and 0.23, respectively. The agreement between microbiological culture and qPCR at the animal level was almost perfect ($\kappa = 0.82$) (**Table 2**).

Validation of IS*6110* Quantitative Real-Time PCR for the Detection of *Mycobacterium tuberculosis* Complex

Because microbiological culture is considered an imperfect test for bTB diagnosis in which SE may be affected by several factors (7, 8, 16), the combination of culture and IS*6110* qPCR was validated to detect MTC positive samples or animals. In this sense, culture-negative and PCR-positive samples obtained in our study could be considered as MTC positives. This way, the four IS*6110* qPCR-positive and culture-negative lymph node samples were further subjected to Sanger sequencing, and the presence of MTC DNA was evidenced in all of them. Consequently, the diagnostic estimates of the direct qPCR for MTC detection were evaluated, considering as MTC-corrected positive samples, culture-positive samples, and those in which MTC was revealed by Sanger sequencing. For tissue samples, 60 of the 77 MTC-corrected positive samples were successfully amplified by means of qPCR targeting IS*6110* with a corrected SE of 77.9% (95% CI: 68.7–87.2%), SP of 100% (95% CI: 100–100%), and reliability of 97.5% (95% CI: 96.4–98.7%). The PPV and NPV values were increased to 100% (95% CI: 100–100%) and 97.3% (95% CI: 96–98.6%), respectively. The PLR and NLR were 160 and 0.22, respectively, with a level of agreement between assays almost perfect ($\kappa = 0.86$) (**Table 3**).

At the animal level, 48 of the 62 MTC-corrected positive animals were also positive for qPCR targeting IS*6110* with a corrected SE and SP of 77.4% (95% CI: 67–87.8%) and 100%

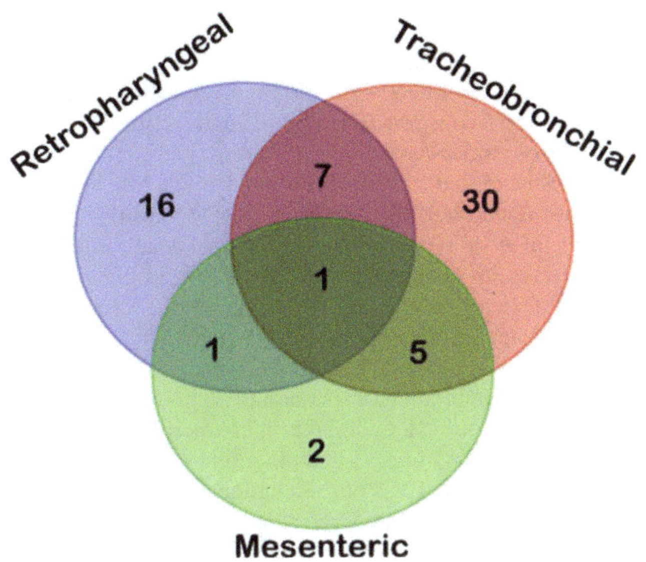

FIGURE 2 | Venn diagram depicted the topographical distribution of positive lymph nodes ($n = 77$) according to their results obtained upon analyzing samples by microbiological culture, qPCR-IS*6110*, and Sanger sequencing. Most positive cattle were disclosed in tracheobronchial lymph node, followed by retropharyngeal and mesenteric lymph nodes, with most positive animals presenting only one positive lymph node highlighting the choice of tissue is a cornerstone for performing an accurate direct diagnosis of MTC.

TABLE 4 | Assessment of the microbiological culture and direct qPCR targeting IS*6110* results obtained upon analyzing 687 lymph nodes belonging to 230 cattle, according to the presence or absence of tuberculosis-like lesions.

		Microbiological culture			
		+	–	Total	
NTBL	qPCR +	36	1	37	661
	qPCR –	17	607	624	
TBL	qPCR +	20	3	23	26
	qPCR –	0	3	3	

+, Positive; –, Negative; qPCR, real-time PCR; 95% CI, 95% confidence level; NTBL, non-tuberculosis-like lesion; TBL, tuberculosis-like lesion.

(95% CI: 100–100%), respectively, and reliability of 93.9% (90.8–97.0%). The measures of PPV and NPV were 100% (95% CI: 100–100%) and 92.3% (95% CI: 88.4–96.2%). The PLR and NLR were 100.2 and 0.2, respectively, and the κ value was 0.83 (almost perfect agreement of both assays) (**Table 3**).

Finally, according to the distribution of MTC-corrected positive results for the lymph nodes (77), the majority of MTC-corrected positive animals (48) were detected in only one lymph node (tracheobronchial = 30; retropharyngeal = 16; mesenteric = 2), 13 animals in two lymph nodes (retropharyngeal–tracheobronchial = 7; tracheobronchial–mesenteric = 5; retropharyngeal–mesenteric = 1), and one animal in the three lymph nodes, as showed in **Figure 2** (**Table 4**).

Bacteriology and Quantitative Real-Time PCR Results Distribution According to Tuberculosis-Like Lesion

Analyzing MTC and qPCR results together with the presence of TBL, 26 of 687 tissue samples (3.8%) showed TBL, and 20 of these 26 samples (76.9%) resulted in both culture and qPCR positive. The remaining six were negative to culture, being three of them also negative to qPCR. In contrast, the other three were positive to qPCR and subsequently confirmed by Sanger sequencing.

Thirty-six of 661 NTBL tissue samples (5.4%) were positive to either microbiological or qPCR assays, 17 were only culture-positive (2.6%), and 1 only qPCR positive (0.2%). Of note, this culture-negative and qPCR-positive sample was confirmed as positive after Sanger sequencing. Thus, 607 NTBL tissue samples (91.8%) were negative for both techniques (**Table 3**).

DISCUSSION

bTB is one of the oldest and most relevant zoonoses worldwide, where its eradication is the main objective of the EU. As a consequence, rapid, cost-effective, and sensitive tools for the diagnosis of different pathogens belonging to MTC play a pivotal role in controlling and preventing its transmission in countries where it is still especially present in dairy and meat cattle herds (13, 15, 28). Therefore, direct qPCR from tissue samples could work as an accurate and rapid diagnostic alternative in animal health (7, 11, 13, 23), which could be implemented by public health agencies not only to reduce the turnaround time on reaching a confirmatory diagnosis compared with microbiological culture but also to shorten the time of exposure to MTC, facilitating the decision-making process. In this context, the main objective of the present study was to evaluate a qPCR targeting IS*6110* to detect MTC directly from fresh tissue bovine lymph node samples.

In the present study, the direct qPCR targeting IS*6110* showed an apparent SE and SP for individual tissue samples of 76.7 and 99.3%, respectively, when compared with microbiological culture. In addition, the agreement between both assays was almost perfect (κ = 0.83). Several factors make it challenging to run a direct detection of MTC, such as the paucibacillary nature of this complex, the extremely hardy disruption of mycobacterial cells, or the extensive necrosis, fibrosis, and mineralization associated with TBL, interfering all of them with mycobacterial DNA isolation and leading to false-negative results, which limits the final diagnosis performance (19, 29, 30). In our case, samples were individually homogenized before the process to reach a uniform distribution of MTC in the whole matrix but also trying to restrict a dilution effect beyond the detection limit of the qPCR. Despite that, 20 samples were positive to microbiological culture but negative for qPCR. It is well-known that the yield and quality of DNA after extraction could depend on multiple factors (11, 15); consequently, DNA isolation was repeated in all qPCR-negative samples increasing proteinase K digestion up to 12 h at 56°C (overnight incubation), obtaining three additional qPCR-positive samples, and slightly improving SE from 71.2 to 76.7%. A similar approach was conducted to improve diagnostic

SE and SP of direct qPCR targeting mpb70 from 88.4 and 92.3 to 94.5 and 96.0%, respectively (11). These results suggest that DNA extraction protocol is certainly relevant, impacting directly on diagnostic SE of direct qPCR from fresh tissue samples.

Several alternative methods have been previously performed to improve diagnostic SE of direct qPCR from tissues. Thus, nested-PCR targeting TbD1 (24) or IS*6110* (17) have been suggested as a method to improve the detection of MTC in bovine tissue samples with a diagnostic SE and SP ranging from 76.0 to 98.2% and from 88.7 to 100%, respectively. Nevertheless, a nested-PCR requires two different amplification steps, increasing the concern about cross-contamination, which could negatively affect diagnostic SP values. On the other hand, Parra et al. (22) used a manual extraction method with capture probes targeting 16S-23S internally transcribed spacer region to isolate a higher yield of mycobacterial DNA from tissue homogenate samples obtaining a diagnostic SE ranging from 61.1% for samples with NTBL to 80.6% for TBL samples, with an average SE of 73.8%. In this sense, Taylor et al. (19) reported an increase of diagnostic SE from 70.1 to 91.2% targeting *IS*1081 and carrying out DNA isolation only from TBL, ruling out positive samples without readily macroscopic lesions. In our case, 23 of 26 lymph nodes with TBL (88.5%) were amplified targeting IS*6110*; nevertheless, when all samples were considered, both TBL and NTBL samples, an SE of 76.7% was obtained, highlighting the potential of using this target for qPCR screening not only in TBL but also in NTBL.

Previous studies targeting mpb70 (11) or IS*6110* (7) have reported higher SE and SP results than those herein reported; however, it is noteworthy to mention that in those studies, there was a high proportion of the evaluated samples with TBL (39.8 and 100%, respectively). This feature evidences that animals included in those studies were in more advanced stages of bTB infection (15, 31). Unlikely, in the present study, most of the tissue samples lacked TBL (661/687), with only 3.6% of them presenting TBL, which points to animals were sampled in earlier stages of the infection. In addition, qPCR targeting IS*6110* showed a moderate diagnostic SE and high SP. These results highlight the diagnostic potential of direct qPCR from fresh tissue to detect MTC at early stages of infection and, therefore, when the mycobacterial load is lower.

Regarding the topographical distribution of the lesions, most of the TBL samples were disclosed in the tracheobronchial lymph node, followed by retropharyngeal and mesenteric lymph nodes, with most positive animals presenting only one affected lymph node (77.4%). One of the strengths of the present study is that a detailed evaluation of the topographical distribution of the results was made, as the choice of tissue samples at the abattoir is a key player for carrying out an accurate direct diagnosis of MTC. In addition, the diagnosis from a pool of lymph nodes from reactor animals with TBL or NTBL is probably to have a dilution impact on the results. According to our results, most of the true positive animals reacted in one single lymph node, highlighting that not only tracheobronchial and retropharyngeal lymph nodes but also mesenteric lymph node, which is uncommonly sampled during postmortem inspection in bTB surveillance systems at the slaughterhouse, should be evaluated and collected for TB diagnosis. These results turn out to be relevant in areas with a low TB prevalence scenario to enhance the diagnostic accuracy of direct detection methods.

Although microbiological culture is considered the *gold standard* for bTB confirmation, this technique is time-consuming and imperfect, inducing false-negative results (8), and SE and SP will always be biased (7, 32); therefore, combination with other techniques is required to truly identify MTC positive samples. Thereby, three of six samples with TBL and culture-negative were detected as positive for direct qPCR and confirmed by Sanger sequencing, displaying a SE and SP of 77.9 and 100%, respectively, for MTC detection. It is worthy of note that the other three culture-negative and qPCR-negative TBL samples presented pyogranulomatous lesions and Ziehl–Neelsen negative results when examined under the light microscope (data not shown). These results suggest that other microorganisms may be involved in the production of these lesions, as has already been demonstrated in pigs (33), which could be taken into account for future studies.

Several factors impact the success of microbiological cultures, such as decontamination process (8) or encapsulation of the granulomas (34); however, DNA amplification of MTC can be successfully performed from fibrotic and encapsulated granulomas. Our results highlight that direct qPCR can detect more positive samples from fresh lymph nodes tissue with TBL than microbiological culture (23 vs. 20), resulting in a faster and effective confirmatory method for MTC during official postmortem inspection at the slaughterhouse. Nonetheless, microbiological culture remains a required method to mycobacterial isolation and molecular epidemiology studies so far (7).

Finally, direct qPCR targeting IS*6110* was also used to run the diagnostic performance of all animals included in this study, showing diagnostic SE and SP values of 77.0 and 99.4%, respectively, which are very close to those previously reported for microbiological culture (7). In addition, predictive values of 97.9% PPV and 92.3% NPV, together with PLR and NLR of 130.2 and 0.23, respectively, point to a qPCR-positive animal could be considered as true positive. Previous reports on animals have indicated either a barely higher SE for qPCR targeting IS*6110* (7) or lower SE for *IS*1081 (16) compared with the diagnostic SE herein reported. In addition, if diagnostic estimates for MTC detection were considered, SE and SP values could be increased up to 77.4 and 100%, respectively. The disparities among studies may be attributed to differences in the approach for data analysis, epidemiologic situation, or the sample size. On the other hand, gross postmortem examination is a critical stage for the detection of bTB-infected animals at slaughterhouses. Nevertheless, the number of reactors with TBL is currently reduced at the slaughterhouse due to the success of surveillance and control programs decreasing bTB prevalence in cattle herds. Therefore, in the present framework, qPCR assay targeting IS*6110* might work as a suitable complementary method to confirm bTB in reactor animals with either TBL or NTBL, decreasing the number of samples subjected to microbiological culture and, hence, the overall associated cost as well as the turnaround time, <48 h, for confirming bTB infection.

CONCLUSION

The present study revealed that qPCR targeting IS*6110* is an efficient confirmatory test that may be implemented in bTB surveillance and control programs, shortening turnaround time to keep decision-makers noticed promptly, as well as reducing economic costs.

AUTHOR CONTRIBUTIONS

JS-C and ÁG-R performed all experiments in this study and Animal Health and Production Laboratory of Córdoba supported with microbiological culture and technical assistance. ÁG-R, JS-C, IR-T, EV, FJ-M, FL-M, FC-T, and LG-G were involved in obtaining and processing tissue samples. LC, IL, JG-L, and CT designed the study. JS-C and ÁG-R wrote the manuscript down with the invaluable insights of JG-L, IL, IR-T, IR-G, FJ-M, LG-G, FC-T, LC, CT, and AM. IL and JG-L directed and supervised the whole study. All authors contributed to the article and approved the submitted version.

FUNDING

This work was supported by the investigation project New measures and techniques to control Bovine Tuberculosis in Andalusia (Financial support for Operational Groups of the European Innovation Partnership for Agricultural Productivity and Sustainability, EIP-AGRI; GOP2I-CO-16-0010). ÁG-R and JS-C have been hired under a research contract from this project. JG-L was supported by a Ramón y Cajal contract of the Spanish Ministry of Economy and Competitiveness (RYC-2014-16735).

ACKNOWLEDGMENTS

We appreciate the technical support offered by the Animal Health and Production Laboratory of Córdoba (Spain).

REFERENCES

1. Aranaz A, De Juan L, Montero N, Sánchez C, Galka M, Delso C, et al. Bovine tuberculosis (*Mycobacterium bovis*) in wildlife in Spain. *J Clin Microbiol.* (2004) 42:2602–8. doi: 10.1128/JCM.42.6.2602-2608.2004
2. Alexander KA, Laver PN, Michel AL, Williams M, van Helden PD, Warren RM, et al. Novel *Mycobacterium tuberculosis* complex pathogen, M. *Mungi Emerg Infect Dis.* (2010) 16:1296–9. doi: 10.3201/eid1608.100314
3. Palmer M V. *Mycobacterium bovis*: characteristics of wildlife reservoir hosts. *Transbound Emerg Dis.* (2013) 60:1–3. doi: 10.1111/tbed.12115
4. Pesciaroli M, Alvarez J, Boniotti MB, Cagiola M, Di Marco V, Marianelli C, et al. Tuberculosis in domestic animal species. *Res Vet Sci.* (2014) 97:S78–85. doi: 10.1016/j.rvsc.2014.05.015
5. Houben RMGJ, Dodd PJ. The global burden of latent tuberculosis infection: a re-estimation using mathematical modelling. *PLOS Med.* (2016) 13:e1002152. doi: 10.1371/journal.pmed.1002152
6. Anon. EN EN Working Document on Eradication of Bovine Tuberculosis in the EU. Available online at: https://www.visavet.es/bovinetuberculosis/data/wd/SANCO-10067-2013_Eradication_campaigns_Task_Force.pdf (accessed December 17, 2020).
7. Courcoul A, Moyen J-L, Brugère L, Faye S, Hénault S, Gares H, et al. Estimation of sensitivity and specificity of bacteriology, histopathology and PCR for the confirmatory diagnosis of bovine tuberculosis using latent class analysis. *PLoS ONE.* (2014) 9:e90334. doi: 10.1371/journal.pone.0090334
8. Corner, Gormley E, Pfeiffer DU. Primary isolation of *Mycobacterium bovis* from bovine tissues: conditions for maximising the number of positive cultures. *Vet Microbiol.* (2012) 156:162–71. doi: 10.1016/j.vetmic.2011.10.016
9. Yates GF, Price-Carter M, Bland K, Joyce MA, Khan F, Surrey M, et al. Comparison of the BBL mycobacteria growth indicator tube, the BACTEC 12B, and solid media for the isolation of *Mycobacterium bovis*. *J Vet Diagnostic Investig.* (2017) 29:508–12. doi: 10.1177/1040638717697763
10. Hines N, Payeur JB, Hoffman LJ. Comparison of the recovery of *Mycobacterium bovis* isolates using the BACTEC MGIT 960 system, BACTEC 460 system, and Middlebrook 7H10 and 7H11 solid media. *J Vet Diagnostic Investig.* (2006) 18:243–50. doi: 10.1177/104063870601800302
11. Lorente-Leal V, Liandris E, Castellanos E, Bezos J, Domínguez L, de Juan L, et al. Validation of a real-time PCR for the detection of *Mycobacterium tuberculosis* complex members in Bovine tissue samples. *Front Vet Sci.* (2019) 6:61. doi: 10.3389/fvets.2019.00061
12. Barandiaran S, Aguirreburualde MSP, Marfil MJ, Vivot MM, Aznar N, Zumárraga M, et al. Bayesian assessment of the accuracy of a PCR-based rapid diagnostic test for bovine tuberculosis in swine. *Front Vet Sci.* (2019) 6:204. doi: 10.3389/fvets.2019.00204
13. Babafemi EO, Cherian BP, Banting L, Mills GA, Ngianga K. Effectiveness of real-time polymerase chain reaction assay for the detection of *Mycobacterium tuberculosis* in pathological samples: a systematic review and meta-analysis. *Syst Rev.* (2017) 6:215. doi: 10.1186/s13643-017-0608-2
14. Silva E. Evaluation of an enzyme-linked immunosorbent assay in the diagnosis of bovine tuberculosis. *Vet Microbiol.* (2001) 78:111–17. doi: 10.1016/S0378-1135(00)00282-0
15. de la Rua-Domenech R, Goodchild AT, Vordermeier HM, Hewinson RG, Christiansen KH, Clifton-Hadley RS. Ante mortem diagnosis of tuberculosis in cattle: a review of the tuberculin tests, γ-interferon assay and other ancillary diagnostic techniques. *Res Vet Sci.* (2006) 81:190–210. doi: 10.1016/j.rvsc.2005.11.005
16. Pucken V-B, Knubben-Schweizer G, Döpfer D, Groll A, Hafner-Marx A, Hörmansdorfer S, et al. Evaluating diagnostic tests for bovine tuberculosis in the southern part of Germany: a latent class analysis. *PLoS ONE.* (2017) 12:e0179847. doi: 10.1371/journal.pone.0179847
17. Costa P, Ferreira AS, Amaro A, Albuquerque T, Botelho A, Couto I, et al. Enhanced detection of tuberculous mycobacteria in animal tissues using a semi-nested probe-based real-time PCR. *PLoS ONE.* (2013) 8:e81337. doi: 10.1371/journal.pone.0081337
18. Thacker TC, Harris B, Palmer MV, Waters WR. Improved specificity for detection of *Mycobacterium bovis* in fresh tissues using IS6110 real-time PCR. *BMC Vet Res.* (2011) 7:50. doi: 10.1186/1746-6148-7-50
19. Taylor GM, Worth DR, Palmer S, Jahans K, Hewinson RG. Rapid detection of *Mycobacterium bovis* DNA in cattle lymph nodes with visible lesions using PCR. *BMC Vet Res.* (2007) 3:12. doi: 10.1186/1746-6148-3-12
20. Mishra A, Singhal A, Chauhan DS, Katoch VM, Srivastava K, Thakral SS, et al. Direct detection and identification of *Mycobacterium tuberculosis* and *Mycobacterium bovis* in bovine samples by a novel nested PCR assay: Correlation with conventional techniques. *J Clin Microbiol.* (2005) 43:5670–8. doi: 10.1128/JCM.43.11.5670-5678.2005
21. Algammal AM, Wahdan A, Elhaig MM. Potential efficiency of conventional and advanced approaches used to detect *Mycobacterium bovis* in cattle. *Microb Pathog.* (2019) 134:103574. doi: 10.1016/j.micpath.2019.103574
22. Parra A, García N, García A, Lacombe A, Moreno F, Freire F, et al. Development of a molecular diagnostic test applied to experimental abattoir

surveillance on bovine tuberculosis. *Vet Microbiol.* (2008) 127:315–24. doi: 10.1016/j.vetmic.2007.09.001

23. Cardoso-Toset F, Luque I, Amarilla SP, Gómez-Gascón L, Fernández L, Huerta B, et al. Evaluation of rapid methods for diagnosis of tuberculosis in slaughtered free-range pigs. *Vet J.* (2015) 204:232–4. doi: 10.1016/j.tvjl.2015.01.022
24. Araújo CP, Osório ALAR, Jorge KSG, Ramos CAN, Filho AFS, Vidal CES, et al. Detection of *Mycobacterium bovis* in bovine and bubaline tissues using nested-PCR for TbD1. *PLoS ONE.* (2014) 9:e91023. doi: 10.1371/journal.pone.0091023
25. Corner LA, Trajstman AC. An evaluation of 1-hexadecylpyridinium chloride as a decontaminant in the primary isolation of *Mycobacterium bovis* from bovine lesions. *Vet Microbiol.* (1988) 18:127–34. doi: 10.1016/0378-1135(88)90058-2
26. Thierry D, Brisson-Noel A, Vincent-Levy-Frebault V, Nguyen S, Guesdon JL, Gicquel B. Characterization of a *Mycobacterium tuberculosis* insertion sequence, IS6110, and its application in diagnosis. *J Clin Microbiol.* (1990) 28:2668–73. doi: 10.1128/jcm.28.12.2668-2673.1990
27. Martínez-Guijosa J, Romero B, Infantes-Lorenzo JA, Díez E, Boadella M, Balseiro A, et al. Environmental DNA: a promising factor for tuberculosis risk assessment in multi-host settings. *PLoS ONE.* (2020) 15:e0233837. doi: 10.1371/journal.pone.0233837
28. Che' Amat A, González-Barrio D, Ortiz JA, Díez-Delgado I, Boadella M, Barasona JA, et al. Testing Eurasian wild boar piglets for serum antibodies against *Mycobacterium bovis. Prev Vet Med.* (2015) 121:93–8. doi: 10.1016/j.prevetmed.2015.05.011
29. Liebana E, Johnson L, Gough J, Durr P, Jahans K, Clifton-Hadley R, et al. Pathology of naturally occurring bovine tuberculosis in England and Wales. *Vet J.* (2008) 176:354–60. doi: 10.1016/j.tvjl.2007.07.001
30. Liebana E, Aranaz A, Mateos A, Vilafranca M, Gomez-Mampaso E, Tercero JC, et al. Simple and rapid detection of *Mycobacterium tuberculosis* complex organisms in bovine tissue samples by PCR. *J Clin Microbiol.* (1995) 33:33–6. doi: 10.1128/jcm.33.1.33-36.1995
31. Corner. Post mortem diagnosis of *Mycobacterium bovis* infection in cattle. *Vet Microbiol.* (1994) 40:53–63. doi: 10.1016/0378-1135(94)90046-9
32. Toft, N., Jørgensen, E., and Højsgaard, S. Diagnosing diagnostic tests: evaluating the assumptions underlying the estimation of sensitivity and specificity in the absence of a gold standard. *Prev. Vet. Med.* (2005) 68, 19–33. doi: 10.1016/j.prevetmed.2005.01.006
33. Cardoso-Toset F, Gómez-Laguna J, Amarilla SP, Vela AI, Carrasco L, Fernández-Garayzábal JF, et al. Multi-etiological nature of tuberculosis-like lesions in condemned pigs at the slaughterhouse. *PLoS ONE.* (2015) 10:e0139130. doi: 10.1371/journal.pone.0139130
34. Menin Á, Fleith R, Reck C, Marlow M, Fernandes P, Pilati C, et al. Asymptomatic cattle naturally infected with *Mycobacterium bovis* present exacerbated tissue pathology and bacterial dissemination. *PLoS ONE.* (2013) 8:e53884. doi: 10.1371/journal.pone.0053884

20

Heterogeneity of Pulmonary Granulomas in Cattle Experimentally Infected with *Mycobacterium bovis*

***Mitchell V. Palmer*[1]*, *Tyler C. Thacker*[2], *Carly Kanipe*[1,3] and *Paola M. Boggiatto*[1]**

[1] *Bacterial Diseases of Livestock Research Unit, National Animal Disease Center, Agricultural Research Service, United States Department of Agriculture, Ames, IA, United States,* [2] *National Veterinary Services Laboratories, Animal and Plant Health Inspection Service, Ames, IA, United States,* [3] *Immunobiology Graduate Program, College of Veterinary Medicine, Iowa State University, Ames, IA, United States*

***Correspondence:**
Mitchell V. Palmer
mitchell.palmer@usda.gov

Mycobacterium bovis is the cause of tuberculosis in most animals, most notably cattle. The stereotypical lesion of bovine tuberculosis is the granuloma; a distinct morphological lesion where host and pathogen interact and disease outcome (i.e., dissemination, confinement, or resolution) is determined. Accordingly, it is critical to understand host-pathogen interactions at the granuloma level. Host-pathogen interactions within individual granulomas at different stages of disease have not been examined in cattle. We examined bacterial burden and cytokine expression in individual pulmonary granulomas from steers at 30, 90, 180, and 270 days after experimental aerosol infection with *M. bovis*. Bacterial burdens within individual granulomas examined 30 days after infection were greater and more heterogenous (variable) than those examined 90 to 270 days after infection. Bacterial burdens did not correlate with expression of IFN-γ, TNF-α, TGF-β, granuloma stage, or lung lesion score, although there was a modest positive correlation with IL-10 expression. Granuloma stage did have modest positive and negative correlations with TNF-α and IL-10, respectively. Heterogeneity and mean expression of IFN-γ, IL-10 and TNF-α did not differ significantly over time, however, expression of TGF-β at 90 days was significantly greater than that seen at 30 days after infection.

Keywords: cytokine, granuloma, *in situ* hybridization, *Mycobacterium bovis*, pathology, tuberculosis

INTRODUCTION

Bacteria of the genus *Mycobacterium* are Gram-positive, acid-fast bacilli. Among the many mycobacterial species, several are important human and animal pathogens such as *Mycobacterium tuberculosis* and *Mycobacterium bovis* (1). Tuberculosis in humans is primarily caused by *M. tuberculosis*; however, the zoonotic pathogen, *M. bovis*, which most commonly affects cattle can also produce tuberculosis in humans (2). The *M. tuberculosis* (*M. tb.*) complex includes *M. tuberculosis*, *M. bovis*, *M. africanum*, *M. microti*, *M. caprae*, *M. canetii*, *M. pinnipedii*, *M. orygis*, *M. suricattae*, *M. mungi*, the dassie bacillus and the chimpanzee bacillus (3–9). Of all these species, *M. bovis* has the broadest host range, which includes most mammalian species, most notably cattle [bovine tuberculosis, (bTB)].

The hallmark lesion of tuberculosis, regardless of host or tissue, is the granuloma. A granuloma resulting from infection with a member of the *M. tb.* complex may also be referred to as a tuberculoid granuloma (10).

The tuberculoid granuloma is a morphologically distinctive microscopic lesion dominated by a modified epithelial-like (epithelioid) macrophage, with lesser numbers of lymphocytes and multinucleated giant cells. In humans and animals, granulomas represent the host-pathogen interface where disease outcome (i.e., dissemination, confinement, or resolution) is determined; therefore, it is critical to understand host-pathogen interactions at the granuloma level (11–13). The granuloma paradox, however, is that although it is crucial for controlling and containing infection, it also contributes to early proliferation of bacilli (14–17).

The pathogenesis of bovine tuberculosis recapitulates many aspects of human tuberculosis; indeed, cattle have been used a model of human tuberculosis (18, 19). In humans and cattle, tiny residues, $<5\,\mu$m, of evaporated droplets (droplet nuclei) can be generated by an infected host while coughing, or in the case of humans, talking or singing (20–22). Such nuclei remain airborne for hours, and once inhaled can be deposited in the terminal bronchioles and alveoli. Resident alveolar macrophages phagocytose the bacilli, which in turn induces the production of cytokines, chemokines and enzymes. Expression of both pro- (e.g., IFN-γ, TNF-α,) and anti-inflammatory (e.g., IL-10, TGF-β) cytokines activate innate immune cells such as neutrophils, monocytes, macrophages and dendritic cells (14, 23). A coordinated exchange of cells between the lung and draining lymph nodes ensues as dendritic cells containing bacilli migrate from the lung to the lymph nodes. There, naïve T cells are activated through antigen presentation. Activated T cells home to the site of infection and cytokine and chemokine signals attract and activate monocytes and macrophages. As cells accumulate, the granuloma forms. The typical tuberculoid granuloma has a central region of caseous necrosis, surrounded by a zone of epithelioid macrophages and multinucleated giant cells, with the outermost zone containing increasing numbers of lymphocytes and occasional plasma cells. As infection persists, a partial to complete fibrous capsule may be produced. In addition to typical granuloma morphology, granulomas may be non-necrotizing or highly mineralized.

In cattle the heterogenous nature of bovine tuberculoid granulomas has been described in terms of morphology, as well as cellular composition and cytokine expression (24–27). Comparisons have also been made between tuberculoid granulomas arising in different organs from the same animal (25, 27). What has been less studied are granuloma changes over the course of disease, from early to late infection, including the bacterial burden within individual granulomas. Research in non-human primate (NHP) models of human tuberculosis reveals that individual granulomas are microenvironments in which local immune responses drive the bacterial burden, disease progression, and overall disease status (12, 28) indicative of disease control at the granuloma level.

The objective of the current study was to describe individual granuloma changes, in terms of morphologic stages, bacterial burdens and cytokine composition at increasing intervals after experimental aerosol infection. We hypothesized that granuloma heterogeneity may be reflected not only in morphology, but also in bacterial burden, and the concomitant cytokine environment.

MATERIALS AND METHODS

Mycobacterium bovis Aerosol Challenge

Mycobacterium bovis strain 10-7428 was used in this experiment. This field strain was of low passage (<3) and had been shown previously to be virulent in the calf aerosol model (29). Inoculum was prepared using standard techniques (30) in Middlebrook's 7H9 liquid media (Becton Dickinson, Franklin Lakes, NJ, USA) supplemented with 10% oleic acid-albumin-dextrose complex (OADC; Difco, Detroit, MI, USA) plus 0.05% Tween 80 (Sigma Chemical Co., St. Louis, MO, USA). Mid log-phase growth bacilli were pelleted by centrifugation at 750 X g, washed twice with phosphate buffered saline (PBS) (0.01 M, pH 7.2) and stored at-80^0 C until used. Frozen stock was warmed to room temperature and diluted to the appropriate cell density in 2 ml of PBS. Bacilli were enumerated by serial dilution plate counting on Middlebrook's 7H11 selective media (Becton Dickinson). A single dose was determined to be 1.12 X 10^4 CFU per steer.

Aerosol infection of steers with virulent *M. bovis* has been described in detail previously (24, 29, 31). Briefly, 20 Holstein steers (9 months of age) were obtained from a source with no history of *M. bovis* infection. Steers were infected with a single dose of virulent *M. bovis* strain 10-7428 by nebulization of inoculum into a mask (Equine AeroMask®, Trudell Medical International, London, ON, Canada) covering the nostrils and mouth. All experimental animal procedures were conducted in accordance with recommendations in the Care and Use of Laboratory Animals of the National Institutes of Health and the Guide for the Care and Use of Agricultural Animals in Research and Teaching (32, 33). Animal-related procedures were also approved by the USDA-National Animal Disease Center Animal Care and Use Committee.

Sample Collection

Five steers each were euthanized at 30, 90, 180, and 270 days after infection. Steers were humanely euthanized by intravenous administration of sodium pentobarbital. Tissues were examined for gross lesions and processed for microscopic analysis as described previously (29). Each lung lobe was examined separately and sectioned at 0.5 - 1.0 cm intervals. Lesions suspected to be granulomas were dissected out and processed as individual samples. In cases where numerous granulomas were present, a maximum of 5 granulomas each from five lung lobes were collected for a total of 25 granulomas per steer.

Individual granulomas were divided with one half being processed for mycobacterial isolation, as described below, and the other half processed for microscopic evaluation by formalin fixation. Individual granulomas and other tissue samples ($\leq$0.5 cm in width) were fixed by immersion in 10% neutral buffered formalin ($\geq$ 20 volumes fixative to 1 volume tissue) for approx. 24 h and transferred to 70% ethanol, followed by standard paraffin embedding techniques. Paraffin embedded samples were cut in 4 μm thick sections, transferred to Superfrost Plus™ charged microscope slides (Thermo Fisher Scientific, Pittsburg, PA) and stained with hematoxylin and eosin (H&E). For all individual granulomas, adjacent sections were stained by the Ziehl-Neelsen technique for visualization of acid-fast bacilli (AFB) and numerous near adjacent unstained sections were used for *in situ* hybridization (ISH).

Lesion Scoring

Lungs and lymph nodes (mediastinal and tracheobronchial) were evaluated using a semiquantitative gross pathology scoring system described previously (34). Lung lobes (left cranial, left caudal, right cranial, right caudal, middle and accessory) were assessed individually based on the following scoring system: 0, no visible lesions; 1, no external gross lesions, but lesions seen on slicing; 2, <5 gross lesions of <10 mm in diameter; 3, >5 gross lesions of <10 mm in diameter; 4, >1 distinct gross lesion of >10 mm in diameter; 5, gross coalescing lesions. Cumulative mean scores were then calculated for each entire lung.

Granuloma Bacterial Burden

Quantitative assessment of mycobacterial burden of individual granulomas was evaluated as described elsewhere (35). Only granulomas from the right and left caudal lobes, for a total of 10 granulomas per steer, were processed. Briefly, granulomas were homogenized in phenol red nutrient broth using a blender. Logarithmic dilutions (10^0-10^9) of homogenates in PBS were plated in 100 ml aliquots on Middlebrook 7H11 selective agar plates (Becton Dickinson) and incubated for 8 weeks at 37 °C. Isolates were confirmed to be *M. bovis* by IS6110 real time PCR as described elsewhere (36).

Microscopic Examination

All individual granulomas were staged according to criteria described previously (24, 25, 37, 38). Stage I (initial) granulomas were characterized by accumulations of epithelioid macrophages admixed with low numbers of lymphocytes and neutrophils. Multinucleated giant cells were sometimes present, but necrosis was absent. When present, AFB were seen within macrophages or multinucleated giant cells. Stage II (solid) granulomas were characterized by accumulations of epithelioid macrophages surrounded by a thin, incomplete fibrous capsule. Infiltrates of neutrophils, lymphocytes and multinucleated giant cells were sometimes present. Necrosis was minimal to mild and centrally located. When present, AFB were seen within macrophages or multinucleated giant cells. Stage III (necrotic) granulomas were characterized by necrotic cores, some with small foci of dystrophic mineralization, surrounded by a zone of epithelioid macrophages admixed with multinucleated giant cells and lymphocytes. As distance from the necrotic core increased, the relative number of lymphocytes also increased and the number of epithelioid macrophages and multinucleated giant cells decreased. The entire granuloma was surrounded by a thin to moderate fibrous capsule. When present, AFB were seen within the necrotic core and, to a lesser extent, within macrophages and multinucleated giant cells. Stage IV (necrotic and mineralized) granulomas were characterized by a variably thick fibrous capsule surrounding irregular multicentric granulomas with multiple necrotic cores, often with foci of dystrophic mineralization. Epithelioid macrophages and multinucleated giant cells surrounded necrotic areas; these cellular infiltrates were bordered by a zone of large numbers of lymphocytes. When present, AFB were seen most often within the necrotic core.

mRNA Chromogenic ISH

Only granulomas from the right and left caudal lobes, for a total of 10 granulomas per steer, were processed for ISH. ISH was performed on individual granulomas from 30, 90- and 270-days post-infection. RNAscope® ZZ probe technology (Advanced Cell Diagnostics, Newark, CA) was used to perform mRNA ISH in formalin-fixed paraffin-embedded (FFPE) tissue sections using the RNAscope® 2.5 HD Reagents – RED kit (Advanced Cell Diagnostics) on samples from 30, 90 and 270 days after infection. Proprietary ZZ probes complementary to mRNA sequences of interest were used for visualization of mRNA transcripts for the following cytokines: IFN-γ (Cat. No. 315581), TNF-α, (Cat. No. 316151), TGF-β (Cat. No. 427271) and IL-10 (Cat. No. 420941). A positive control probe targeted the *Bos taurus*-specific *cyclophilin B* (*PPIB*) housekeeping gene (Cat. No. 319451), while a probe targeting *dapB* of *Bacillus subtilis* (Cat. No. 310043) was used as a negative control. The RNAscope® labeling technique has been shown to be capable of single mRNA molecule detection (39).

Formalin-fixed paraffin embedded tissue pretreatment was performed with manual antigen retrieval according to the manufacturer's instructions. Slides were baked in a dry oven for 1 hr at 60°C to promote tissue-to-slide adherence, deparaffinized and rehydrated in fresh xylenes and 100% ethanol, and air dried. RNAscope® hydrogen peroxide (Advanced Cell Diagnostics) was next applied to each tissue section for 10 min at room temperature (RT, 20^0 C) to block endogenous peroxidase activity, followed by rinsing with fresh distilled water (dH_2O). Disruption of formalin cross-linking and unmasking of antigenic epitopes was achieved by submerging slides in a boiling 1X RNAscope® target retrieval solution (Advanced Cell Diagnostics) for 15 min, followed by rinsing with fresh dH_2O and 100% ethanol. Once slides had completely air dried, a hydrophobic barrier was drawn around each tissue using an ImmEdge® pen (Vector Laboratories, Burlingame, CA), and slides were stored at RT overnight with desiccants. The following day, RNAscope® Protease Plus was applied to each tissue section and incubated in a humidifying tray at 40°C in a HybEZ™ Hybridization System oven (Advanced Cell Diagnostics) for 30 min. Slides were then rinsed with fresh dH_2O before proceeding to probe hybridization.

Probe hybridization, amplification, and detection were performed according to manufacturer's instructions. All incubations were carried out in a humidifying tray either at RT or in a HybEZ™ oven at 40°C. Between each incubation step, slides were washed with fresh 1X Wash Buffer (Advanced Cell Diagnostics). To allow binding of the ZZ probe to target mRNA, customized probe prewarmed to 40°C was applied to each tissue section and incubated at 40°C for 2 hrs. Branched amplification and detection of the probe with Fast Red chromogen (Advanced

Cell Diagnostics) was achieved by incubating slides with kit reagents (Advanced Cell Diagnostics) as follows: AMP 1 (30 min), AMP 2 (15 min), AMP 3 (30 min), and AMP 4 (15 min) at 40°C; AMP 5 (30 min) and AMP 6 (15 min) at RT; and a 60:1 solution of RED-A: RED-B (Advanced Cell Diagnostics) at RT for 10 min.

Following RED detection, slides were rinsed with fresh dH_2O before being transferred to a 1:1 Gill's hematoxylin I:dH_2O (American MasterTech, Lodi, CA) counterstain. Slides were submerged in hematoxylin solution for 2 min, rinsed with fresh dH_2O thrice, submerged in 0.02% ammonia water for bluing, and dry baked at 40°C for 20 min or until completely dry. Tissue dehydration was not completed due to the alcohol-sensitive nature of the Fast Red chromogen. To mount the tissue samples, slides were dipped in fresh xylenes, 1–2 drops of aqueous EcoMount mounting medium (Biocare Medical, Pacheco, CA) was applied to each tissue section, and a #1 thickness cover slip was applied over top of the tissue section. Slides were dried at RT in the dark overnight before microscopic examination.

Morphometry

Slides were scanned at 40X magnification and digitized using the Aperio ScanScope XT workstation (Aperio Technology, Inc., Vista, CA, USA). Digitized images of individual granulomas were analyzed using image analysis software (HALO™, Indica Labs, Inc., Corrales, NM). Using the RNA ISH HALO™ module, the chromogenic reaction of Fast Red was identified and the signal (i.e., red dots) quantified. The RNA ISH module algorithm identifies both cells and signal allowing the quantification of signal number per area occupied by cells within the granuloma (i.e., signal/total cell area). The entire section of each granuloma was analyzed.

Statistical Analysis

Mean values for lesion scores, tissue weights and cytokine expression at each time point were evaluated using one-way analysis of variance, followed by Tukey's *post-hoc* multiple comparison test (GraphPad Prism 8.0, GraphPad Software, San Diego, CA, USA) to compare differences between means. Correlations between multiple variables were analyzed using Pearson correlation coefficients (GraphPad Prism 8.0). For all analyses a p-value < 0.05 was considered significant.

RESULTS

Gross Lesions, Lesion Scores and Granuloma Stages

Gross lesions were seen in lungs of all infected steers at all time points. The spread and variability (i.e., SD) of lung lesion scores within groups was similar and the means did not differ significantly (**Figure 1**). Granulomas examined at 30 days post-infection were predominantly stage I (**Figure 2**). At 90, 180- and 270-days post-infection all 4 granuloma stages were represented, albeit to varying degrees (**Figure 2**).

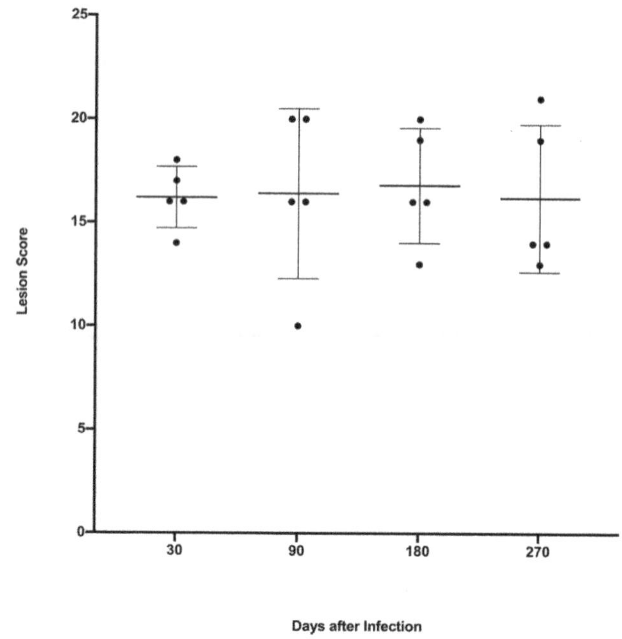

FIGURE 1 | Lung lesion scores from calves experimentally infected with *M. bovis* and examined at various time points after infection. Values are expressed as individual scores with mean ± SD.

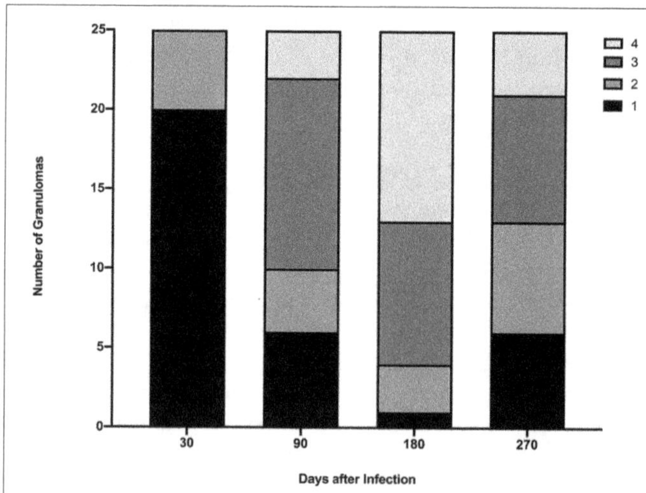

FIGURE 2 | Granuloma stages collected from lungs of steers euthanized 30, 90, 180, and 270 days after experimental infection with *M. bovis*. A maximum of 5 granulomas were collected from each of 5 lung lobes (right cranial, left cranial, right caudal and middle, left caudal, and accessory).

Bacterial Burden of Individual Granulomas

As a group, steers examined 30 days after infection had a significantly higher bacterial burden ($p < 0.0001$) than cattle examined at 90, 180 and 270 days after infection (**Figure 3**). Additionally, as groups, the bacterial burdens of cattle examined 90, 180 and 270 days after infection did not differ significantly from each other (**Figure 3**). Examination of individual granulomas revealed the bacterial burdens of

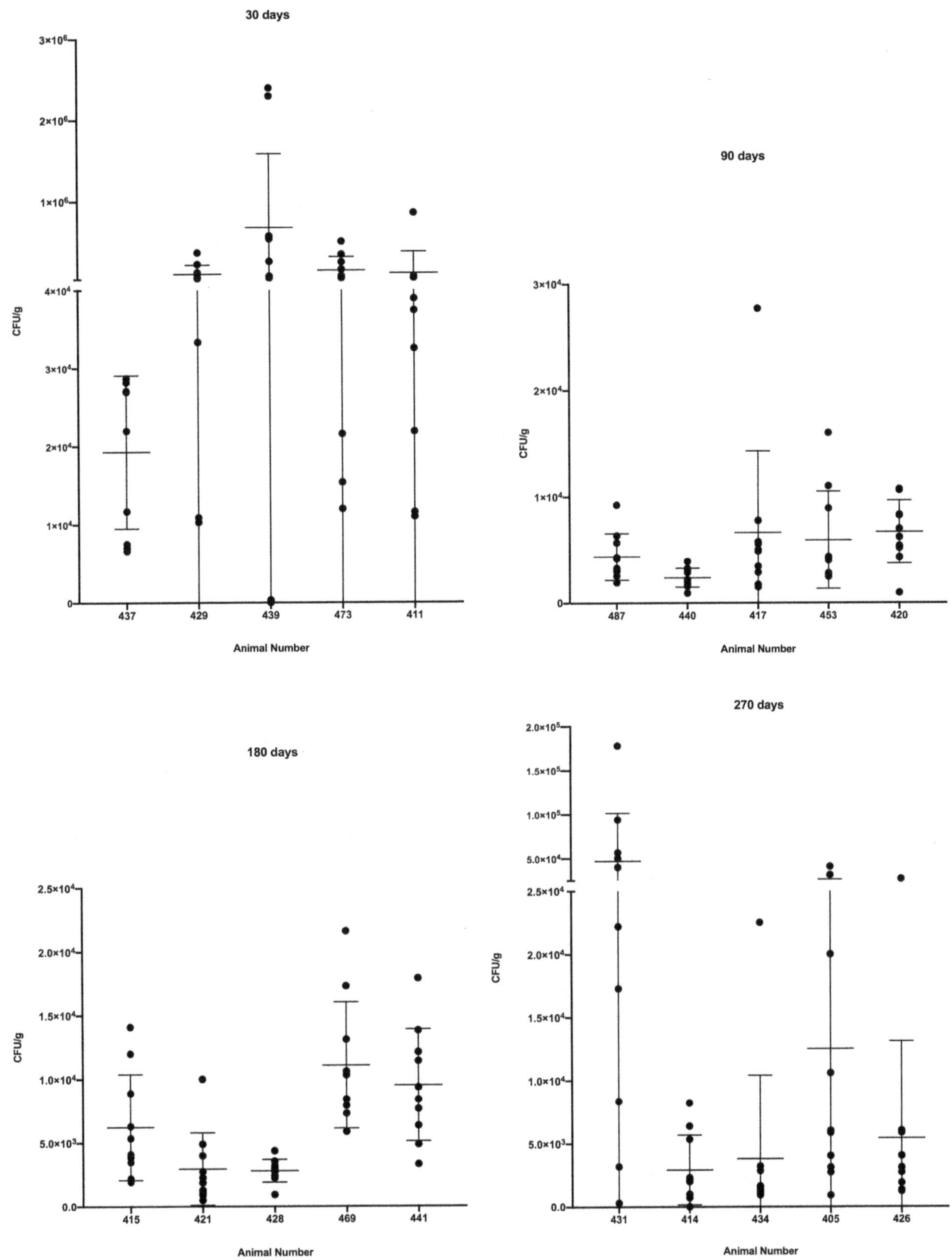

FIGURE 3 | Bacterial burden in colony-forming units/g (CFU/g) in individual granulomas from steers experimentally infected with *M. bovis* and examined at 30, 90, 180, and 270 days after infection. Values represent CFU/g within individual granulomas from right and left caudal lobes with individual animal means ± SD.

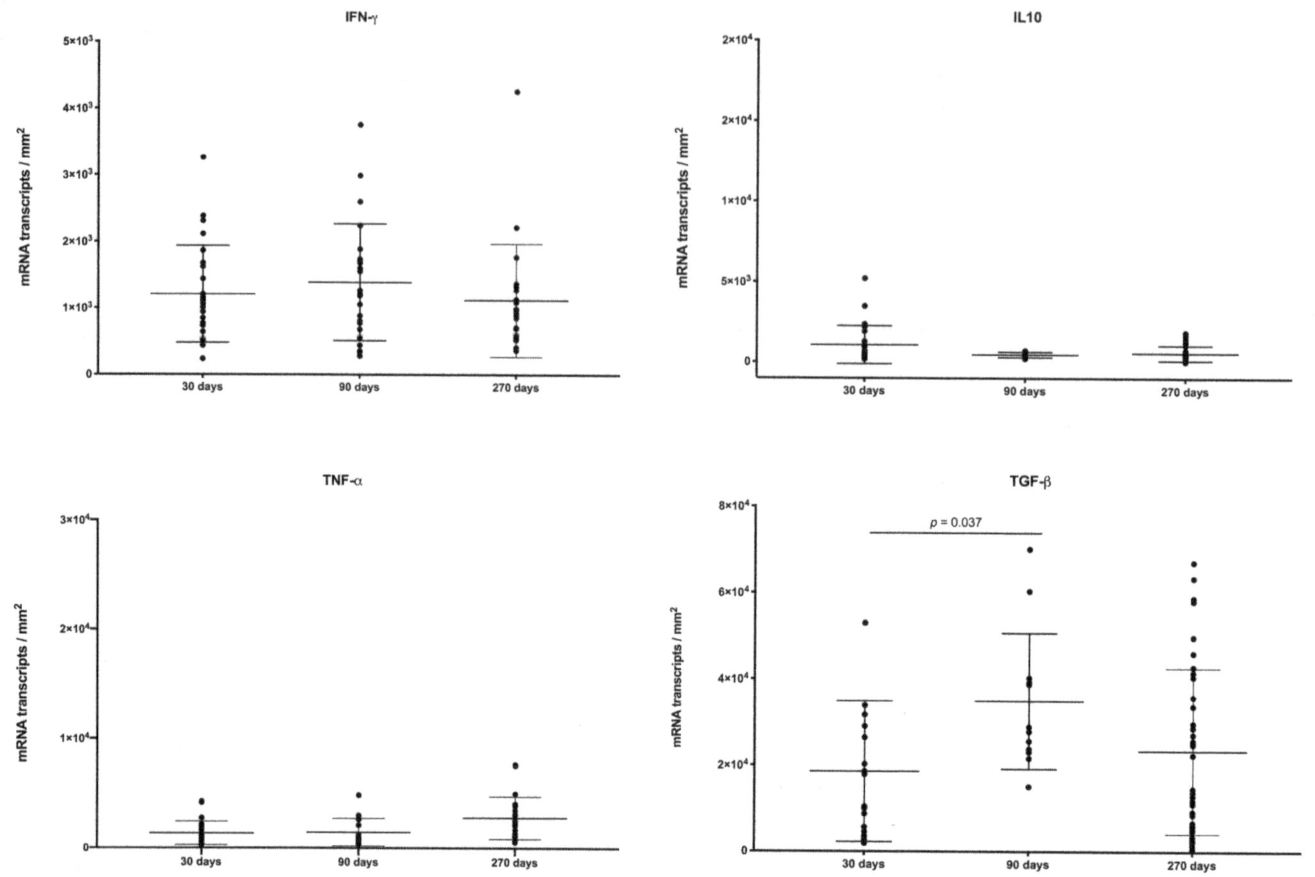

FIGURE 4 | Expression of IFN-γ, IL-10, TNF-α, and TGF-β, as measured by *in-situ* hybridization in individual granulomas from right and left caudal lung lobes of steers experimentally infected with *M. bovis* and examined at 30, 90, and 270 days after infection. Values represent mRNA transcripts/mm^2 with group means ± SD.

granulomas in all animals at all time points were heterogenous with varying degrees of dispersion. The burden range was high, as a number of granulomas from animals examined 30 days post-infection had bacterial burdens $>10^5$ CFU/g while a single granuloma from steer #439, 30 days post-infection contained no culturable *M. bovis* (i.e., sterile granuloma). Although no additional sterile granulomas were noted, a single granuloma with <100 CFU/g was seen in steer #414 at 270 days post-infection.

In situ Hybridization

The balance of pro- and anti-inflammatory cytokines likely contribute to the dynamic nature of granulomas over the course of infection (40). We assessed the expression of various cytokines within granulomas from different time points after infection. Individual granuloma cytokine expression was heterogenous and the variability was greater for IFN-γ and TGF-β compared to IL-10 and TNF-α (**Figure 4**). However, we observed no significant differences in mean expression of IFN-γ, IL-10 or TNF-α at any time points examined, with the exception of TGF-β where expression was significantly greater at 90 days compared to 30 days.

Correlations

When all timepoints were combined, there a was marginally positive correlation between bacterial burden and IL-10 expression; otherwise at any individual time point there was no correlation between bacterial burden and gene expression for any cytokine (**Table 1**). Granuloma stage was marginally positive correlated with TNF-α, and negatively correlated with IL-10 gene expression when all time-points were combined; however, no correlation was seen at individual time points (**Supplementary Tables 1–3**). No correlation was noted between lung lesion score and bacterial burden at any time point.

Cytokine gene expression using all time-points combined showed marginal positive correlations between IFN-γ and both IL-10 and TNF-α (**Table 1**). These marginal positive correlations were also seen at 30 days post-infection (**Supplementary Table 1**), however, only the positive correlation between IFN-γ and TNF-α carried over to the 90-day post-infection time point (**Supplementary Table 2**). No correlations between cytokine gene expression were noted at 270 days post-infection (**Supplementary Table 3**).

TABLE 1 | Pearson correlation coefficients (r) for cytokine expression, bacterial burden (CFU/g) and granuloma stage in pulmonary granulomas examined at all time-points combined (30, 90, 180, and 270 days after infection) from calves experimentally infected with aerosolized *M. bovis*.

	IFN-γ	IL-10	TNF-α	TGF-β	CFU/g
IL-10	0.35[a]	–	–	–	–
	0.007[b]				
TNF-α	0.26	0.03	–	–	–
	0.043	0.790			
TGF-β	0.079	-0.042	−0.127	–	–
	0.556	0.757	0.346		
CFU/g	−0.085	0.250	−0.148	−0.055	–
	0.484	**0.032**	0.248	0.676	
Granuloma Stage	−0.04	−0.35	0.36	0.203	−0.129
	0.714	**0.003**	**0.003**	0.121	0.138

[a] *Pearson coefficient (r).*
[b] *p-value (<0.05 are highlighted in bold text).*

DISCUSSION

Prior studies in cattle have described the morphological heterogeneity of tuberculoid granulomas in both experimental and natural infections (26, 37, 41, 42). The present study examined bacterial burdens of individual pulmonary tuberculoid granulomas at 30, 90, 180 and 270 days after experimental aerosol infection and revealed heterogeneity in bacterial burdens at all time points. Heterogeneity of both morphology and bacterial burdens of individual granulomas has not been examined in cattle. Such heterogeneity suggests that bovine pulmonary tuberculoid granulomas may have their own behavior and trajectory as has been demonstrated in NHP models of human tuberculosis (12, 28). In spite of this independence, as a group the bacterial burden at 30 days was significantly greater than later time points. A decrease in bacterial burden beyond 30 days after infection is consistent with previous studies in cattle demonstrating evidence of a delayed type hypersensitivity (DTH) response to *M. bovis* antigens 3–4 weeks after infection (43–46). The present data would suggest that after the time required for a DTH adaptive immune response to develop there is an overall 1-2 log decrease in bacterial burdens. Nevertheless, there was only a single granuloma from which no *M. bovis* was isolated. Such sterile granulomas are not uncommon in NHP models of human tuberculosis (11, 12, 40). The NHP model has also demonstrated a higher bacterial burden in lesions arising at earlier time points and a significant reduction in bacterial burden after the onset of adaptive immunity, consistent with the findings in this study (12).

Previous studies of tuberculoid granulomas of cattle have suggested that bacterial burdens are increased in late stage IV granulomas, while others have found no correlation between bacterial numbers and granuloma stage (26, 41). Those studies, however, estimated bacterial burden by enumerating AFB observed in microscopic tissue sections. In the current study, we saw no correlation between bacterial burden and granuloma stage and there was not an observable increase in bacterial burdens in granulomas collected at later time points. To the contrary, we found bacterial burdens higher at 30 days post-infection than at later time points. Bacterial burdens did not correlate with expression of IFN-γ, TNF-α, TGF-β, granuloma stage, or lung lesion score, although there was a modest positive correlation with IL-10 expression. Granuloma stage did have modest positive and negative correlations with TNF-α and IL-10, respectively.

Considered a key cytokine, IFN-γ is critical to macrophage activation and pivotal in a protective Th1 response to mycobacteria. Therefore, an interesting finding of the present study was the steady state of IFN-γ expression over time, which did not correlate with either bacterial burden or granuloma stage. Prior studies in cattle have produced inconclusive results in terms of IFN-γ expression in granulomas. Some of these differences may be in technique, inoculation dose, duration of disease, or tissue (i.e., lymph nodes vs. lung). Previous cattle studies using IHC to measure IFN-γ protein within granulomas showed no difference in expression based on granuloma stage; however, there was increased IFN-γ expression in calves receiving a higher dose (1,000 CFU vs. 1 CFU) (42). A separate study using IHC showed an increase in IFN-γ protein immunolabeling between stages I and IV (41). Yet, another study, also using IHC, showed IFN-γ in granulomas of all stages, with a qualitative, but not significant decrease in labeling in late stage IV granulomas compared to earlier stages (47). A study using mRNA extracted from formalin-fixed paraffin-embedded lymph node cross sections showed no significant differences in expression levels of IFN-γ, TNF-α or IL-10 at 5, 12, and 19 weeks after infection and no correlation between lesion severity and individual cytokine expression (48). Supporting the present findings, a study using ISH methods similar to those used here, demonstrated that IFN-γ expression did not differ between stage I and stage IV granulomas examined at a single time point (150 days) after experimental infection (24).

In contrast to IFN-γ expression, there was a mild, but not significant trend of increasing TNF-α gene expression from 30 to 270-days post-infection. Increasing TNF-α levels, may be associated with the increased presence of necrosis within granulomas as they progress from stage I, non-necrotizing granulomas to stage IV granulomas with significant necrosis. Necrosis is a consistent feature of many tuberculoid granulomas, regardless of mycobacterial species, host species or target organ, intimating the importance of this process in the pathogenesis of tuberculosis. Tissue destruction facilitates spread of disease as bacilli gain entrance to vascular elements, which carry them to distant sites. Other studies using granulomas from cattle collected at a single time-point after experimental infection, or from naturally infected cattle of unknown disease duration have shown decreasing trends, increasing trends, or no difference, respectively, between TNF-α expression in granulomas of stage I to IV. (24, 41, 47, 49).

In tuberculosis, TNF-α has been shown to be critical, with low levels associated with fatal disease; however, excessive TNF-α induces a hyper-inflammatory environment (50, 51). TNF-α induces cytokine production by macrophages, activates macrophages for killing, and modulates macrophage apoptosis (52). Considered pro-inflammatory, cytokines such as TNF-α and IFN-γ if left uncontrolled can lead to excessive tissue damage, increased inflammation, and deteriorating disease status. To balance inflammation and tissue destruction, IL-10 deactivates macrophages, resulting in diminished Th1 cytokine production and decreased production of reactive nitrogen and oxygen species (53). The present study suggests that early in infection, when bacterial burdens are higher and inflammation is increasing, IL-10 production is stimulated. This stimulation appears less critical at later time points when bacterial burdens are lower. In mice, overexpression of IL-10 is associated with increased bacterial burdens, while in humans with tuberculosis, elevated levels of IL-10 have been associated with more active disease and more severe clinical signs (54, 55).

Examinations of TGF-β expression in granulomas from experimentally infected cattle have yielded conflicting results. In one study of lymph node granulomas from experimentally infected cattle examined 29 weeks after infection TGF-β expression was greater in more advanced granulomas compared to early stage granulomas (37). Two other studies found lower expression in late stage granulomas compared to early stage granulomas (49, 56). TGF-β is a key cytokine implicated in fibrinogenesis and new collagen synthesis. In macaques, TGF-β has been suggested as a critical driver of tissue repair in active tuberculosis (57). As more advanced granulomas are often characterized by a peripheral fibrous capsule, the presence of increased TGF-β expression at 90 days compared to 30 days, as seen in the present study, is consistent with a role in fibrosis.

In NHPs positron emission tomography-computed tomography (PET-CT) imaging has allowed serial imaging during the course of infection producing a dynamic map of individual granuloma activity that can be correlated with postmortem exam findings (11, 12). The present study in cattle attempted to follow the course of infection by examining individual animals at increasing intervals after infection. This method yields multiple snap shots of granuloma activity at defined time points, but does not allow observation of individual granuloma development, activity and disease progression within an animal. Thus, a shortcoming of the present study is that we are unaware of the state of individual granulomas before or after the defined time points. Nevertheless, examination of individual pulmonary granulomas of cattle did reveal significant heterogeneity in bacterial burdens, however it is less clear how bacterial burdens relate to granuloma development or cytokine production within granulomas.

ETHICS STATEMENT

The animal study was reviewed and approved by USDA-National Animal Disease Center Animal Care and Use Committee.

AUTHOR CONTRIBUTIONS

MP and TT: experiment design. MP and CK: sample collection and experiments. MP and PB data analysis. MP: manuscript preparation. MP, TT, CK, and PB: manuscript editing. All authors contributed to the article and approved the submitted version.

FUNDING

The authors disclosed receipt of the following financial support for the research, authorship, and/or publication of this article: Research funds were provided by the United States Department of Agriculture, Agricultural Research Service Project (CRIS #5030-32000-222).

ACKNOWLEDGMENTS

The authors thank clinical veterinarian, Dr. Rebecca Cox and animal caretakers, Lisa Ashburn, Hannah Shroeder, Robin Zeisneiss and David Lubbers for excellent animal care, and Shelly Zimmerman, Allison Lasley and Jayne Wiarda for excellent technical assistance.

REFERENCES

1. Sizemore C, Lacourciere K, Parker T. The many hosts of mycobacteria: an interdisciplinary approach to understanding mycobacterial diseases. In: Mukundan H, Chambers MA, Waters RW, Larsen MH, editors. *Tuberculosis, Leprosy and Mycobacterial Diseases of Man and Animals*. Boston, MA: CABI. (2015).
2. Langer A, LoBue PA. Public health significance of zoonotic tuberculosis in animals and humans. In: Thoen CO, Steele JH, Kaneene JB, editors. *Zoonotic Tuberculosis: Mycobacterium bovis and other Pathogenic Mycobacteria*. Ames: Wiley Blackwell. (2014) p. 21–34.
3. Rodriguez-Campos S, Smith NH, Boniotti MB, Aranaz A. Overview and phylogeny of *Mycobacterium tuberculosis* complex organisms: implications

for diagnostics and legislation of bovine tuberculosis. *Res Vet Sci.* (2014) 97:S5–19. doi: 10.1016/j.rvsc.2014.02.009

4. Coscolla M, Gagneux S. Consequences of genomic diversity in *Mycobacterium tuberculosis*. *Semin Immunol.* (2014) 26:431–44. doi: 10.1016/j.smim.2014.09.012
5. Cousins DV, Bastida R, Cataldi A, Quse V, Redrobe S, Dow S, et al. Tuberculosis in seals caused by a novel member of the *Mycobacterium tuberculosis* complex: *Mycobacterium pinnipedii* sp. nov. *Int J Syst Evol Microbiol.* (2003) 53:1305–14. doi: 10.1099/ijs.0.02401-0
6. Cousins DV, Francis BR, Gow BL, Collins DM, McGlashan CH, Gregory A, et al. Tuberculosis in captive seals: bacteriological studies on an isolate belonging to the *Mycobacterium tuberculosis* complex. *Res Vet Sci.* (1990) 48:196–200. doi: 10.1016/S0034-5288(18)30990-1
7. Cousins DV, Peet RL, Gaynor WT, Williams SN, Gow BL. Tuberculosis in imported hyrax (*Procavia capensis*) caused by an unusual variant belonging to the *Mycobacterium tuberculosis* complex. *Vet Microbiol.* (1994) 42:135–45. doi: 10.1016/0378-1135(94)90013-2
8. Parsons SD, Drewe JA, Gey van Pittius NC, Warren RM, van Helden PD. Novel cause of tuberculosis in meerkats, South Africa. *Emerg Infect Dis.* (2013) 19:2004–7. doi: 10.3201/eid1912.130268
9. Alexander KA, Laver PN, Michel AL, Williams M, van Helden PD, Warren RM, et al. Novel *Mycobacterium tuberculosis* complex pathogen, *M.* Mungi. *Emerg Infect Dis.* (2010) 16:1296–9. doi: 10.3201/eid1608.100314
10. Myers RK, McGavin MD, Zachary JF. Cellular adaptations, injury, and death: Morphologic, biochemical, and genetic bases. In: Zachary JF, McGavin MD, editors. *Pathologic Basis of Veterinary Disease.* St. Louis: Elsevier Mosby. (2012) p. 122–4.
11. Lin PL, Coleman T, Carney JP, Lopresti BJ, Tomko J, Fillmore D, et al. Radiologic responses in cynomolgous macaques for assessing tuberculosis chemotherapy regimens. *Antimicrob Agents Chemother.* (2013) 57:4237–44. doi: 10.1128/AAC.00277-13
12. Lin PL, Ford CB, Coleman MT, Myers AJ, Gawande R, Ioerger T, et al. Sterilization of granulomas is common in active and latent tuberculosis despite within-host variability in bacterial killing. *Nat Med.* (2014) 20:75–9. doi: 10.1038/nm.3412
13. Gideon HP, Skinner JA, Baldwin N, Flynn JL, Lin PL. Early whole blood transcriptional signatures are associated with severity of lung inflammation in cynomolgus macaques with *Mycobacterium tuberculosis* infection. *J Immunol.* (2016) 197:4817–28. doi: 10.4049/jimmunol.1601138
14. Cicchese JM, Evans S, Hult C, Joslyn LR, Wessler T, Millar JA, et al. Dynamic balance of pro- and anti-inflammatory signals controls disease and limits pathology. *Immunol Rev.* (2018) 285:147–67. doi: 10.1111/imr.12671
15. Davis JM, Ramakrishnan L. The role of the granuloma in expansion and dissemination of early tuberculous infection. *Cell.* (2009) 136:37–49. doi: 10.1016/j.cell.2008.11.014
16. Ramakrishnan L. Revisiting the role of the granuloma in tuberculosis. *Nat Rev Immunol.* (2012) 12:352–66. doi: 10.1038/nri3211
17. Flynn JL. Mutual attraction: does it benefit the host or the bug? *Nat Immunol.* (2004) 5:778–9. doi: 10.1038/ni0804-778
18. Waters WR, Palmer MV. *Mycobacterium bovis* infection of cattle and white-tailed deer: translational research of relevance to human tuberculosis. *ILAR J.* (2015) 56:26–43. doi: 10.1093/ilar/ilv001
19. Waters WR, Maggioli MF, McGill JL, Lyashchenko KP, Palmer MV. Relevance of bovine tuberculosis research to the understanding of human disease: historical perspectives, approaches, and immunologic mechanisms. *Vet Immunol Immunopathol.* (2014) 159:113–32. doi: 10.1016/j.vetimm.2014.02.009
20. Wells WF, Ratcliffe HL,Grumb C. On the mechanics of droplet nuclei infection; quantitative experimental air-borne tuberculosis in rabbits. *Am J Hyg.* (1948) 47:11–28.
21. Loudon RG, Roberts RM. Droplet expulsion from the respiratory tract. *Am Rev Respir Dis.* (1967) 95:435–42.
22. Loudon RG, Roberts RM. Singing and the dissemination of tuberculosis. *Am Rev Respir Dis.* (1968) 98:297–300.
23. Etna MP, Giacomini E, Severa M, Coccia EM. Pro- and anti-inflammatory cytokines in TB: a two-edged sword in TB pathogenesis. *Semin Immunol.* (2014) 26:543–51. doi: 10.1016/j.smim.2014.09.011
24. Palmer MV, Thacker TC,Waters WR. Analysis of cytokine gene expression using a novel chromogenic in-situ hybridization method in pulmonary granulomas of cattle infected experimentally by aerosolized *Mycobacterium bovis*. *J Comp Pathol.* (2015) 153:150–9. doi: 10.1016/j.jcpa.2015.06.004
25. Palmer MV, Thacker TC,Waters WR. Differential cytokine gene expression in granulomas from lungs and lymph nodes of cattle experimentally infected with aerosolized *Mycobacterium bovis*. *PLoS ONE.* (2016) 11:e0167471. doi: 10.1371/journal.pone.0167471
26. Palmer MV, Waters WR, Thacker TC. Lesion development and immunohistochemical changes in granulomas from cattle experimentally infected with *Mycobacterium bovis*. *Vet Pathol.* (2007) 44:863–74. doi: 10.1354/vp.44-6-863
27. Shu D, Heiser A, Wedlock DN, Luo D, de Lisle GW, Buddle BM. Comparison of gene expression of immune mediators in lung and pulmonary lymph node granulomas from cattle experimentally infected with *Mycobacterium bovis*. *Vet Immunol Immunopathol.* (2014) 160:81–9. doi: 10.1016/j.vetimm.2014.03.017
28. Cadena AM, Fortune SM, Flynn JL. Heterogeneity in tuberculosis. *Nat Rev Immunol.* (2017) 17:691–702. doi: 10.1038/nri.2017.69
29. Waters WR, Thacker TC, Nelson JT, DiCarlo DM, Maggioli MF, Greenwald R, et al. Virulence of two strains of *Mycobacterium bovis* in cattle following aerosol infection. *J Comp Pathol.* (2014) 151:410–9. doi: 10.1016/j.jcpa.2014.08.007
30. Larsen MH, Biermann K, Jacobs WR Jr. Laboratory maintenance of *Mycobacterium tuberculosis*. *Curr Protoc Microbiol.* (2007) 6:10A.1.1–10A.1.8. doi: 10.1002/9780471729259.mc10a01s6
31. Palmer MV, Waters WR,Whipple DL. Aerosol delivery of virulent *Mycobacterium bovis* to cattle. *Tuberculosis.* (2002) 82:275–82. doi: 10.1054/tube.2002.0341
32. Garber JC. *Guide for the Care and Use of Laboratory Animals.* Washington, DC: The National Academies Press (2011) 1–246.
33. Federation of Animal Science Societies. *Guide for the Care and Use of Agricultural Animals in Research and Teaching.* Champaign, IL: Federation of Animal Science Societies (2010).
34. Vordermeier HM, Chambers MA, Cockle PJ, Whelan AO, Simmons J, Hewinson RG. Correlation of ESAT-6-specific gamma interferon production with pathology in cattle following *Mycobacterium bovis* BCG vaccination against experimental bovine tuberculosis. *Infect Immun.* (2002) 70:3026–32. doi: 10.1128/IAI.70.6.3026-3032.2002
35. Waters WR, Palmer MV, Nonnecke BJ, Thacker TC, Scherer CF, Estes DM, et al. Failure of a *Mycobacterium tuberculosis* DeltaRD1 DeltapanCD double deletion mutant in a neonatal calf aerosol *M.* bovis challenge model: comparisons to responses elicited by M. bovis bacille calmette guerin. *Vaccine.* (2007) 25:7832–40. doi: 10.1016/j.vaccine.2007.08.029
36. Thacker TC, Harris B, Palmer MV, Waters WR. Improved specificity for detection of *Mycobacterium bovis* in fresh tissues using IS6110 real-time PCR. *BMC Vet Res.* (2011) 7:50. doi: 10.1186/1746-6148-7-50
37. Wangoo A, Johnson L, Gough J, Ackbar R, Inglut S, Hicks D, et al. Advanced granulomatous lesions in *Mycobacterium bovis*-infected cattle are associated with increased expression of type I procollagen, gamma delta (WC1+) T cells and CD 68+ cells. *J Comp Pathol.* (2005) 133:223–34. doi: 10.1016/j.jcpa.2005.05.001
38. Johnson L, Gough J, Spencer Y, Hewinson G, Vordermeier M, Wangoo A. Immunohistochemical markers augment evaluation of vaccine efficacy and disease severity in bacillus Calmette-Guerin (BCG) vaccinated cattle challenged with *Mycobacterium bovis*. *Vet Immunol Immunopathol.* (2006) 111:219–29. doi: 10.1016/j.vetimm.2006.01.016
39. Wang F, Flanagan J, Su N, Wang LC, Bui S, Nielson A, et al. RNAscope[?]: a novel *in situ* RNA analysis platform for formalin-fixed, paraffin-embedded tissues. *J Mol Diagn.* (2012) 14:22–9. doi: 10.1016/j.jmoldx.2011.08.002
40. Gideon HP, Phuah J, Myers AJ, Bryson BD, Rodgers MA, Coleman MT, et al. Variability in tuberculosis granuloma T cell responses exists, but a balance of pro- and anti-inflammatory cytokines is associated with sterilization. *PLoS Pathog.* (2015) 11:e1004603. doi: 10.1371/journal.ppat.1004603
41. Tulu B, Martineau HM, Zewude A, Desta F, Jolliffe DA, Abebe M, et al. Cellular and cytokine responses in granulomas of asymptomatic cattle

naturally infected with *Mycobacterium bovis* in Ethiopia. *Infect Immun.* (2020) 88:e00507-20. doi: 10.1128/IAI.00507-20

42. Johnson L, Dean G, Rhodes S, Hewinson G, Vordermeier M, Wangoo A. Low-dose *Mycobacterium bovis* infection in cattle results in pathology indistinguishable from that of high-dose infection. *Tuberculosis.* (2007) 87:71–6. doi: 10.1016/j.tube.2006.04.002
43. Waters WR, Palmer MV, Nonnecke BJ, Thacker TC, Scherer CF, Estes DM, et al. Efficacy and immunogenicity of *Mycobacterium bovis* DeltaRD1 against aerosol *M.* bovis infection in neonatal calves. *Vaccine.* (2009) 27:1201–9. doi: 10.1016/j.vaccine.2008.12.018
44. Dean GS, Rhodes SG, Coad M, Whelan AO, Cockle PJ, Clifford DJ, et al. Minimum infective dose of *Mycobacterium bovis* in cattle. *Infect Immun.* (2005) 73:6467–71. doi: 10.1128/IAI.73.10.6467-6471.2005
45. Rhodes SG, Palmer N, Graham SP, Bianco AE, Hewinson RG,Vordermeier HM. Distinct response kinetics of gamma interferon and interleukin-4 in bovine tuberculosis. *Infect Immun.* (2000) 68:5393–400. doi: 10.1128/IAI.68.9.5393-5400.2000
46. Thom ML, Hope JC, McAulay M, Villarreal-Ramos B, Coffey TJ, Stephens S, et al. The effect of tuberculin testing on the development of cell-mediated immune responses during *Mycobacterium bovis* infection. *Vet Immunol Immunopathol.* (2006) 114:25–36. doi: 10.1016/j.vetimm.2006.07.001
47. Aranday-Cortes E, Bull NC, Villarreal-Ramos B, Gough J, Hicks D, Ortiz-Pelaez A, et al. Upregulation of IL-17A, CXCL9 and CXCL10 in early-stage granulomas induced by *Mycobacterium bovis* in cattle. *Transbound Emerg Dis.* (2013) 60:525–37. doi: 10.1111/j.1865-1682.2012.01370.x
48. Witchell J, Maddipatla SV, Wangoo A, Vordermeier M, Goyal M. Time dependent expression of cytokines in *Mycobacterium bovis* infected cattle lymph nodes. *Vet Immunol Immunopathol.* (2010) 138:79–84. doi: 10.1016/j.vetimm.2010.07.004
49. Aranday-Cortes E, Hogarth PJ, Kaveh DA, Whelan AO, Villarreal-Ramos B, Lalvani A, et al. Transcriptional profiling of disease-induced host responses in bovine tuberculosis and the identification of potential diagnostic biomarkers. *PLoS ONE.* (2012) 7:e30626. doi: 10.1371/journal.pone.0030626
50. Dorhoi A, Kaufmann SH. Tumor necrosis factor alpha in mycobacterial infection. *Semin Immunol.* (2014) 26:203–9. doi: 10.1016/j.smim.2014.04.003
51. Flynn JL, Goldstein MM, Chan J, Triebold KJ, Pfeffer K, Lowenstein CJ, et al. Tumor necrosis factor-alpha is required in the protective immune response against *Mycobacterium tuberculosis* in mice. *Immunity.* (1995) 2:561–72. doi: 10.1016/1074-7613(95)90001-2
52. Flynn JL, Chan J, Lin PL. Macrophages and control of granulomatous inflammation in tuberculosis. *Mucosal Immunol.* (2011) 4:271–8. doi: 10.1038/mi.2011.14
53. Beamer GL, Flaherty DK, Assogba BD, Stromberg P, Gonzalez-Juarrero M, de Waal Malefyt R, et al. Interleukin-10 promotes *Mycobacterium tuberculosis* disease progression in CBA/J mice. *J Immunol.* (2008) 181:5545–50. doi: 10.4049/jimmunol.181.8.5545
54. Bonecini-Almeida MG, Ho JL, Boechat N, Huard RC, Chitale S, Doo H, et al. Down-modulation of lung immune responses by interleukin-10 and transforming growth factor beta (TGF-beta) and analysis of TGF-beta receptors I and II in active tuberculosis. *Infect Immun.* (2004) 72:2628–34. doi: 10.1128/IAI.72.5.2628-2634.2004
55. Verbon A, Juffermans NP, van Deventer SJ, Speelman P, VanDeutekom HV. Serum concentrations of cytokines in patients with active tuberculosis (TB) and after treatment. *Clin Exp Immunol.* (1999) 115:110–3. doi: 10.1046/j.1365-2249.1999.00783.x
56. Salguero FJ, Gibson S, Garcia-Jimenez W, Gough J, Strickland TS, Vordermeier HM, et al. Differential cell composition and cytokine expression within lymph node granulomas from BCG-vaccinated and non-vaccinated cattle experimentally infected with *Mycobacterium bovis. Transbound Emerg Dis.* (2017) 64:1734–49. doi: 10.1111/tbed.12561
57. DiFazio RM, Mattila JT, Klein EC, Cirrincione LR, Howard M, Wong EA, et al. Active transforming growth factor-beta is associated with phenotypic changes in granulomas after drug treatment in pulmonary tuberculosis. *Fibrogenesis Tissue Repair.* (2016) 9:6. doi: 10.1186/s13069-016-0043-3

21

RNA-Seq Transcriptome Analysis of Peripheral Blood from Cattle Infected with *Mycobacterium bovis* Across an Experimental Time Course

Kirsten E. McLoughlin[1], Carolina N. Correia[1], John A. Browne[1], David A. Magee[1], Nicolas C. Nalpas[1†], Kevin Rue-Albrecht[1†], Adam O. Whelan[2†], Bernardo Villarreal-Ramos[2‡], H. Martin Vordermeier[2‡], Eamonn Gormley[3], Stephen V. Gordon[3,4] and David E. MacHugh[1,4]*

[1] Animal Genomics Laboratory, UCD School of Agriculture and Food Science, UCD College of Health and Agricultural Sciences, University College Dublin, Dublin, Ireland, [2] TB Immunology and Vaccinology Team, Department of Bacteriology, Animal and Plant Health Agency, Weybridge, United Kingdom, [3] UCD School of Veterinary Medicine, UCD College of Health and Agricultural Sciences, University College Dublin, Dublin, Ireland, [4] UCD Conway Institute of Biomolecular and Biomedical Research, University College Dublin, Dublin, Ireland

***Correspondence:**
David E. MacHugh
david.machugh@ucd.ie

†Present address:
Nicolas C. Nalpas, Quantitative Proteomics and Proteome Centre Tübingen, Interfaculty Institute for Cell Biology, University of Tübingen, Tübingen, Germany
Kevin Rue-Albrecht, MRC WIMM Centre for Computational Biology, University of Oxford, Oxford, United Kingdom
Adam O. Whelan, Biomedical Sciences, Defence Science and Technology Laboratory, Salisbury, United Kingdom
‡Bernardo Villarreal-Ramos and H. Martin Vordermeier have positions as Ser Cymru II Professors of Immunology at the Institute of Biological, Environmental & Rural Sciences, Aberystwyth University, Aberystwyth, United Kingdom

Bovine tuberculosis, caused by infection with members of the *Mycobacterium tuberculosis* complex, particularly *Mycobacterium bovis*, is a major endemic disease affecting cattle populations worldwide, despite the implementation of stringent surveillance and control programs in many countries. The development of high-throughput functional genomics technologies, including RNA sequencing, has enabled detailed analysis of the host transcriptome to *M. bovis* infection, particularly at the macrophage and peripheral blood level. In the present study, we have analysed the transcriptome of bovine whole peripheral blood samples collected at −1 week pre-infection and +1, +2, +6, +10, and +12 weeks post-infection time points. Differentially expressed genes were catalogued and evaluated at each post-infection time point relative to the −1 week pre-infection time point and used for the identification of putative candidate host transcriptional biomarkers for *M. bovis* infection. Differentially expressed gene sets were also used for examination of cellular pathways associated with the host response to *M. bovis* infection, construction of *de novo* gene interaction networks enriched for host differentially expressed genes, and time-series analyses to identify functionally important groups of genes displaying similar patterns of expression across the infection time course. A notable outcome of these analyses was identification of a 19-gene transcriptional biosignature of infection consisting of genes increased in expression across the time course from +1 week to +12 weeks post-infection.

Keywords: biomarker, cattle, gene expression, host-pathogen interaction, immune response, time series, tuberculosis, *Mycobacterium bovis*

INTRODUCTION

Bovine tuberculosis (BTB) is caused by *Mycobacterium bovis* and other intracellular bacterial pathogens of the *Mycobacterium tuberculosis* complex (MTBC), which display 99.9% DNA sequence identity at the genome level (1–3). Each member of the MTBC has a distinctive host spectrum, such that tuberculosis (TB) affects a wide range of mammals including humans (4). In addition, BTB has been classified as the fourth most important disease of livestock in terms of zoonotic and economic impact globally (5, 6). It has also been conservatively estimated that BTB costs $3 billion annually and imposes a large financial burden on farmers with infected herds (7, 8). Furthermore, as a zoonosis, *M. bovis* infection has important implications for human health; transmission from cattle to humans does occur and is responsible for a small but significant number of human TB cases, particularly in developing countries (9–11).

Tuberculous mycobacteria—primarily *M. bovis* and *M. tuberculosis*, the main cause of human TB—are generally inhaled from the environment within aerosol droplets and are phagocytosed by host alveolar macrophages (AMs); therefore, infection is normally initiated within, and restricted to, lung tissues (12–15). Tuberculous mycobacteria have evolved a wide range of mechanisms to modulate, suppress, and manipulate specific host immune mechanisms, including inhibition of phagosomal maturation, detoxification of reactive oxygen and nitrogen species (ROS and RNS), repair of ROS- and RNS-induced cellular damage, resistance to antimicrobial and cytokine defences, modulation of antigen presentation, and induction of cellular necrosis and inhibition of apoptosis (16–19). Tuberculous disease is characterised by lesions located at the site of infection, which are formed when AMs and other immune cells engage and eliminate most of the bacilli. The remaining intact mycobacterial cells are confined in granulomas that act to contain the infection, but may, under certain conditions, actually facilitate expansion and dissemination of mycobacteria to spread infection (20–22).

In Ireland, a test and slaughter policy for BTB was introduced in the early 1950s as part of the national BTB eradication scheme (23, 24). This policy includes compulsory screening of all animals using the single intradermal comparative tuberculin test alone or in conjunction with an *in vitro* enzyme-linked immunosorbent assay-based interferon γ (IFN-γ) release assay (IGRA) that increases the sensitivity of diagnosis (25). However, limitations of current diagnostic methods prevent early and accurate detection and subsequent removal of all infected animals from a herd, thereby contributing to the ongoing persistence of BTB, which continues to impact cattle production in Ireland, the United Kingdom, and other countries (24, 26). Therefore, the most important objective of an effective BTB control strategy—to identify and remove all infected cattle from a herd regardless of the stage of infection—is substantially hindered by current diagnostic technologies. Novel methods of BTB diagnosis are urgently required to augment current test procedures in conjunction with appropriate wildlife reservoir control measures (27).

In recent years, the availability of a well-annotated bovine genome sequence combined with high-throughput functional genomics technologies has provided an unprecedented opportunity to gain a deeper understanding of host–pathogen interaction, identify blood-derived RNA-based biomarkers, and develop new diagnostic methods for BTB caused by infection with *M. bovis* (28–33).

Previous transcriptomics studies of the host immune response to *M. bovis* have been performed using blood-derived RNA obtained from both naturally and experimentally infected animals, as it has been shown that host immune responses occurring in peripheral blood reflect those at the primary site of disease in BTB (34). In this regard, the dynamic transcriptome of circulating blood, which contains a large pool of "biosensors" in the form of RNA transcripts, can reflect physiological and pathological events occurring elsewhere in different tissues and organs, thereby providing a comprehensive overview of the status of the immune system (35, 36). In addition, peripheral blood has provided information on the pathobiology of many diseases; it is accessible and easily collected, making it ideally suited for the development of diagnostic biomarker tests based on transcriptional profiling (37–39).

For the experimental work described here, RNA sequencing (RNA-seq) was used to study the bovine whole peripheral blood transcriptome in response to infection with *M. bovis* across a large-scale 14-week animal infection time course. The main objectives of the study were to examine the host peripheral blood transcriptional responses across the early stages of *M. bovis* infection and identify differentially expressed (DE) genes across the infection time course that represent promising candidate biomarkers for BTB. In addition, we aimed to identify host canonical pathways and interaction networks enriched for DE genes, which may shed light on the immunobiology of *M. bovis* infection in cattle. We also used time-series analysis and Gene Ontology (GO) information to identify functionally important groups of DE genes across the infection time course.

MATERIALS AND METHODS

Overview of Animal Infection Time Course Experiment

Animal resources for the present study were obtained from a 26-week vaccination and challenge experiment of age- and sex-matched cattle infected with *M. bovis* (40–44). Ten male age-matched Holstein–Friesian calves (4–6 months old) were sourced from farms known to be free of BTB disease. The animals used for the experimental work described here were the naive control group (non-vaccinated) for a vaccine efficacy study (40). **Figure 1** shows the experimental schedule used by Dean et al. (40) and details the sampling time points for the 10 non-vaccinated control cattle used for the research work described here.

Inoculation With *M. bovis* Strain AF2122/97

The challenge strain, *M. bovis* AF2122/97 (2, 45), was delivered endobronchially at 2×10^3 colony-forming units per animal using the following procedure described by Whelan et al. (46).

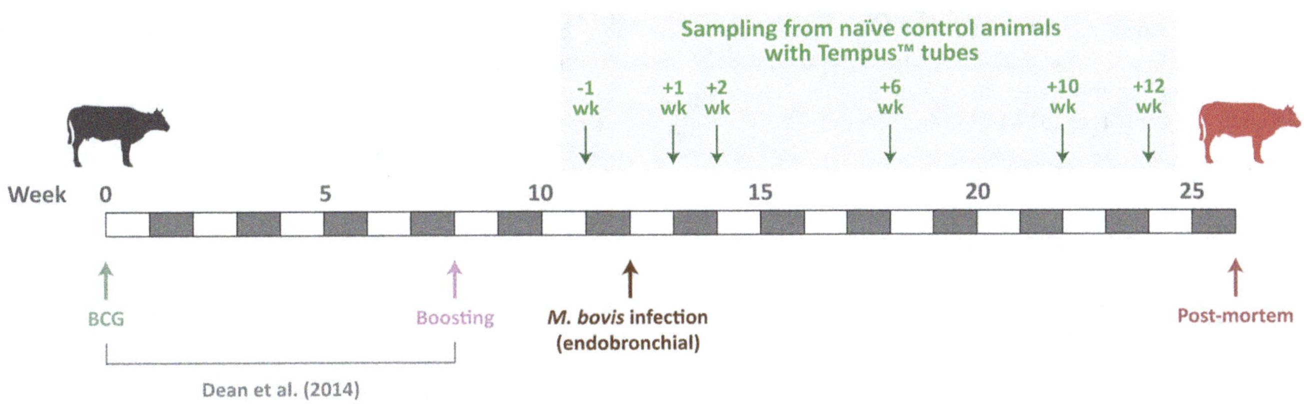

FIGURE 1 | Schedule for the *M. bovis* infection time-course experiment. Sampling time points for the 10 non-vaccinated control cattle used are indicated by green arrows.

Prior to endobronchial inoculation animals were sedated with Rompun® (Bayer Animal Health, Newbury, UK) according to the manufacturer's instructions. Following this, an LSVP 22 VGS89x14 endoscope (Veterinary Endoscopy Services, Welshpool, UK) lubricated with Vet-Lubigel (Millpledge Veterinary, Clarborough, UK) was inserted through a nostril into the trachea and placed above the bronchial opening to the cardiac lobe and the main bifurcation between left and right lobes. A cannula of 1.8-mm internal diameter (Veterinary Endoscopy Services) was inserted through the endoscope and used to deliver the *M. bovis* AF2122/97 inoculum in 2 mL of phosphate-buffered saline (PBS). Following this, an additional 2 mL of PBS was then used to wash the cannula, and the cannula and endoscope were withdrawn. For each individual animal, a new sterile cannula was used, the internal channel of the endoscope, through which the cannula was inserted, was rinsed with 20 mL of PBS, and the outside of the endoscope was cleaned thoroughly with sterilising tissue wipes (Medichem International, Sevenoaks, UK).

Individual responses to infection across the time course and disease pathology for the animals used in this study have been described in detail previously and include whole-blood IFN-γ assay, evaluation of peripheral blood mononuclear cell (PBMC) cytokine responses by intracellular cytokine staining, gross (visible) pathology and histopathology, and evaluation of bacterial load in lymph nodes (40, 41).

Peripheral Blood Collection and Total RNA Extraction

Approximately 3 mL of *ex vivo* peripheral blood was sampled from all 10 naive control animals at −1 week pre-infection and then at +1, +2, +6, +10, and +12 weeks post-infection (**Figure 1**). All blood samples were obtained during the morning (between 7:00 and 10:00 A.M.) of each collection day and directly collected into Tempus™ blood RNA tubes (Applied Biosystems®/Thermo Fisher Scientific, Warrington, UK). Immediately after blood collection at each time point, Tempus™ tube samples for each animal were vortexed for ~10 s to ensure complete red blood cell lysis. Tempus™ tube blood lysate samples for animals at each of the nine time points were then stored at −80°C until they were used for total RNA extraction and purification.

The Tempus™ Spin RNA Isolation Kit (Applied Biosystems®/Thermo Fisher Scientific) was used for total RNA extraction and purification using the following protocol provided by the manufacturer. Tempus™ tube blood lysate samples were thawed at room temperature prior to RNA extraction and purification. Once thawed, for each sample, ~3 mL of blood lysate was transferred to a 50-mL plastic centrifuge tube, and PBS was added to a final volume of 12 mL. Each sample was then mixed by vortexing for 30 s and then centrifuged at 3,000 × *g* for 30 min at 4°C. The supernatant was then removed, and the remaining RNA-containing pellet was resuspended with a brief vortex in 400 μL of the proprietary RNA Purification Resuspension Solution. Following this, the resuspended RNA sample was pipetted into the RNA purification filter inserted into a 1.5-mL microcentrifuge tube for waste collection. The RNA purification filter/microcentrifuge tube was then centrifuged at 16,000 × *g* for 30 s, and the liquid waste and microcentrifuge tube discarded. The RNA purification filter was then placed in a clean microcentrifuge tube, 500 μL of proprietary RNA Purification Wash Solution 1 was added, followed by another centrifugation step at 16,000 × *g* for 30 s and disposal of the liquid waste and microcentrifuge tube. This step was then repeated using 500 μL of proprietary RNA Purification Wash Solution 2 with a centrifugation step at 16,000 × *g* for 30 s. A final wash step was then performed with 500 μL of RNA Purification Wash Solution 2 and centrifugation at 16,000 × *g* for 30 s followed by disposal of the liquid waste and microcentrifuge tube. The RNA purification filter was then placed in a clean microcentrifuge tube and centrifuged at 16,000 × *g* for 30 s to dry the membrane. The RNA purification filter was then inserted into a clean RNase-free collection microcentrifuge tube and 100 μL of Nucleic Acid Purification Elution Solution was added and incubated for 2 min followed by centrifugation at

16,000 × g for 30 s; the RNA eluate was then pipetted back onto the filter membrane, and the centrifugation step was repeated. Approximately 90 μL of the final RNA eluate was then pipetted (avoiding particulate material) into a new labelled RNase-free collection microcentrifuge for long-term storage at −80°C.

RNA Quality Checking and Quantification

RNA quantity and quality checking were performed using a NanoDrop™ 1000 spectrophotometer (Thermo Fisher Scientific, Waltham, MA, USA) and an Agilent 2100 Bioanalyzer using an RNA 6000 Nano LabChip kit (Agilent Technologies, Cork, Ireland). The majority of samples displayed a 260/280 ratio > 1.8 and RNA integrity numbers >8.0 (**Supplementary Table 1** in **Supplementary Material 1**). RNA quality and quantity checking revealed that three samples did not have measurable quantities of RNA, and these were excluded from downstream RNA-seq library preparation (15, ID 6520, +2 weeks; 21, ID 6522, +2 weeks; and 27, ID 6526, + 2 weeks).

Strand-Specific RNA-Seq Library Preparation and Sequencing

For RNA-seq library preparation, 1 μg of total RNA from each sample was used to prepare individually barcoded strand-specific RNA-seq libraries. Two rounds of poly(A)$^+$ RNA purification were performed for all RNA samples using the Dynabeads® mRNA DIRECT™ Micro Kit (Ambion®/Thermo Fisher Scientific, Austin, TX, USA) according to the manufacturer's instructions. The purified poly(A)$^+$ RNA was then used to generate strand-specific RNA-seq libraries using the ScriptSeq™ v2 RNA-Seq Library Preparation Kit, the ScriptSeq™ Index PCR Primers (sets 1–4), and the FailSafe™ PCR enzyme system (all sourced from Epicentre®/Illumina® Inc., Madison, WI, USA) according to the manufacturer's instructions. RNA-seq libraries were purified using the Agencourt® AMPure® XP system (Beckman Coulter Genomics, Danvers, MA, USA) according to the manufacturer's instructions for double size selection (0.75× followed by 1.0× ratio). RNA-seq libraries were quantified using a Qubit® fluorometer and Qubit® dsDNA HS Assay Kit (Invitrogen™/Thermo Fisher Scientific, Carlsbad, CA, USA), whereas library quality cheques were performed using an Agilent 2100 Bioanalyzer and High Sensitivity DNA Kit (Agilent Technologies Ltd.). Individually barcoded RNA-seq libraries were pooled in equimolar quantities, and the quantity and quality of the final pooled libraries (three pools in total) were assessed as described previously. RNA-seq library sample barcode index sequences are detailed in **Supplementary Table 1** (**Supplementary Material 1**).

Prior to high-throughput sequencing, the content of several RNA-seq libraries was validated using conventional Sanger dideoxy sequencing. Library inserts from 16 libraries were cloned using the Zero Blunt® TOPO® PCR Cloning Kit according to the manufacturer's instructions (Invitrogen™/Thermo Fisher Scientific). Sanger sequencing of 36 plasmid inserts from these selected libraries confirmed that the RNA-seq libraries contained inserts derived from bovine mRNA. Plasmid sequencing was outsourced (Source Bioscience Ltd., Dublin, Ireland), and sequences generated were validated using BLAST searching of the DNA sequence database (47). Cluster generation and high-throughput sequencing of the pooled RNA-seq libraries were performed using an Illumina® HiSeq™ 2000 Sequencing System at the MSU Research Technology Support Facility (RTSF) Genomics Core (https://rtsf.natsci.msu.edu/genomics; Michigan State University, MI, USA). Each of the three pooled libraries was sequenced independently on five lanes split across multiple Illumina® flow cells. The pooled libraries were sequenced as paired-end 2 × 100 nucleotide reads using Illumina® version 5.0 sequencing kits. Additionally, after exploratory data analysis (**Supplementary Figures 1, 2**), it was decided to remove animal ID 6522 completely from the analysis and proceed with 52 RNA-seq sample data sets (**Supplementary Table 1** in **Supplementary Material 1**). All RNA-seq data generated for this study have been deposited in the European Nucleotide database with experiment series accession numbers (PRJEB27764 and PRJEB44470).

Bioinformatics Analyses of RNA-Seq Data

Except where indicated, bioinformatics procedures and analyses were performed on a 32-core Compute Server running Linux Ubuntu (version 12.04.2) hosted at the UCD Research IT Data Centre (stampede.ucd.ie) and administered by the UCD Animal Genomics Group. All of the bioinformatics workflow/pipeline components including Linux Bash, Perl, and R scripts used were deposited in a GitHub repository (https://github.com/kmcloughlin1/RNA-sequencing) and were modified from published methods described by our group (48). **Supplementary Figure 3** shows a schematic of the complete RNA-seq bioinformatics workflow and the downstream tools used for time-series analysis and various systems biology methods.

Deconvolution (filtering and segregation of sequence reads based on the unique RNA-seq library barcode index sequences; **Supplementary Table 1** in **Supplementary Material 1**) was performed by the MSU RTSF Genomics Core using a pipeline that simultaneously demultiplexed and converted pooled sequence reads to discrete FASTQ files for each RNA-seq sample with no barcode index mismatches permitted. The RNA-seq FASTQ sequence read data were then downloaded from the MSU RTSF Genomics Core FTP server, and a custom Perl script was used to filter out paired-end reads containing adapter sequence contamination (with up to three mismatches allowed) and to remove poor quality paired-end reads (i.e., one or both reads containing 25% of bases with a Phred quality score <20). The quality of individual RNA-seq sample library files was then reassessed postfiltering using the FastQC software package (version 0.10.1) (49).

Paired-end reads, from each filtered individual library, were aligned to the *Bos taurus* reference genome (UMD3.1.73) (50) using the STAR aligner software package (version 2.3.0) (51). For each library, raw counts for each gene based on the sense strand data were obtained using the featureCounts software from the Subread package (version 1.3.5-p4) (52). The featureCounts parameters were set to unambiguously assign uniquely aligned paired-end reads in a stranded manner to the exons of genes within the UMD3.1.73 *B. taurus* reference genome annotation. The gene count outputs were then used to perform differential gene expression analysis using the edgeR Bioconductor package (version 3.2.4) (53) within an R-based pipeline that was customised to perform the following functions:

1. Use biomaRt (54) to generate a detailed bovine gene annotation for downstream analyses, then filter out all bovine rRNA genes.
2. Filter out genes displaying expression levels below a minimal detection threshold of one count per million in at least $n = 9$ individual libraries (where n = smallest group of biological replicates).
3. Calculate normalisation factors for each library using the trimmed mean of M values method (55).
4. Identify DE genes between the pre-infection animal group (−1 week) and each of the post-infection animal groups (+1, +2, +6, +10, and +12 weeks) using a paired-sample approach with the edgeR package. Differential expression was evaluated by fitting a negative binomial generalised linear model for each gene.
5. Correct for multiple testing using the Benjamini–Hochberg method (56) with a false discovery rate (FDR) threshold of ≤0.05.

Systems Analyses of RNA-Seq Gene Expression Data

The Ingenuity® Pathway Analysis (IPA) software package (57) with the Ingenuity® Knowledge Base (Qiagen Corp., Redwood City, CA, USA; release date July 2014; www.ingenuity.com) was used to identify overrepresented (enriched) canonical pathways and construction of biological interaction networks for sets of DE genes at each post-infection time point (+1, +2, +6, +10, and +12 weeks) compared to the pre-infection time point (−1 week). For identification of overrepresented canonical pathways, a multiple testing correction (Benjamini–Hochberg method) was applied with an FDR threshold ≤0.05. The IPA Biomarker Filter tool was also used to identify and prioritise molecular biomarker candidates such that only experimentally observed and high-confidence predicted biological relationships were included. All the IPA data sources were used for three mammalian species in the IPA Knowledge Base (*Homo sapiens, Mus musculus, Rattus norvegicus*). Biological interaction networks were ranked according to Network Score values generated algorithmically by IPA and based on the hypergeometric distribution and calculated with the right-tailed Fisher exact test (58).

Time-Series Analysis of RNA-Seq Gene Expression Data

Time-series analysis of gene expression data from the animal infection time-course experiment was performed using the Short Time-series Expression Miner (STEM) software package (59). The computational procedure for selecting model profiles that are representative and distinct is described by Ernst et al. (60). The software package implements a method for clustering short time-series expression data that can differentiate between real and random patterns of temporal gene expression changes and assigns each gene to the model profile that most closely matches the temporal gene expression profile for that gene as determined by the correlation coefficient. A permutation test is then used to determine which model profiles have a statistically significant number of genes assigned compared to random expectations from the mean number assigned to each profile based on the permuted data (59). STEM also incorporates GO enrichment functionality for biological interpretation of time-series gene expression data.

RESULTS AND DISCUSSION

RNA-Seq Summary Statistics

Deconvolution and filtering of sequence reads to remove adaptor-dimer contamination yielded a mean of 20.6 ± 2.0 million reads per individual barcoded RNA-seq sample library ($n = 52$ libraries and ± SD); this corresponded to a mean of 82% reads that passed this filtering step. These filtered reads were then aligned to the *B. taurus* UMD3.1.73 genome build. This yielded a mean of 15.4 ± 1.7 million filtered reads (91.5%) that uniquely mapped to this bovine genome build with a mean mapped length of 195.6 ± 0.6 bp; a mean of 0.77 ± 0.19 million reads (4.6%) that mapped to multiple genomic locations and 0.67 ± 0.17 million reads (3.9%) that did not map to any genomic location. Further analysis demonstrated that a mean of 63.1% of the filtered uniquely mapping reads (9.7 ± 1.1 million reads) were assigned to Ensembl gene IDs for the UMD3.1.73 genome build and 36.9% (5.7 ± 0.86 million reads) were ambiguous or could not be assigned to an annotated genomic region. **Supplementary Table 2** (**Supplementary Material 1**) and **Supplementary Figure 4** show the RNA-seq summary statistics. Filtering of the RNA-seq data using 52 samples (60 minus the three technical dropouts and the animal ID 6522 samples at −1, +1, +6, +10, and +12 weeks) produced 12,406 genes suitable for downstream differential expression analysis.

Multidimensional scaling plots (**Supplementary Figure 5**) demonstrated that it was not possible to differentiate the infected animals from non-infected animals during the early stages of the animal infection time course (+1 week post-infection vs. −1 week pre-infection, and +2 weeks vs. −1 week pre-infection). Conversely, discrimination of infected and non-infected animals was partially observed at +6 weeks post-infection and was clearly evident at +10 weeks post-infection, but this pattern of discrimination effectively disappeared by +12 weeks post-infection. Previous work by our group has shown that microarray and RNA-seq gene expression data sets from peripheral blood leukocytes (PBLs) can be used to unambiguously discriminate *M. bovis*–infected from non-infected control cattle (28, 31). However, it is important to note that the *M. bovis*–infected animals used for these earlier studies were heavily infected animals, which were maintained for ongoing disease surveillance and potency testing of diagnostic reagents.

Differentiation of *M. bovis*–Infected and Non-infected Control Groups: Toward the Development of Transcriptomics-Based Biomarkers

The concept and the implications regarding biomarker identification and biosignature development for infectious disease have been explored thoroughly by Chaussabel et al. (36, 61, 62). In particular, these researchers emphasise that leukocytes present in peripheral blood convey valuable information about the status of the immune system that can be translated to biomarkers and onward to sensitive and specific biosignatures of infection. In addition, peripheral blood is easily accessible and can be stabilised and processed for high-throughput transcriptomics analyses using RNA-seq and other massively parallel gene expression technologies such as microarrays. It is also notable that development of transcriptional biomarkers in cattle is relatively straightforward because very low levels of globin gene transcripts (*HBA* and *HBB*) are observed in bovine peripheral blood compared to other mammalian species (63, 64).

Statistical analysis of the RNA-seq gene expression data with a B-H FDR adjusted $P \leq 0.05$ demonstrated that differential gene expression was evident between each of the five post-infection time points (+1, +2, +6, +10, and +12 weeks) and the −1 week pre-infection time point (**Figure 2A**). Relatively small numbers of DE genes were detected at +1 week (37 exhibited increased and 20 exhibited

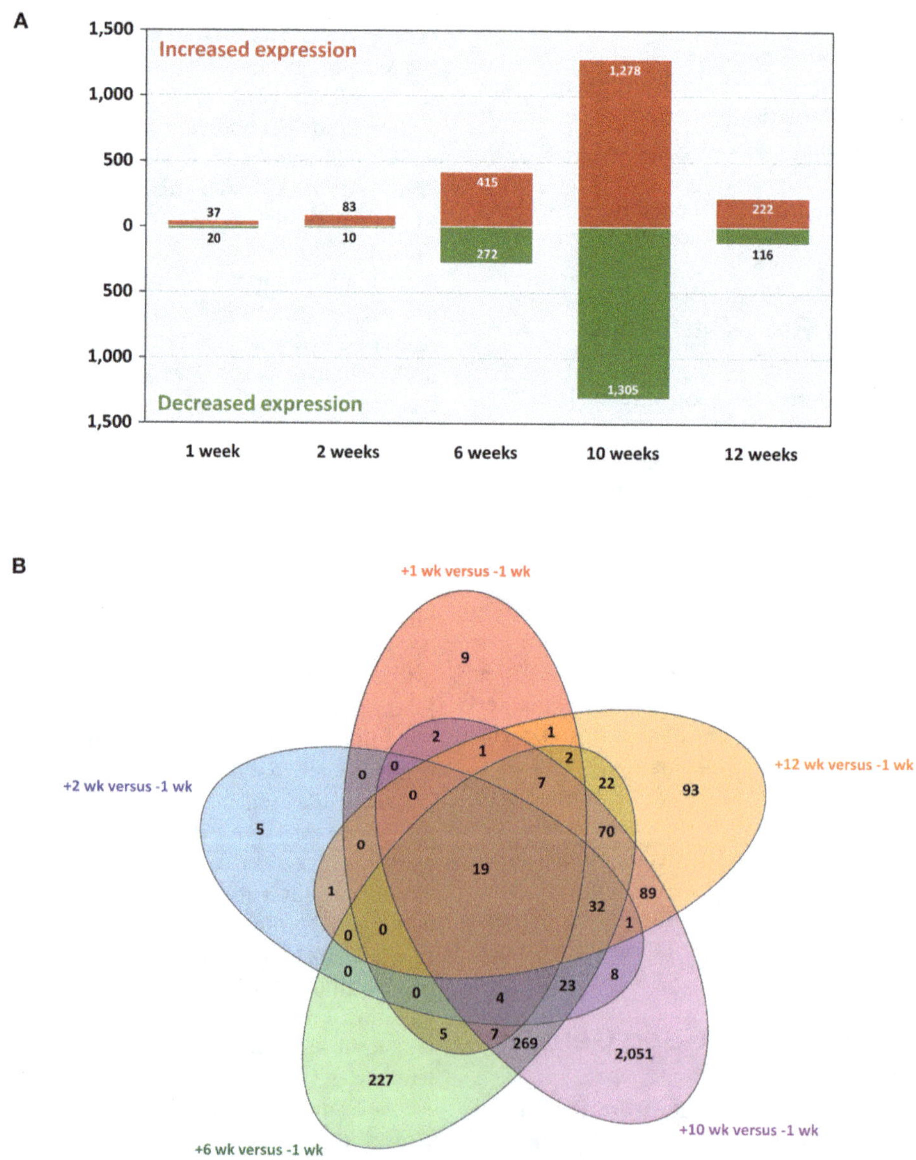

FIGURE 2 | Statistically significant differentially expressed genes. Five post-infection time points are shown relative to the −1 week pre-infection time point (B-H FDR adjusted $P \leq 0.05$). **(A)** Bar graph showing numbers of genes with increased and decreased expression and **(B)** Venn diagram showing the overlaps of DE genes for every multiple-time-point comparison.

decreased expression) and +2 weeks (83 increased and 10 decreased); however, the numbers of DE genes were substantially greater at +6 weeks (415 increased and 272 decreased), +10 weeks (1,278 increased and 1,305 decreased), and +12 weeks (222 increased and 116 decreased). **Supplementary Tables 3–7** (**Supplementary Material 2**) provide detailed information on the differential expression analysis results at each of the five post-infection time points relative to the −1 week pre-infection time point for the complete set of 12,406 filtered genes. **Figure 2B** also shows a Venn diagram for the significant DE genes at each of the five post-infection time points (relative to the −1 week pre-infection control time point). In addition, **Table 1** provides detailed information for 19 genes shown in **Figure 3** that were significantly DE across all the five post-infection time points compared to the −1 week pre-infection control time point.

As shown in **Figure 3**, there is a striking concordance between the patterns of expression for these 19 genes across the infection time course and earlier PBL microarray and RNA-seq studies published by our group (28, 31). These results provide good support for the hypothesis that a biosignature of *M. bovis* infection can be generated using transcriptomics data from cattle with early- and later-stage BTB. It also provides evidence that putative transcriptional biomarkers, identified using an experimental challenge with a relatively high *M. bovis* infectious dose, can be translated as diagnostic tools for use in naturally infected animals. Diagnostic biosignature development focusing on smaller panels of transcriptomics-based biomarkers has been used with notable success for human TB. In this case, research work has focused on specificity and differentiating active TB from latent TB and also TB disease from non-infected controls and diseases with similar pathology but distinct aetiology such as sarcoidosis, pneumonia, and lung cancer (35, 39, 65–71).

Previous work on *M. tuberculosis* and human immunodeficiency virus infection in humans has shown that *CXCR4* is upregulated in blood monocytes and bronchoalveolar lavage cells from human patients with pulmonary TB (72–74). In addition, a loss-of-function mutation in the murine *Thbd* gene that impairs activated protein C production results in uncontrolled lung inflammation in mice infected with *M. tuberculosis*, highlighting the importance of the *THBD* gene in mammalian TB disease (75). Galietti et al. have also shown that *M. tuberculosis*- and *M. bovis*-infected, but not *M. avium*-infected, human monocytes showed increased expression of the CDKN1A protein encoded by *CDKN1A* (76). A range of studies have shown that levels of the protein product of the *PLAUR* gene are elevated in serum from human patients infected with *M. tuberculosis* (77–81). Increased expression of the *OSM* gene and induction of matrix metalloproteinases, which contribute to tissue damage characteristic of TB, have been demonstrated in *M. tuberculosis*-infected human monocytes (82). High expression of *OSM* was also observed in the blood transcriptome of patients presenting with high mycobacterial load sputum (83). In addition, the *OSM* gene is located within a candidate QTL region for TB susceptibility identified using admixture mapping in humans (84).

Ten of the 19 genes that showed consistently increased expression across all post-infection time points were observed to overlap with results from RNA-seq of an *in vitro* infection time-course experiment using bovine AMs stimulated with *M. bovis* (48). *FOSB* and *NR4A1* were upregulated in AMs at 2 hpi; *CXCL8*, *NR4A1*, *PLAUR*, and *RGS16* were upregulated at 6 hpi; *EVI2A*, *CXCL8*, *FOSB*, *HBEGF*, *OSM*, *PLAUR*, *RGS16*, and *THBD* were upregulated at 24 hpi; the eight genes observed at 24 hpi plus the *CDKN1A* gene were also upregulated at 48 hpi.

One of the most notable putative transcriptional biomarkers represented in the panel of 19 genes and in the independent PBL studies is *CXCL8* (previously known as *IL8*). CXCL8 is a chemokine encoded by the *CXCL8* gene, which is a strong neutrophil chemoattractant and also chemotactic for monocytes and T cells (85, 86); it has been observed to exhibit increased expression for different mycobacterial infections in a range of mammalian systems (87–95). CXCL8 enhances killing of mycobacteria by neutrophils and macrophages (96, 97), and these immune cells also secrete CXCL8 when stimulated by *M. tuberculosis* (98). In this regard, Godaly and Young showed that *M. bovis* bacillus Calmette–Guérin (BCG) induces CXCL8 secretion by human neutrophils via MyD88-dependent signalling through TLR2 and TLR4 (99). Also, stimulation of human lung fibroblasts *in vitro* using conditioned medium from *M. tuberculosis*-infected monocytes caused prolonged expression of *CXCL8* mRNA and >10-fold increase in CXCL8 secretion (88).

With regard to the *CXCL8* mRNA transcript as a biomarker of infection, Alessandri et al. were able to detect significantly elevated levels of the CXCL8 cytokine in plasma from patients with pulmonary TB (87). More recently, based on reversion of IGRA test results in a Chinese cohort, it has been proposed that decreased serum levels of CXCL8 are associated with clearance of *M. tuberculosis* infection (100). In addition, using microarray and reverse transcriptase–qualitative polymerase chain reaction technologies, Widdison et al. have shown that *M. tuberculosis*- and *M. bovis*-infected bovine AMs express high levels of *CXCL8* transcripts compared to non-infected control cells (90). In support of this, using RNA-seq, we have shown that *CXCL8* increases in expression in bovine AMs infected with either *M. tuberculosis* or *M. bovis* across a 48-h time course (101). *CXCL8* has also been shown to be significantly increased in expression after *in vitro* PPD-b stimulation of PBMCs from cattle infected with *M. bovis* (102) and bovine monocyte-derived macrophages (103). *CXCL8* also exhibited increased expression in PBL (28) but decreased expression in non-stimulated PBMCs from *M. bovis*-infected cattle (104). Also, Almeida de Souza et al. have shown that antimycobacterial treatment reduces high plasma levels of CXCL8 and other CXC chemokines detected in plasma from human patients with active TB (91), and Huang et al. have also demonstrated that AMs and PBMCs from TB patients express CXCL8 at significantly higher levels than healthy controls (94). Interestingly, the potential specificity of increased *CXCL8* gene expression as a biomarker for *M. bovis* infection in cattle is illustrated by recent results obtained by Alonso-Hearn et al. (105). Using similar RNA-seq methodology, they observed significantly decreased expression of *CXCL8* in peripheral blood from cattle infected with *M. avium* subsp. *paratuberculosis*, the causative agent of Johne disease. Finally, it is important to note that several primary studies and meta-analyses

TABLE 1 | Nineteen genes that exhibited statistically significant differential expression for each of the five post-infection time points vs. the −1 week pre-infection control time point.

Ensembl ID	Gene symbol	Gene name	+1 week post-infection		+2 weeks post-infection		+6 weeks post-infection		+10 weeks post-infection		+12 weeks post-infection	
			Fold-change	B-H FDR *P*-value	Fold-change	B-H FDR *P*-value	Fold-change	B-H FDR *P*-value	Fold-change	B-H FDR *P*-value	Fold-change	B-H FDR *P*-value
ENSBTAG00000000306	*ITK*	IL-2–inducible T-cell kinase	+1.28	0.006848	+1.36	0.000235	+1.23	0.009551	+1.37	0.000001	+1.35	0.000044
ENSBTAG00000000507	*NR4A1*	Nuclear receptor subfamily 4, group A, member 1	+2.51	0.026721	+3.52	0.000214	+4.49	0.000000	+11.04	0.000000	+2.51	0.007555
ENSBTAG00000001060	*CXCR4*	Chemokine (C-X-C motif) receptor 4	+1.99	0.004449	+2.05	0.003150	+2.13	0.000126	+3.09	0.000000	+2.30	0.000037
ENSBTAG00000002758	*THBD*	Thrombomodulin	+1.89	0.033131	+2.01	0.015038	+2.76	0.000001	+3.10	0.000000	+1.86	0.012975
ENSBTAG00000003553	*ZFP36L2*	ZFP36 ring finger protein-like 2	+1.52	0.035631	+1.58	0.020932	+1.69	0.000259	+1.87	0.000001	+1.52	0.011716
ENSBTAG00000003650	*NR4A2*	Nuclear receptor subfamily 4, group A, member 2	+2.49	0.029283	+3.49	0.000308	+4.32	0.000001	+9.96	0.000000	+2.59	0.006347
ENSBTAG00000004305	*RGS16*	Regulator of G-protein signalling 16	+2.42	0.037004	+3.09	0.000829	+2.84	0.000682	+4.84	0.000000	+2.27	0.028004
ENSBTAG00000006806	*KRT17*	Keratin 17	+5.57	0.003229	+7.94	0.000098	+10.26	0.000001	+14.58	0.000000	+4.16	0.010868
ENSBTAG00000008182	*FOSB*	FBJ murine osteosarcoma viral oncogene homologue B	+2.50	0.004449	+4.02	0.000001	+5.05	0.000000	+6.27	0.000000	+2.93	0.000079
ENSBTAG00000008353	*CDKN1A*	Cyclin-dependent kinase inhibitor 1A (p21, Cip1)	+1.71	0.049537	+2.24	0.000142	+2.59	0.000000	+3.73	0.000000	+2.03	0.000391
ENSBTAG00000009354	*EVI2A*	Ecotropic viral integration site 2A	+1.34	0.002116	+1.26	0.047028	+1.43	0.000003	+1.57	0.000000	+1.37	0.000092
ENSBTAG00000013125	*PLAUR*	Plasminogen activator, urokinase receptor	+3.52	0.001379	+5.30	0.000001	+5.96	0.000000	+13.03	0.000000	+3.81	0.000049
ENSBTAG00000016163	*OSM*	Oncostatin M	+2.44	0.029283	+4.03	0.000023	+3.83	0.000003	+6.79	0.000000	+2.61	0.004204
ENSBTAG00000019716	*CXCL8*	Chemokine (C-X-C motif) ligand 8	+3.09	0.001379	+6.56	0.000000	+5.93	0.000000	+14.19	0.000000	+4.87	0.000000
ENSBTAG00000021766	*HBEGF*	Heparin-binding EGF-like growth factor	+3.94	0.001379	+4.18	0.000308	+5.45	0.000001	+9.77	0.000000	+3.00	0.007067
ENSBTAG00000031707	*FRMD6*	FERM domain containing 6	+1.29	0.013896	+1.28	0.022194	+1.36	0.000059	+1.41	0.000001	+1.44	0.000001
ENSBTAG00000035224	—	Uncharacterized protein	+6.24	0.002116	+5.88	0.001857	+7.06	0.000071	+22.21	0.000000	+6.64	0.000304
ENSBTAG00000037608	—	Uncharacterized protein	+2.94	0.030981	+3.43	0.005467	+4.08	0.000066	+9.59	0.000000	+3.07	0.006033
ENSBTAG00000039037	*SERPINB4*	Serpin peptidase inhibitor, clade B	+3.50	0.017337	+4.90	0.000308	+5.58	0.000006	+12.68	0.000000	+4.24	0.000868

Linear mean fold-change values are shown for each gene at each post-infection time point vs. the −1 week pre-infection control time point.

			Animal infection time course - RNA-seq (versus -1 wk)					PBL study	PBL study
			+1 wk	+2 wk	+6 wk	+10 wk	+12 wk	RNA-seq	Microarray
ENSBTAG00000000306	*ITK*	IL2-inducible T-cell kinase	1.28	1.36	1.23	1.37	1.35	1.68	
ENSBTAG00000000507	*NR4A1*	Nuclear receptor subfamily 4, group A, member 1	2.51	3.52	4.49	11.04	2.51	4.04	1.56
ENSBTAG00000001060	*CXCR4*	Chemokine (C-X-C motif) receptor 4	1.99	2.05	2.13	3.09	2.30	3.23	2.48
ENSBTAG00000002758	*THBD*	Thrombomodulin	1.89	2.01	2.76	3.10	1.86	1.50	1.29
ENSBTAG00000003553	*ZFP36L2*	ZFP36 ring finger protein-like 2	1.52	1.58	1.69	1.87	1.52	4.06	
ENSBTAG00000003650	*NR4A2*	Nuclear receptor subfamily 4, group A, member 2	2.49	3.49	4.32	9.96	2.59	7.32	3.22
ENSBTAG00000004305	*RGS16*	Regulator of G-protein signaling 16	2.42	3.09	2.84	4.84	2.27	2.84	1.55
ENSBTAG00000006806	*KRT17*	Keratin 17	5.57	7.94	10.26	14.58	4.16	40.23	5.39
ENSBTAG00000008182	*FOSB*	FBJ murine osteosarcoma viral oncogene homolog B	2.50	4.02	5.05	6.27	2.93		
ENSBTAG00000008353	*CDKN1A*	Cyclin-dependent kinase inhibitor 1A (p21, Cip1)	1.71	2.24	2.59	3.73	2.03	3.01	2.14
ENSBTAG00000009354	*EVI2A*	Ecotropic viral integration site 2A	1.34	1.26	1.43	1.57	1.37		
ENSBTAG00000013125	*PLAUR*	Plasminogen activator, urokinase receptor	3.52	5.30	5.96	13.03	3.81	6.91	4.52
ENSBTAG00000016163	*OSM*	Oncostatin M	2.44	4.03	3.83	6.79	2.61	4.37	
ENSBTAG00000019716	*CXCL8*	chemokine (C-X-C motif) ligand 8	3.09	6.56	5.93	14.19	4.87	5.41	1.70
ENSBTAG00000021766	*HBEGF*	Heparin-binding EGF-like growth factor	3.94	4.18	5.45	9.77	3.00	10.02	
ENSBTAG00000031707	*FRMD6*	FERM domain containing 6	1.29	1.28	1.36	1.41	1.44	2.48	1.30
ENSBTAG00000035224	---	Uncharacterized protein	6.24	5.88	7.06	22.21	6.64		
ENSBTAG00000037608	---	Uncharacterized protein	2.94	3.43	4.08	9.59	3.07	7.83	
ENSBTAG00000039037	*SERPINB4*	Serpin peptidase inhibitor, clade B	3.50	4.90	5.58	12.68	4.24	10.13	

Lowest expression increase — Highest expression increase

FIGURE 3 | Heat map showing linear fold-change values for the panel of 19 consistently DE genes across the *M. bovis* infection course. Linear fold-change values for the post-infection time points are shown relative to the −1 week pre-infection time point. Also shown are the equivalent results obtained using RNA-seq and Affymetrix® GeneChip® Bovine Genome Array technologies by McLoughlin et al. (31).

have provided evidence that a single-nucleotide polymorphism (rs4073) at the human *CXCL8* gene locus is associated with resistance/susceptibility to *M. tuberculosis* infection (106–109).

Functional Biology of Peripheral Blood Gene Expression Across the Infection Time Course

Of the 12,406 genes (50.40% of total *B. taurus* reference genes) that were suitable for differential expression analysis, 10,703 genes (86.27%) were mapped to molecules in the IPA Knowledge Base. IPA was used to identify overrepresented canonical pathways and construct biological interaction networks for sets of DE genes at each post-infection time point (+1, +2, +6, +10, and +12 weeks) compared to the pre-infection control time point (−1 week). Only DE genes that were significant after a multiple testing correction was applied (Benjamini–Hochberg method, FDR threshold ≤0.05) were used. The gene expression data for the panel of 19 genes (**Table 1**) were also analysed using IPA and to identify enriched canonical pathways and biological interaction networks. However, these analyses did not reveal any notable functionally relevant pathways or networks (results not shown).

+1 Week Post-infection Time Point

Forty-eight of the 57 DE genes detected between sample groups at +1 week post-infection and −1 week pre-infection were mapped to the IPA Knowledge Base (84.21%); however, no statistically significant canonical pathways were detected for this gene expression contrast. Four biological interaction networks were generated from this 57-DE-gene set using the IPA Knowledge Base. **Supplementary Figure 6** shows the highest-ranked network, which is associated with embryonic development, organismal development, and reproductive system development and function, and has the ubiquitin C protein encoded by the *UBC* gene as a central hub.

+2 Weeks Post-infection Time Point

Eighty-one of the 93 DE genes detected between sample groups at +2 weeks post-infection and −1 week pre-infection were mapped to the IPA Knowledge Base (87.10%). **Supplementary Table 8** (**Supplementary Material 3**) details the overrepresented IPA canonical pathways for this DE gene set. The top-ranked canonical pathway at +2 weeks post-infection was the *Glucocorticoid Receptor Signalling* pathway with eight genes displaying increased expression (*CDKN1A*, *CXCL8*, *DUSP1*, *FOS*, *IL10*, *PLAUR*, *PTGS2*, and *SGK1*) out of a total of 275 members of this pathway ($P = 1.05 \times 10^{-5}$). The main effects of glucocorticoid steroid hormones signalling through the cytosolic nuclear receptor subfamily 3, group C, member 1 (glucocorticoid receptor) (NR3C1) protein on the immune system are to upregulate expression of anti-inflammatory genes and downregulate expression of proinflammatory genes

(110, 111). Therefore, glucocorticoid receptor signalling activity evident in the peripheral blood transcriptome during the early stages of *M. bovis* infection may reflect perturbation of homeostasis (112) and possible modulation of host cellular mechanisms at the site of infection in the lungs.

Nine biological interaction networks were generated from this 81-DE-gene set using the IPA Knowledge Base. **Figure 4** shows the highest-ranked network, which was centred on increased expression of the *IL10, CXCL2, CXCR4*, and *CXCR2* genes with *Cellular Movement, Haematological System Development and Function*, and *Immune Cell Trafficking* as the top IPA disease and function categories. In this regard, IL-10, an inhibitory and anti-inflammatory pleiotropic cytokine with a major role in suppression of macrophage and dendritic cell functions, has been hypothesised as a target for modulation and manipulation by mycobacterial pathogens (113, 114). Also, IL-10 is linked to chronic mycobacterial infection in the mouse model (115–117). It has been shown that mycobacterial RNA induces IL-10 production in infected cells through TLR3-mediated activation of the PI3K/AKT signalling pathway (118) and that *M. tuberculosis* infection of THP-1 cells induces *IL10* expression through perturbation of the histone deacetylases HDAC6 and HDAC11 (119). In addition, it has been observed that increased levels of IL-10 cytokine in TB patients lead to impaired T-cell function, thereby contributing to an inefficient host immune response (120).

+6 Weeks Post-infection Time Point

Six hundred twenty-six of the 687 DE genes detected between sample groups at +6 weeks post-infection and −1 week pre-infection were mapped to the IPA Knowledge Base (91.12%). **Supplementary Table 9** (**Supplementary Material 3**) details the overrepresented IPA canonical pathways for this DE gene set. Twenty-five biological interaction networks were generated from this 626-DE-gene set using the IPA Knowledge Base, and **Supplementary Figure 7** shows the highest-ranked network, which contains mostly down-regulated focus molecules associated with DNA replication, recombination and repair, and control of gene expression and the cell cycle.

+10 Weeks Post-infection Time Point

For the +10 weeks post-infection vs. −1 week pre-infection contrast, 2,247 of the 2,583 DE genes were mapped to the IPA Knowledge Base (86.99%). **Supplementary Table 10** (**Supplementary Material 3**) details the overrepresented IPA canonical pathways for this DE gene set. The top-ranked canonical pathway was the *Protein Ubiquitination Pathway*, with 40 of 64 entities present in the pathway containing 255 members ($P = 1.36 \times 10^{-11}$) exhibiting decreased expression relative to the −1 week pre-infection group. In this regard, it is noteworthy that *M. tuberculosis* has recently been demonstrated to suppress innate immunity by exploiting the host ubiquitination system (121–124).

Twenty-five biological interaction networks were generated from this 2,247-DE-gene set using the IPA Knowledge Base. **Figure 5** shows the highest-ranked network, which was centred on the amyloid β (A4) precursor protein encoded by the *APP* gene (previously known as *ABPP*) as a central hub, and the top IPA disease and function categories represented were *Antigen Presentation, Carbohydrate Metabolism*, and *Cardiovascular Disease*. Currently, there are few published research works demonstrating differential expression of the *APP* gene during TB in vertebrates (125, 126); however, the presence of this network at +10 weeks post-infection suggests that the represented genes and gene products may have roles in BTB development and host–pathogen interactions. In addition, using RNA-seq, the *APP* gene was also significantly increased in expression in PBL from *M. bovis*–infected cattle compared to non-infected controls (31).

+12 Weeks Post-infection Time Point

There was a marked decrease in the number of DE genes at +12 weeks compared to +10 weeks post-infection, which may reflect control of the infection by the immune system at this stage of the time course. Two hundred ninety-three of the 338 DE genes detected between sample groups at +12 weeks post-infection and −1 week pre-infection were mapped to the IPA Knowledge Base (86.69%). **Supplementary Table 11** (**Supplementary Material 3**) details the overrepresented IPA canonical pathways for this DE gene set. The top-ranked canonical pathway was *T Cell Receptor Signalling* with 12 molecules detected from a total of 97 pathway members ($P = 8.96 \times 10^{-9}$). These 12 genes (*CAMK4, CD247, CD3D, CD3E, CD3G, CD8A, CD8B, FOS, ITK, LCK, PRKCQ*, and *ZAP70*) all displayed increased expression relative to −1 week pre-infection, pointing towards the presence of mycobacterial antigen presentation and T-cell activation via T-cell receptor (TCR) signal transduction (12, 127, 128).

Nineteen biological interaction networks were generated from this 293-DE-gene set using the IPA Knowledge Base, and **Figure 6** shows the highest-ranked network, which was centred on increased expression of the CXCR4, PTGS2, and KLF4 proteins, and the top IPA disease and function categories represented were *Cellular Development, Haematological System Development and Function*, and *Cell-mediated Immune Response*. As described above, the *CXCR4* gene is known to be upregulated in blood monocytes and bronchoalveolar lavage cells from human patients with pulmonary TB (74). In addition, the *PTGS2* gene (previously known as *COX-2*) encodes prostaglandin-endoperoxide synthase 2, a key enzyme in prostaglandin biosynthesis, which is known to be triggered in macrophages—via a TLR2-dependent mechanism—by ESAT-6 proteins secreted by virulent *M. tuberculosis* and *M. bovis* (129). In this regard, it has been hypothesised that induction of PTGS2 may facilitate intracellular mycobacterial survival through inhibition of p53-dependent apoptosis (130). Conversely, it has also been shown that PTGS2 enhances bactericidal activity in *M. tuberculosis*–infected macrophages through promotion of autophagy (131).

The *KLF4* gene encodes a zinc finger–containing transcription factor that regulates macrophage polarisation, displaying increased expression in M2 macrophages and strongly decreased expression in M1 macrophages (132). Integrative network analyses of transcriptome, protein–protein interaction, and transcription factor–binding site data have shown that KLF4 is an important regulator of lung cell gene expression during the early events of *M. tuberculosis* infection in mice (133). It has

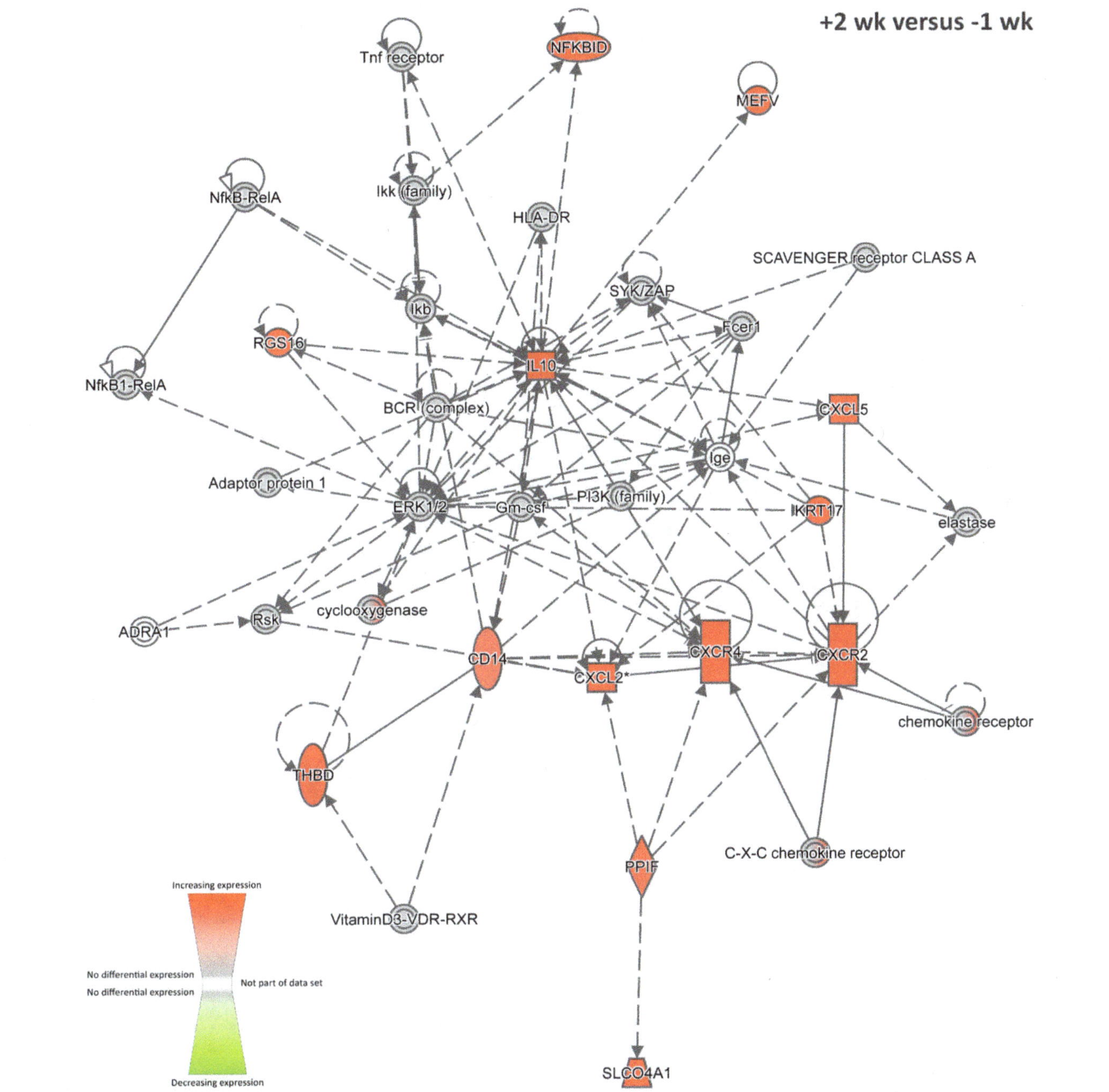

FIGURE 4 | The top-ranked biological interaction network generated using IPA for +2 weeks post-infection. Differential gene expression is represented with a red–green colour scale. This network consisted of 13 focus molecules (IPA Network Score = 24), and the top IPA Disease and Function categories represented were *Cellular Movement*, *Haematological System Development and Function*, and *Immune Cell Trafficking*. A detailed legend for IPA biological interaction networks including a key for node shapes and edge classifications is available.

also been shown that nitric oxide (NO) and KLF4 epigenetically modify class II transactivator protein causing repression of major histocompatibility complex (MHC) class II expression during *M. bovis* BCG infection of murine macrophages (134). Furthermore, downregulation of microRNA-26a during *M. tuberculosis* infection of murine macrophages upregulates KLF4, in turn promoting increased arginase and decreased activity of inducible NO synthase, as well as preventing trafficking of *M. tuberculosis* to lysosomes (135). Taken together, these results support the hypothesis that increased expression of *KLF4* facilitates mycobacterial evasion of host immune surveillance.

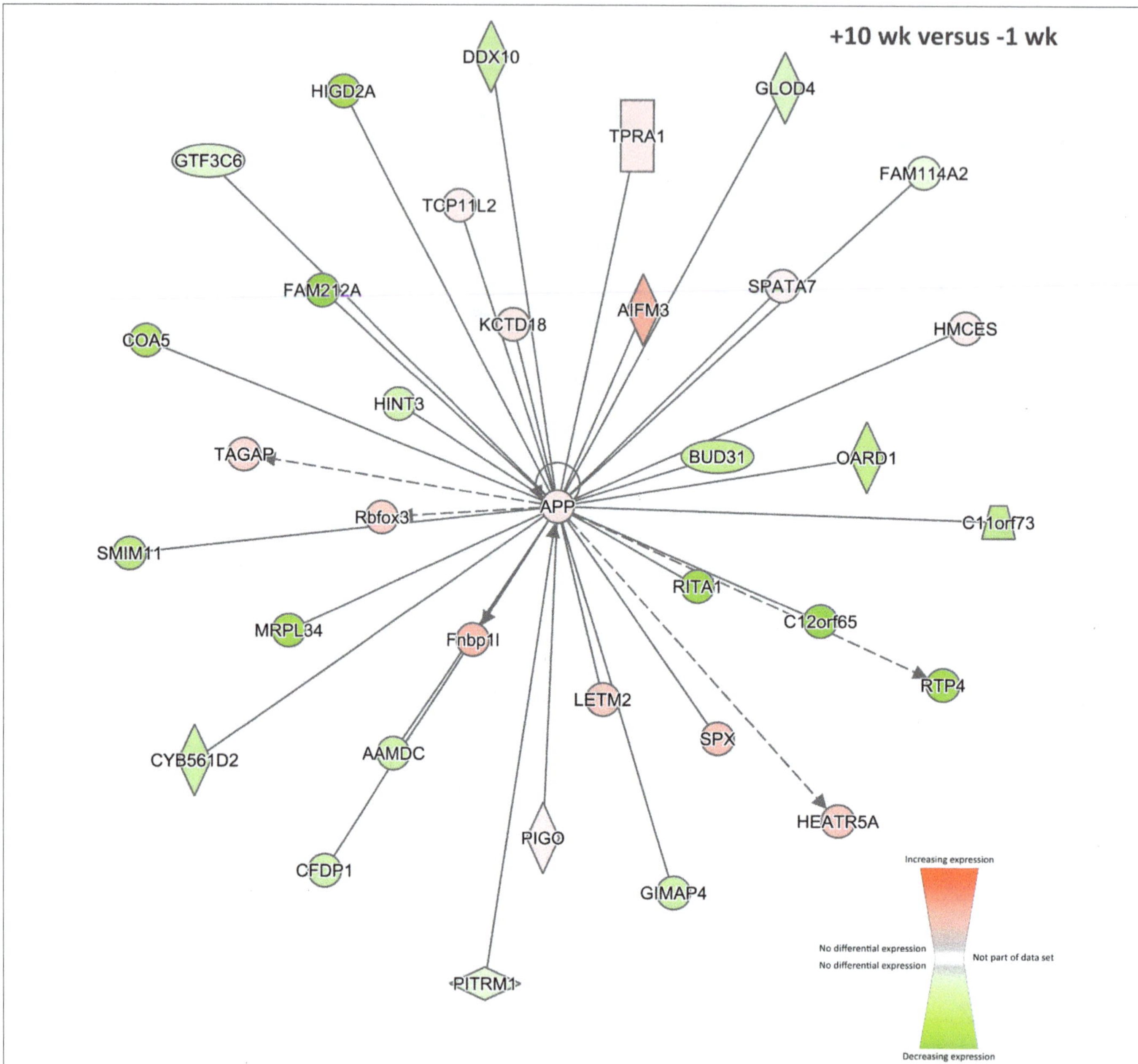

FIGURE 5 | The top-ranked biological interaction network generated using IPA for +10 weeks post-infection. Differential gene expression is represented with a red–green colour scale. This network consisted of 35 focus molecules (IPA Network Score = 39), and the top IPA Disease and Function categories represented were *Antigen Presentation*, *Carbohydrate Metabolism*, and *Cardiovascular Disease*. A detailed legend for IPA biological interaction networks including a key for node shapes and edge classifications is available.

Time-Series Analysis

The STEM tool was designed specifically for analyses of short time-series data sets (3–8 time points) (59, 60) similar to the RNA-gene expression data set obtained from the *M. bovis* animal infection time-course experiment described here. Time-series analysis can be a powerful technique for uncovering networks of coregulated genes in longitudinal time-course experiments (136–138), particularly for gene expression data associated with host immunobiological responses to infection (139–142).

For the present study, STEM time-series analyses of differential gene expression across the *M. bovis* infection time course demonstrated that large groups of genes exhibited comparable patterns of gene expression across the five post-infection time points (+1, +2, +6, +10, and +12 weeks post-infection) relative to the −1 week pre-infection time point. Two different STEM analyses were performed based on (a) expression data for all detectable expressed genes across the infection time course, which corresponded to 4,103 genes (*STEM analysis 1*)

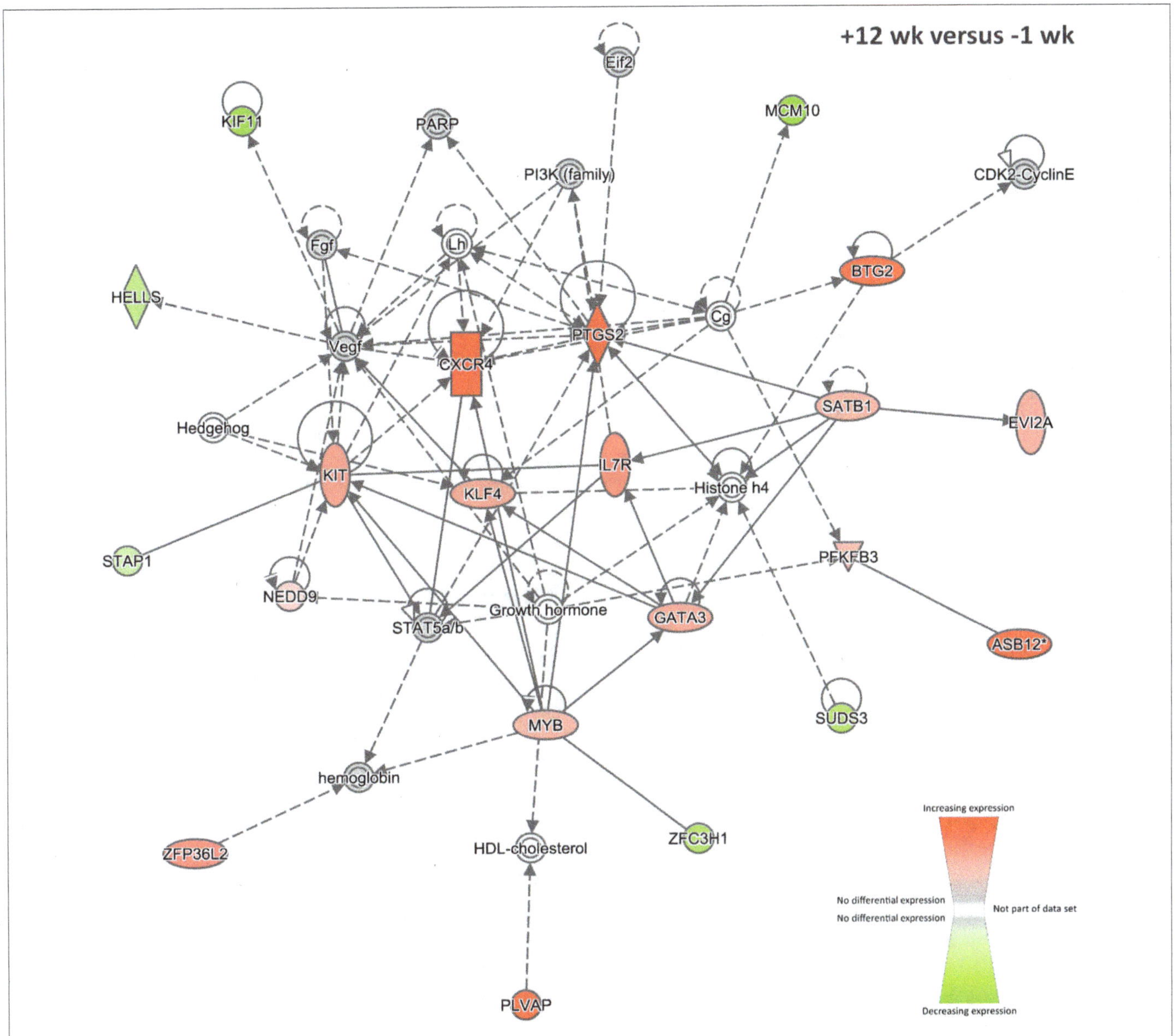

FIGURE 6 | The top-ranked biological interaction network generated using IPA for +12 weeks post-infection. Differential gene expression is represented with a red–green colour scale. This network consisted of 21 focus molecules (IPA Network Score = 33), and the top IPA Disease and Function categories represented were *Cellular Development*, *Haematological System Development and Function*, and *Cell-mediated Immune Response*. A detailed legend for IPA biological interaction networks including a key for node shapes and edge classifications is available.

and (b) the union set of DE genes from all post-infection time points vs. −1 week pre-infection, which corresponded to 2,935 genes (*STEM analysis 2*). **Supplementary Figure 8** shows the top 50 time-series model profiles obtained for *STEM analysis 1* and *STEM analysis 2*.

The top-ranked time-series profiles (by *P*-value) obtained using the two different STEM analyses were very similar. For example, as shown in **Supplementary Table 12** (**Supplementary Material 4**), the first-ranked STEM model profile for *STEM analysis 1* (profile 40; **Figure 7**) was enriched for the *signal transduction*, *single organism signalling*, *cell communication*, *regulation of multicellular organismal process*, and *cellular response to stimulus* GO terms. This profile was also similar to the second-ranked model profile for *STEM analysis 2* (profile 40; **Supplementary Figure 9**), which was enriched for many of the same GO terms (*signal transduction*, *single organism signalling*, *cell communication*; see **Supplementary Table 13**, **Supplementary Material 4**). The third-ranked model profile for *STEM analysis 1* (profile 23; **Supplementary Figure 9**) was highly similar to the first-ranked model profile for *STEM analysis*

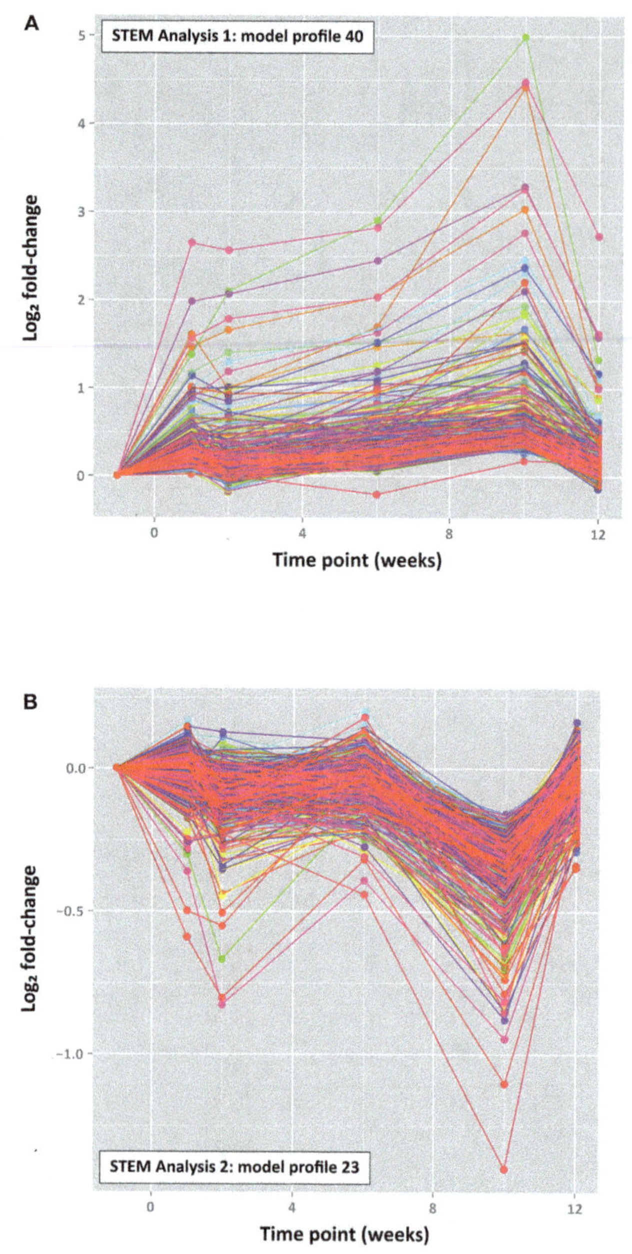

FIGURE 7 | Top-ranked STEM time series profiles. **(A)** The first-ranked model profile (profile 40) for *STEM analysis 1* (4,103 filtered genes) (303 genes assigned; 80.7 genes expected; FDR-adjusted $P = 3.2 \times 10^{-99}$) and **(B)** the first-ranked model profile (profile 23) for *STEM analysis 2* (2,935 filtered genes) (516 genes assigned; 108.9 genes expected; FDR-adjusted $P = 1.6 \times 10^{-187}$). The coloured lines in each model profile represent individual genes.

2 (profile 23; **Figure 7**) with exactly the same overrepresented GO terms (*mitochondrial inner membrane, organelle inner membrane, mitochondrial part, mitochondrial membrane, mitochondrial envelope*; **Supplementary Tables 14, 15, Supplementary Material 4**).

It is interesting to note that STEM profile 40 in each analysis is characterised by a cluster of ~300 genes associated with cell signalling and cellular response to stimuli, which exhibited increasing expression across the four time points with a peak at +10 weeks, followed by a substantial decrease at +12 weeks (**Figure 7**). Conversely, STEM profile 23 (516 genes for *STEM analysis 2*) is characterised by genes associated with mitochondrial components, particularly the mitochondrial membrane, which displayed an oscillating pattern of expression with a marked decrease at +1 week 10 post-infection (**Figure 7**).

These time-dependent patterns of gene expression in peripheral blood may reflect pathogenesis of early BTB disease during the infection time course with concomitant host cellular responses to *M. bovis* infection, disruption of homeostasis, and changing cellular, tissue, and organismal energy requirements (143–145). In addition, it is important to note that although these longitudinal patterns of gene expression may be due to coregulation of genes in the same cluster, they are likely to also reflect fluctuations in peripheral blood cell type populations comparable to those previously observed for comparisons of *M. bovis*-infected and control non-infected cattle (28, 104).

CONCLUSIONS

The results presented here provide good support for the hypothesis that the peripheral blood transcriptome constitutes a source of gene expression biomarkers for BTB caused by *M. bovis* infection in cattle. This is particularly apparent for the panel of 19 genes exhibiting consistently, statistically significantly increased expression across the infection time course, the majority of which (16 genes) were also significantly increased in PBL harvested from an independent cohort of field-infected cattle. However, the sensitivity and specificity of putative transcriptional biosignatures of *M. bovis* infection will need to be verified and validated using larger panels of cattle naturally infected with *M. bovis* and also populations of animals infected with a range of viral and bacterial pathogens.

ETHICS STATEMENT

The animal study was reviewed and approved by Animal & Plant Health Agency (APHA), Animal Use Ethics Committee (UK Home Office PCD number 70/6905).

AUTHOR CONTRIBUTIONS

DMac, SG, EG, KM, AW, BV-R, and HV conceived and designed the project and organised bovine sample collection. KM, NN, DMag, and JB performed RNA extraction and RNA-seq library generation. KM, NN, KR-A, CC, and DMac performed the analyses. KM, CC, and DMac wrote the manuscript. All authors reviewed and approved the final manuscript.

FUNDING

This work was supported by Investigator Grants from Science Foundation Ireland (Nos. SFI/08/IN.1/B2038 and SFI/15/IA/3154), Research Grants from the Department of Agriculture, Food and the Marine (Nos. RSF 06 405 and 17/RD/US-ROI/52), a Department for Environment, Food & Rural Affairs Project Grant (No. SE3224), a European Union Framework 7 Project Grant (No. KBBE-211602-MACROSYS), a Brazilian Science Without Borders—CAPES Grant (No. BEX-13070-13-4), and the UCD Wellcome Trust funded Computational Infection Biology PhD Programme (Grant no. 097429/Z/11/Z).

ACKNOWLEDGMENTS

The authors would like to thank all members of the Animal Services Unit of the APHA, Weybridge for their exemplary care of the animals used in these experiments.

REFERENCES

1. Cole ST, Brosch R, Parkhill J, Garnier T, Churcher C, Harris D, et al. Deciphering the biology of *Mycobacterium tuberculosis* from the complete genome sequence. *Nature.* (1998) 393:537–44. doi: 10.1038/31159
2. Garnier T, Eiglmeier K, Camus JC, Medina N, Mansoor H, Pryor M, et al. The complete genome sequence of *Mycobacterium bovis*. *Proc Natl Acad Sci USA.* (2003) 100:7877–82. doi: 10.1073/pnas.1130426100
3. Brites D, Loiseau C, Menardo F, Borrell S, Boniotti MB, Warren R, et al. A new phylogenetic framework for the animal-adapted *Mycobacterium tuberculosis* complex. *Front Microbiol.* (2018) 9:2820. doi: 10.3389/fmicb.2018.02820
4. Malone KM, Gordon SV. *Mycobacterium tuberculosis* complex members adapted to wild and domestic animals. *Adv Exp Med Biol.* (2017) 1019:135–54. doi: 10.1007/978-3-319-64371-7_7
5. Perry BD, Randolph TF, McDermott JJ, Sones KR, Thornton PK. *Investing in Animal Health Research to Alleviate Poverty.* Nairobi: ILRI (International Livestock Research Institute) (2002).
6. Perry B, Grace D. The impacts of livestock diseases and their control on growth and development processes that are pro-poor. *Philos Trans R Soc Lond B Biol Sci.* (2009) 364:2643–55. doi: 10.1098/rstb.2009.0097
7. Steele JH. Introduction (Part 2 Regional and Country Status Reports). In: Thoen CO, Steele JH, editors, *Mycobacterium bovis Infection in Animals and Humans.* Ames, IA: Iowa State University Press (1995). p. 169–72.
8. Waters WR, Palmer MV, Buddle BM, Vordermeier HM. Bovine tuberculosis vaccine research: historical perspectives and recent advances. *Vaccine.* (2012) 30:2611–22. doi: 10.1016/j.vaccine.2012.02.018
9. Olea-Popelka F, Muwonge A, Perera A, Dean AS, Mumford E, Erlacher-Vindel E, et al. Zoonotic tuberculosis in human beings caused by *Mycobacterium bovis* – a call for action. *Lancet Infect Dis.* (2017) 17:e21–e5. doi: 10.1016/S1473-3099(16)30139-6
10. Kanipe C, Palmer MV. *Mycobacterium bovis* and you: a comprehensive look at the bacteria, its similarities to *Mycobacterium tuberculosis*, and its relationship with human disease. *Tuberculosis.* (2020) 125:102006. doi: 10.1016/j.tube.2020.102006
11. Luciano SA, Roess A. Human zoonotic tuberculosis and livestock exposure in low- and middle-income countries: a systematic review identifying challenges in laboratory diagnosis. *Zoonoses Public Health.* (2020) 67:97–111. doi: 10.1111/zph.12684
12. O'Garra A, Redford PS, McNab FW, Bloom CI, Wilkinson RJ, Berry MP. The immune response in tuberculosis. *Annu Rev Immunol.* (2013) 31:475–527. doi: 10.1146/annurev-immunol-032712-095939
13. Domingo M, Vidal E, Marco A. Pathology of bovine tuberculosis. *Res Vet Sci.* (2014) 97:S20–9. doi: 10.1016/j.rvsc.2014.03.017
14. Pai M, Behr MA, Dowdy D, Dheda K, Divangahi M, Boehme CC, et al. Tuberculosis. *Nat Rev Dis Primers.* (2016) 2:16076. doi: 10.1038/nrdp.2016.76
15. Scriba TJ, Coussens AK, Fletcher HA. Human immunology of tuberculosis. *Microbiol Spectr.* (2016) 4. doi: 10.1128/9781555819569.ch11
16. de Chastellier C. The many niches and strategies used by pathogenic mycobacteria for survival within host macrophages. *Immunobiology.* (2009) 214:526–42. doi: 10.1016/j.imbio.2008.12.005
17. Cambier CJ, Falkow S, Ramakrishnan L. Host evasion and exploitation schemes of *Mycobacterium tuberculosis*. *Cell.* (2014) 159:1497–509. doi: 10.1016/j.cell.2014.11.024
18. Schorey JS, Schlesinger LS. Innate immune responses to tuberculosis. *Microbiol Spectr.* (2016) 4. doi: 10.1128/microbiolspec.TBTB2-0010-2016
19. Awuh JA, Flo TH. Molecular basis of mycobacterial survival in macrophages. *Cell Mol Life Sci.* (2017) 74:1625–48. doi: 10.1007/s00018-016-2422-8
20. Martinot AJ. Microbial offense vs host defense: who controls the TB granuloma? *Vet Pathol.* (2018) 55:14–26. doi: 10.1177/0300985817705177
21. Pagan AJ, Ramakrishnan L. The formation and function of granulomas. *Annu Rev Immunol.* (2018) 36:639–65. doi: 10.1146/annurev-immunol-032712-100022
22. Cassidy JP. TB or not TB? The granuloma is the question. *Vet Pathol.* (2019) 56:508–9. doi: 10.1177/0300985819844815
23. More SJ, Good M. Understanding and managing bTB risk: perspectives from Ireland. *Vet Microbiol.* (2015) 176:209–18. doi: 10.1016/j.vetmic.2015.01.026
24. More SJ. Can bovine TB be eradicated from the Republic of Ireland? Could this be achieved by 2030? *Ir Vet J.* (2019) 72:3. doi: 10.1186/s13620-019-0140-x
25. Gormley E, Doyle MB, Fitzsimons T, McGill K, Collins JD. Diagnosis of *Mycobacterium bovis* infection in cattle by use of the gamma-interferon (Bovigam) assay. *Vet Microbiol.* (2006) 112:171–9. doi: 10.1016/j.vetmic.2005.11.029
26. Allen AR, Skuce RA, Byrne AW. Bovine tuberculosis in Britain and Ireland - a perfect storm? The confluence of potential ecological and epidemiological impediments to controlling a chronic infectious disease. *Front Vet Sci.* (2018) 5:109. doi: 10.3389/fvets.2018.00109
27. Vordermeier HM, Jones GJ, Buddle BM, Hewinson RG, Villarreal-Ramos B. Bovine tuberculosis in cattle: vaccines, DIVA tests, and host biomarker discovery. *Annu Rev Anim Biosci.* (2016) 4:87–109. doi: 10.1146/annurev-animal-021815-111311
28. Killick KE, Browne JA, Park SD, Magee DA, Martin I, Meade KG, et al. Genome-wide transcriptional profiling of peripheral blood leukocytes from cattle infected with *Mycobacterium bovis* reveals suppression of host immune genes. *BMC Genomics.* (2011) 12:611. doi: 10.1186/1471-2164-12-611
29. Aranday-Cortes E, Hogarth PJ, Kaveh DA, Whelan AO, Villarreal-Ramos B, Lalvani A, et al. Transcriptional profiling of disease-induced host responses in bovine tuberculosis and the identification of potential diagnostic biomarkers. *PLoS ONE.* (2012) 7:e30626. doi: 10.1371/journal.pone.0030626
30. Blanco FC, Soria M, Bianco MV, Bigi F. Transcriptional response of peripheral blood mononuclear cells from cattle infected with *Mycobacterium bovis*. *PLoS ONE.* (2012) 7:e41066. doi: 10.1371/journal.pone.0041066

31. McLoughlin KE, Nalpas NC, Rue-Albrecht K, Browne JA, Magee DA, Killick KE, et al. RNA-seq transcriptional profiling of peripheral blood leukocytes from cattle infected with *Mycobacterium bovis*. *Front Immunol.* (2014) 5:396. doi: 10.3389/fimmu.2014.00396
32. Klepp LI, Eirin ME, Garbaccio S, Soria M, Bigi F, Blanco FC. Identification of bovine tuberculosis biomarkers to detect tuberculin skin test and IFNγ release assay false negative cattle. *Res Vet Sci.* (2019) 122:7-14. doi: 10.1016/j.rvsc.2018.10.016
33. Wiarda JE, Boggiatto PM, Bayles DO, Waters WR, Thacker TC, Palmer MV. Severity of bovine tuberculosis is associated with innate immune-biased transcriptional signatures of whole blood in early weeks after experimental *Mycobacterium bovis* infection. *PLoS ONE.* (2020) 15:e0239938. doi: 10.1371/journal.pone.0239938
34. Rhodes SG, Buddle BM, Hewinson RG, Vordermeier HM. Bovine tuberculosis: immune responses in the peripheral blood and at the site of active disease. *Immunology.* (2000) 99:195–202. doi: 10.1046/j.1365-2567.2000.00944.x
35. Blankley S, Berry MP, Graham CM, Bloom CI, Lipman M, O'Garra A. The application of transcriptional blood signatures to enhance our understanding of the host response to infection: the example of tuberculosis. *Philos Trans R Soc Lond B Biol Sci.* (2014) 369:20130427. doi: 10.1098/rstb.2013.0427
36. Chaussabel D. Assessment of immune status using blood transcriptomics and potential implications for global health. *Semin Immunol.* (2015) 27:58-66. doi: 10.1016/j.smim.2015.03.002
37. Correia CN, Nalpas NC, McLoughlin KE, Browne JA, Gordon SV, MacHugh DE, et al. Circulating microRNAs as potential biomarkers of infectious disease. *Front Immunol.* (2017) 8:118. doi: 10.3389/fimmu.2017.00118
38. Faherty O'Donnell SL, Correia CN, MacHugh DE. CHAPTER 4: MicroRNAs and mycobacterial infections in humans and domestic animals. In: Peplow PV, Martinez B, Calin GA, Esquela-Kerscher A, editors. *MicroRNAs in Diseases and Disorders: Emerging Therapeutic Targets.* Cambridge, MK: The Royal Society of Chemistry (2019). p. 105–32. doi: 10.1039/9781788016421-00105
39. Maertzdorf J, McEwen G, Weiner III J, Tian S, Lader E, Schriek U, et al. Concise gene signature for point-of-care classification of tuberculosis. *EMBO Mol Med.* (2016) 8:86–95. doi: 10.15252/emmm.201505790
40. Dean G, Whelan A, Clifford D, Salguero FJ, Xing Z, Gilbert S, et al. Comparison of the immunogenicity and protection against bovine tuberculosis following immunization by BCG-priming and boosting with adenovirus or protein based vaccines. *Vaccine.* (2014) 32:1304-10. doi: 10.1016/j.vaccine.2013.11.045
41. Dean GS, Clifford D, Whelan AO, Tchilian EZ, Beverley PC, Salguero FJ, et al. Protection induced by simultaneous subcutaneous and endobronchial vaccination with BCG/BCG and BCG/adenovirus expressing antigen 85A against *Mycobacterium bovis* in cattle. *PLoS ONE.* (2015) 10:e0142270. doi: 10.1371/journal.pone.0142270
42. Metcalfe HJ, Steinbach S, Jones GJ, Connelley T, Morrison WI, Vordermeier M, et al. Protection associated with a TB vaccine is linked to increased frequency of Ag85A-specific CD4(+) T cells but no increase in avidity for Ag85A. *Vaccine.* (2016) 34:4520–5. doi: 10.1016/j.vaccine.2016.07.055
43. Jones GJ, Coad M, Khatri B, Bezos J, Parlane NA, Buddle BM, et al. Tuberculin skin testing boosts interferon gamma responses to DIVA reagents in *Mycobacterium bovis*-infected cattle. *Clin Vaccine Immunol.* (2017) 24:e00551-16. doi: 10.1128/CVI.00551-16
44. Salguero FJ, Gibson S, Garcia-Jimenez W, Gough J, Strickland TS, Vordermeier HM, et al. Differential cell composition and cytokine expression within lymph node granulomas from BCG-vaccinated and non-vaccinated cattle experimentally infected with *Mycobacterium bovis*. *Transbound Emerg Dis.* (2017) 64:1734–49. doi: 10.1111/tbed.12561
45. Malone KM, Farrell D, Stuber TP, Schubert OT, Aebersold R, Robbe-Austerman S, et al. Updated reference genome sequence and annotation of *Mycobacterium bovis* AF2122/97. *Genome Announc.* (2017) 5:e00157-17. doi: 10.1128/genomeA.00157-17
46. Whelan A, Court P, Xing Z, Clifford D, Hogarth PJ, Vordermeier M, et al. Immunogenicity comparison of the intradermal or endobronchial boosting of BCG vaccinates with Ad5-85A. *Vaccine.* (2012) 30:6294-300. doi: 10.1016/j.vaccine.2012.07.086
47. Johnson M, Zaretskaya I, Raytselis Y, Merezhuk Y, McGinnis S, Madden TL. NCBI BLAST: a better web interface. *Nucleic Acids Res.* (2008) 36:W5-9. doi: 10.1093/nar/gkn201
48. Nalpas NC, Magee DA, Conlon KM, Browne JA, Healy C, McLoughlin KE, et al. RNA sequencing provides exquisite insight into the manipulation of the alveolar macrophage by tubercle bacilli. *Sci Rep.* (2015) 5:13629. doi: 10.1038/srep13629
49. Andrews S. *FastQC - A Quality Control Tool for High Throughput Sequence Data.* (2016). Available online at: http://www.bioinformatics.babraham.ac.uk/projects/fastqc/
50. Zimin AV, Delcher AL, Florea L, Kelley DR, Schatz MC, Puiu D, et al. A whole-genome assembly of the domestic cow, *Bos taurus*. *Genome Biol.* (2009) 10:R42. doi: 10.1186/gb-2009-10-4-r42
51. Dobin A, Davis CA, Schlesinger F, Drenkow J, Zaleski C, Jha S, et al. STAR: ultrafast universal RNA-seq aligner. *Bioinformatics.* (2013) 29:15-21. doi: 10.1093/bioinformatics/bts635
52. Liao Y, Smyth GK, Shi W. featureCounts: an efficient general purpose program for assigning sequence reads to genomic features. *Bioinformatics.* (2014) 30:923–30. doi: 10.1093/bioinformatics/btt656
53. Robinson MD, McCarthy DJ, Smyth GK. edgeR: a Bioconductor package for differential expression analysis of digital gene expression data. *Bioinformatics.* (2010) 26:139–40. doi: 10.1093/bioinformatics/btp616
54. Durinck S, Moreau Y, Kasprzyk A, Davis S, De Moor B, Brazma A, et al. BioMart and Bioconductor: a powerful link between biological databases and microarray data analysis. *Bioinformatics.* (2005) 21:3439-40. doi: 10.1093/bioinformatics/bti525
55. Robinson MD, Oshlack A. A scaling normalization method for differential expression analysis of RNA-seq data. *Genome Biol.* (2010) 11:R25. doi: 10.1186/gb-2010-11-3-r25
56. Benjamini Y, Hochberg Y. Controlling the false discovery rate - a practical and powerful approach to multiple testing. *J R Stat Soc Ser B Methodol.* (1995) 57:289–300. doi: 10.1111/j.2517-6161.1995.tb02031.x
57. Kramer A, Green J, Pollard J Jr, Tugendreich S. Causal analysis approaches in ingenuity pathway analysis. *Bioinformatics.* (2014) 30:523-30. doi: 10.1093/bioinformatics/btt703
58. Agresti A. A survey of exact inference for contingency tables. *Statist Sci.* (1992) 7:131–53. doi: 10.1214/ss/1177011454
59. Ernst J, Bar-Joseph Z. STEM: a tool for the analysis of short time series gene expression data. *BMC Bioinformatics.* (2006) 7:191. doi: 10.1186/1471-2105-7-191
60. Ernst J, Nau GJ, Bar-Joseph Z. Clustering short time series gene expression data. *Bioinformatics.* (2005) 1:i159–68. doi: 10.1093/bioinformatics/bti1022
61. Chaussabel D, Quinn C, Shen J, Patel P, Glaser C, Baldwin N, et al. A modular analysis framework for blood genomics studies: application to systemic lupus erythematosus. *Immunity.* (2008) 29:150-64. doi: 10.1016/j.immuni.2008.05.012
62. Chaussabel D, Pascual V, Banchereau J. Assessing the human immune system through blood transcriptomics. *BMC Biol.* (2010) 8:84. doi: 10.1186/1741-7007-8-84
63. Hossain MA, Yamato O, Yamasaki M, Otsuka Y, Maede Y. Relation between reticulocyte count and characteristics of erythrocyte 5'-nucleotidase in dogs, cats, cattle and humans. *J Vet Med Sci.* (2003) 65:193-197. doi: 10.1292/jvms.65.193
64. Correia CN, McLoughlin KE, Nalpas NC, Magee DA, Browne JA, Rue-Albrecht K, et al. RNA sequencing (RNA-seq) reveals extremely low levels of reticulocyte-derived globin gene transcripts in peripheral blood from horses (Equus caballus) and cattle (*Bos taurus*). *Front Genet.* (2018) 9:278. doi: 10.3389/fgene.2018.00278
65. Berry MP, Graham CM, McNab FW, Xu Z, Bloch SA, Oni T, et al. An interferon-inducible neutrophil-driven blood transcriptional signature in human tuberculosis. *Nature.* (2010) 466:973–7. doi: 10.1038/nature09247
66. Maertzdorf J, Weiner, J. III., Mollenkopf HJ, Bornot TB, Network BT, et al. Common patterns and disease-related signatures in tuberculosis and sarcoidosis. *Proc Natl Acad Sci USA.* (2012) 109:7853–8. doi: 10.1073/pnas.1121072109
67. Cliff JM, Kaufmann SH, McShane H, van Helden P, O'Garra A. The human immune response to tuberculosis and its treatment: a view

from the blood. *Immunol Rev.* (2015) 264:88–102. doi: 10.1111/imr.12269

68. Blankley S, Graham CM, Turner J, Berry MP, Bloom CI, Xu Z, et al. The transcriptional signature of active tuberculosis reflects symptom status in extra-pulmonary and pulmonary tuberculosis. *PLoS ONE.* (2016) 11:e0162220. doi: 10.1371/journal.pone.0162220
69. Sweeney TE, Braviak L, Tato CM, Khatri P. Genome-wide expression for diagnosis of pulmonary tuberculosis: a multicohort analysis. *Lancet Respir Med.* (2016) 4:213–24. doi: 10.1016/S2213-2600(16)00048-5
70. Leong S, Zhao Y, Joseph NM, Hochberg NS, Sarkar S, Pleskunas J, et al. Existing blood transcriptional classifiers accurately discriminate active tuberculosis from latent infection in individuals from south India. *Tuberculosis.* (2018) 109:41–51. doi: 10.1016/j.tube.2018.01.002
71. Estévez O, Anibarro L, Garet E, Pallares Á, Barcia L, Calviño L, et al. An RNA-seq based machine learning approach identifies latent tuberculosis patients with an active tuberculosis profile. *Front Immunol.* (2020) 11:1470. doi: 10.3389/fimmu.2020.01470
72. Hoshino Y, Tse DB, Rochford G, Prabhakar S, Hoshino S, Chitkara N, et al. *Mycobacterium tuberculosis*-induced CXCR4 and chemokine expression leads to preferential X4 HIV-1 replication in human macrophages. *J Immunol.* (2004) 172:6251–8. doi: 10.4049/jimmunol.172.10.6251
73. Rosas-Taraco AG, Arce-Mendoza AY, Caballero-Olin G, Salinas-Carmona MC. *Mycobacterium tuberculosis* upregulates coreceptors CCR5 and CXCR4 while HIV modulates CD14 favoring concurrent infection. *AIDS Res Hum Retroviruses.* (2006) 22:45–51. doi: 10.1089/aid.2006.22.45
74. Shankar EM, Vignesh R, Ellegard R, Barathan M, Chong YK, Bador MK, et al. HIV-*Mycobacterium tuberculosis* co-infection: a 'danger-couple model' of disease pathogenesis. *Pathog Dis.* (2014) 70:110–8. doi: 10.1111/2049-632X.12108
75. Weijer S, Wieland CW, Florquin S, van der Poll T. A thrombomodulin mutation that impairs activated protein C generation results in uncontrolled lung inflammation during murine tuberculosis. *Blood.* (2005) 106:2761–8. doi: 10.1182/blood-2004-12-4623
76. Galietti F, Bollo E, Cappia S, Dondo A, Pregel P, Nicali R, et al. p53 expression in cultured blood human monocytes infected with mycobacterial strains. *Panminerva Med.* (2001) 43:249–55.
77. Juffermans NP, Dekkers PE, Verbon A, Speelman P, van Deventer SJ, van der Poll T. Concurrent upregulation of urokinase plasminogen activator receptor and CD11b during tuberculosis and experimental endotoxemia. *Infect Immun.* (2001) 69:5182–5. doi: 10.1128/IAI.69.8.5182-5185.2001
78. Eugen-Olsen J, Gustafson P, Sidenius N, Fischer TK, Parner J, Aaby P, et al. The serum level of soluble urokinase receptor is elevated in tuberculosis patients and predicts mortality during treatment: a community study from Guinea-Bissau. *Int J Tuberc Lung Dis.* (2002) 6:686–92.
79. Ostrowski SR, Ravn P, Hoyer-Hansen G, Ullum H, Andersen AB. Elevated levels of soluble urokinase receptor in serum from mycobacteria infected patients: still looking for a marker of treatment efficacy. *Scand J Infect Dis.* (2006) 38:1028–32. doi: 10.1080/00365540600868305
80. Djoba Siawaya JF, Bapela NB, Ronacher K, Veenstra H, Kidd M, Gie R, et al. Immune parameters as markers of tuberculosis extent of disease and early prediction of anti-tuberculosis chemotherapy response. *J Infect.* (2008) 56:340–7. doi: 10.1016/j.jinf.2008.02.007
81. Araujo Z, Macias-Segura N, Lopez-Ramos JE, De Waard JH, Vanegas M, Patarroyo MA, et al. Diagnostic accuracy of combinations of serological biomarkers for identifying clinical tuberculosis. *J Infect Dev Ctries.* (2018) 12:429–41. doi: 10.3855/jidc.9554
82. O'Kane CM, Elkington PT, Friedland JS. Monocyte-dependent oncostatin M and TNF-alpha synergize to stimulate unopposed matrix metalloproteinase-1/3 secretion from human lung fibroblasts in tuberculosis. *Eur J Immunol.* (2008) 38:1321–30. doi: 10.1002/eji.200737855
83. Dupnik KM, Bean JM, Lee MH, Jean Juste MA, Skrabanek L, Rivera V, et al. Blood transcriptomic markers of *Mycobacterium tuberculosis* load in sputum. *Int J Tuberc Lung Dis.* (2018) 22:950–8. doi: 10.5588/ijtld.17.0855
84. Daya M, van der Merwe L, Gignoux CR, van Helden PD, Moller M, Hoal EG. Using multi-way admixture mapping to elucidate TB susceptibility in the South African Coloured population. *BMC Genomics.* (2014) 15:1021. doi: 10.1186/1471-2164-15-1021
85. Zhang Y, Broser M, Cohen H, Bodkin M, Law K, Reibman J, et al. Enhanced interleukin-8 release and gene expression in macrophages after exposure to *Mycobacterium tuberculosis* and its components. *J Clin Invest.* (1995) 95:586–92. doi: 10.1172/JCI117702
86. Gerszten RE, Garcia-Zepeda EA, Lim YC, Yoshida M, Ding HA, Gimbrone, et al. MCP-1 and IL-8 trigger firm adhesion of monocytes to vascular endothelium under flow conditions. *Nature.* (1999) 398:718–23. doi: 10.1038/19546
87. Alessandri AL, Souza AL, Oliveira SC, Macedo GC, Teixeira MM, Teixeira AL. Concentrations of CXCL8, CXCL9 and sTNFR1 in plasma of patients with pulmonary tuberculosis undergoing treatment. *Inflamm Res.* (2006) 55:528–33. doi: 10.1007/s00011-006-5136-9
88. O'Kane CM, Boyle JJ, Horncastle DE, Elkington PT, Friedland JS. Monocyte-dependent fibroblast CXCL8 secretion occurs in tuberculosis and limits survival of mycobacteria within macrophages. *J Immunol.* (2007) 178:3767–76. doi: 10.4049/jimmunol.178.6.3767
89. Sawant KV, McMurray DN. Guinea pig neutrophils infected with *Mycobacterium tuberculosis* produce cytokines which activate alveolar macrophages in noncontact cultures. *Infect Immun.* (2007) 75:1870–7. doi: 10.1128/IAI.00858-06
90. Widdison S, Watson M, Piercy J, Howard C, Coffey TJ. Granulocyte chemotactic properties of *M. tuberculosis* versus *M. bovis*-infected bovine alveolar macrophages. *Mol Immunol.* (2008) 45:740–9. doi: 10.1016/j.molimm.2007.06.357
91. Almeida de Souza C, Abramo C, Alves CC, Mazzoccoli L, Ferreira AP, Teixeira HC. Anti-mycobacterial treatment reduces high plasma levels of CXC-chemokines detected in active tuberculosis by cytometric bead array. *Mem Inst Oswaldo Cruz.* (2009) 104:1039–41. doi: 10.1590/S0074-02762009000700018
92. Lee HM, Shin DM, Kim KK, Lee JS, Paik TH, Jo EK. Roles of reactive oxygen species in CXCL8 and CCL2 expression in response to the 30-kDa antigen of *Mycobacterium tuberculosis*. *J Clin Immunol.* (2009) 29:46–56. doi: 10.1007/s10875-008-9222-3
93. Andersson M, Lutay N, Hallgren O, Westergren-Thorsson G, Svensson M, Godaly G. *Mycobacterium bovis* bacilli Calmette-Guerin regulates leukocyte recruitment by modulating alveolar inflammatory responses. *Innate Immun.* (2012) 18:531–40. doi: 10.1177/1753425911426591
94. Huang KH, Wang CH, Lee KY, Lin SM, Lin CH, Kuo HP. NF-kappaB repressing factor inhibits chemokine synthesis by peripheral blood mononuclear cells and alveolar macrophages in active pulmonary tuberculosis. *PLoS ONE.* (2013) 8:e77789. doi: 10.1371/journal.pone.0077789
95. Domingo-Gonzalez R, Prince O, Cooper A, Khader SA. Cytokines and chemokines in *Mycobacterium tuberculosis* infection. *Microbiol Spectr.* (2016) 4. doi: 10.1128/microbiolspec.TBTB2-0018-2016
96. Nibbering PH, Pos O, Stevenhagen A, Van Furth R. Interleukin-8 enhances nonoxidative intracellular killing of *Mycobacterium fortuitum* by human granulocytes. *Infect Immun.* (1993) 61:3111–6. doi: 10.1128/IAI.61.8.3111-3116.1993
97. Krupa A, Fol M, Dziadek BR, Kepka E, Wojciechowska D, Brzostek A, et al. Binding of CXCL8/IL-8 to *Mycobacterium tuberculosis* modulates the innate immune response. *Mediators Inflamm.* (2015) 2015:124762. doi: 10.1155/2015/124762
98. Kasahara K, Sato I, Ogura K, Takeuchi H, Kobayashi K, Adachi M. Expression of chemokines and induction of rapid cell death in human blood neutrophils by *Mycobacterium tuberculosis*. *J Infect Dis.* (1998) 178:127–137. doi: 10.1086/515585
99. Godaly G, Young DB. *Mycobacterium bovis* bacille Calmette Guerin infection of human neutrophils induces CXCL8 secretion by MyD88-dependent TLR2 and TLR4 activation. *Cell Microbiol.* (2005) 7:591–601. doi: 10.1111/j.1462-5822.2004.00489.x
100. Xin H, Zhang H, Cao X, Li X, Li M, Feng B, et al. Serum level of IL-8 is associated with reversion of QuantiFERON-TB gold in-tube tests. *J Infect.* (2019) 78:292–8. doi: 10.1016/j.jinf.2018.08.010
101. Malone KM, Rue-Albrecht K, Magee DA, Conlon K, Schubert OT, Nalpas NC, et al. Comparative 'omics analyses differentiate *Mycobacterium tuberculosis* and *Mycobacterium bovis* and reveal distinct macrophage responses to infection with the human and bovine tubercle bacilli. *Microb Genom.* (2018) 4:e000163. doi: 10.1099/mgen.0.000163

102. Meade KG, Gormley E, O'Farrelly C, Park SD, Costello E, Keane J, et al. Antigen stimulation of peripheral blood mononuclear cells from *Mycobacterium bovis* infected cattle yields evidence for a novel gene expression program. *BMC Genomics.* (2008) 9:447. doi: 10.1186/1471-2164-9-447
103. Taraktsoglou M, Szalabska U, Magee DA, Browne JA, Sweeney T, Gormley E, et al. Transcriptional profiling of immune genes in bovine monocyte-derived macrophages exposed to bacterial antigens. *Vet Immunol Immunopathol.* (2011) 140:130–9. doi: 10.1016/j.vetimm.2010.12.002
104. Meade KG, Gormley E, Doyle MB, Fitzsimons T, O'Farrelly C, Costello E, et al. Innate gene repression associated with *Mycobacterium bovis* infection in cattle: toward a gene signature of disease. *BMC Genomics.* (2007) 8:400. doi: 10.1186/1471-2164-8-400
105. Alonso-Hearn M, Canive M, Blanco-Vazquez C, Torremocha R, Balseiro A, Amado J, et al. RNA-Seq analysis of ileocecal valve and peripheral blood from Holstein cattle infected with Mycobacterium avium subsp. paratuberculosis revealed dysregulation of the CXCL8/IL8 signaling pathway. *Sci Rep.* (2019) 9:14845. doi: 10.1038/s41598-019-51328-0
106. Ma X, Reich RA, Wright JA, Tooker HR, Teeter LD, Musser JM, et al. Association between interleukin-8 gene alleles and human susceptibility to tuberculosis disease. *J Infect Dis.* (2003) 188:349–55. doi: 10.1086/376559
107. Lindenau JD, Guimarães LS, Friedrich DC, Hurtado AM, Hill KR, Salzano FM, et al. Cytokine gene polymorphisms are associated with susceptibility to tuberculosis in an Amerindian population. *Int J Tuberc Lung Dis.* (2014) 18:952–7. doi: 10.5588/ijtld.14.0060
108. Yu Z, Wit W, Xiong L, Cheng Y. Associations of six common functional polymorphisms in interleukins with tuberculosis: evidence from a meta-analysis. *Pathog Dis.* (2019) 77:ftz053. doi: 10.1093/femspd/ftz053
109. Chen J, Ma A. Associations of polymorphisms in interleukins with tuberculosis: evidence from a meta-analysis. *Immunol Lett.* (2020) 217:1–6. doi: 10.1016/j.imlet.2019.10.012
110. Rogatsky I, Ivashkiv LB. Glucocorticoid modulation of cytokine signaling. *Tissue Antigens.* (2006) 68:1–12. doi: 10.1111/j.1399-0039.2006.00599.x
111. Busillo JM, Cidlowski JA. The five Rs of glucocorticoid action during inflammation: ready, reinforce, repress, resolve, and restore. *Trends Endocrinol Metab.* (2013) 24:109–19. doi: 10.1016/j.tem.2012.11.005
112. D'Attilio L, Santucci N, Bongiovanni B, Bay ML, Bottasso O. Tuberculosis, the disrupted immune-endocrine response and the potential thymic repercussion as a contributing factor to disease physiopathology. *Front Endocrinol.* (2018) 9:214. doi: 10.3389/fendo.2018.00214
113. Redford PS, Murray PJ, O'Garra A. The role of IL-10 in immune regulation during *M. tuberculosis* infection. *Mucosal Immunol.* (2011) 4:261–70. doi: 10.1038/mi.2011.7
114. Hmama Z, Pena-Diaz S, Joseph S, Av-Gay Y. Immunoevasion and immunosuppression of the macrophage by *Mycobacterium tuberculosis. Immunol Rev.* (2015) 264:220–32. doi: 10.1111/imr.12268
115. Turner J, Gonzalez-Juarrero M, Ellis DL, Basaraba RJ, Kipnis A, Orme IM, et al. *In vivo* IL-10 production reactivates chronic pulmonary tuberculosis in C57BL/6 mice. *J Immunol.* (2002) 169:6343–51. doi: 10.4049/jimmunol.169.11.6343
116. Huynh JP, Lin CC, Kimmey JM, Jarjour NN, Schwarzkopf EA, Bradstreet TR, et al. Bhlhe40 is an essential repressor of IL-10 during *Mycobacterium tuberculosis* infection. *J Exp Med.* (2018) 215:1823–38. doi: 10.1084/jem.20171704
117. Ouyang W, O'Garra A. IL-10 family cytokines IL-10 and IL-22: from basic science to clinical translation. *Immunity.* (2019) 50:871–91. doi: 10.1016/j.immuni.2019.03.020
118. Bai W, Liu H, Ji Q, Zhou Y, Liang L, Zheng R, et al. TLR3 regulates mycobacterial RNA-induced IL-10 production through the PI3K/AKT signaling pathway. *Cell Signal.* (2014) 26:942–50. doi: 10.1016/j.cellsig.2014.01.015
119. Wang X, Wu Y, Jiao J, Huang Q. *Mycobacterium tuberculosis* infection induces IL-10 gene expression by disturbing histone deacetylase 6 and histone deacetylase 11 equilibrium in macrophages. *Tuberculosis.* (2018) 108:118–23. doi: 10.1016/j.tube.2017.11.008
120. Harling K, Adankwah E, Guler A, Afum-Adjei Awuah A, Adu-Amoah L, Mayatepek E, et al. Constitutive STAT3 phosphorylation and IL-6/IL-10 co-expression are associated with impaired T-cell function in tuberculosis patients. *Cell Mol Immunol.* (2019) 16:275–87. doi: 10.1038/cmi.2018.5
121. Wang J, Li BX, Ge PP, Li J, Wang Q, Gao GF, et al. *Mycobacterium tuberculosis* suppresses innate immunity by coopting the host ubiquitin system. *Nat Immunol.* (2015) 16:237–45. doi: 10.1038/ni.3096
122. Franco LH, Nair VR, Scharn CR, Xavier RJ, Torrealba JR, Shiloh MU, et al. The ubiquitin ligase Smurf1 functions in selective autophagy of *Mycobacterium tuberculosis* and anti-tuberculous host defense. *Cell Host Microbe.* (2017) 21:59–72. doi: 10.1016/j.chom.2016.11.002
123. Chai Q, Wang X, Qiang L, Zhang Y, Ge P, Lu Z, et al. A *Mycobacterium tuberculosis* surface protein recruits ubiquitin to trigger host xenophagy. *Nat Commun.* (2019) 10:1973. doi: 10.1038/s41467-019-09955-8
124. Chai Q, Wang L, Liu CH, Ge B. New insights into the evasion of host innate immunity by *Mycobacterium tuberculosis. Cell Mol Immunol.* (2020) 17:901–13. doi: 10.1038/s41423-020-0502-z
125. Wang JP, Rought SE, Corbeil J, Guiney DG. Gene expression profiling detects patterns of human macrophage responses following *Mycobacterium tuberculosis* infection. *FEMS Immunol Med Microbiol.* (2003) 39:163–72. doi: 10.1016/S0928-8244(03)00223-2
126. Keller C, Hoffmann R, Lang R, Brandau S, Hermann C, Ehlers S. Genetically determined susceptibility to tuberculosis in mice causally involves accelerated and enhanced recruitment of granulocytes. *Infect Immun.* (2006) 74:4295–309. doi: 10.1128/IAI.00057-06
127. Harding CV, Boom WH. Regulation of antigen presentation by *Mycobacterium tuberculosis*: a role for Toll-like receptors. *Nat Rev Microbiol.* (2010) 8:296–307. doi: 10.1038/nrmicro2321
128. Harriff MJ, Purdy GE, Lewinsohn DM. Escape from the phagosome: the explanation for MHC-I processing of mycobacterial antigens? *Front Immunol.* (2012) 3:40. doi: 10.3389/fimmu.2012.00040
129. A SK, Bansal K, Holla S, Verma-Kumar S, Sharma P, Balaji KN. ESAT-6 induced COX-2 expression involves coordinated interplay between PI3K and MAPK signaling. *Mol Immunol.* (2012) 49:655–63. doi: 10.1016/j.molimm.2011.11.011
130. Dutta NK, Mehra S, Martinez AN, Alvarez X, Renner NA, Morici LA, et al. The stress-response factor SigH modulates the interaction between *Mycobacterium tuberculosis* and host phagocytes. *PLoS ONE.* (2012) 7:e28958. doi: 10.1371/journal.pone.0028958
131. Xiong W, Wen Q, Du X, Wang J, He W, Wang R, et al. Novel function of cyclooxygenase-2: suppressing mycobacteria by promoting autophagy via the protein kinase B/mammalian target of rapamycin pathway. *J Infect Dis.* (2018) 217:1267–79. doi: 10.1093/infdis/jiy033
132. Liao X, Sharma N, Kapadia F, Zhou G, Lu Y, Hong H, et al. Kruppel-like factor 4 regulates macrophage polarization. *J Clin Invest.* (2011) 121:2736–49. doi: 10.1172/JCI45444
133. Yaqubi M, Mohammadnia A, Fallahi H. Transcription factor regulatory network for early lung immune response to tuberculosis in mice. *Mol Med Rep.* (2015) 12:2865–71. doi: 10.3892/mmr.2015.3721
134. Ghorpade DS, Holla S, Sinha AY, Alagesan SK, Balaji KN. Nitric oxide and KLF4 protein epigenetically modify class II transactivator to repress major histocompatibility complex II expression during *Mycobacterium bovis* bacillus Calmette-Guerin infection. *J Biol Chem.* (2013) 288:20592–606. doi: 10.1074/jbc.M113.472183
135. Sahu SK, Kumar M, Chakraborty S, Banerjee SK, Kumar R, Gupta P, et al. MicroRNA 26a (miR-26a)/KLF4 and CREB-C/EBPβ regulate innate immune signaling, the polarization of macrophages and the trafficking of *Mycobacterium tuberculosis* to lysosomes during infection. *PLoS Pathog.* (2017) 13:e1006410. doi: 10.1371/journal.ppat.1006410
136. Bar-Joseph Z. Analyzing time series gene expression data. *Bioinformatics.* (2004) 20:2493–503. doi: 10.1093/bioinformatics/bth283
137. Bar-Joseph Z, Gitter A, Simon I. Studying and modelling dynamic biological processes using time-series gene expression data. *Nat Rev Genet.* (2012) 13:552–64. doi: 10.1038/nrg3244
138. Oh S, Song S, Dasgupta N, Grabowski G. The analytical landscape of static and temporal dynamics in transcriptome data. *Front Genet.* (2014) 5:35. doi: 10.3389/fgene.2014.00035
139. Blanc M, Hsieh WY, Robertson KA, Watterson S, Shui G, Lacaze P, et al. Host defense against viral infection involves interferon

mediated down-regulation of sterol biosynthesis. *PLoS Biol.* (2011) 9:e1000598. doi: 10.1371/journal.pbio.1000598

140. Jorgensen HB, Buitenhuis B, Rontved CM, Jiang L, Ingvartsen KL, Sorensen P. Transcriptional profiling of the bovine hepatic response to experimentally induced *E. coli* mastitis. *Physiol Genomics.* (2012) 44:595–606. doi: 10.1152/physiolgenomics.00084.2011
141. Dimitrakopoulou K, Vrahatis AG, Wilk E, Tsakalidis AK, Bezerianos A. OLYMPUS: an automated hybrid clustering method in time series gene expression. Case study: host response after Influenza A (H1N1) infection. *Comput Methods Programs Biomed.* (2013) 111:650–61. doi: 10.1016/j.cmpb.2013.05.025
142. Maslove DM, Wong HR. Gene expression profiling in sepsis: timing, tissue, translational considerations. *Trends Mol Med.* (2014) 20:204–13. doi: 10.1016/j.molmed.2014.01.006
143. Neill SD, Bryson DG, Pollock JM. Pathogenesis of tuberculosis in cattle. *Tuberculosis.* (2001) 81:79–86. doi: 10.1054/tube.2000.0279
144. Cassidy JP. The pathogenesis and pathology of bovine tuberculosis with insights from studies of tuberculosis in humans and laboratory animal models. *Vet Microbiol.* (2006) 112:151–161. doi: 10.1016/j.vetmic.2005.11.031
145. Waters WR, Maggioli MF, McGill JL, Lyashchenko KP, Palmer MV. Relevance of bovine tuberculosis research to the understanding of human disease: historical perspectives, approaches, immunologic mechanisms. *Vet Immunol Immunopathol.* (2014) 159:113–32. doi: 10.1016/j.vetimm.2014.02.009

Permissions

All chapters in this book were first published by Frontiers; hereby published with permission under the Creative Commons Attribution License or equivalent. Every chapter published in this book has been scrutinized by our experts. Their significance has been extensively debated. The topics covered herein carry significant findings which will fuel the growth of the discipline. They may even be implemented as practical applications or may be referred to as a beginning point for another development.

The contributors of this book come from diverse backgrounds, making this book a truly international effort. This book will bring forth new frontiers with its revolutionizing research information and detailed analysis of the nascent developments around the world.

We would like to thank all the contributing authors for lending their expertise to make the book truly unique. They have played a crucial role in the development of this book. Without their invaluable contributions this book wouldn't have been possible. They have made vital efforts to compile up to date information on the varied aspects of this subject to make this book a valuable addition to the collection of many professionals and students.

This book was conceptualized with the vision of imparting up-to-date information and advanced data in this field. To ensure the same, a matchless editorial board was set up. Every individual on the board went through rigorous rounds of assessment to prove their worth. After which they invested a large part of their time researching and compiling the most relevant data for our readers.

The editorial board has been involved in producing this book since its inception. They have spent rigorous hours researching and exploring the diverse topics which have resulted in the successful publishing of this book. They have passed on their knowledge of decades through this book. To expedite this challenging task, the publisher supported the team at every step. A small team of assistant editors was also appointed to further simplify the editing procedure and attain best results for the readers.

Apart from the editorial board, the designing team has also invested a significant amount of their time in understanding the subject and creating the most relevant covers. They scrutinized every image to scout for the most suitable representation of the subject and create an appropriate cover for the book.

The publishing team has been an ardent support to the editorial, designing and production team. Their endless efforts to recruit the best for this project, has resulted in the accomplishment of this book. They are a veteran in the field of academics and their pool of knowledge is as vast as their experience in printing. Their expertise and guidance has proved useful at every step. Their uncompromising quality standards have made this book an exceptional effort. Their encouragement from time to time has been an inspiration for everyone.

The publisher and the editorial board hope that this book will prove to be a valuable piece of knowledge for researchers, students, practitioners and scholars across the globe.

List of Contributors

Smaragda Tsairidou, Elizabeth J. Glass, John A. Woolliams and Andrea B. Doeschl-Wilson
The Roslin Institute and Royal (Dick) School of Veterinary Studies, University of Edinburgh, Edinburgh, United Kingdom

Adrian Allen, Andrew W. Byrne and Robin A. Skuce
Agri-Food and Biosciences Institute, Belfast, United Kingdom

Mike Coffey
Scotland's Rural College, Midlothian, United Kingdom

Georgios Banos
The Roslin Institute and Royal (Dick) School of Veterinary Studies, University of Edinburgh, Edinburgh, United Kingdom
Scotland's Rural College, Midlothian, United Kingdom

Osvaldo Anacleto
The Roslin Institute and Royal (Dick) School of Veterinary Studies, University of Edinburgh, Edinburgh, United Kingdom
Institute of Mathematical and Computer Sciences, University of São Paulo, São Paulo, Brazil

Bryce M. Buddle
Ag Research, Hopkirk Research Institute, Palmerston North, New Zealand

Hans Martin Vordermeier
Animal and Plant Health Agency, Addlestone, United Kingdom

Mark A. Chambers
Animal and Plant Health Agency, Addlestone, United Kingdom
Faculty of Health & Medical Sciences, School of Veterinary Medicine, University of Surrey, Guildford, United Kingdom

Lin-Mari de Klerk-Lorist
Veterinary Wildlife Services, Kruger National Park, Department of Agriculture, Forestry and Fisheries, Pretoria, South Africa

Megan Cross
Department of Fisheries and Wildlife, Michigan State University, East Lansing, MI, United States

Alex Heeren
Sierra Nevada Research Institute, University of California, Merced, CA, United States

Louis J. Cornicelli
Minnesota Department of Natural Resources, Division of Fish and Wildlife, St. Paul, MN, United States

David C. Fulton
U.S. Geological Survey, Minnesota Cooperative Fish and Wildlife Research Unit, University of Minnesota, St. Paul, MN, United States

Syeda A. Hadi and Srinand Sreevatsan
Department of Pathobiology and Diagnostic Investigation, College of Veterinary Medicine, Michigan State University, East Lansing, MI, United States

Wade R. Waters and Mitchell Palmer
National Animal Disease Center, Agricultural Research Service, United States Department of Agriculture, Ames, IA, United States

Konstantin P. Lyashchenko
Chembio Diagnostic Systems Inc., Medford, NY, United States

A. R. Allen, R. A. Skuce and A. W. Byrne
Veterinary Science Division, Agri-Food and Biosciences Institute, Belfast, United Kingdom

Héléna Ladreyt
French School of Veterinary Services (ENSV), Lyon, France

Mathilde Saccareau
Mathematical Modelling of Infectious Diseases Unit, Institut Pasteur, Paris, France
Epidemiology Unit, Paris-Est University, Laboratory for Animal Health, French Agency for Food, Environment and Occupational Health and Safety (ANSES), Maisons-Alfort, France

Aurélie Courcoul and Benoit Durand
Epidemiology Unit, Paris-Est University, Laboratory for Animal Health, French Agency for Food, Environment and Occupational Health and Safety (ANSES), Maisons-Alfort, France

Mitchell V. Palmer
Infectious Bacterial Diseases of Livestock Research Unit, National Animal Disease Center, Agricultural Research Service, United States Department of Agriculture, Ames, IA, United States

Fikre Fekadu and Takele Beyene Tufa
College of Veterinary Medicine and Agriculture, Addis Ababa University, Bishoftu, Ethiopia

Tariku Jibat Beyene
College of Veterinary Medicine and Agriculture, Addis Ababa University, Bishoftu, Ethiopia
Centre for Outcomes Research and Epidemiology, Department of Diagnostic Medicine, Pathobiology, College of Veterinary Medicine, Kansas State University, Manhattan, KS, United States

Ashenafi Feyisa Beyi
College of Veterinary Medicine and Agriculture, Addis Ababa University, Bishoftu, Ethiopia
Department of Veterinary Microbiology and Preventive Medicine, College of Veterinary Medicine, Iowa State University, Ames, IA, United States

Bedaso Mammo Edao
College of Veterinary Medicine and Agriculture, Addis Ababa University, Bishoftu, Ethiopia
Department of Veterinary Medicine, University of Cambridge, Cambridge, United Kingdom

Fanos Tadesse Woldemariyam
College of Veterinary Medicine and Agriculture, Addis Ababa University, Bishoftu, Ethiopia
Faculty of Bioscience Engineering, KU Leuven, Leuven, Belgium

Fanta Desissa Gutema
College of Veterinary Medicine and Agriculture, Addis Ababa University, Bishoftu, Ethiopia
Faculty of Veterinary Medicine, Ghent University, Ghent, Belgium

Édouard Réveillaud and Pascal Hendrikx
Anses, Unit of Coordination and Support to Surveillance, Maisons-Alfort, France

Stéphanie Desvaux and Jean Hars
French Hunting and Wildlife Agency (ONCFS), Studies and Research Department, Auffargis, France

Maria-Laura Boschiroli
University Paris-Est–Anses, French Reference Laboratory for Tuberculosis, Maisons-Alfort, France

Éva Faure
National Hunters Federation (FNC), Issy-les-Moulineaux, France

Alexandre Fediaevsky, Lisa Cavalerie, Fabrice Chevalier and Pierre Jabert
French General Directorate for Food (DGAL), Animal Health Unit, Paris, France

Sylvie Poliak
French Association of Directors and Managers of Public Veterinary Laboratories of Analyses (Adilva), Paris, France

Isabelle Tourette
French National Federation of Animal Health Defense Associations (GDS France), Paris, France

Céline Richomme
Anses, Nancy Laboratory for Rabies and Wildlife, Malzéville, France

Klaas Frankena
Adaptation Physiology Group, Department of Animal Sciences, Wageningen University, Wageningen, Netherlands
Quantitative Veterinary Epidemiology Group, Department of Animal Sciences, Wageningen University, Wageningen, Netherlands

Mart C. M. de Jong
Quantitative Veterinary Epidemiology Group, Department of Animal Sciences, Wageningen University, Wageningen, Netherlands

Liesbeth Jacobs and Tonny van Dijk
Thermofisher Scientific, Prionics Lelystad B.V., Lelystad, Netherlands

Margaret Good
Discipline of Zoology, School of Natural Sciences, Trinity College Dublin, The University of Dublin, Dublin, Ireland
Independent Researcher and Private Consultant, Dun Laoghaire, Co. Dublin, Ireland

Anthony Duignan
Department of Agriculture, Food and the Marine, Dublin, Ireland

Jenny-Ann L. M. L. Toribio
The University of Sydney, Farm Animal Health, Sydney School of Veterinary Science, Sydney, NSW, Australia

Elva Borja
The University of Sydney, Farm Animal Health, Sydney School of Veterinary Science, Sydney, NSW, Australia
Vet Essentials, Suva, Fiji

Leo F. Borja, Ronil Prasad and Tomasi Tunabuna
Ministry of Agriculture, Koronivia Research Station, Koronivia, Fiji

Melinda K. Cosgrove and Daniel J. O'Brien
Wildlife Disease Laboratory, Michigan Department of Natural Resources, Lansing, MI, United States

David S. L. Ramsey
Department of Environment, Land, Water and Planning, Arthur Rylah Institute for Environmental Research, Heidelberg, VIC, Australia

Rebecca Callaby, Stella Mazeri, Adrian Muwonge and Barend M. de C Bronsvoort
The Roslin Institute, Royal (Dick) School of Veterinary Studies, University of Edinburgh, Midlothian, United Kingdom

Robert F. Kelly and Ian G. Handel
The Roslin Institute, Royal (Dick) School of Veterinary Studies, University of Edinburgh, Midlothian, United Kingdom
Royal (Dick) School of Veterinary Studies, University of Edinburgh, Midlothian, United Kingdom

Nkongho F. Egbe
Microbiology and Parasitology Unit, Faculty of Allied Medical Science, University of Calabar, Calabar, Nigeria

Diana J. L. Williams
Veterinary Parasitology, Institute of Infection and Global Health and School of Veterinary Science, Liverpool, United Kingdom

Ngu Ngwa Victor
School of Veterinary Medicine and Sciences, University of Ngaoundere, Ngaoundere, Cameroon

Vincent N. Tanya
Cameroon Academy of Sciences, Yaoundé, Cameroon

Melissa Sander
Tuberculosis Reference Laboratory Bamenda, Hospital Roundabout, Bamenda, Cameroon

Lucy Ndip
Laboratory of Emerging Infectious Diseases, University of Buea, Buea, Cameroon

Richard Ngandolo
Laboratoire de Recherches Vétérinaires et Zootechniques de Farcha, N'Djamena, Chad

Kenton L. Morgan
Institute of Ageing and Chronic Disease and School of Veterinary Science, University of Liverpool, Neston, United Kingdom

Kathy Orloski
U.S. Department of Agriculture, Animal and Plant Health Inspection Service, Veterinary Services, Centers for Epidemiology and Animal Health, Fort Collins, CO, United States

Suelee Robbe-Austerman and Tod Stuber
National Veterinary Services Laboratories, U.S. Department of Agriculture, Animal and Plant Health Inspection Service, Veterinary Services, Ames, IA, United States

Bill Hench and Mark Schoenbaum
U.S. Department of Agriculture, Animal and Plant Health Inspection Service, Veterinary Services, Fort Collins, CO, United States

John B. Kaneene
Center for Comparative Epidemiology, College of Veterinary Medicine, Michigan State University, East Lansing, MI, United States

Paulo Alex Carneiro
Center for Comparative Epidemiology, College of Veterinary Medicine, Michigan State University, East Lansing, MI, United States
Amazonas State Federal Institute, Manaus, Brazil

Taiana T. Silva-Pereira and Ana Marcia Sa Guimaraes
Laboratory of Applied Research in Mycobacteria, Department of Microbiology, Institute of Biomedical Sciences, University of São Paulo, São Paulo, Brazil

Robert B. Abramovitch
Department of Microbiology and Molecular Genetics, Michigan State University, East Lansing, MI, United States

Cristina Kraemer Zimpel
Laboratory of Applied Research in Mycobacteria, Department of Microbiology, Institute of Biomedical Sciences, University of São Paulo, São Paulo, Brazil
Department of Microbiology and Molecular Genetics, Michigan State University, East Lansing, MI, United States

Taynara Nunes Pasquatti
Dom Bosco Catholic University, Campo Grande, Brazil

Haruo Takatani and Christian B. D. G. Silva
Agência de Defesa Agropecuaria Do Amazonas, Manaus, Brazil

Alberto M. R. Davila
Computational and Systems Biology Laboratory, Oswaldo Cruz Institute and Graduate Program in Biodiversity and Health, FIOCRUZ, Rio de Janeiro, Brazil

Flabio R. Araujo
Embrapa Gado de Corte, Campo Grande, Brazil

Sreenidhi Srinivasan, Christian Herrera and Vivek Kapur
Department of Animal Science, The Pennsylvania State University, University Park, PA, United States
The Huck Institutes of the Life Sciences, The Pennsylvania State University, University Park, PA, United States

Andrew J. K. Conlan and James Wood
Disease Dynamics Unit, Department of Veterinary Medicine, University of Cambridge, Cambridge, United Kingdom

Laurel A. Easterling
School of Veterinary Medicine, University of Pennsylvania, Philadelphia, PA, United States

Premanshu Dandapat
Indian Veterinary Research Institute, Eastern Regional Station, Kolkata, India

Maroudam Veerasami
Cisgen Biotech Discoveries Pvt Ltd, Chennai, India

Gobena Ameni
Aklilu Lemma Institute of Pathobiology, Addis Ababa University, Addis Ababa, Ethiopia

Naresh Jindal
Department of Veterinary Public Health and Epidemiology, Lala Lajpat Rai University of Veterinary and Animal Sciences, Hisar, India

Gopal Dhinakar Raj
Translational Research Platform for Veterinary Biological, Tamil Nadu University of Veterinary and Animal Sciences, Chennai, India

Nick Juleff
The Bill & Melinda Gates Foundation, Seattle, WA, United States

Douwe Bakker
Technical Consultant and Independent Researcher, Lelystad, Netherlands

Martin Vordermeier
Animal and Plant Health Agency, Addlestone, United Kingdom
Centre for Bovine Tuberculosis, Institute for Biological, Environmental and Rural Sciences, University of Aberystwyth, Aberystwyth, United Kingdom

David J. Kelly
Discipline of Zoology, School of Natural Sciences, Trinity College Dublin, The University of Dublin, Dublin, Ireland

Enda Mullen
National Parks and Wildlife Service, Department of Housing, Local Government and Heritage, Dublin, Ireland

Érica Bravo Sales, Antônio Augusto Fonseca Jr, Cristina Magalhães Gonçalves and Natanael Lamas Dias
Laboratório Federal de Defesa Agropecuária de Minas Gerais, Pedro Leopoldo, Minas Gerais, Brazil

Andrey Pereira Lage and Giovanna Ivo Andrade
Escola de Veterinária, Universidade Federal de Minas Gerais, Belo Horizonte, Minas Gerais, Brazil

Philip Noel Suffys and Harrison Magdinier Gomes
FioCruz, Rio de Janeiro, Rio de Janeiro, Brazil

José Soares Ferreira Neto, Ana Marcia de Sá Guimarães and Marcos Bryan Heinemann
Universidade de São Paulo, São Paulo, São Paulo, Brazil

José María Sánchez-Carvajal, Inés Ruedas-Torres, Fernanda Larenas-Muñoz, Irene Magdalena Rodríguez-Gómez, Librado Carrasco and Jaime Gómez-Laguna
Department of Anatomy and Comparative Pathology and Toxicology, University of Córdoba, Córdoba, Spain

Ángela Galán-Relaño, Lidia Gómez-Gascón, Alfonso Maldonado and Carmen Tarradas
Department of Animal Health, University of Córdoba, Córdoba, Spain

Eduardo Vera
Department of Anatomy and Comparative Pathology and Toxicology, University of Córdoba, Córdoba, Spain
Department of Animal Health, University of Córdoba, Córdoba, Spain

Francisco Jurado-Martos, Fernando Cardoso-Toset and Inmaculada Luque
CICAP—Food Research Centre, Córdoba, Spain

Paola M. Boggiatto
Bacterial Diseases of Livestock Research Unit, National Animal Disease Center, Agricultural Research Service, United States Department of Agriculture, Ames, IA, United States

Tyler C. Thacker
National Veterinary Services Laboratories, Animal and Plant Health Inspection Service, Ames, IA, United States
Infectious Bacterial Diseases of Livestock Research Unit, National Animal Disease Center, Agricultural Research Service, United States Department of Agriculture, Ames, IA, United States

Carly Kanipe
Bacterial Diseases of Livestock Research Unit, National Animal Disease Center, Agricultural Research Service, United States Department of Agriculture, Ames, IA, United States
Immunobiology Graduate Program, College of Veterinary Medicine, Iowa State University, Ames, IA, United States

Kirsten E. McLoughlin, Carolina N. Correia, John A. Browne, David A. Magee, Nicolas C. Nalpas and Kevin Rue-Albrecht
Animal Genomics Laboratory, UCD School of Agriculture and Food Science, UCD College of Health and Agricultural Sciences, University College Dublin, Dublin, Ireland

Adam O. Whelan, Bernardo Villarreal-Ramos and H. Martin Vordermeier
TB Immunology and Vaccinology Team, Department of Bacteriology, Animal and Plant Health Agency, Weybridge, United Kingdom

Eamonn Gormley
UCD School of Veterinary Medicine, UCD College of Health and Agricultural Sciences, University College Dublin, Dublin, Ireland

Stephen V. Gordon
UCD School of Veterinary Medicine, UCD College of Health and Agricultural Sciences, University College Dublin, Dublin, Ireland
UCD Conway Institute of Biomolecular and Biomedical Research, University College Dublin, Dublin, Ireland

David E. MacHugh
Animal Genomics Laboratory, UCD School of Agriculture and Food Science, UCD College of Health and Agricultural Sciences, University College Dublin, Dublin, Ireland
UCD Conway Institute of Biomolecular and Biomedical Research, University College Dublin, Dublin, Ireland

Index

www.ingramcontent.com/pod-product-compliance
Lightning Source LLC
LaVergne TN
LVHW061510220926
848485LV00017B/793